Encyclopedia of Medicine and Life Science

Volume I

Encyclopedia of Medicine and Life Science
Volume I

Edited by **Allen Richardson**

FOSTER ACADEMICS
New Jersey

Published by Foster Academics,
61 Van Reypen Street,
Jersey City, NJ 07306, USA
www.fosteracademics.com

Encyclopedia of Medicine and Life Science: Volume I
Edited by Allen Richardson

International Standard Book Number: 978-1-63242-163-0 (Hardback)

Printed in China.

Contents

Preface

The vast field of life sciences comprises of the fields of science that consist of the scientific study of living organisms like microorganisms, animals, plants and human beings. It also includes related matters like bioethics. While biology remains the central focus of the life sciences, technological developments in biotechnology and molecular biology have led to a mushrooming of specializations and interdisciplinary subjects. Life science is a field that is helpful in improving the standard and quality of life. There are applications for life sciences in medicine, health, agriculture as well as in pharmaceutical and food science industries. There is considerable overlap between many of the topics of study in the life sciences. Life sciences also encompass the fields of life systems technologies, food processing, biotechnology, biomedical technologies, environmental science and bio-medical devices. Organizations and institutions also devote the bulk of their efforts in the various stages of research, development, technology transfer and commercialization. Most life scientists are largely involved in research and development and work in the laboratory or field. There are many opportunities available even in distantly related areas such as administration, management, illustrating, service work, teaching, financial support, legal support, writing, sales and even photography.

This book is an attempt to compile and collate all available research on new ideas in life sciences under one umbrella. I am grateful to those who put their hard work, effort and expertise into these research projects as well as those who were supportive in this endeavour.

Editor

1

The Molecular Genetics and Cellular Mechanisms Underlying Pulmonary Arterial Hypertension

Rajiv D. Machado

School of Life Sciences, Faculty of Science, University of Lincoln, Brayford Pool, Lincoln LN6 7TS, UK

Correspondence should be addressed to Rajiv D. Machado; rmachado@lincoln.ac.uk

Academic Editors: J. A. Castro and B. Witzenbichler

Pulmonary arterial hypertension (PAH) is an incurable disorder clinically characterised by a sustained elevation of mean arterial pressure in the absence of systemic involvement. As the adult circulation is a low pressure, low resistance system, PAH represents a reversal to a foetal state. The small pulmonary arteries of patients exhibit luminal occlusion resultant from the uncontrolled growth of endothelial and smooth muscle cells. This vascular remodelling is comprised of hallmark defects, most notably the plexiform lesion. PAH may be familial in nature but the majority of patients present with spontaneous disease or PAH associated with other complications. In this paper, the molecular genetic basis of the disorder is discussed in detail ranging from the original identification of the major genetic contributant to PAH and moving on to current next-generation technologies that have led to the rapid identification of additional genetic risk factors. The impact of identified mutations on the cell is examined, particularly, the determination of pathways disrupted in disease and critical to pulmonary vascular maintenance. Finally, the application of research in this area to the design and development of novel treatment options for patients is addressed along with the future directions PAH research is progressing towards.

1. Pulmonary Vascular Development

Three distinct models have been put forward in an attempt to shed light on the processes underlying the development of the pulmonary vascular bed and, in particular, the respective roles played by the key morphological events of vasculogenesis and angiogenesis. Vasculogenesis is defined by recruitment and differentiation of the endothelial progenitor cells into mature endothelial cells which proliferate, migrate, differentiate, and organise into a vascular plexus that forms the foundation for the early vascular system. Angiogenesis is the process of branching growth from existing vessels. Favouring angiogenesis as the predominant mechanism in pulmonary vascular development, Parera et al. suggest that expansion of the lung bud is resultant upon the formation of new capillary structures from previously established vessels [1]. By contrast, Hall et al. support vasculogenesis as the central process driving the generation of arteries and veins from the central vascular plexus [2]. Finally, deMello and Reid implicate both processes in vascular development, positing the theory that the early events involve the differentiation of mesenchymal cells to endothelial populations that is succeeded by angiogenic mechanisms impacting on endothelial cells derived from preexistent vessels [3].

The development of the pulmonary vascular system and circulation depends on an array of genetic factors working in a tightly regulated spatiotemporal fashion. These elements include transcription factors and cytokines amongst others. Among the key factors known to regulate vessel formation are the vascular endothelial growth factor (VEGF), transforming growth factor beta (TGF-β) family members, and angiopoietins along with several growth factor receptors [4]. Of these VEGF is intrinsic to pulmonary vascular development. Transgenic mouse studies wherein VEGF alleles have been conditionally ablated in the lung epithelium results in a phenotype exhibiting the near complete loss of the pulmonary capillary network [5]. In humans, heterozygous loss of VEGF leads to embryonic death and marked abnormalities of vascularisation [6]. VEGF is instrumental in generation of the vasoactive metabolites nitric oxide (NO) and prostacyclin

(PGI_2) via activation of endothelial nitric oxide synthase and prostacyclin synthase, respectively. Both metabolites are critical in the regulation of vascular tone [7, 8]. The TGF-β receptors and ligands are involved in lung morphogenesis and formation of the pulmonary circulatory system with the cytoplasmic mediators, the Smads, playing a role in pulmonary artery endothelial cell (PAEC) proliferation, and migration [9]. The angiopoietin family along with their receptor Tie-2 are important in endothelial cell migration and in the control of vascular maintenance and remodelling. Defects in these proteins results in extreme vascular abnormalities [10].

1.1. Haemodynamic and Structural Adaptation in Foetal and Neonatal Pulmonary Circulation. The site of blood oxygenation in the foetus is the placenta. At this stage of life the patent foramen ovale (FO) and the patent ductus arteriosis (DA) are open. The flow of blood from the placenta is, thus, directed away from the foetal lungs. Oxygenated blood is directed to the chambers of the heart via the foramen ovale. Negligible quantities of blood enter the lungs as the high resistance of foetal pulmonary vasculature encourages diversion through the ductus arteriosis. The resistance relates to the morphology of the muscular arteries and arterioles, in which the smooth muscle layer is thick and the lumen narrow [11–14]. Upon birth, the lungs are employed in blood oxygenation. A fall in pulmonary vascular resistance soon follows as a consequence of pulmonary artery and arteriole dilatation concomitant with an increase in systemic pressure. Upon systemic pressure surpassing that of pulmonary vascular resistance the foramen ovale shuts, soon followed by the contraction of the ductus arteriosis [15, 16] (Figures 1(a) and 1(b)).

1.2. Haemodynamic and Structural Features of Postnatal and Adult Circulation. The closure of the ductus arteriosis and, subsequently, the foramen ovale generates a dramatic increase of blood flow through the lungs (Figure 1(c)). During the first two or three weeks of life, significant structural changes to the muscular arteries and arterioles occur. Considerable luminal widening with accompanying medial thinning is exhibited. A more gradated decrease in media width progresses over one and a half years until the pulmonary vasculature reaches a steady adult state. Critical to the significant decrease in the postnatal circulation and, indeed, the maintenance of the adult circulation is the change in functional outcomes of signalling pathways comprising key vasoactive elements. The adult pulmonary circulation reflects its structural features by being a low-pressure system of between 7 and 15 mm Hg with an average of approximately 9 mm Hg [17–20].

2. Pulmonary Arterial Hypertension

Pulmonary arterial hypertension (PAH) represents a dramatic reversal of the physiological adult circulation to a disease state bearing features of foetal high vascular resistance. Whilst the disorder is uncommon with an incidence calculated at 1-2 cases per million per year, it is progressive and typified by high morbidity and mortality. PAH is clinically diagnosed when mean pulmonary artery pressure is maintained at >25 mm Hg at rest or 30 mm Hg during exercise with normal pulmonary capillary wedge pressure and elevated pulmonary vascular resistance [21]. Diagnostic protocols include patients having a Doppler echocardiogram to determine right heart size and function, left ventricular diastolic and systolic function, and putative causes of pulmonary hypertension [22]. Prior to a treatment course being decided patients require right heart catheterization to measure hemodynamic parameters, for example, pulmonary arterial pressure and vascular resistance [23]. PAH afflicts both adults and children but, in the main, occurs in the 3rd to 4th decade of life. For reasons that are yet to be fully explained the disease exhibits a sex bias affecting twice as many females than males [24]. A proportion of PAH patients, approximately 10%, have a family history of disease which in certain cases has been observed to be transmitted through multiple generations [25]. Due to the advent of contemporary therapies, patient life expectancy has been improved but the disease remains incurable. In the absence of heart-lung transplantation the disease, typically, remains fatal with death occurring due to the strain imposed on the right side of the heart. A significantly lower number of male offspring of PAH affected women has been noted, suggestive of selective male foetal wastage. The condition appears to affect all racial and ethnic groups equivalently [24].

2.1. Classification of Pulmonary Hypertension (PH). As defined by the 2008 World Health Organization symposium on pulmonary hypertension, there exist 5 major classes. These comprise: Group 1. PAH; Group 2. PH associated with left heart disease; Group 3. PH associated with alveolar hypoxia and/or other disorders of the respiratory system; Group 4. Thromboembolic disease resulting in PH; Group 5. PH with unclear multifactorial mechanisms. PAH itself is sub-divided into 5 additional categories comprising idiopathic PAH (IPAH), heritable PAH (HPAH), which identifies patients with multiple affected family members and/or an identified germ-line mutation, PAH associated with known risk factors for disease, PAH associated with additional diseases (APAH) which may include HIV infection, systemic sclerosis, and congenital heart disease. The final class is persistent pulmonary hypertension of the newborn [26].

2.2. Functional Classes of Pulmonary Arterial Hypertension. The World Health Organization, in addition to the clinical classification of PH, has developed a four tier classification system that segregates patients on the basis of disease severity with Class I being the mildest and Class IV the most severe form of disease. Patients falling within Class I comprise individuals with PH that is not accompanied by constraints on physical activity. Moreover, normal physical activity does not result in dyspnoea, fatigue, syncope, or chest pain. Class II patients have PH with mild limitation of physical activity whereas Class III patients are severely impaired in the ability to perform physically exerting tasks. Class IV patients present with symptoms if any physical activity is performed; these individuals are representative of end stage disease with clear

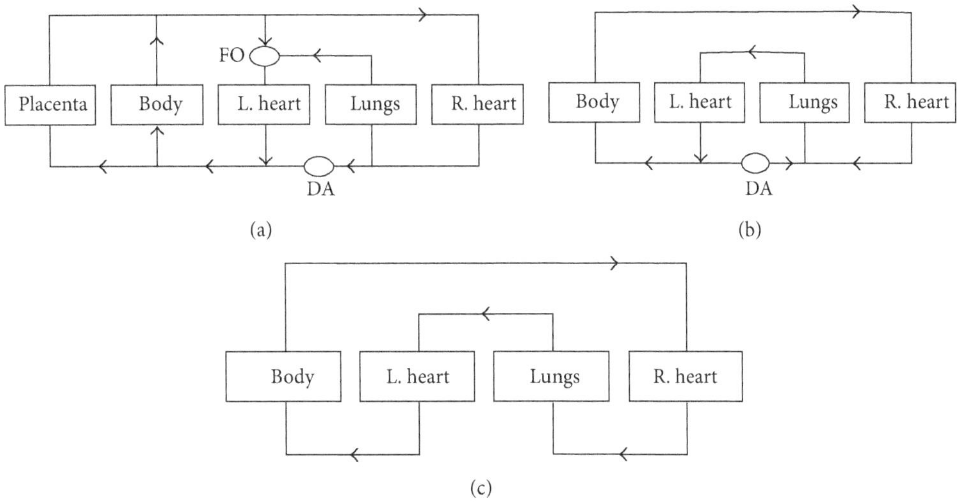

FIGURE 1: Development of the circulatory system. Systemic and pulmonary circulation in the (a) foetus, (b) neonate, and (c) adult. The arrows refer to the direction of blood flow through the anatomical compartments, depicted by the labelled rectangular boxes. The oval shapes labelled FO and DA refer to the foramen ovale and ductus arteriosus, respectively.

indications of heart failure. Additionally, shortness of breath and general fatigue are evident in a resting state [27].

2.3. Histopathology of PAH. PAH is associated with the development of vascular lesions and aberrant vascular remodelling. While a series of lesions are typically observed in PAH, these can be present as heterogeneous populations both within and between families suggesting that the initial causal factor generating lesion types is the same. The arterial circulation is predominantly impacted upon although there is evidence of limited venous remodelling. A frequent pathological observation in PAH is medial hypertrophy of the muscular pulmonary arteries and muscularization of the arterioles. Accompanying this is a duplication of the elastic lamina and a characteristic thickening of the medial smooth muscle (Figure 2). Affected vessels are similar to foetal muscular arteries albeit in an adult circulation system. A hallmark pathological finding in PAH is the plexiform lesion present in approximately a third of patient lung tissue. Plexiform lesions are typically associated with end-stage PAH but are not emblematic of the disease as they are also observed with other disorders arising with PH. Situated in muscular arteries, usually of an external diameter between 100–200 μm, they typically arise at the origin of pulmonary arterioles and display aberrations of the media and intimal lining. The lesion is defined by the segmental destruction of the medial cell wall layer. The lesion typically presents with a profusion of smooth muscle cells, myofibroblasts, macrophages, and proliferating endothelial cells. The upregulation of growth factors, such as vascular endothelial growth factor (VEGF) and its receptor, has been described in the endothelial cells within the plexiform lesion [28–30]. The initiating factors and, indeed, cell type responsible for the generation of plexiform lesions remain a source of uncertainty. While debate continues as to the source of lesional formation being smooth muscle cells or endothelial cells an important observation has been the report of endothelial cells within lesions being monoclonal, suggestive of neoplastic expansion. Furthermore, plexiform endothelial cells from idiopathic patients have been shown to exhibit microsatellite instability in DNA repair genes, proapoptotic genes and in the *TGF-β* gene, which is also a central feature of cancer cells and is described as the "two hit" tumour suppressor gene hypothesis [31]. Contrastingly, however, cells obtained by microdissection of plexiform lesions from lungs of HPAH subjects exhibited no evidence of similar somatic mutations. These data indicate that microsatellite instability is unlikely to underpin both categories of PAH [32]. The arterial lumen, proximal to the lesion, is obstructed by eccentric or concentric intimal fibroelastosis. Distally, the artery is markedly dilatated and thin-walled.

2.4. Disease Pathogenesis

2.4.1. Endothelial Cell Abnormalities. Imbalances in vasoactive metabolites are a central feature of the vascular endothelium of PAH patients. Vasocontrictive agents, for example, thromboxane and endothelin-1, are found to be significantly upregulated in pulmonary arteries [33, 34]. By contrast, the vasodilators prostacyclin, nitric oxide, and the nitric oxide messenger cyclic guanosine monophosphate are present at much reduced levels. Through unclear mechanisms, the upstream catalysts of these proteins, prostacyclin synthase, and nitric oxide synthase, respectively, are also greatly diminished in patient lung tissue [35, 36].

2.4.2. Inflammation. Inflammation has long been recognised as having a role in the development of PAH. Evidence of heightened levels of inflammatory cytokines in patient tissue include tumour necrosis factor, IL-6, IL-1β, and monocyte chemoattractant protein 1 [37, 38]. Vascular lesions in PAH patient lung display classic inflammatory features which include the presence of macrophages, monocytes, and T

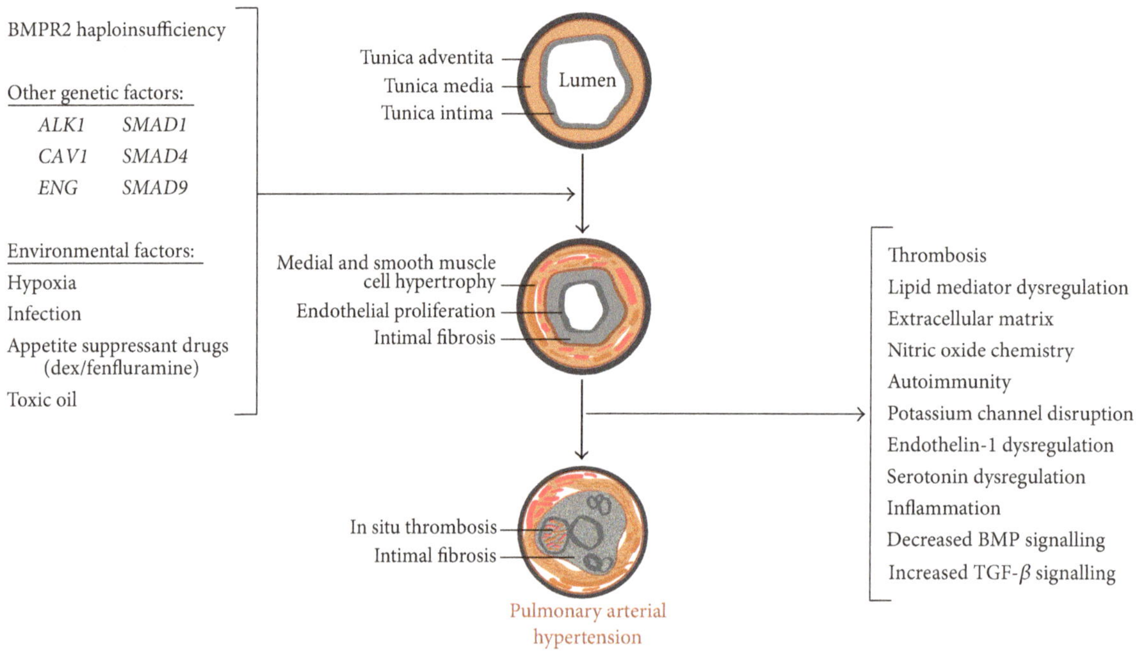

FIGURE 2: Cause and effect in pulmonary arterial hypertension. Schematic representing the genetic and environmental factors involved in the aetiology of PAH and the biochemical readouts associated with PAH presentation. *BMPR2* haploinsufficiency remains the major genetic contributant to disease pathogenesis. The central depiction of a section through a pulmonary artery shows the hallmark features at each stage of PAH progression.

and B lymphocytes [39]. Inflammatory chemokines are also found at elevated levels in PAH patients, in particular the chemotactic protein FKN, RANTES, and chemokine ligand 5 [40].

2.4.3. Voltage-Gated Potassium Channels. Intracellular calcium levels are regulated by voltage-gated potassium channels which act by regulating membrane potential and controlling the release of calcium. Intracellular calcium is integral in driving contraction of pulmonary artery smooth muscle cells (PASMCs) and promoting hypertrophy. Calcium levels in PAH smooth muscle cells have been shown to be elevated likely as a direct consequence of the observed reduction in transcript for potassium channels and low current in patients by comparison to controls. The paucity of potassium channels has been posited as a potential explanation for the vasoconstriction and uncontrolled proliferation observed in patients [41].

2.4.4. Serotonin and the Serotonin Transporter. IPAH patients exhibit elevated levels of serotonin (5-HT) which persist post heart-lung transplantation. This finding indicates a causal role for 5-HT in the pathogenesis of PAH [42]. 5-HT, stored primarily in the platelets, is a potent vasoconstricting agent and mitogen which promotes smooth muscle cell proliferation. The mitogenic effects of 5-HT are mediated by the serotonin transporter, 5-HTT [43]. Indeed, chemical inhibition of 5-HTT results in a loss of 5-HT induced cell proliferation. 5-HTT is expressed at high levels on PASMCs and increased production of 5-HTT in PASMCs is capable of triggering spontaneous PAH [44].

2.4.5. The Warburg Phenotype. Cancer cells display dysmorphic mitochondria and a glycolytic shift in metabolism which is believed to confer resistance to apoptosis [45]. This cellular phenomenon, known as the Warburg phenotype, has also been observed in PASMCs and PAECs from human PAH patients as well as in a rodent model of PAH [46]. This link to a cancer phenotype appears to be associated with depleted levels of the tumour suppressor gene and antioxidant enzyme SOD2. SOD2 scavenges super-oxide, converting it to hydrogen peroxide in the mitochondria, a critical step in the regulation of cell proliferation. Significant downregulation of SOD2 is observed in the pulmonary arteries and plexiform lesions of PAH patients [47].

2.4.6. Extracellular Matrix. Mitogens in the extracellular matrix (ECM) are released and tenascin-C upregulated due to the abnormal degradation of the ECM by matrix metalloproteinases and elastases in patients. Tenascin-C has a proproliferative effect on smooth muscle cells as it enhances the response to mitogenic agents. Studies have shown that inhibition of these substances reduced vascular remodelling and the severity of disease thereby indicating their importance in smooth muscle homestasis [48] (Figure 2).

3. Genetics and Genomics of PAH

Heritable PAH was first reported by Dresdale et al. in 1951 [49]. In families, the disease segregates in an autosomal dominant manner and with markedly reduced penetrance as indicated by the absence of overt disease symptoms in multiple obligate carriers. Although all examined pedigrees suggest that HPAH is a single gene disorder, the reduced penetrance, sex bias, and disparity of age of disease onset both within and between families serve to highlight complex traits of inheritance [50]. Using microsatellite based genotyping and standard linkage analysis in multiple families, a locus for the causative gene was identified by two independent groups in 1997 [51, 52]. Nichols et al. employed 6 large pedigrees for linkage studies and isolated a minimal linkage interval of 25 cM with a maximum LOD score of 6.97 [52]. This large region was saturated with further markers of high informativity and haplotype mapping was conducted in several additional kindreds to refine the linkage peak by the fine mapping of recombination events amongst affected individuals. These genetic analyses facilitated the refinement of the original 25 cM interval to a more tractable 4.8 cM located on chromosome 2q33 [53]. Although typically a late-onset autosomal dominant disease, microsatellite data generated during the course of the linkage investigation did not provide evidence of shared disease haplotypes in US and UK populations that would be indicative of the presence of founder mutations.

3.1. Transcript Mapping and Positional Cloning of the Gene Underlying HPAH. To derive a clear appreciation of the actual size of the interval and unambiguously position polymorphic markers and, critically, expressed sequence elements a physical map was created employing contigs comprising YACs, BACs, and PACs. These studies established the interval as being 5.8 Mb and harbouring within it 79 transcriptional units [53]. Characterized genes with likely biological relevance to PAH were prioritized for analysis by direct Sanger sequencing. Screening of a number of candidate genes culminated in the identification of independent heterozygous mutations, in numerous familial cases, of the gene *BMPR2* [54, 55]. *BMPR2* encodes the transmembrane bone morphogenetic receptor type II of the TGF-β superfamily of signalling molecules. TGF-β molecules are indispensible in a multitude of cellular activities which include proliferation, apoptosis, migration and differentiation [56]. Shortly after the identification of *BMPR2* defects in PAH families, mutation analysis was extended to a cohort of patients with sporadic onset of disease. All cases were rigorously screened to ensure the absence of a family history, associated disease and exposure to known risk factors. Initial investigations revealed the presence of *BMPR2* mutations in 26% of patients thereby expanding a role for this gene in the wider spectra of PH. Thereafter, several international studies have been conducted on IPAH patients with mutation detection rates ranging from 11–40% [57–60].

3.2. BMPR2 Structure and Function. *BMPR2* is a relatively large gene, consisting of 13 coding exons arrayed over 190 kb of genomic DNA with a transcriptional start site at base pair position −1148 relative to the initiation codon adenine. It has an unusually long 3′ UTR of approximately 11 kb [61]. The transcript encodes a protein of 1038 amino acids comprising an extracellular ligand binding domain (exons 2 and 3), a single pass transmembrane domain (exons 4 and 5), a highly conserved catalytic kinase domain (exons 6 to 11) and a cytoplasmic domain (exons 12 and 13) of uncertain functional relevance. Of note, this cytoplasmic tail is unique in length amongst other TGF-β receptors all of which contain short intracellular tracts. Exon 12 is removed by alternative splicing to render a naturally occurring shorter receptor species which while, as is the case with the long form, is ubiquitously expressed at the transcript level, the protein product has not been extensively tested to determine functionality [62].

The BMP signalling pathway is a highly regulated system controlled on multiple layers and in a cell-specific manner by a variety of mechanisms that include competitive ligand binding, intracellular inhibition of receptor types and cell-specific utilisation of different receptor combinations to generate myriad signalling outcomes. In its basic form, signalling is initiated at the cell surface when extracellular ligand is bound by a heterotetrameric complex comprising BMPR-II and a type-I partner receptor which may be BMPR1A or BMPR1B [63]. As an illustration of pathway specificity, in pulmonary endothelial cells, BMPR-II binds the type I receptor ALK-1 which is predominantly expressed in the endothelium in order to transduce signal in response to the ligand BMP9 [64]. When brought together upon binding ligand the constitutively kinase active BMPR-II transphosphorylates the GS domain of its type I partner thus activating its catalytic domain. The type I receptor, next, contacts and phosphorylates cytoplasmic effector molecules, for example, the receptor Smad proteins (R-Smads). BMP signalling is differentiated from TGF-β pathways by the fact that each activate a different subset of R-Smads. In the case of the BMPs, these are R-Smad1, 5, and 8 whereas the TGF-β receptors phosphorylate Smads 2 and 3. Common to both systems is Smad4 which binds the activated R-Smads and chaperones them to the nucleus where, in combination with nuclear cofactors they act, in complex, to regulate the transcription of a target set of genes [63]. More recently, it has become evident that signalling routed through this pathway is far more complex than previously thought. Several Smad independent pathways have emerged from the characterization of BMPR-II interacting proteins, for example, Tctex-1, LIMK-1, RACK-1, tenascin-1, that regulate cellular processes which include actin cytoskeletal dynamics and maintenance of the extracellular matrix [65–68]. An important pathway regulated by BMP signalling is that of p38MAPK [69]. Increasingly, an understanding has grown of the mechanisms governing p38MAPK activation downstream of BMPR-II and, indeed, Smad activation itself. Optimal signalling through either downstream pathway appears to be dependent on endocytosis of receptor complexes. Smad signalling requires receptor internalization through clathrin-coated pits whereas p38MAPK activation is reliant on receptor complexes being endocytosed through a caveolae mediated route [70]. The mode of receptor oligomerization is also considered vital in determination of downstream pathway activation. Receptor complexes may either be preassembled or induced by ligand; in the former instance Smad signalling is the favoured pathway whereas ligand recruitment of receptor complexes, the more common mechanism, leads to alkaline phosphatase activation via the p38MAPK pathway [71].

3.3. The BMPR2 Mutation Spectrum in HPAH. Mutations in *BMPR2* have been now reported in a multitude of ethnic groups as a result of a systematic survey of exons, intron-exon junctions, and, less frequently, noncoding regions including the 5′ and 3′ UTR and putative promoter region. In the main, point mutations in the gene have been examined using Sanger sequencing and/or denaturing high-performance liquid chromatography (DHPLC). Large scale gene rearrangements have been screened for using multiplex ligation-dependent probe amplification (MLPA) technology in addition to conventional Southern blotting. These independent investigations, when combined, identify deleterious variation in 70% of subjects with affected relatives, with more likelihood to be found when gene screening routinely advances to analysis of intronic and regulatory regions. More unexpectedly, mutations of genes encoding BMPR-II and, indeed, other members of the TGF-β superfamily have been detected in PAH associated with other conditions or risk factors, for example exposure to the appetite suppressant drugs fenfluramine and dex-fenfluramine. The distribution and class of mutation in hereditary and spontaneous disease is largely indistinguishable. In both HPAH and IPAH, mutations are arrayed across the gene, albeit at extremely low frequency in exons 5 and 13, and comprise all categories including missense, nonsense, frame-shift, splice-site, small deletions and insertions, as well as larger gene rearrangements. To date, over 300 independent mutations of *BMPR2* have been identified [72]. In the main, the variant level of severity has been inferred by confirmation of segregation amongst affecteds and carriers in families, degree of evolutionary conservation across species and occurrence in key functional domains. However, representative examples of mutant alleles, impacting upon the major receptor domains, have been taken forward by several research groups to *in vitro* functional analysis of the effect of identified patient specific mutations on downstream signalling pathways.

3.3.1. Haploinsufficiency Is the Primary Molecular Mechanism of Disease. Mutations of *BMPR2* likely to cause premature truncation of the open reading frame constitute large gene deletions and duplications (~6%), splice-site mutation (~9%), frame-shift (~24%), and nonsense defects (~29%). Thus, 70% of all identified mutations in HPAH would be predicted to lead to aberrantly truncated mutant alleles [72, 73]. Truncating mutations have been detected across the gene but spare the terminal exon 13. The effect of truncating point mutations on messenger RNA was assessed using patient cell lines harbouring this class of mutation. The level of the transcript under physiological conditions was estimated by means of quantitative polymerase chain reaction (qPCR) assays. As predicted, upon the addition of puromycin, a well known inhibitor of the nonsense mediated decay (NMD) pathway, transcript levels increased significantly. These data indicate that the majority of mutations predicting premature truncation are detected by the NMD surveillance machinery and removed from the cell by degradation of the mutant harbouring allele [74]. Taken together with the evidence of large and whole gene deletions of *BMPR2*, these observations firmly establish haploinsufficiency as the central molecular mechanism of disease in familial and sporadic forms of PAH [75] (Figure 2). While the vast majority of truncating mutations typically impact upon the coding region an interesting exception is found in the form of a double substitution of contiguous bases approximately 900 base pairs upstream of the start site of translation. The GC < AT mutation was identified in a large kindred and observed to segregate with the disease phenotype. *In silico* analysis of the region of sequence harbouring this variation suggested the introduction of a new translational start site stronger than the wild-type which, if employed, would lead to the incorporation of a premature termination codon in exon 1 of the gene. As this event would be predicted to produce a transcript susceptible to NMD, allele-specific polymerase chain reaction was employed to test transcript levels from patient cell lines before and after the application of NMD inhibitors. The resultant data indicated a consequent restoration of mutant message indicating that NMD was being triggered. The detection of this novel mutation serves to emphasise the likely presence of pathogenic variation contained within noncoding sequence not typically screened [61].

3.3.2. Amino Acid Substitution in HPAH. Missense mutations underlying amino acid substitutions impact primarily on areas of the receptor that are of pivotal catalytic and/or structural importance. As such, this form of mutation has been found to be largely restricted to those exons and, indeed, residues that are pre-requisites for BMPR-II signalling activity. The majority of missense mutations have been identified in exons 2 and 3 encoding the extracellular domain, and exons 6 to 11, encoding the kinase domain. Only a handful of missense mutations have been identified in exon 12, responsible for the long cytoplasmic tail [72, 73].

3.3.3. Mutations of the BMPR-II Extracellular Domain. Three dimensional structural studies reveal that the extracellular domains of the TGF-β receptors, including BMPR-II, are highly organised structures which bear resemblance to a class of toxins known as the three finger toxin family. This complex fold is substantially dependent on the formation of five disulphide bridges themselves dependent on 10 cysteine residues spread across the proximal exons. The importance of these particular residues is indicated by the fact that they are invariant in the majority of type II receptor species [76]. Of note, amino acid substitutions within this domain predominantly affect the conserved cysteine residues, testimony to their importance to receptor integrity. *In vitro* studies using tagged constructs bearing cysteine mutations demonstrated that the subcellular localisation of the encoded mutant proteins was cytosolic by contrast to the plasma membrane positioning of the wild-type receptor. These results point to the likelihood of normal membrane trafficking being compromised as a consequence of protein misfolding leading to the trapping of mutant receptors in the cytoplasm [77].

3.3.4. Kinase Domain Defects in PAH. The kinase domain of BMPR-II belongs, along with the other TGF-β receptors, to the extensive and highly evolutionarily conserved eukaryotic protein kinase (EUK) superfamily. Eukaryotic kinases share structural and functional features as well as the phosphate group transfer mechanism. EUKs are composed of 12 subdomains each with specific functional characteristics necessary to effect the step-wise processes required for a successful catalytic outcome. Broadly, the N-terminal end of the receptor is responsible for adenosine triphosphate binding while subdomains in the distal half are required for substrate recognition of initiation of substrate phosphorylation. Within these subdomains are distinctive patterns of conserved residues and, further, as revealed by X-ray crystallography, invariant residues which are indispensible to function [78]. Missense mutations typically cluster within the more highly conserved subdomains and conserved residues. This is best illustrated by recurrent PAH-specific mutation at position 491 in the amino acid chain. Within the kinase domain this residue is critical to activity as it forms an ion pair with a conserved glutamic acid at position 386. By contrast, few variants, the majority of which may be described as being of unknown significance, arise in the weakly conserved regions of the kinase domain, for example, subdomain IV, which does not appear to play a major role in kinase function or structure [72, 73]. All noncysteine substitutions of the kinase domain are localised correctly to the plasma membrane due to the structural integrity of the receptor being preserved. Transient transfection of a large series of mutant receptors harbouring kinase domain defects indicate the loss of kinase function by their inability to activate a Smad binding element upstream of a luciferase reporter gene. In many cases the receptor was effectively kinase dead by comparison to wild-type controls. Intriguingly, it was also noted that transfection of both cysteine and noncysteine receptors lowered luciferase readouts to below base-line levels implying a dominant negative effect on the wild-type receptor. This was hypothesised as being a result of sequestration of the wild-type partner by mutant receptors into signalling defective complexes. However, it is often the case that assays of this nature do not accurately reflect the *in vivo* situation making over interpretation of the data unwise [77, 79].

3.3.5. Mutations of the Cytoplasmic Terminus. Approximately 15% of the mutation load in PAH is confined to the cytoplasmic tail region with the vast majority of recorded mutations in this domain truncating in nature [72, 73]. Of interest, the small number of missense mutations observed in patients are clearly distinct from the rest of the spectrum. These mutant receptors appear broadly analogous to wild-type in the ability to translocate to the cell-surface and activate luciferase reporters [77, 79]. To investigate the pathogenicity of these variants, research streams turned to identifying Smad-independent pathways, regulated by the cytoplasmic domain, that were potentially of significance in disease precipitation and progression. To facilitate this objective, a number of studies focussed on developing an understanding of the role of the cytoplasmic tail in signalling by the identification of protein interacting partners. Amongst the interacting proteins identified were the cytoskeletal proteins Tctex-1, a light chain of the macromolecular motor cytoplasmic dynein and LIMK-1, a regulator of actin polymerization. Tctex-1 was discovered to be a kinase substrate of BMPR-II; the presence of mutation in the cytoplasmic tail attenuated this process. Mutations in this domain resulted in the constitutive activation of LIMK-1 resulting in abnormalities in actin dynamics [65, 66]. More recently, studies conducted on a transgenic mouse harbouring a cytoplasmic domain mutation (p.R899X), which due to massive overexpression of the transgene acts in a dominant negative manner, demonstrated augmented levels of Rho/Rho-kinase. Moreover, in certain cell populations this resulted in increased production of IL-6 which, when suppressed, ameliorated symptoms of disease. No perturbation of the Smad signalling pathway was observed suggesting that activation of Rho-kinase may represent an additional disease pathway specifically related to the cytoplasmic tail [80].

3.3.6. Pathway Dysregulation as a Result of BMPR-II Mutation. The single pathway disrupted by all mutation irrespective of position is that of the proproliferative kinase p38MAPK which is found to be upregulated by BMPR-II mutation. p38MAPK has been linked, *in vitro*, to the abnormal proliferation of PAH cells as this cellular defect can be reversed in the presence of specific p38MAPK inhibitors [77].

TGF-β signalling in normal PASMCs exerts an antiproliferative response. By contrast, BMPR-II defects in human and experimental PAH appear to induce an upregulation in TGF-β signalling in concert with a proproliferative effect on PASMCs. As examination of the canonical TGF-β pathway did not uncover evidence of dysregulation, it was speculated that Smad-independent signalling might play a role. Assessment of mutant cell lines with identified *BMPR2* mutation led to the discovery of an elevation in the expression and activity of TGF-β activated kinase (TAK-1). As the downstream substrates of TAK-1 include p38MAPK and ERK-1, it has been posited that the increased pool of TAK-1, responding to TGF-β stimulation, drives the uncontrolled proliferation of mutant cells by activation of its substrates [81]. Davies et al. drew a link between BMPR-II dysfunction and misdirected NF-κB signalling leading, in turn, to an increased production of IL-6 and PASMC proliferation in response to abnormally elevated TGF-β stimulation [82].

3.3.7. Atypical BMPR2 Mutations in APAH. The majority of mutations observed in studies conducted on PAH associated with other conditions and/or risk factors, primarily appetite suppressant drugs, demonstrate a marked dissimilarity to the HPAH mutation spectrum. In contrast to HPAH, over 90% of these variants are missense mutations which display a different profile to the amino acid substitutions in hereditary and spontaneous disease. Whereas cysteine residues are predominantly mutated in HPAH, these residues are spared in PAH associated with congenital heart disease and anorexigen intake. Moreover, many of the identified substitutions occur in regions of the receptor that make a limited contribution to the functional and structural integrity of the receptor, for example exon 5 of the gene. *In vitro* reporter based studies aimed at determining the effect of a series of these reported APAH mutations on BMPR-II signalling activity concluded that their ability to activate the reporter gene was comparable to wild-type. Hence, interpretation of the mechanisms by which these variants trigger PAH is problematic. It is feasible that these alleles represent low penetrance risk factors that require additional environmental insults and genetic modifiers to precipitate disease [72, 73].

3.3.8. Recurrent BMPR2 Mutations in HPAH. Mutations observed on multiple occasions in unrelated cases accounts for approximately 40% of observed variation in HPAH and are comprised of at least 25 independent defects. While large-scale systematic studies have not been performed to determine whether these mutations arise from common founder haplotypes, those mutations which have been analysed (c.994C>T (p.R332X), c.2579delT (p.N861fsX10) and c.2695C>T (p.R899X)) by microsatellite marker haplotyping clearly confirm that in each case the mutation was harboured in a distinct haplotype with no evidence of marker sharing between patients [72, 73]. These results support the hypothesis of a recurrent mutation process in favour of the presence of ancestral mutations ascertained in multiple individuals. Moreover, the majority of the observed recurrent mutations occur at CpG islands and, thus, likely arise as a result of spontaneous deamination of methylated cytosines with subsequent conversion to thymidine, a relatively common mutational mechanism. Recurrent frameshift mutations as a result of small insertions and deletions are typically found in regions of low sequence complexity, potentially implicating replication slippage as a cause for mutation at those positions. Investigation of isolated populations, notably that of Finland, also failed to uncover evidence of founder mutations indicating that if it does exist it is most likely uncommon [83].

3.3.9. Genotype-Phenotype Correlations. Analyses of a relationship between mutation class and position with broad disease parameters including age of onset, hemodynamic function in patients, and survival failed to yield data indicative of a meaningful correlation. More recently, research into putative correlations has endeavoured to interrogate more subtle aspects of phenotype. Elliott et al. attempted to assess the relationship between *BMPR2* sequence variation and vasoreactivity, an important clinical consideration in the treatment of patients using vasodilators such as prostacyclin analogues. A total of 67 familial and idiopathic patients were investigated for *BMPR2* nonsynonymous variation, of which 27 patients proved positive for variation with 22 harbouring bona fide pathogenic mutations. Vasoreactivity was evaluated between the sets of patients with and without variation using stringent clinical criteria. None of the mutation carriers were found to be vasoreactive by contrast to 35% of patients with no form of variation. These results are a compelling indication of a correlation between defective BMPR-II signalling and vascular tone and responsiveness [84].

In a Chinese study comprising 305 individuals, the presence of *BMPR2* mutations was noted to be associated with higher risk of mortality once adjusted for age and gender. The effect was most prominent in the male group but did not reach statistical significance in females which the authors attributed to the more complex disease aetiology in women [85].

In seeking to explore the reasons behind the remarkably low penetrance in *BMPR2* mutation carriers Cogan et al. examined the role played by alternatively spliced isoforms of the gene. A comparative analysis was conducted between lymphocytes from 47 affected mutation carriers versus 35 unaffected mutation carriers. Patients were determined to have a significantly higher ratio of the allele lacking exon 12 to the full-length transcript by comparison to carriers. Scrutiny of exon 12 revealed the presence of an exonic splice enhancer capable of binding serine/arginine-rich splicing factor 2 (SRSF2) which promotes exon inclusion. SRSF2 levels were found to be lower in patients than carriers and, theoretically would be anticipated to result in an elevation of levels of the shorter isoform [86].

3.4. Locus Heterogeneity in PAH

3.4.1. ALK and Endoglin. PAH, infrequently, may copresent with the vascular disorder hereditary haemorrhagic telangiectasia (HHT) wherein patients have PAH clinically and histopathologically identical to the hereditary form of disease, although PAH can also develop as a direct consequence of the pathophysiology of HHT. HHT, or Rendu-Osler-Weber syndrome, is an autosomal dominant disease with an incidence of approximately 1/10,000 in Europe. HHT is characterised by abnormal vascular development and a range of distinctive clinical complications. An early, common symptom is epistaxes (nosebleeds), observed in up to 90% of affected individuals. Other clinical manifestations may include telangiectases, red to violet lesions that develop on digits; the facial, nasal, and buccal mucosa; and the gastrointestinal (GI) tract. Haemorrhage from the GI bed, noted in 20–40% of patients, is progressive and can result in chronic anaemia [87].

Arteriovenous malformations (AVMs) engineer a direct communication between the arterial and venous systems that bypasses the capillary bed. AVMs have been detected in the pulmonary circulation in 25% of HHT cases; the hepatic circulation in 8–16% of patients and the cerebral circulation in 15% of the affected population. AVMs are considered to be a major contributant to morbidity and mortality in HHT patients [87].

Although the primary pathophysiological defect in HHT has yet to be determined, genetic linkage studies have revealed molecular heterogeneity in HHT and the identity of two loci. The disease genes at chromosome 9q34 and 12q13 have been identified as encoding the TGF-β pathway receptors *endoglin* and *ALK1*, respectively [88, 89]. Non-linkage to chromosome 9 and 12, in two HHT pedigrees, has suggested the likelihood of a third, as yet unidentified, locus [90]. *Endoglin* is a 14 exon gene, expressed at high levels on human vascular endothelial cells. Disparate mutations have been recorded in *endoglin* and appear to correlate to a severe clinical phenotype, with a high incidence of pulmonary AVMs (PAVMs) [91].

ALK1 is organised into 10 exons with the first translated methionine within exon 2. Families, with segregating *ALK1* mutations, tend to exhibit late-onset and milder disease manifestation. PAVMs have never been reported in patients bearing mutations in this gene. The molecular basis of dominance, in both *endoglin* and *ALK1*, is widely accepted as being that of haploinsufficiency [92].

ALK-1 and endoglin are type I and type III receptors respectively operating within the TGF-β pathway. This biological link with BMPR-II suggested a common molecular aetiology in patients with PAH-HHT. Five pedigrees in which both diseases were cosegregating were analysed for mutations in the three genes encoding these receptors. Screening of the coding regions and intron/exon boundaries revealed the presence of two truncating mutations and three missense mutations in *ALK1*, thereby identifying a second gene predisposing to the development of pulmonary hypertension [93]. Since the original report of *ALK1* as an underlying factor in PAH, several groups have analysed additional cohorts and thereby built on the mutation spectrum of the gene. These studies now reveal that 20% of all known *ALK1* mutations lead to the onset of PAH and, of these, 81% are distinct to defects causing HHT alone. Of the identified mutations, amino acid substitutions constitute the predominant class and affect functionally key domains of the receptor, in particular the kinase domain and NANDOR box [94]. More recently, evidence has emerged of *ALK1* mutations causing PAH in the absence of HHT. However, it must be noted that these subjects, in the main, have early-onset or childhood PAH thus retaining the possibility that HHT could develop at a later stage [95]. *Endoglin* mutation may also represent a rare cause of PAH-HHT with four defects detected in patients thus far. All *endoglin* mutations would be expected to lead to premature truncation of the transcript [73].

3.4.2. SMADs 1, 4, and 9. The discovery of mutations in three members of the TGF-β family leading to susceptibility to PAH emphasizes the role played by this signalling pathway in the maintenance of the pulmonary architecture. A number of recent studies have sought to expand on these findings by examining members of the downstream pathway for deleterious variation in patients in whom the known risk factors have been eliminated. By means of a direct sequencing approach in a limited cohort of 23 Japanese cases, Shintani et al. isolated a mutation in the BMP-specific receptor Smad gene *SMAD9* (p.C202X) predicting the incorporation of a premature truncation codon [96]. In the largest candidate gene study conducted in PAH a total of 324 idiopathic and associated PAH patients, previously excluded for mutations in *BMPR2*, *ALK1*, and *endoglin*, were screened for *SMAD1*, *-4*, *-5*, and *-9* by Sanger sequencing. This analysis resulted in the detection of 4 variants in the IPAH panel consisting of 198 cases, each of which was absent in a panel of 1000 controls and 60 fully sequenced exomes. These variants in *SMAD1* (p.V3A), *SMAD4* (p.N13S; c.1448-6T>C), and *SMAD9* (p.K43E) may define an additional 2.2% of the IPAH population with a genetic background to disease. However, whilst significant, it was found that the impact of these variants on functional outcomes was less extreme than classical *BMPR2* mutation. Therefore, they fall into the category of variants of unknown significance that, potentially, require other environmental and genetic factors to prove pathogenic. Alternatively, these defects may impact upon Smad-independent pathways, the investigation of which was not within the scope of this study [97]. Of interest, *SMAD9* had previously been associated with disease precipitation and progression due to the onset of manifest PAH in a *Smad9* knock-out mouse model. The *SMAD9* defects in the human studies are thus especially convincing in the light of the mouse model exhibiting clinical and histopathological features of PAH near identical to that observed in patients [98]. Two amino acid substitutions of the type I receptor *BMPR1B* (p.S160N and p.F392L) were recently identified upon the screening of a panel of 43 IPAH patients. *In vitro* and reporter assays indicated that the downstream effect of these variants was to induce increased production of Smad9 associated with or responsible for an increase in transcriptional activity suggestive of a gain-of-function mechanism. As both the human studies, on the basis of functional analyses, when combined with heterozygous loss of Smad9 in the mouse, suggested haploinsufficiency as the molecular mechanism for disease, the conclusions drawn by Chida et al. appear to contradict the preceding three reports. Further functional testing is required to fully elucidate the pathogenicity of these variants [99].

3.4.3. Caveolin-1. Homozygous *Caveolin-1* (*Cav1*) knock-out mice develop moderate PAH indicating a role for this gene in the aetiology of disease [100]. Next-generation sequencing technologies, in particular full exome sequencing, have transformed the field of disease gene identification by facilitating the rapid analysis of the entire exome in patient samples. By taking advantage of this methodology Austin et al. successfully identified a second causal gene in familial PAH, namely the human orthologue of *Cav1*. The analysis of 4 members of a multi-generational family led to the detection of a truncating mutation in *CAV1* (c.474delA), a finding which was consolidated by the subsequent demonstration of mutation segregation amongst the other affected members of the family. The *CAV1* variant was observed in unaffected members of this family and this was interpreted as, potentially, being due to incomplete penetrance in a similar vein to mutations of *BMPR2*. Analysis of a replication cohort by Sanger sequencing led to the identification of a second premature truncation (c.473delC) in a single IPAH case lending plausibility to the likelihood of the gene representing a rare inherited risk factor in familial PAH [101].

3.5. Modifying Factors Conferring Risk of Disease. Although PAH is an oligogenic disease, family studies demonstrate clinical features reminiscent of a complex disorder, for example, gender bias and reduced penetrance. This concept is lent strength by the existence of several pairs of monozygotic twins discordant for disease [73]. These observations suggest the existence of genetic modifier genes either promoting or protecting against disease. This hypothesis has been subject to much investigation in the form of examination of annotated variation in candidate genes believed to be involved in disease pathogenesis. Amongst others, these include the genes encoding the angiotensin converting enzyme (ACE), the serotonin transporter (at least four independent investigations), endoglin, prostaglandin synthase, and the voltage gated potassium channel subunit Kv1.5 [102–109]. The confounding factor affecting all these studies is the small sample size employed in each case which would not have the statistical power to detect modifying variation of small or moderate effect size. Moreover, validation of initial observations by means of a replication study in an independent cohort has not been attempted. Confirmation by replication studies is now acknowledged as being an essential component of any case control association analysis. In its absence these studies remain incomplete and conclusions drawn, whilst tantalising, have to be treated with some caution. In recent times, the development and wide-spread utilisation of the HapMap resource has revolutionised genome-wide association studies (GWAS). This form of analysis obviates the inefficient interrogation of limited variable loci in a few genes and, combined with the advances in genotyping technology, allows for a rapid examination of several hundred thousand independent loci in large sample sets. The relative lack of success of the candidate gene approach makes a GWAS a much more appealing study design option and one with potential to yield important new insights. Sample size remains an important consideration and due to the low incidence and prevalence of PAH, it is clear global cooperation is required to obtain case groups in excess of 1000 samples.

3.6. Animal Models of PH. The Fawn-Hooded rat (FHR) is a spontaneous model of pulmonary hypertension when exposed to mildly hypoxic conditions. While the trait appears to be hereditary there are phenotypic distinctions between PH in this animal and the human condition [110].

Five artificially generated mouse models harbouring *BMPR2* mutation have been reported and routinely employed in the study of the consequences of *BMPR2* disruption on the molecular and phenotypic level. The value of these animal models is twofold. Even in the absence of manifest disease symptoms murine models carrying domain specific *BMPR2* defects provide an invaluable and sustainable source of mutant cell lines that may be employed for interrogation of the BMP pathway in the disease cell and, further, can be characterized on the phenotypic level to gain an insight into the impact of mutation on cellular function. The ultimate goal is that these models go on to recapitulate the disease phenotype, in full or in part, to support the development of research targeted at providing therapeutic options for patients. Two mouse models were generated by utilisation of homologous recombination knock-out methodologies aimed at the removal of exon 2 and exons 4 and 5, respectively. In both instances the mutation proved to be homozygous lethal with the mutant animals dying *in utero*. Whilst both animal models displayed numerous developmental anomalies, cardiac defects particularly of the outflow tract were especially notable in the exon 2 knock-out mouse. In the heterozygous state, these mice were healthy and did not develop measureable features of disease. However, by comparison to wild-type mice, the mutant carriers displayed a significantly higher susceptibility to disease when exposed to environmental risk factors, for example exposure to hypoxia and the inflammatory agent 5-lipooxygenase [111, 112]. A widely used model is a mouse harbouring a point mutation (p.R899X) in exon 12 of the *BMPR2* gene generated by a knock-in strategy. Analogous to the knock-out mice, mutant animals are nonviable in the homozygous condition and asymptomatic in the heterozygous state [113].

Transgenic mouse models are produced through overexpression of a mutant allele introduced as a cDNA construct. As such, they less accurately reflect the genetic architecture of the human mutant carrier. Two transgenic mouse models have been developed to overexpress the point mutations c.504insT and c.2695C>T, driven by the smooth muscle specific promoter SM22, both of which predict incorporation of a premature termination codon [114, 115]. In nature, these mutations would be expected to be lost via the NMD pathway. However, as the NMD process is contingent on the presence of intronic regions, these mutant alleles are spared and expressed in protein form. The presence in the cell of multiple copies of these mutant alleles led to the spontaneous development of aspects of disease. Mice displayed increased pulmonary artery pressure and vessel muscularization. It may be hypothesised that these disease alleles behave in a dominant-negative fashion by acting as a trap for wild type receptors thereby diminishing the available pool of receptors capable of forming active complexes. The precipitation of overt pulmonary hypertension in the transgenic mice lends support for a threshold model of disease. While *BMPR2* haploinsufficiency is a major factor in predisposition to disease, it is not in itself enough to trigger disease in the majority of mutation carriers. Additional factors would appear to be required for disease to manifest and, foremost among these, is the inexplicable loss of wild type receptor in the cells of patients with severe disease. Together with the observations made on the transgenic mouse models, it is likely that a progressive reduction of BMPR-II levels is what is required for a disease state to occur [116].

4. Treatment Options in PAH

Treatment for PAH, while much improved in recent times, remains ameliorative and, in general, PAH continues to be a disease distinguished by high morbidity and mortality. All patients are required to undergo a test for vasoreactivity, typically with adenosine or epoprostenol delivered intravenously and/or inhaled nitric oxide. The patient's response is considered positive when the mean pulmonary artery pressure is lowered by 10 mm Hg and remains less than 40 mm Hg with no alteration in cardiac output and systemic pressure. Patients exhibiting a positive response are usually first administered calcium channel blocker treatments; unfortunately the vast majority of patients are nonresponsive and require alternative medical interventions. Calcium channel blockers including diltiazem and nifedipine are delivered at low initial doses and gradually augmented to the maximum level tolerated. After time, the efficacy of this form of treatment decreases and other options need to be explored [117].

4.1. Prostacyclin Analogues. The study of cellular pathways disrupted in the progression of PAH has pinpointed three cellular systems that have proven to be amenable to therapeutic intervention. The prostacyclin metabolic pathway is known to be dysregulated in PAH as indicated by reduced expression of prostacyclin synthase in the pulmonary arteries and of prostacyclin metabolites in the urine. Prostacyclin is a multifunctional prostanoid that functions as a powerful vasodilatory agent, an inhibitor of proliferation and platelet aggregation, all hallmark features of the PAH pulmonary circulation [118]. There are three prostacyclin analogues commonly used in patient care, namely epoprostenol, treprostinil, and iloprost. Epoprostenol is continuously administered intravenously at a starting dose of 2 ng/kg/min with an optimal level between 25–40 ng/kg/min [23]. Several substantial studies testify to the efficacy of the treatment in alleviating haemodynamic abnormalities in patients when compared against older, conventional therapies. Improvements were noted in mean arterial pressure, exercise capacity as measured by a 6 minute walk test, and pulmonary vascular resistance. Sitbon et al. conducted a longitudinal study of 178 patients with severe PAH over a five year period and noted survival rates of 85%, 70%, 63%, and 55% over 1, 2, 3, and 5 years [119]. Epoprostenol has been associated with side effects of varying severity that may range from diarrhoea to thrombosis [120]. Treprostinil is also associated with significant improvements in hemodynamic and symptomatic outcomes in patients when infused subcutaneously. As a monotherapy, treprostinil delivers better survival rates than epoprostenol with survival at 88% at one year and 70% at four years by comparison to 69% and 38% [121]. While the adverse effects of this treatment are broadly similar to intravenous injection of epoprostenol, when treprostinil is used intravenously it has potential to lead to a heightened risk of gram negative blood stream infections as well as life threatening catheter infections [122]. Unlike epoprostenol and treprostinil, iloprost is a stable prostacyclin analogue that remains effective for a longer period of time. It also provides the considerable advantage of obviating catheter related complications as it can be inhaled in aerosolized form. A large multi-centre trial, comprising 207 patients with severe PAH (Class III and IV), demonstrated that iloprost therapy resulted in an improvement of at least one functional class [123]. Deleterious effects of iloprost usage are generally mild by comparison to the other commonly employed prostacyclin analogues.

4.2. Endothelin-1 Blocking Agents. Endothelin-1 has long been considered to be involved in the aetiology of PAH. It is significantly upregulated in the circulation of PAH patients leading to the development of agents capable of blocking its effects, most prominently bosentan, sitaxsentan, and ambrisentan. Unusually, bosentan is an endothelin antagonist that is capable of blocking both ETA and ETB receptors. Kaplan-Meir survival curves indicated that survival rates of patients treated with bosentan were 96% and 89% in years 1 and 2, respectively [124]. These estimates compared favourably with patients undergoing epoprostenol. Bosentan improves symptoms, haemodynamics, and exercise capacity but can lead to dangerous side effects which include liver problems and hypotension. Male subjects may be at risk of infertility and testicular atrophy [125]. Ambrisentan is a specific ETA receptor antagonist that has been shown by place controlled trials of randomized patients to effect sustained improvements in pulmonary haemodynamics and exercise capacity. While possible testicular atrophy remains a significant side effect, unlike bosentan, the risk of liver damage is low [126].

4.3. Combined Therapy. When monotherapy begins to fail to improve symptoms and quality of life in patients a combinatorial strategy is next employed. These, typically, consist of the dual administration of a prostacyclin analogue with an endothelial antagonist. Whilst anecdotal evidence does point to improvements in functional readouts, reduced toxicity, and efficacy of treatment, thus far only a few clinical trials have been run to validate these observations. A placebo controlled study of 405 PAH patients revealed that a combination of bosentan with tadalafil, more known for its usage in treating erectile dysfunction, drove a quantifiable improvement in exercise capacity allied to retardation of clinical worsening [127]. In an analysis of 267 PAH patients, compared to patients treated with placebo while on intravenous epoprostenol, those given sildenafil showed significant improvements in cardiac outputs and mean pulmonary arterial pressure [128].

4.4. Therapy for End-Stage Disease. The majority of patients even when benefiting from the highest levels of contemporary PAH therapy will progressively worsen to a critical life-threatening stage. At this time invasive procedures, often atrial septostomy followed by lung transplantation are typically the last remaining options. An atrial septostomy is a procedure designed to introduce a shunt, or conduit, between the right and left atria. This adaptation reduces the blood volume in the right side of the heart and, as a consequence, reduces the work-load in pumping blood to the lungs and improves the ventricular function of the heart. While this procedure provides a measure of clinical stability, it is considered only a precursor to eventual lung transplantation. Lung transplantation, which may be single lung transplantation, double lung transplantation, or heart and lung transplantation, is considered the last therapeutic resort for PAH patients. Following transplantation, patient survival rates have been reported as 66%, 57%, 47%, and 27% at years 1, 3, 5, and 10, respectively [129]. The type of lung transplantation chosen for recipient patients varies internationally from centre to centre.

4.5. Current Approaches to Therapy. Recent data released by the Registry to Evaluate Early and Long-term Pulmonary Arterial Hypertension, a longitudinal study of patients from North America, and the French Network on Pulmonary Hypertension, underlines the fact that even with recent improvements in therapeutic protocols, survival figures over three years is still unacceptably modest [130, 131]. Research into PAH has noticeably attempted to address this continuing problem by seeking to translate pathway based studies to therapeutic options. While palliative care has been undoubtedly important in transforming the patient's quality of life, there is increasingly a sense of urgency to employ the growing understanding of defects in the BMP pathway to create directed therapy protocols with the potential to permanently halt or reverse the progression of this disease. To do so, such treatments would be expected to demonstrably remove clinical features of PAH, for example vascular lesions by reverse vascular modelling, and promote the restoration of homeostatic balance between vasoconstrictive and vasodilatory agents.

4.6. Gene Therapy. The confounding factors present in the application of gene therapy to human disease are numerous and have stalled the application of this technology to PAH until recently. Complications inherent in gene-based therapies include insertional mutagenesis as well as practical limitations, for example, vector design and delivery, the short duration a beneficial outcome will last and, perhaps, most pertinently in PAH the correct cellular target. Reynolds et al. sought to overcome some of these impediments in a recent study on gene delivery in two experimental rat models of PAH: PAH induced by chronic hypoxia and monocrotaline (MCT)-induced PH. Both rat populations recapitulated the hallmark features of disease, namely raised pulmonary vascular pressure and evidence of vascular modelling. Although neither model harboured *BMPR2* mutation, both had diminished levels of the encoded protein, an as yet unexplained phenomena also observed in PAH patients negative for mutations of the gene. The authors specifically targeted the pulmonary endothelium with a *BMPR2* adenoviral gene delivery vehicle by the linkage of a bispecific antibody to the angiotensin-converting enzyme. BMPR-II expression was detected in and confined to the pulmonary arterioles and alveolar capillaries. Receptor expression was absent in the cardiac sections tested indicating successful and specific delivery to the lung. Introducing the vector to the endothelial layer of pulmonary arteries resulted in a marked improvement in pulmonary haemodynamics including mean pulmonary arterial pressure and right ventricular systolic pressure. Of interest, these changes while positive, were less impressive in the monocrotaline model and did not reach statistical significance. In both models there was clear evidence of a reduction in abnormal vascular remodelling most likely due to a concurrent decrease in the uncontrolled expansion of the endothelial and smooth muscle layers. Recent studies have drawn a clear link between the elevation of TGF-β expression and activity in the lung tissue of PAH patients with disease pathogenesis. In the case of the experimental rat models, this disease trait was identified in the MCT treated mouse but was absent in the hypoxia induced model, in itself evidence of the fact that whilst of utility animal models do not fully mirror the human disease state. Nonetheless, the depression of TGF-β activity is a much sought after therapeutic goal and the upregulation of BMPR-II signalling activity via adenoviral delivery was found to quench the exuberant TGF-β response in the MCT rat model. In follow-up studies conducted on human pulmonary microvascular endothelial cells *in vitro*, this study noted that the restoration of BMPR-II levels and, by extension, rescue of BMP signalling blocked TGF-β induced endothelial-mesenchymal transition. This is certainly an important observation but its mechanistic significance in the aetiology of PAH remains to be fully investigated. The primary impact of this particular study is that both rat models, with markedly different initiating factors precipitating disease and substantially distinct phenotypic responses to environmental insults, nonetheless responded to BMPR-II levels being heightened in the correct cell type. These data suggest that the common denominator between different categories of PAH is the level of BMPR-II, likely in the endothelial layer, dropping below a threshold level whereupon the disease state overtly manifests. On a therapy level, this gene delivery option if applicable to humans may benefit a wide spectrum of PH sufferers including those without *BMPR2* mutation [132].

As described previously, prostaglandin enhancement is a vital form of treatment in PAH on account of the disruption of this pathway in the progression of the disease. Yet, this form of treatment loses efficacy over time and, moreover, is associated with several potential complications. Patient quality of life is much impaired when prostacyclin is delivered by use of integrated catheters administering continuous intravenous medication and, additionally, the risk of catheter related infection is significant. PAH was induced in the mouse by prolonged exposure to hypoxic conditions and these animals were employed in a study of the potential feasibility of Prostaglandin I_2 Synthase (hPGIS) gene delivery in the attenuation and/or reversal of disease symptoms. Moreover, Kataoka et al. investigated the efficiency and effect of an adeno-associated virus (AAV) vector in gene delivery and, further, extended these investigations to different AAV serotypes. Two AAV vectors, type I and type II carrying the hPGIS transcript, were injected into the thigh skeletal tissue of hypoxia induced (10% O_2) PAH mice which had been exposed to the risk condition for 8 weeks. Both treatments resulted in a decrease of right ventricular systolic pressure, the ratio of right ventricular weight to body weight, and the ratio of RV weight to left ventricular plus septal weight, measures that all reached statistical significance. Additionally, the treatment resulted in a reversal of thickening of the medial wall of pulmonary arterioles. In conclusion, both vector systems were equally effective in halting and, indeed, reversing aspects of the pathogenic PAH phenotype [133].

Yet, it is equally apparent that major obstacles need be overcome. It is unclear, given the present technological constraints, whether this form of treatment is indeed the Holy Grail for sufferers of PAH. The questions that need to be explicated consist of, but are not confined to, whether a gene delivery system that can maintain extended periods of expression is an achievable aim in the foreseeable future. In addition, can a swift change in the cellular environment by, for example, restoring BMPR-II levels, effect a long-term alteration in the framework of the cells comprising the pulmonary circulation? Most importantly, the basic science affected by treatment such as this needs to be fully explored. Are other non-disease systems impacted by treatment and in what way? These and many more considerations remain to be interrogated.

5. Future Directions

There is still genetic variation to be uncovered in all forms of PAH. This will be greatly aided by the advent of next-generation sequencing and genotyping systems which will facilitate the discovery of rare and common variation underlying disease. Significant effort needs to be applied in fully elucidating the epidemiology of this condition, in particular to aid genetic counselling of patients. Treatment options, in light of the molecular breakthroughs achieved thus far, must aim higher and execute treatments that become more than simply palliative but, instead, curative.

References

[1] M. C. Parera, M. van Dooren, M. van Kempen et al., "Distal angiogenesis: a new concept for lung vascular morphogenesis," *American Journal of Physiology*, vol. 288, no. 1, pp. L141–L149, 2005.

[2] S. M. Hall, A. A. Hislop, and S. G. Haworth, "Origin, differentiation, and maturation of human pulmonary veins," *American Journal of Respiratory Cell and Molecular Biology*, vol. 26, no. 3, pp. 333–340, 2002.

[3] D. E. deMello and L. M. Reid, "Embryonic and early fetal development of human lung vasculature and its functional implications," *Pediatric and Developmental Pathology*, vol. 3, no. 5, pp. 439–449, 2000.

[4] C. Galambos and D. E. deMello, "Molecular mechanisms of pulmonary vascular development," *Pediatric and Developmental Pathology*, vol. 10, no. 13, pp. 1–17, 2007.

[5] H. Yamamoto, E. Jun Yun, H. P. Gerber, N. Ferrara, J. A. Whitsett, and T. H. Vu, "Epithelial-vascular cross talk mediated by VEGF-A and HGF signaling directs primary septae formation during distal lung morphogenesis," *Developmental Biology*, vol. 308, no. 1, pp. 44–53, 2007.

[6] P. Carmeliet, V. Ferreira, G. Breier et al., "Abnormal blood vessel development and lethality in embryos lacking a single VEGF allele," *Nature*, vol. 380, no. 6573, pp. 435–439, 1996.

[7] L. Morbidelli, C. H. O. Chang, J. G. Douglas, H. J. Granger, F. Ledda, and M. Ziche, "Nitric oxide mediates mitogenic effect of VEGF on coronary venular endothelium," *American Journal of Physiology*, vol. 270, no. 1, part 2, pp. H411–H415, 1996.

[8] H. He, V. J. Venema, X. Gu, R. C. Venema, M. B. Marrero, and R. B. Caldwell, "Vascular endothelial growth factor signals endothelial cell production of nitric oxide and prostacyclin through Flk-1/KDR activation of c-Src," *The Journal of Biological Chemistry*, vol. 274, no. 35, pp. 25130–25135, 1999.

[9] M. Southwood, T. K. Jeffery, X. Yang et al., "Regulation of bone morphogenetic protein signalling in human pulmonary vascular development," *Journal of Pathology*, vol. 214, no. 1, pp. 85–95, 2008.

[10] C. Suri, P. F. Jones, S. Patan et al., "Requisite role of angiopoietin-1, a ligand for the TIE2 receptor, during embryonic angiogenesis," *Cell*, vol. 87, no. 7, pp. 1171–1180, 1996.

[11] J. Rasanen, D. C. Wood, S. Weiner, A. Ludomirski, and J. C. Huhta, "Role of the pulmonary circulation in the distribution of human fetal cardiac output during the second half of pregnancy," *Circulation*, vol. 94, no. 5, pp. 1068–1073, 1996.

[12] A. M. Rudolph, "Aortopulmonary transposition in the fetus: speculation on pathophysiology and therapy," *Pediatric Research*, vol. 61, no. 3, pp. 375–380, 2007.

[13] T. Kiserud, "Physiology of the fetal circulation," *Seminars in Fetal and Neonatal Medicine*, vol. 10, no. 6, pp. 493–503, 2005.

[14] S. K. Sinha and S. M. Donn, "Fetal-to-neonatal maladaptation," *Seminars in Fetal and Neonatal Medicine*, vol. 11, no. 3, pp. 166–173, 2006.

[15] A. J. Moss, G. Emmanouilides, and E. R. Duffie Jr., "Closure of the ductus arteriosus in the newborn infant," *Pediatrics*, vol. 32, pp. 25–30, 1963.

[16] B. Van Overmeire and S. Chemtob, "The pharmacologic closure of the patent ductus arteriosus," *Seminars in Fetal and Neonatal Medicine*, vol. 10, no. 2, pp. 177–184, 2005.

[17] S. G. Haworth, S. M. Hall, M. Chew, and K. Allen, "Thinning of fetal pulmonary arterial wall and postnatal remodelling: ultrastructural studies on the respiratory unit arteries of the pig," *Virchows Archiv A*, vol. 411, no. 2, pp. 161–171, 1987.

[18] S. G. Haworth and A. A. Hislop, "Pulmonary vascular development: normal values of peripheral vascular structure," *American Journal of Cardiology*, vol. 52, no. 5, pp. 578–583, 1983.

[19] A. Hislop, "Developmental biology of the pulmonary circulation," *Paediatric Respiratory Reviews*, vol. 6, no. 1, pp. 35–43, 2005.

[20] S. G. Haworth and A. A. Hislop, "Lung development—the effects of chronic hypoxia," *Seminars in Neonatology*, vol. 8, no. 1, pp. 1–8, 2003.

[21] J. R. Runo and J. E. Loyd, "Primary pulmonary hypertension," *The Lancet*, vol. 361, no. 9368, pp. 1533–1544, 2003.

[22] N. Galiè, M. M. Hoeper, M. Humbert et al., "Guidelines for the diagnosis and treatment of pulmonary hypertension: the Task Force for the Diagnosis and Treatment of Pulmonary Hypertension of the European Society of Cardiology (ESC) and the European Respiratory Society (ERS), endorsed by the International Society of Heart and Lung Transplantation (ISHLT)," *European Heart Journal*, vol. 30, no. 20, pp. 2493–2537, 2009.

[23] V. V. McLaughlin, S. L. Archer, D. B. Badesch et al., "ACCF/AHA 2009 Expert Consensus Document on Pulmonary Hypertension. A Report of the American College of Cardiology Foundation Task Force on Expert Consensus Documents and the American Heart Association Developed in Collaboration With the American College of Chest Physicians;

American Thoracic Society, Inc.; and the Pulmonary Hypertension Association," *Journal of the American College of Cardiology*, vol. 53, no. 17, pp. 1573–1619, 2009.

[24] J. E. Loyd, M. G. Butler, T. M. Foroud, P. M. Conneally, J. A. Phillips III, and J. H. Newman, "Genetic anticipation and abnormal gender ratio at birth in familial primary pulmonary hypertension," *American Journal of Respiratory and Critical Care Medicine*, vol. 152, no. 1, pp. 93–97, 1995.

[25] E. D. Austin, J. E. Loyd, and J. A. Phillips III, "Genetics of pulmonary arterial hypertension," *Seminars in Respiratory and Critical Care Medicine*, vol. 30, no. 4, pp. 386–398, 2009.

[26] G. Simonneau, I. M. Robbins, M. Beghetti et al., "Updated clinical classification of pulmonary hypertension," *Journal of the American College of Cardiology*, vol. 54, no. 1, supplement, pp. S43–S54, 2009.

[27] G. Simonneau, N. Galiè, L. J. Rubin et al., "Clinical classification of pulmonary hypertension," *Journal of the American College of Cardiology*, vol. 43, no. 12, supplement, pp. 5S–12S, 2004.

[28] J. E. Loyd, J. B. Atkinson, G. G. Pietra, R. Virmani, and J. H. Newman, "Heterogeneity of pathologic lesions in familial primary pulmonary hypertension," *American Review of Respiratory Disease*, vol. 138, no. 4, pp. 952–957, 1988.

[29] R. M. Tuder, M. Chacon, L. Alger et al., "Expression of angiogenesis-related molecules in plexiform lesions in severe pulmonary hypertension: evidence for a process of disordered angiogenesis," *Journal of Pathology*, vol. 195, no. 3, pp. 367–374, 2001.

[30] R. M. Tuder, B. Groves, D. B. Badesch, and N. F. Voelkel, "Exuberant endothelial cell growth and elements of inflammation are present in plexiform lesions of pulmonary hypertension," *American Journal of Pathology*, vol. 144, no. 2, pp. 275–285, 1994.

[31] M. E. Yeager, G. R. Halley, H. A. Golpon, N. F. Voelkel, and R. M. Tuder, "Microsatellite instability of endothelial cell growth and apoptosis genes within plexiform lesions in primary pulmonary hypertension," *Circulation Research*, vol. 88, no. 1, pp. E2–E11, 2001.

[32] R. D. Machado, V. James, M. Southwood et al., "Investigation of second genetic hits at the BMPR2 locus as a modulator of disease progression in familial pulmonary arterial hypertension," *Circulation*, vol. 111, no. 5, pp. 607–613, 2005.

[33] B. W. Christman, C. D. McPherson, J. H. Newman et al., "An imbalance between the excretion of thromboxane and prostacyclin metabolites in pulmonary hypertension," *The New England Journal of Medicine*, vol. 327, no. 2, pp. 70–75, 1992.

[34] K. G. Kreymborg, S. Uchida, P. Gellert et al., "Identification of right heart-enriched genes in a murine model of chronic outflow tract obstruction," *Journal of Molecular and Cellular Cardiology*, vol. 49, no. 4, pp. 598–605, 2010.

[35] J. Wharton, J. W. Strange, G. M. O. Møller et al., "Antiproliferative effects of phosphodiesterase type 5 inhibition in human pulmonary artery cells," *American Journal of Respiratory and Critical Care Medicine*, vol. 172, no. 1, pp. 105–113, 2005.

[36] C. E. Sparacino-Watkins, Y. C. Lai, and M. T. Gladwin, "Nitrate-nitrite-nitric oxide pathway in pulmonary arterial hypertension therapeutics," *Circulation*, vol. 125, no. 23, pp. 2824–2826, 2012.

[37] M. Humbert, G. Monti, F. Brenot et al., "Increased interleukin-1 and interleukin-6 serum concentrations in severe primary pulmonary hypertension," *American Journal of Respiratory and Critical Care Medicine*, vol. 151, no. 5, pp. 1628–1631, 1995.

[38] T. Itoh, N. Nagaya, H. Ishibashi-Ueda et al., "Increased plasma monocyte chemoattractant protein-1 level in idiopathic pulmonary arterial hypertension," *Respirology*, vol. 11, no. 2, pp. 158–163, 2006.

[39] R. M. Tuder and N. F. Voelkel, "Pulmonary hypertension and inflammation," *Journal of Laboratory and Clinical Medicine*, vol. 132, no. 1, pp. 16–24, 1998.

[40] P. M. Hassoun, L. Mouthon, J. A. Barberà et al., "Inflammation, growth factors, and pulmonary vascular remodeling," *Journal of the American College of Cardiology*, vol. 54, no. 1, supplement, pp. S10–S19, 2009.

[41] X. J. Yuan, J. Wang, M. Juhaszova, S. P. Gaine, and L. J. Rubin, "Attenuated K+ channel gene transcription in primary pulmonary hypertension," *The Lancet*, vol. 351, no. 9104, pp. 726–727, 1998.

[42] P. Herve, L. Drouet, C. Dosquet et al., "Primary pulmonary hypertension in a patient with a familial platelet storage pool disease: role of serotonin," *American Journal of Medicine*, vol. 89, no. 1, pp. 117–120, 1990.

[43] M. R. MacLean, P. Herve, S. Eddahibi, and S. Adnot, "5-Hydroxytryptamine and the pulmonary circulation: receptors, transporters and relevance to pulmonary arterial hypertension," *British Journal of Pharmacology*, vol. 131, no. 2, pp. 161–168, 2000.

[44] C. Guignabert, M. Izikki, L. I. Tu et al., "Transgenic mice overexpressing the 5-hydroxytryptamine transporter gene in smooth muscle develop pulmonary hypertension," *Circulation Research*, vol. 98, no. 10, pp. 1323–1330, 2006.

[45] J. P. Bayley and P. Devilee, "The Warburg effect in 2012," *Current Opinion in Oncology*, vol. 24, no. 1, pp. 62–67, 2012.

[46] S. L. Archer, E. D. Michelakis, B. Thébaud et al., "A central role for oxygen-sensitive K+ channels and mitochondria in the specialized oxygen-sensing system," *Novartis Foundation Symposium*, vol. 272, pp. 157–171, 2006.

[47] S. L. Archer, M. Gomberg-Maitland, M. L. Maitland, S. Rich, J. G. N. Garcia, and E. K. Weir, "Mitochondrial metabolism, redox signaling, and fusion: a mitochondria-ROS-HIF-1α-Kv1.5 O2-sensing pathway at the intersection of pulmonary hypertension and cancer," *American Journal of Physiology*, vol. 294, no. 2, pp. H570–H578, 2008.

[48] M. Rabinovitch, "Pathobiology of pulmonary hypertension: extracellular matrix," *Clinics in Chest Medicine*, vol. 22, no. 3, pp. 433–449, 2001.

[49] D. T. Dresdale, M. Schultz, and R. J. Michtom, "Primary pulmonary hypertension. I. Clinical and hemodynamic study," *The American Journal of Medicine*, vol. 11, no. 6, pp. 686–705, 1951.

[50] S. Rich, D. R. Dantzker, S. M. Ayres et al., "Primary pulmonary hypertension. A national prospective study," *Annals of Internal Medicine*, vol. 107, no. 2, pp. 216–223, 1987.

[51] J. H. Morse, A. C. Jones, R. J. Barst et al., "Mapping of familial primary pulmonary hypertension locus (PPH1) to chromosome 2q31-q32," *Circulation*, vol. 95, no. 12, pp. 2603–2606, 1997.

[52] W. C. Nichols, D. L. Koller, B. Slovis et al., "Localization of the gene for familial primary pulmonary hypertension to chromosome 2q31-32," *Nature Genetics*, vol. 15, no. 3, pp. 277–280, 1997.

[53] R. D. Machado, M. W. Pauciulo, N. Fretwell et al., "A physical and transcript map based upon refinement of the critical interval for PPH1, a gene for familial primary pulmonary hypertension," *Genomics*, vol. 68, no. 2, pp. 220–228, 2000.

[54] K. B. Lane, R. D. Machado, M. W. Pauciulo et al., "Heterozygous germline mutations in BMPR2, encoding a TGF-β receptor, cause familial primary pulmonary hypertension," *Nature Genetics*, vol. 26, no. 1, pp. 81–84, 2000.

[55] Z. Deng, J. H. Morse, S. L. Slager et al., "Familial primary pulmonary hypertension (Gene PPH1) is caused by mutations in the bone morphogenetic protein receptor-II gene," *American Journal of Human Genetics*, vol. 67, no. 3, pp. 737–744, 2000.

[56] K. Miyazono, Y. Kamiya, and M. Morikawa, "Bone morphogenetic protein receptors and signal transduction," *Journal of Biochemistry*, vol. 147, no. 1, pp. 35–51, 2010.

[57] J. R. Thomson, R. D. Machado, M. W. Pauciulo et al., "Sporadiac primary pulmonary hypertension is associated with germline mutations of the gene encoding BMPR-II, a receptor member of the TGF-β family," *Journal of Medical Genetics*, vol. 37, no. 10, pp. 741–745, 2000.

[58] R. Koehler, E. Grünig, M. W. Pauciulo et al., "Low frequency of BMPR2 mutations in a German cohort of patients with sporadic idiopathic pulmonary arterial hypertension," *Journal of Medical Genetics*, vol. 41, no. 12, article e127, 2004.

[59] H. Morisaki, N. Nakanishi, S. Kyotani, A. Takashima, H. Tomoike, and T. Morisaki, "BMPR2 mutations found in Japanese patients with familial and sporadic primary pulmonary hypertension," *Human Mutation*, vol. 23, no. 6, p. 632, 2004.

[60] J. H. Newman, R. C. Trembath, J. A. Morse et al., "Genetic basis of pulmonary arterial hypertension: current understanding and future directions," *Journal of the American College of Cardiology*, vol. 43, no. 12, supplement, pp. 33S–39S, 2004.

[61] M. A. Aldred, R. D. Machado, V. James, N. W. Morrell, and R. C. Trembath, "Characterization of the BMPR2 5′-untranslated region and a novel mutation in pulmonary hypertension," *American Journal of Respiratory and Critical Care Medicine*, vol. 176, no. 8, pp. 819–824, 2007.

[62] F. Liu, F. Ventura, J. Doody, and J. Massague, "Human type II receptor for bone morphogenic proteins (BMPs): extension of the two-kinase receptor model to the BMPs," *Molecular and Cellular Biology*, vol. 15, no. 7, pp. 3479–3486, 1995.

[63] J. Massague, "TGF-beta signal transduction," *Annual Review of Biochemistry*, vol. 67, pp. 753–791, 1998.

[64] L. David, J. J. Feige, and S. Bailly, "Emerging role of bone morphogenetic proteins in angiogenesis," *Cytokine and Growth Factor Reviews*, vol. 20, no. 3, pp. 203–212, 2009.

[65] R. D. Machado, N. Rudarakanchana, C. Atkinson et al., "Functional interaction between BMPR-II and Tctex-1, a light chain of dynein, is isoform-specific and disrupted by mutations underlying primary pulmonary hypertension," *Human Molecular Genetics*, vol. 12, no. 24, pp. 3277–3286, 2003.

[66] V. C. Foletta, M. A. Lim, J. Soosairaiah et al., "Direct signaling by the BMP type II receptor via the cytoskeletal regulator LIMK1," *Journal of Cell Biology*, vol. 162, no. 6, pp. 1089–1098, 2003.

[67] A. Zakrzewicz, M. Hecker, L. M. Marsh et al., "Receptor for activated C-kinase 1, a novel interaction partner of type II bone morphogenetic protein receptor, regulates smooth muscle cell proliferation in pulmonary arterial hypertension," *Circulation*, vol. 115, no. 23, pp. 2957–2968, 2007.

[68] K. Ihida-Stansbury, D. M. McKean, K. B. Lane et al., "Tenascin-C is induced by mutated BMP type II receptors in familial forms of pulmonary arterial hypertension," *American Journal of Physiology*, vol. 291, no. 4, pp. L694–L702, 2006.

[69] A. Nohe, E. Keating, P. Knaus, and N. O. Petersen, "Signal transduction of bone morphogenetic protein receptors," *Cellular Signalling*, vol. 16, no. 3, pp. 291–299, 2004.

[70] A. Hartung, K. Bitton-Worms, M. M. Rechtman et al., "Different routes of bone morphogenic protein (BMP) receptor endocytosis influence BMP signaling," *Molecular and Cellular Biology*, vol. 26, no. 20, pp. 7791–7805, 2006.

[71] A. Nohe, S. Hassel, M. Ehrlich et al., "The mode of bone morphogenetic protein (BMP) receptor oligomerization determines different BMP-2 signaling pathways," *The Journal of Biological Chemistry*, vol. 277, no. 7, pp. 5330–5338, 2002.

[72] R. D. Machado, O. Eickelberg, C. G. Elliott et al., "Genetics and genomics of pulmonary arterial hypertension," *Journal of the American College of Cardiology*, vol. 54, no. 1, supplement, pp. S32–S42, 2009.

[73] R. D. Machado, M. A. Aldred, V. James et al., "Mutations of the TGF-β type II receptor BMPR2 in pulmonary arterial hypertension," *Human Mutation*, vol. 27, no. 2, pp. 121–132, 2006.

[74] E. D. Austin, J. A. Phillips, J. D. Cogan et al., "Truncating and missense BMPR2 mutations differentially affect the severity of heritable pulmonary arterial hypertension," *Respiratory Research*, vol. 10, article 87, 2009.

[75] R. D. Machado, M. W. Pauciulo, J. R. Thomson et al., "BMPR2 haploinsufficiency as the inherited molecular mechanism for primary pulmonary hypertension," *American Journal of Human Genetics*, vol. 68, no. 1, pp. 92–102, 2001.

[76] J. Greenwald, W. H. Fischer, W. W. Vale, and S. Choe, "Three-finger toxin fold for the extracellular ligand-binding domain of the type II activin receptor serine kinase," *Nature Structural Biology*, vol. 6, no. 1, pp. 18–22, 1999.

[77] N. Rudarakanchana, J. A. Flanagan, H. Chen et al., "Functional analysis of bone morphogenetic protein type II receptor mutations underlying primary pulmonary hypertension," *Human Molecular Genetics*, vol. 11, no. 13, pp. 1517–1525, 2002.

[78] S. K. Hanks and T. Hunter, "Protein kinases 6. The eukaryotic protein kinase superfamily: kinase (catalytic) domain structure and classification," *The FASEB Journal*, vol. 9, no. 8, pp. 576–596, 1995.

[79] A. Nishihara, T. Watabe, T. Imamura, and K. Miyazono, "Functional heterogeneity of bone morphogenetic protein receptor-II mutants found in patients with primary pulmonary hypertension," *Molecular Biology of the Cell*, vol. 13, no. 9, pp. 3055–3063, 2002.

[80] T. Yasuda, Y. Tada, N. Tanabe, K. Tatsumi, and J. West, "Rho-kinase inhibition alleviates pulmonary hypertension in transgenic mice expressing a dominant-negative type II bone morphogenetic protein receptor gene," *American Journal of Physiology*, vol. 301, no. 5, pp. 667–674, 2011.

[81] M. T. Nasim, T. Ogo, H. M. Chowdhury et al., "BMPR-II deficiency elicits pro-proliferative and anti-apoptotic responses through the activation of TGFbeta-TAK1-MAPK pathways in PAH," *Human Molecular Genetics*, vol. 21, no. 11, pp. 2548–2558, 2012.

[82] R. J. Davies, A. M. Holmes, J. Deighton et al., "BMP type II receptor deficiency confers resistance to growth inhibition by TGF-beta in pulmonary artery smooth muscle cells: role of proinflammatory cytokines," *American Journal of Physiology*, vol. 302, no. 6, pp. L604–L615, 2012.

[83] M. Sankelo, J. A. Flanagan, R. Machado et al., "BMPR2 mutations have short lifetime expectancy in primary pulmonary

hypertension," *Human Mutation*, vol. 26, no. 2, pp. 119–124, 2005.

[84] C. G. Elliott, E. W. Glissmeyer, G. T. Havlena et al., "Relationship of BMPR2 mutations to vasoreactivity in pulmonary arterial hypertension," *Circulation*, vol. 113, no. 21, pp. 2509–2515, 2006.

[85] D. Liu, W. H. Wu, Y. M. Mao et al., "BMPR2 mutations influence phenotype more obviously in male patients with pulmonary arterial hypertension," *Circulation*, vol. 5, no. 5, pp. 511–518, 2012.

[86] J. Cogan, E. Austin, L. Hedges et al., "Role of BMPR2 alternative splicing in HPAH penetrance," *Circulation*, vol. 126, no. 15, pp. 1907–1916, 2012.

[87] J. McDonald, P. Bayrak-Toydemir, and R. E. Pyeritz, "Hereditary hemorrhagic telangiectasia: an overview of diagnosis, management, and pathogenesis," *Genetics in Medicine*, vol. 13, no. 7, pp. 607–616, 2011.

[88] K. A. McAllister, K. M. Grogg, D. W. Johnson et al., "Endoglin, a TGF-β binding protein of endothelial cells, is the gene for hereditary haemorrhagic telangiectasia type 1," *Nature Genetics*, vol. 8, no. 4, pp. 345–351, 1994.

[89] D. W. Johnson, J. N. Berg, M. A. Baldwin et al., "Mutations in the activin receptor-like kinase 1 gene in hereditary haemorrhagic telangiectasia type," *Nature Genetics*, vol. 13, no. 2, pp. 189–195, 1996.

[90] G. M. F. Wallace and C. L. Shovlin, "A hereditary haemorrhagic telangiectasia family with pulmonary involvement is unlinked to the known HHT genes, endoglin and ALK-1," *Thorax*, vol. 55, no. 8, pp. 685–690, 2000.

[91] C. L. Shovlin and M. Letarte, "Hereditary haemorrhagic telangiectasia and pulmonary arteriovenous malformations: issues in clinical management and review of pathogenic mechanisms," *Thorax*, vol. 54, no. 8, pp. 714–729, 1999.

[92] S. A. Abdalla, N. Pece-Barbara, S. Vera et al., "Analysis of ALK-1 and endoglin in newborns from families with hereditary hemorrhagic telangiectasia type 2," *Human Molecular Genetics*, vol. 9, no. 8, pp. 1227–1237, 2000.

[93] R. E. Harrison, J. A. Flanagan, M. Sankelo et al., "Molecular and functional analysis identifies ALK-1 as the predominant cause of pulmonary hypertension related to hereditary haemorrhagic telangiectasia," *Journal of Medical Genetics*, vol. 40, no. 12, pp. 865–871, 2003.

[94] S. A. Abdalla, U. Cymerman, D. Rushlow et al., "Novel mutations and polymorphisms in genes causing hereditary hemorrhagic telangiectasia," *Human Mutation*, vol. 25, no. 3, pp. 320–321, 2005.

[95] A. Chida, M. Shintani, H. Yagi et al., "Outcomes of childhood pulmonary arterial hypertension in BMPR2 and ALK1 mutation carriers," *American Journal of Cardiology*, vol. 110, no. 4, pp. 586–593, 2012.

[96] M. Shintani, H. Yagi, T. Nakayama, T. Saji, and R. Matsuoka, "A new nonsense mutation of SMAD8 associated with pulmonary arterial hypertension," *Journal of Medical Genetics*, vol. 46, no. 5, pp. 331–337, 2009.

[97] M. T. Nasim, T. Ogo, M. Ahmed et al., "Molecular genetic characterization of SMAD signaling molecules in pulmonary arterial hypertension," *Human Mutation*, vol. 32, no. 12, pp. 1385–1389, 2011.

[98] Z. Huang, D. Wang, K. Ihida-Stansbury, P. L. Jones, and J. F. Martin, "Defective pulmonary vascular remodeling in Smad8 mutant mice," *Human Molecular Genetics*, vol. 18, no. 15, pp. 2791–2801, 2009.

[99] A. Chida, M. Shintani, T. Nakayama et al., "Missense mutations of the BMPR1B (ALK6) gene in childhood idiopathic pulmonary arterial hypertension," *Circulation Journal*, vol. 76, no. 6, pp. 1501–1508, 2012.

[100] N. A. Maniatis, V. Shinin, D. E. Schraufnagel et al., "Increased pulmonary vascular resistance and defective pulmonary artery filling in caveolin-1-/- mice," *American Journal of Physiology*, vol. 294, no. 5, pp. L865–L873, 2008.

[101] E. D. Austin, L. Ma, C. LeDuc et al., "Whole exome sequencing to identify a novel gene (caveolin-1) associated with human pulmonary arterial hypertension," *Circulation*, vol. 5, no. 3, pp. 336–343, 2012.

[102] W. T. Abraham, M. V. Raynolds, D. B. Badesch et al., "Angiotensin-converting enzyme DD genotype in patients with primary pulmonary hypertension: increased frequency and association with preserved haemodynamics," *Journal of the Renin-Angiotensin-Aldosterone System*, vol. 4, no. 1, pp. 27–30, 2003.

[103] M. M. Hoeper, A. Tacacs, U. Stellmacher, and R. Lichtinghagen, "Lack of association between angiotensin converting enzyme (ACE) genotype, serum ACE activity, and haemodynamics in patients with primary pulmonary hypertension," *Heart*, vol. 89, no. 4, pp. 445–446, 2003.

[104] A. A. Aldashev, A. S. Sarybaev, A. S. Sydykov et al., "Characterization of high-altitude pulmonary hypertension in the Kyrgyz: association with angiotensin-converting enzyme genotype," *American Journal of Respiratory and Critical Care Medicine*, vol. 166, no. 10, pp. 1396–1402, 2002.

[105] S. Eddahibi, M. Humbert, E. Fadel et al., "Serotonin transporter overexpression is responsible for pulmonary artery smooth muscle hyperplasia in primary pulmonary hypertension," *The Journal of Clinical Investigation*, vol. 108, no. 8, pp. 1141–1150, 2001.

[106] R. D. Machado, R. Koehler, E. Glissmeyer et al., "Genetic association of the serotonin transporter in pulmonary arterial hypertension," *American Journal of Respiratory and Critical Care Medicine*, vol. 173, no. 7, pp. 793–797, 2006.

[107] E. D. Willers, J. H. Newman, J. E. Loyd et al., "Serotonin transporter polymorphisms in familial and idiopathic pulmonary arterial hypertension," *American Journal of Respiratory and Critical Care Medicine*, vol. 173, no. 7, pp. 798–802, 2006.

[108] C. V. Remillard, D. D. Tigno, O. Platoshyn et al., "Function of Kv1.5 channels and genetic variations of KCNA5 in patients with idiopathic pulmonary arterial hypertension," *American Journal of Physiology*, vol. 292, no. 5, pp. C1837–C1853, 2007.

[109] R. Koehler, H. Olschewski, M. Hoeper, B. Janssen, and E. Grünig, "Serotonin transporter gene polymorphism in a cohort of German patients with idiopathic pulmonary arterial hypertension or chronic thromboembolic pulmonary hypertension," *Chest*, vol. 128, no. 6, supplement, p. 619, 2005.

[110] J. Rehman and S. L. Archer, "A proposed mitochondrial-metabolic mechanism for initiation and maintenance of pulmonary arterial hypertension in fawn-hooded rats: the warburg model of pulmonary arterial hypertension," *Advances in Experimental Medicine and Biology*, vol. 661, pp. 171–185, 2010.

[111] H. Beppu, M. Kawabata, T. Hamamoto et al., "BMP type II receptor is required for gastrulation and early development of mouse embryos," *Developmental Biology*, vol. 221, no. 1, pp. 249–258, 2000.

[112] E. C. Délot, M. E. Bahamonde, M. Zhao, and K. M. Lyons, "BMP signaling is required for septation of the outflow tract of the

mammalian heart," *Development*, vol. 130, no. 1, pp. 209–220, 2003.

[113] P. Caruso, Y. Dempsie, H. C. Stevens et al., "A role for miR-145 in pulmonary arterial hypertension: evidence from mouse models and patient samples," *Circulation Research*, vol. 111, no. 3, pp. 290–300, 2012.

[114] J. West, K. Fagan, W. Steudel et al., "Pulmonary hypertension in transgenic mice expressing a dominant-negative BMPRII gene in smooth muscle," *Circulation Research*, vol. 94, no. 8, pp. 1109–1114, 2004.

[115] J. West, J. Harral, K. Lane et al., "Mice expressing BMPR2R899X transgene in smooth muscle develop pulmonary vascular lesions," *American Journal of Physiology*, vol. 295, no. 5, pp. L744–L755, 2008.

[116] C. Atkinson, S. Stewart, P. D. Upton et al., "Primary pulmonary hypertension is associated with reduced pulmonary vascular expression of type II bone morphogenetic protein receptor," *Circulation*, vol. 105, no. 14, pp. 1672–1678, 2002.

[117] R. J. Barst, J. S. R. Gibbs, H. A. Ghofrani et al., "Updated evidence-based treatment algorithm in pulmonary arterial hypertension," *Journal of the American College of Cardiology*, vol. 54, no. 1, supplement, pp. S78–S84, 2009.

[118] N. Galiè, A. Manes, and A. Branzi, "Prostanoids for pulmonary arterial hypertension," *American Journal of Respiratory Medicine*, vol. 2, no. 2, pp. 123–137, 2003.

[119] O. Sitbon, M. Humbert, H. Nunes et al., "Long-term intravenous epoprostenol infusion in primary pulmonary hypertension: prognostic factors and survival," *Journal of the American College of Cardiology*, vol. 40, no. 4, pp. 780–788, 2002.

[120] A. K. Doran, D. D. Ivy, R. J. Barst, N. Hill, S. Murali, and R. L. Benza, "Guidelines for the prevention of central venous catheter-related blood stream infections with prostanoid therapy for pulmonary arterial hypertension," *International Journal of Clinical Practice. Supplement*, no. 160, pp. 5–9, 2008.

[121] V. V. McLaughlin, A. Shillington, and S. Rich, "Survival in primary pulmonary hypertension: the impact of epoprostenol therapy," *Circulation*, vol. 106, no. 12, pp. 1477–1482, 2002.

[122] Centers for Disease Control and Prevention CDC, "Bloodstream infections among patients treated with intravenous epoprostenol or intravenous treprostinil for pulmonary arterial hypertension—seven sites, United States, 2003—2006," *Morbidity and Mortality Weekly Report (MMWR)*, vol. 56, no. 8, pp. 170–172, 2007.

[123] H. Olschewski, G. Simonneau, N. Galiè et al., "Inhaled iloprost for severe pulmonary hypertension," *The New England Journal of Medicine*, vol. 347, no. 5, pp. 322–329, 2002.

[124] N. Galiè, L. Rubin, M. Hoeper et al., "Treatment of patients with mildly symptomatic pulmonary arterial hypertension with bosentan (EARLY study): a double-blind, randomised controlled trial," *The Lancet*, vol. 371, no. 9630, pp. 2093–2100, 2008.

[125] L. J. Rubin, D. B. Badesch, R. J. Barst et al., "Bosentan therapy for pulmonary arterial hypertension," *The New England Journal of Medicine*, vol. 346, no. 12, pp. 896–903, 2002.

[126] N. Galiè, H. Olschewski, R. J. Oudiz et al., "Ambrisentan for the treatment of pulmonary arterial hypertension: results of the ambrisentan in pulmonary arterial hypertension, randomized, double-Blind, placebo-controlled, multicenter, efficacy (ARIES) study 1 and 2," *Circulation*, vol. 117, no. 23, pp. 3010–3019, 2008.

[127] J. K. Olsson, R. T. Zamanian, J. A. Feinstein, and R. L. Doyle, "Surgical and interventional therapies for pulmonary arterial hypertension," *Seminars in Respiratory and Critical Care Medicine*, vol. 26, no. 4, pp. 417–428, 2005.

[128] G. Simonneau, L. J. Rubin, N. Galiè et al., "Addition of sildenafil to long-term intravenous epoprostenol therapy in patients with pulmonary arterial hypertension: a randomized trial," *Annals of Internal Medicine*, vol. 149, no. 8, pp. 521–530, 2008.

[129] E. P. Trulock, L. B. Edwards, D. O. Taylor, M. M. Boucek, B. M. Keck, and M. I. Hertz, "Registry of the International Society for Heart and Lung Transplantation: twenty-third official adult lung and heart-lung transplantation report—2006," *Journal of Heart and Lung Transplantation*, vol. 25, no. 8, pp. 880–892, 2006.

[130] R. L. Benza, D. P. Miller, M. Gomberg-Maitland et al., "Predicting survival in pulmonary arterial hypertension: insights from the registry to evaluate early and long-term pulmonary arterial hypertension disease management (REVEAL)," *Circulation*, vol. 122, no. 2, pp. 164–172, 2010.

[131] M. Humbert, O. Sitbon, A. Chaouat et al., "Survival in patients with idiopathic, familial, and anorexigen-associated pulmonary arterial hypertension in the modern management era," *Circulation*, vol. 122, no. 2, pp. 156–163, 2010.

[132] A. M. Reynolds, M. D. Holmes, S. M. Danilov, and P. N. Reynolds, "Targeted gene delivery of BMPR2 attenuates pulmonary hypertension," *European Respiratory Journal*, vol. 39, no. 2, pp. 329–343, 2012.

[133] M. Kataoka, T. Kawakami, Y. Tamura et al., "Gene transfer therapy by either type 1 or type 2 adeno-associated virus expressing human prostaglandin I2 synthase gene is effective for treatment of pulmonary arterial hypertension," *Journal of Cardiovascular Pharmacology and Therapeutics*. In press.

2

The Role of Inflammatory Cytokines, the RANKL/OPG Axis, and the Immunoskeletal Interface in Physiological Bone Turnover and Osteoporosis

M. Neale Weitzmann[1,2]

[1] *Atlanta Department of Veterans Affairs Medical Center, Decatur, GA 30033, USA*
[2] *Division of Endocrinology and Metabolism and Lipids, Department of Medicine, Emory University School of Medicine, 101 Woodruff Circle, 1305 WMRB, Atlanta, GA 30322, USA*

Correspondence should be addressed to M. Neale Weitzmann; mweitzm@emory.edu

Academic Editors: G. Da Silva Xavier and E. Hajduch

Although it has long been recognized that inflammation, a consequence of immune-driven processes, significantly impacts bone turnover, the degree of centralization of skeletal and immune functions has begun to be dissected only recently. It is now recognized that formation of osteoclasts, the bone resorbing cells of the body, is centered on the key osteoclastogenic cytokine, receptor activator of NF-κB ligand (RANKL). Although numerous inflammatory cytokines are now recognized to promote osteoclast formation and skeletal degradation, with just a few exceptions, RANKL is now considered to be the final downstream effector cytokine that drives osteoclastogenesis and regulates osteoclastic bone resorption. The biological activity of RANKL is moderated by its physiological decoy receptor, osteoprotegerin (OPG). New discoveries concerning the sources and regulation of RANKL and OPG in physiological bone turnover as well as under pathological (osteoporotic) conditions continue to be made, opening a window to the complex regulatory processes that control skeletal integrity and the depth of integration of the skeleton within the immune response. This paper will examine the interconnection between bone turnover and the immune system and the implications thereof for physiological and pathological bone turnover.

1. Introduction

Mineralized bone consists of a protein matrix comprising predominantly, but not exclusively, collagen type I fibers that are layered down in oriented linear bundles. This protein matrix scaffold is coated with a layer of mineral, predominantly calcium phosphate in the form of crystals of hydroxyapatite [1].

The skeleton forms in early life, mainly through endochondral ossification in which bone is initially patterned in mineralized cartilage followed by replacement of the cartilage template by mineralized bone. Some skeletal components including certain bones of the skull such as the calvaria are formed without a cartilage intermediate through direct matrix and mineralization deposition, a process referred to as intramembranous ossification [2].

The skeleton achieves its final shape and ultimate form through bone modeling, a process involving the coordinated activity of bone synthesizing osteoblasts and bone resorbing osteoclasts. This process of selective bone deposition and removal sculpts the skeleton to achieve final shape and optimal load bearing capacity [3, 4]. Bone modeling continues until early adulthood in humans at which time peak bone mineral density (BMD) and bone size are achieved. Thereafter, the skeleton undergoes a process of bone renewal referred to as remodeling. In remodeling bone resorbing osteoclasts and bone forming osteoblasts work in unison to resorb damaged or worn bones and resynthesize new bones, as well as allowing for growth and expansion of the marrow cavity and increase in trabecular thickness. Initially, the process of bone remodeling is homeostatic, as the rate of osteoclastic bone resorption is matched by the rate of osteoblastic bone formation. The net result is bone repair without net gain or loss of bone mass, and in principle bone remodeling has the capacity to replace approximately 25 percent of trabecular bone and 3% of cortical bone each year [3, 4].

In reality, this capacity of the skeleton to regenerate in a homeostatic manner is short-lived, and both men and women start losing bone by their fourth decade of life. After menopause bone loss is greatly intensified for a time in women where a rapid phase of bone loss ensues for 5–10 years as a consequence of estrogen decline. Men experience a slower linear loss of bone mass as a consequence of a progressive decline in sex steroids [3].

This persistent loss of bone density and mass with age leads to osteopenia (low bone mass) and ultimately culminates in osteoporosis, a condition that greatly increases the risk of a bone fracture. Although younger males (between the ages of 15 to 49) are almost 3 times more likely to sustain a fracture than females [5], in older populations fracture incidence is significantly higher in women than men where fragility fractures affect almost one in two older women compared to one in three to four older men [6]. The reason for increased fracture incidence in women is complex but in addition to losing bone faster following the menopause, women also accumulate less skeletal mass than men during growth, particularly in puberty. This results in smaller bones with thinner cortices and with a smaller diameter that have a relatively reduced load bearing capacity [3].

The consequences of fracture can be devastating and are a significant cause of morbidity and mortality [7, 8]. Vertebral fractures can cause severe back pain and disability [9], while hip fractures are usually extremely serious and nearly always result in hospitalization and major surgery. Hip fractures are fatal about 20% of the time and produce permanent disability about half the time [8, 10]. In some studies one-year mortality after hip fracture has been seen to reach as high as 30% [11]. Survivors often suffer tremendous indignity and decline in quality of life due to the need for extensive rehabilitation and protracted nursing home stays that often deprive the aged of their mobility and independence, sometimes permanently [12]. The financial consequences for patients and society of bone fractures are considerable [12]. Total fractures in 2005 were >2 million costing nearly $17 billion, and these costs are projected to rise by almost 50% by 2025 [13].

There have been tremendous advances over the last 2 decades in understanding the processes that regulate physiological bone turnover and in delineating the mechanisms by which multiple pathological conditions collide with the skeleton. A surprisingly large number of these maladies center on inflammation and immune dysregulation associated with natural aging and leading to collateral damage to the skeleton. Furthermore, infections and immunological diseases such as human immunodeficiency virus-1 (HIV-1) and infection/acquired immunodeficiency syndrome (AIDS) are now recognized to take a severe toll on the skeleton, predisposing even relatively young men and women to the consequences of bone fracture.

The immunoskeletal interface involves the centralization of immune and skeletal functions around common cell types and cytokine effectors that control physiological bone mass, but lead to skeleton deterioration under states of prolonged immune activation. Realization of this interconnection of the immune and skeletal systems more than a decade ago has now spawned the emergence of a dedicated field of study, sometimes referred to as "osteoimmunology," different aspects of which have been the subject of a number of excellent review articles including [14–23].

2. Osteoclasts and the Receptor Activator of NF-κB (RANK)/RANK Ligand (RANKL)/Osteoprotegerin (OPG) System

Osteoclasts are the unique cells of the body tasked with resorbing bone. These giant multinucleated cells bind down onto bone surfaces creating a sealing zone and a ruffled-membrane border into which apical proton pumps accumulate hydrogen ions that combine with chloride ions to form hydrochloric acid, which degrades bone mineral. The exposed collagen matrix is attacked by acid resistant endosomal and lysosomal enzymes that cleave collagen fibers effectively removing small quantities of bone [24].

A central enigma in the world of osteoclast biology has been how osteoclasts form and what regulates their differentiation and activity. It has long been recognized that the osteoclast precursors circulate amid the monocyte/macrophage population and differentiate into preosteoclasts that fuse to form giant bone resorbing mature osteoclasts [25]. It was further recognized that inflammatory processes such as rheumatoid arthritis and periodontal infection predispose to osteoclastic bone loss, giving rise to speculation that inflammatory cytokines such as Interleukin (IL) −1, tumor necrosis factor alpha (TNFα), and IL-6 may play critical roles in osteoclast formation [26, 27].

Interestingly, these cytokines when placed on purified monocytes fail to induce significant osteoclast formation suggesting an indirect mechanism of action. Because bone formation and resorption work in unison (are coupled) during bone modeling and remodeling, it was further speculated that osteoblasts may regulate the activity of osteoclasts. Studies from the Suda group in Japan were indeed able to demonstrate that purified osteoblasts treated with vitamin D and cocultured in contact with osteoclast precursors (monocytes) from mouse spleen promoted significant formation of multinucleated cells capable of resorbing pits on dentin, a bone substitute, and hence meeting the functional requirement for designation as osteoclasts [28].

However, the identity of the osteoclastogenic cytokine responsible for osteoclast formation and commonly referred to as osteoclast differentiation factor (ODF) would remain obscure for another decade.

By the late 1980s the technologies of molecular biology and protein biochemistry had evolved sufficiently to set the stage for a series of pivotal discoveries in the field of bone biology. The first, in 1997, was the identification, by two independent groups, of a potent negative inhibitor of osteoclastogenesis named osteoprotegerin (OPG) [29] by Amgen investigators in the USA and osteoclastogenesis inhibitory factor

(OCIF) [30] by investigators in Japan. The following year, using advanced molecular biology approaches, the Amgen group was able to purify and define a ligand to OPG (OPG ligand (OPGL)) that potently stimulated the production of osteoclasts from purified precursors [31]. Almost simultaneously, using an extensive biochemical purification strategy, the Suda group in Japan identified an equivalent ligand to OCIF on the surface of osteoblasts whose potent osteoclastogenic activity they ascribed to the elusive ODF [32]. OPGL and ODF were found to be structurally and functionally identical, potently promoting osteoclast formation in the absence of any other exogenous factors, with the exception of the monocytic survival factor macrophage colony stimulating factor (M-CSF). Interestingly, a factor structurally identical to OPGL and ODF had been previously reported by two independent groups of immunologists and had been named receptor activator of NF-κB ligand (RANKL) [33] and tumor necrosis factor-related activation-induced cytokine (TRANCE) [34]. These groups showed that this factor, expressed by T cells, had immunomodulatory functions through receptors (RANK/TRANCE-receptor) present on dendritic cells [33–35]. Although all these different terms were used interchangeably for some years, in the context of bone biology the preferred terms are now RANKL to describe the osteoclastogenic cytokine, OPG to describe its inhibitor, and RANK to describe the receptor for RANKL.

It is now clear that RANKL is the key final effector osteoclastogenic cytokine and in the presence of a permissive concentration of M-CSF is capable of inducing osteoclast formation and promoting osteoclast resorptive activity in the absence of any other cytokines. OPG functions as a decoy receptor, preventing association of RANKL with RANK receptor [35] and thus moderating osteoclastogenesis and bone resorption (reviewed in [25, 36, 37]).

It is now understood that the osteoclast precursor is a cell expressing one or more markers of the monocyte lineage (typically CD14, cFms (the M-CSF receptor), or CD11b) and RANK. Binding of RANKL to RANK initiates a sequence of signal transduction pathways mediated though TNF receptor-associated factor 6 (TRAF6) and including NF-κB [38–40], c-Jun N-terminal kinase (JNK)/cJun/fos [38, 41–43], and nuclear factor of activated T cells (NFAT) [44–46] that initiate the differentiation of the early osteoclast precursor into a preosteoclast (recognized *in vitro* or *ex vivo* by the expression of the enzyme tartrate resistant acid phosphatase (TRAP)). Preosteoclasts ultimately fuse with each other into mature multinucleated bone resorbing osteoclasts recognized by the expression of key osteoclast markers including TRAP [47], calcitonin receptors [28], cathepsin K [48], pp60c-src [49], matrix metalloproteinase 9 (MMP9) [50], and the alpha V beta 3 integrin chains [51, 52]. Osteoclasts originating from multiple species can further be identified by reactivity to a unique osteoclast-specific monoclonal antibody (121F) [53].

The central role of RANKL in basal osteoclast formation and bone homeostasis has been established in animal models where genetic deletion of RANKL leads to an osteopetrotic phenotype characterized by a complete absence of osteoclasts and a failure of tooth eruption (an osteoclast driven process) [54]. Similarly, the key physiological role of OPG has been established in knock-out (KO) and transgenic overexpression studies in mice where deletion of the OPG gene leads to large numbers of osteoclasts and to severe bone erosions [54, 55]. By contrast transgenic overexpression causes an osteopetrotic phonotype in mice [56].

Consistent with the animal studies activating mutations in the receptor RANK are associated with familial expansile osteolysis, a rare autosomal dominant bone disorder characterized by focal areas of increased bone remodeling [57]. Many forms of Paget's and Juvenile Paget's disease may result from deletions/mutations in the OPG gene (*TNFRSF11B*) [58–60].

Human disease associated with mutations in the RANKL gene is rare, although a novel mutation in the gene for transforming growth factor beta 1 (*TGFβ1*) and a missense change in *TNFSF11* encoding RANKL may both contribute to the bone phenotype associated with Camurati-Engelmann disease [61].

From a therapeutic standpoint several studies have demonstrated the capacity of OPG suppression to ameliorate osteoporotic states and/or improve bone mass in ovariectomized animals (a model of postmenopausal osteoporosis) by means of adenoviral OPG delivery in mice [62], a single intravenous OPG injection in ovariectomized rats [63], weekly treatment of gonadal intact monkeys [64], and a single injection in postmenopausal women [65]. Although OPG has never been successfully translated into an approved therapy for humans, a humanized neutralizing antibody (Denosumab) directed against RANKL is now US Food and Drug Administration (FDA) approved for fracture prevention and amelioration of postmenopausal and other forms of osteoporosis [66, 67].

The evidence is now extremely strong supporting a final effector role of the RANK/RANKL/OPG system in osteoclast formation and the regulation of bone resorption. It is also now clear that inflammatory cytokines such as IL-1, TNFα and M-CSF that have long been associated with osteoclastic bone loss, function by promoting RANKL production by osteoblast precursors (bone marrow stromal cells (BMSC)) and/or mature osteoblasts [68, 69]; and/or by reducing OPG production [70], and/or by upregulating the receptor RANK on osteoclast precursors [71] thus increasing their sensitivity to prevailing RANKL concentrations. IL-1 and TNFα have long been implicated in osteoclast formation in postmenopausal osteoporosis [26, 72] and in animal models thereof (ovariectomy) [73–76]. In a recent study it was further demonstrated that IL-1 mediates the osteoclastogenic effect of TNFα by enhancing stromal cell expression of RANKL and directly stimulating differentiation of osteoclast precursors [69]. TNFα turns out to have another property that is relatively unique among the inflammatory cytokines; TNFα has particularly potent effects on osteoclastogenesis as it not only promotes RANKL production [68] but synergizes with RANKL to amplify osteoclastogenesis [77, 78] and to intensify osteoclastic resorption [79] by integrating with RANKL-induced signal transduction pathways [79, 80]. These effects are likely a consequence of the fact that RANKL is in fact a TNF-superfamily member and functions through many of the same pathways induced by TNFα itself. Although some early studies suggested that TNFα may be capable of direct RANKL-independent osteoclastogenesis [81], the weight of evidence now goes against this theory, and it is likely, given the ability of RANKL to amplify RANKL-induced osteoclastogenesis, that in these studies the mouse-derived osteoclast precursors were endogenously exposed to RANKL *in vivo* and hence were primed to respond to TNFα *ex vivo*.

As a consequence of the inflammatory action of TNFα, its overexpression *in vivo*, as in the case in transgenic mice, leads to inflammation resembling human rheumatoid arthritis with significant focal and systemic bone erosions [82, 83]. Indeed TNFα decoy receptors are now accepted therapies for human rheumatoid arthritis [84].

3. TNFα and the NF-κB Signal Transduction Pathway in Bone Resorption

The molecular action of TNFα is in large measure a consequence of its ability to potently stimulate activation of the NF-κB transcription factor. This pathway is also a major mediator of RANKL-induced signal transduction, and not surprisingly TNFα potently augments RANKL-induced osteoclast formation. The importance of NF-κB to osteoclast development, function, and survival has long been recognized [41, 85–88] and is strongly supported by evidence of osteopetrosis in p50 and p52 NF-κB double KO mice, as a consequence of defective osteoclast differentiation [89]. The NF-κB subunit RelB has further been shown to play a key role in osteoclast differentiation [87] while the p65 NF-κB subunit prevents JNK-mediated apoptosis during RANKL-induced commitment to the osteoclast phenotype [41]. Pharmacological antagonists of NF-κB signaling have been shown to suppress osteoclast activation [86] and to blunt osteoclastic bone resorption and ameliorate bone loss induced by ovariectomy in mice [90], multiple myeloma induced osteoclast formation and activity *in vitro* [91], implant particle-induced osteoclastogenesis [92], and in a rheumatoid arthritis animal model *in vivo* [93].

4. NF-κB and Bone Formation

Surprisingly, when it comes to osteoblasts and bone formation NF-κB signal transduction is quite dissimilar to that of osteoclast formation/bone resorption and is in fact potently inhibitory. It has long been recognized that the p65 NF-κB subunit is inhibitory to vitamin D-stimulated osteoblastic osteocalcin transcription (a measure of osteoblast differentiation) [94]. As a potent stimulator of NF-κB, it is not surprising that several studies have documented inhibitory effects of TNFα on osteoblast formation [95, 96] while in a mouse fracture healing model the pharmacological suppression of TNFα reverses age-related defects in bone formation [97].

Mechanistically, one mechanism by which TNFα suppresses osteoblast differentiation is by suppressing Smad signaling in differentiating osteoblasts, through an NF-κB-mediated process [98]. Smad signals are mediated in part by members of the transforming growth factor beta (TGFβ) superfamily, including TGFβ itself and bone morphogenetic proteins (BMPs). TGFβ and BMPs are key factors needed for directing the commitment of osteoblast precursors, along an osteoblastic trajectory and for their differentiation into mineralizing osteoblasts [99, 100]. BMPs are potent physiological inducers of osteoblast differentiation and angiogenesis [101], and BMP-2 is now employed as a pharmacological tool for promoting bone repair in orthopaedic implants [102].

TGFβ is thought to play important roles in early osteoblast lineage commitment [103] and in the recruitment of bone marrow stromal cells to bone resorptive sites, through a Smad-dependent signaling pathway [104]. TGFβ regulates osteoblast differentiation in a biphasic manner as TGFβ stimulates development and proliferation of early osteoblasts, but inhibits their maturation. How TGFβ and BMPs coordinate osteoblast differentiation is unclear. TGFβ strongly stimulates the synthesis of extracellular matrix proteins [105] but *in vitro* studies show an inhibitory effect on the final mineralization process, which nonetheless does occur *in vivo* despite the presence in the bone microenvironment of high concentrations of TGFβ [106, 107]. One explanation for this apparent contradiction is that the TGFβ receptor is downregulated during osteoblast differentiation following exposure of cells to collagen synthesized by the osteoblasts and enabling osteoblasts to escape from the inhibition of TGFβ [108].

The interface between NF-κB and Smad signaling is poorly understood but studies reveal that NF-κB signaling upregulates the inhibitory Smad, Smad-7 that antagonizes osteoblast differentiation [109]. These data are consistent with studies showing that TNFα promotes systemic bone loss in part, by stimulating proteasomal degradation of BMP proteins by a mechanism involving Smad ubiquitination regulatory factor 1 (Smurf1) [110]. Furthermore, TNFα is reported to inhibit BMP-induced osteoblast differentiation through activating stress-associated protein kinase (SAPK)/JNK signaling [111].

Indeed, it has long been recognized that TNFα contributes to ovariectomy-induced bone loss not only by promoting bone resorption, but also by suppressing the compensatory response in bone formation that is initiated in response to bone resorption, a consequence of the homeostatic coupling process. Indeed, pharmacological suppression of TNFα increases bone formation in the context of ovariectomy [75]. Consistent with these data we have demonstrated that estrogen promotes bone anabolism *in vitro* by antagonizing NF-κB activation in the osteoblastic cell line MC3T3 [112].

In contrast to inflammatory states characterized by high concentrations of TNFα, we recently investigated the effect of physiological endogenous levels of TNFα on basal bone formation *in vivo* using TNFα KO mice, as well as TNFα receptor type I (p55) and type II (p75) KO mice. Our studies demonstrated that mice null for TNFα and the p55 receptor exhibited a significantly elevated bone mineral density (BMD) and bone volume as a consequence of significantly elevated bone formation. Our data suggested that TNFα potently diminished the acquisition of peak bone mass demonstrating the powerful effect of even low concentrations of endogenous TNFα on the bone formation machinery [98]. Consistent with these effects an extensive *in vivo* investigation of NF-κB signaling on basal bone formation has demonstrated that a conditional inactivation of NF-κB signaling in osteoblasts by means of transgenic overexpression of the inhibitor of κB kinase (IKK) increases trabecular bone mass and BMD and reverses ovariectomy-induced bone loss by enhancing bone formation [113].

Like the action of estrogen, a number of natural and nutritional agents that have been associated with bone protective effects by exhibiting stimulatory activities on bone formation and suppressive actions of bone resorption appear to exploit this divergent role of NF-κB signaling on bone cells. We have shown that vitamin K2 [114], Honokiol [115], Zinc [116], and the carotenoid *p*-hydroxycinnamic [117, 118] are all capable of modulating NF-κB activation in osteoblast and osteoclast precursors *in vitro* by antagonizing RANKL- and TNFα-induced NF-κB activation in osteoblasts and osteoclasts, respectively.

5. RANKL and OPG Production under Physiological and Pathological Conditions

5.1. Physiological RANKL Production. Although it is recognized that many cell types have the capacity to produce RANKL and OPG, the major source of both of these factors, especially under basal conditions, has generally been ascribed to osteoblasts, the bone building cells, and their precursors, cells originating from mesenchymal stem cells (MSCs) and sometimes referred to as bone marrow stromal cells (BMSCs). These conclusions however, are primarily based on *in vitro* studies and are now contested by newly emerging *in vivo* data [119]. In a recent *in vivo* study targeted osteoblast deletion in mice was found to lead to osteopenia, as expected; however bone resorption continued normally in the absence of bone formation, and osteoclast number was not significantly impacted. This outcome suggested that osteoblasts and bone formation do not control the extent of bone resorption through production of balsa RANKL *in vivo* as previously believed [120].

This concept of osteoblast-independent sources of RANKL was further illustrated in two recent back-to-back studies in the journal Nature Medicine that have challenged our notions of where basal RANKL originates. Using a state-of-the-art Cre-directed conditional RANKL KO system, mice were generated with specific RANKL gene deletions in MSCs and revealed that RANKL expression in mesenchyme-derived cells was essential for osteoclast formation in growing long bones, but not in vertebrae, or calvaria. Furthermore, tooth eruption was normal in these mice suggesting that the source of RANKL necessary for that process is not MSC derived [119]. MSCs are pluripotent cells that give rise to multiple cell lineage including osteoblasts/osteocytes, chondrocytes, fibroblasts, myocytes, and adipocytes [121]. Because the MSC deletion potentially impacted multiple lineages, further specific deletions of RANKL were performed in late-proliferating chondrocytes, mature osteoblasts, and in osteocytes (terminally differentiated osteoblasts entombed in bone matrix). RANKL derived from hypertrophic chondrocytes was found to be essential for mineralized cartilage resorption (a process central to endochondral bone formation) while osteocytes were necessary for bone remodeling as well as for bone resorption associated with unloading, in a tail-suspension model [119].

Interestingly, although activated T and B cells are well-recognized sources of RANKL, conditional RANKL KO in T and B cells failed to impact bone mass suggesting that RANKL derived from lymphocytes is not involved in the regulation of basal bone remodeling [122]. In another study, purified bone cell cultures *in vitro* revealed that RANKL expression and osteoclast formation by osteocytes are significantly higher than those of osteoblasts and stromal cells. The importance of osteocytes as a source of RANKL was further confirmed using an osteocyte conditional RANKL KO model that revealed that the development of a significant osteopetrosis occurs in the absence of RANKL production by osteocytes [123] suggesting a critical role of osteocyte RANKL in basal bone modeling/remodeling. Taken together these studies reveal an essential role for RANKL expressed by osteocytes and chondrocytes in basal osteoclastogenesis.

5.1.1. RANKL-Independent Osteoclastogenesis. Although there is no doubt as to the importance of the RANK/RANKL/OPG axis in physiological and pathological bone turnover, a number of cytokines have now been identified that directly promote osteoclastogenesis in a RANKL-independent manner and may contribute to bone loss associated with certain pathological conditions, including inflammation.

5.1.2. Osteoclastogenic Factor of Activated T Cells (SOFAT). In 2001 we reported the results of a series of studies examining the mechanisms by which activated T cells promote osteoclastogenesis in inflammatory conditions and the reasons for spontaneous osteoclast formation in cultures of peripheral blood mononuclear cells, a system that is devoid of stromal cells/osteoblasts or exogenous cytokines. These studies found that both $CD4^+$ and $CD8^+$ T cells, when activated by the lectin phytohemagglutinin-P (PHA), potently stimulate human osteoclast formation *in vitro*. Following the discovery of RANKL as the key osteoclastogenic factor we were in fact able to demonstrate that RANKL production was clearly responsible for a significant proportion of the osteoclastogenic activity of the activated T cells. Interestingly, we also documented an intriguing residual osteoclastogenic activity that persisted in the presence of saturating concentrations of OPG and the RANKL inhibitor and that accounted for approximately 30% of the T-cell-dependent effect [124]. Similar data were found for IL-7-induced T-cell-mediated osteoclast formation in culture [125]. We further demonstrated that activated T-cell-conditioned medium had the ability to superinduce osteoclastogenesis in cultures of purified monocytes maximally stimulated by saturating concentrations of RANKL and M-CSF [124]. These data led us to conclude that activated T cells are able to promote osteoclastogenesis via both RANKL-dependent and RANKL-independent mechanisms [124, 125].

It was almost a decade before the exact nature of this controversial RANKL-independent osteoclastogenic cytokine was delineated. Using an intensive biochemical purification strategy we were able to fractionate conditioned medium from human activated T cells by high-performance liquid chromatography (HPLC) and recover biologically active fractions for further resolution by sodium dodecyl sulfate (SDS), and polyacrylamide gel electrophoresis (PAGE) which revealed a major candidate protein that was further characterized by mass spectrometry. With its protein sequence identified the putative factor was cloned and expressed using recombinant DNA technologies. The resulting protein which we termed secreted osteoclastogenic factor of activated T cells (SOFAT) was found to derive from an unusual mRNA splice variant coded by the threonine synthase-like 2 gene (*THNSL-2*) homolog. What was particularly surprising was that *THNSL-2* is a remnant of a gene that codes for threonine synthase in plants and microorganisms but is nonfunctional in higher organisms. Despite this lack of function *THNSL-2* has remained remarkably conserved in mammalian species, suggesting an ongoing functionality. Although the physiological/pathological function of SOFAT remains unknown, recombinant SOFAT was capable of stimulating functional osteoclast formation in the absence of osteoblasts or exogenous RANKL and in a manner that was completely insensitive to saturating concentrations of the RANKL inhibitor osteoprotegerin. Like RANKL, however, SOFATs osteoclastogenic activity was potently amplified by the inflammatory cytokine TNFα [126].

SOFAT had a further function, the capacity to promote IL-6 production from osteoblasts, another activity of formerly unknown source that had been previously documented in activated T-cell-conditioned medium [127].

While the function of SOFAT and its mechanisms of action remain to be characterized, we speculate that SOFAT may act to exacerbate inflammation and/or bone turnover under inflammatory conditions when T cells are activated such as in rheumatoid arthritis, periodontitis, and in conditions of estrogen deficiency, inflammatory disease states that are discussed in detail below.

5.1.3. Homologous to Lymphotoxins Exhibiting Inducible Expression and Competing with Herpes Simplex Virus Glycoprotein D for Herpesvirus Entry Mediator (HVEM), a Receptor Expressed by T Lymphocytes (LIGHT). Homologous to lymphotoxins exhibiting inducible expression and competing with herpes simplex virus glycoprotein D for herpesvirus entry mediator (HVEM), a receptor expressed by T lymphocytes (LIGHT), a member of the TNF superfamily (*TNFSF14*), that is significantly upregulated in the serum of human rheumatoid arthritis patients, is another cytokine expressed by activated T cells as well as monocytes, granulocytes, and immature dendritic cells. LIGHT has the capacity to induce osteoclast formation from both human and murine monocytes in the absence of RANKL and in a manner insensitive to OPG and RANK-Fc (a synthetic soluble decoy receptor of RANKL based on the RANKL receptor). Osteoclastogenesis was however impeded by blocking antibodies to the p75 TNF receptor. Like SOFAT, LIGHT may play an important role in supporting bone loss in patients with rheumatoid arthritis exacerbating RANKL-induced localized or systemic bone loss [128].

5.1.4. TGFβ in Osteoclastic Bone Resorption. Although TGFβ has been shown to stimulate early bone formation (see the aforementioned), several studies have shown a capacity of this cytokine to also promote vitamin D-dependent production of osteoclasts in osteoblast cocultures [129] and to augment *in vitro* RANKL-mediated osteoclast formation [130, 131]. In contrast, TGFβ has also been reported to inhibit osteoclastogenesis [132–134]. These confusing activities may be a consequence of biphasic effects whereby TGFβ stimulates osteoclastogenesis at low doses, but suppresses it at high concentrations [129]. Potential mechanisms of osteoclast inhibition are through production of OPG [135] as well as suppression of RANKL from osteoblasts [136]. It has further been reported that estrogen promotes apoptosis of murine osteoclasts through production of TGFβ [133]. Consistent with this apoptotic capacity we have reported that B cells *in vitro* are inhibitory to osteoclastogenesis as they secrete significant concentrations of TGFβ, leading to apoptosis of osteoclasts and their precursors [134]. This may be further compounded by B cell OPG secretion, potentially amplified, in part, by a cell autonomous effect of TGFβ on B cells.

Under conditions of estrogen deficiency in mice *in vivo* we have further shown that a decline in TGFβ production is permissive for T-cell-driven inflammatory bone loss, as TGFβ is a potent inhibitor of T-cell activation. Consequently, estrogen-induced TGFβ may act to protect the skeleton from the ravages of inflammation [137] (discussed in detail later).

Interestingly, one study has reported direct TGFβ-induced osteoclast formation by a RANKL-independent mechanism [138]. In this study addition of TGFβ to cultures of human monocytes and RAW 264.7 cells (a monocytic cell line that acts as early osteoclast precursors) in the presence of M-CSF but in the absence of RANKL or other inflammatory cytokines induced the formation of functional bone resorbing osteoclasts. Resorption was not suppressed by OPG or by neutralizing antibodies to TNFα, its receptors, or the gp130 chain of IL-6, suggesting that TGFβ acted independently of RANKL, TNFα, or IL-6 production. Furthermore, while RANKL stimulates large osteoclasts, TGFβ induced large numbers of mononucleated preosteoclasts and small mature osteoclasts producing many small resorption lacunae [138].

The significance of TGFβ in the regulation of basal osteoclastogenesis *in vivo* remains unclear with the potential for RANKL-dependent and -independent effects and direct inhibitory effects as well as indirect inhibitory effects through modulation of RANKL and OPG and through suppression of T-cell activation, creating a complex interplay.

5.2. Physiological OPG Production. Like RANKL, based on *in vitro* studies OPG production has traditionally been ascribed to osteoblasts and BMSCs. However, as far back as 1998 it was recognized that human B cells are a significant source of OPG and that modulation of the CD40 costimulatory receptor *in vivo* could markedly stimulate B cell OPG production [139]. These studies were considered of importance for the actions of RANKL in the context of immune function, but given the historical view that osteoblasts were the source of bone active OPG, the significance of these findings was overlooked in terms of a role in bone biology for almost a decade. In 2007 we reported that mice deficient in B cells had significantly elevated basal bone resorption and diminished BMD and volume. The central defect driving this imbalance in bone resorption relative to formation was a bone marrow deficiency in OPG, leading to an imbalance in the RANKL/OPG ratio that was permissive to bone resorption. Transplantation of B cells back into B cell KO mice was able to restore OPG to wild-type (WT) levels and rescue the development of osteoporosis [140].

Using WT mice we were able to quantify B-lineage sources of OPG production and were surprised to find that mature B cells accounted for 45% of total bone marrow OPG production. In addition, B cell precursors, immature B cells, and plasma cells further contributed OPG to the bone microenvironment with the entire B cell linage accounting for 64% of total OPG production [140].

An interesting finding was that as reported previously for human B cells [139], activation of the CD40 costimulatory receptor led to enhanced B cell OPG production. Because the cognate ligand of CD40 (CD40 ligand (CD40L)) is expressed by activated T cells, we further investigated the potential of T cells to regulate basal B cell OPG production using T-cell deficient nude mice, CD40L KO mice, and CD40 KO mice. These models confirmed that bone marrow OPG production is significantly compromised by T-cell deficiency and/or by genetic ablation of CD40 and CD40L costimulatory molecules, with a resulting increase in bone resorption and reduced bone mass [140]. The data were also consistent with a previous study demonstrating that depletion of $CD4^+$ and $CD8^+$ T lymphocytes in mice *in vivo* enhanced osteoclast formation *ex vivo* by a mechanism involving, in part, a pronounced suppression of OPG production [141].

Interestingly, osteopenia is a prominent clinical feature of patients with X-linked hyper-IgM syndrome, an inherited immune deficiency disorder caused by mutations in the gene encoding CD40L. Although the mechanisms for this bone loss are not clear, reduced interferon gamma (IFNγ) production has been reported by T cells [142]. OPG production was not investigated in this model.

Taken together these studies suggest that under basal conditions lymphocytes (both T cells and B cells) play an important stabilizing role and are protective of bone mass. As a consequence disruption of B cell or T cell function may have unfortunate repercussions for physiological bone turnover.

6. Consequences of Pathological Alterations to OPG Production

6.1. HIV-1 Infection and Osteoporosis. The quintessential immunodeficiency disease condition is the collapse of immunity that ensues following infection by the HIV-1 virus and leads to the constellation of pathological events generally referred to as acquired immunodeficiency syndrome (AIDS).

More than a decade ago alterations in skeletal metabolism were reported in AIDS patients on antiretroviral therapy (ART) [143]. The mechanisms responsible however were unclear but appeared to involve multiple underlying factors including ART, a collection of drugs used to suppress viral replication, traditional risk factors for osteoporosis such as smoking, drug use, and alcohol consumption, AIDS pathologies such as hypogonadism and renal disease, and a generalized low body mass index (BMI) that is often correlated with low bone mass [144–146]. In fact, based on this tight association between BMI and BMD, many now believe that low BMI associated with skeletal wasting is likely the most important underlying cause of low BMD in HIV patients [147]. Nonetheless, despite these clinical correlations no clear cause-effect relationship has been established between BMI and BMD in HIV infection, and, in fact, patients without wasting disease and with normal body weight also display reduced BMD at key sites including the lumbar spine and hip [148].

HIV infection itself is now considered a defined risk factor for osteoporosis although use of ART is recognized as an additional contributor to skeletal decline [149, 150]. Attesting to the impact of HIV infection recent studies show that an astounding two of every three patients with HIV infection, naive to ART, are osteopenic with 10% displaying outright osteoporosis [151].

Following initiation of ART, bone loss intensifies during the first 2 years of treatment leading to an additional 2%–6% decline in BMD, a decrease of a magnitude similar to that sustained during the first 2 years of menopause [150].

Until recently the consequences of this bone loss were unclear and the potential impact on patient health controversial. This, in part, was a consequence of the fact that the majority of HIV patients are relatively young and BMD is a poor indicator of fracture risk in younger populations (<55 years of age) [152]. Indeed, the standard clinical definitions of osteopenia and osteoporosis, as defined by the World Health Organization (WHO), are based on a statistical T score derived from BMD (quantified by means of dual-energy X-ray absorptiometry (DEXA or DXA) a bone densitometry technique). Osteopenia is defined as a T score of between -1.0 and -2.5 and osteoporosis as ≥ -2.5. The T score represents the number of standard deviations (SDs) below a mean peak bone mass of an average healthy young adult derived from a reference database and typically further adjusted for race and gender [153]. While DEXA is a convenient and noninvasive technology, the sensitivity of BMD as a predictor of fracture risk is limited by the fact that this index does not take into account the geometrical and material characteristics of bone [154]. Furthermore, cancellous (trabecular) bone only represents 20% of total bone mass, and although both cortical and trabecular bone significantly contribute to structural strength of bone, DEXA provides an integrated measurement of both bone compartments significantly underestimating the contribution of trabecular bone.

Despite fears being raised as to an epidemic of future fragility fractures as the mean age of the HIV demographic continues to trend upward [155] given the uncertainties in how to interpret changes in BMD in younger patients, physicians have been wary of intervening therapeutically in the absence of hard data regarding true fracture incidence. Over the last decade evidence of increased bone fracture has slowly accumulated to a critical mass. Among the first studies to report fragility fractures in HIV-infected patients on ART was from Guaraldi et al. who documented a 49-year-old male AIDS patient with osteopenia and a 51 year old male AIDS patient with osteoporosis, both of whom had suffered fractures after trivial trauma [156].

A central problem in investigating fracture in small cohorts is lack of statistical power owing to the relatively low rate of fracture in the general population and especially in men where fracture incidence remains low and stable (typically below 2%) until advanced age (>70 years of age) [157].

Studies involving ever-increasing population size have progressively cemented the concept that fracture incidence trends higher in HIV-infected populations. These studies include that of Arnsten et al., who studied BMD and incident fractures in 328 men over the age of 49 (mean age 55) with HIV infection and in 231 at risk individuals without HIV infection. BMD was reported to be significantly lower in HIV-infected compared with HIV-uninfected men at the femoral neck and lumbar spine after adjusting for age, weight, race, testosterone level, prednisone, and illicit drug use. Incident fracture rates per 100 person-years were 38% increase in HIV-infected men but fell short of being statistically significant, despite decreased BMD being associated with increased fracture risk [158].

In another fracture study involving a Canadian cohort, a ~2-fold higher fracture rate was observed in 138 HIV-infected women relative to 402 HIV^- controls. Interestingly the study reported that HIV^+ women were more likely to have had fragility fractures despite BMD values that were not different than women from a national population-based cohort [159]. This study may again highlight the major weakness in DEXA in discriminating between BMD and bone quality, the latter being a more important index of load bearing capacity and fracture risk.

In 2008, results from a large population-based analysis of a total of 8525 HIV-infected and 2,208,792 non-HIV-infected patients confirmed previous fears regarding a fracture epidemic by demonstrating a significant escalation in fracture incidence in men beginning at relatively young age (40–49 years) and achieving a dramatic ~4 fold increase in HIV^+ men by 60–69 years of age. In contrast to men, fracture incidence in healthy women is not stable and rises exponentially with age from around 0.5% at 30–39 years of age to ~3.5% by age 70–79. Importantly, HIV-infected women showed increased fracture prevalence relative to seronegative women at virtually every age and achieving an over 2-fold increase between 60 and 69 years of age [157].

This pivotal study has now been validated by other large population-based studies including the United States Department of Veterans Affairs (VA) cohort which comprised 39,375 HIV-infected patients and showed fracture rates of 24%–32% higher than uninfected populations [160] and in the HIV outpatient study (HOPS) study, a cohort of 5826 HIV patients where a 2- to 4-fold higher incidence of fracture was observed in the HIV seropositive population [161].

Not all studies have found increased fracture incidence however; for example, in the Women's Interagency HIV Study involving 1728 HIV-infected and 663 uninfected women the authors reported little difference in fracture incidence rates by HIV status in predominantly premenopausal women. Multivariate models did however reveal that race (white versus African-American), hepatitis C virus infection, and higher serum creatinine were statistically significant predictors of incident fracture [162].

While the bulk of recent data supports a significant decline in BMD and increase in facture incidence in HIV^+ populations the mechanisms responsible remain unclear. One of the hallmarks of HIV-infection is the loss of $CD4^+$ T cells as a consequence of a continuous stimulation of the immune system leading to activation-induced cell death (AICD) that is exacerbated by a failure to effectively restore T cells owing to reduced thymic function in the context of HIV infection [163]. Interestingly, although dramatic depletion of $CD4^+$ T cells is one of the most recognized features of HIV infection, in fact the entire immune system is severely impacted with significant impairment of the B-cell compartment leading to compromised humoral immunity [164, 165]. Because T cells are central regulators of B-cell activity, alterations in T-cell function further drive impairment of B-cell activity. Alterations in the B-cell compartment include a significant decline in B-cell numbers as well as a significant increase in the frequency of immature/transitional B cells [165]. Although the exact causes of diminished B-cell number and alterations in B-cell subpopulations are poorly understood, cytokine imbalances, decreased T-cell function, direct viral exposure, and viral antigens are all likely to play a role [166].

6.2. B-Cell Disruption Drives Bone Loss in an Animal Model of HIV-1 Infection in the HIV-1 Transgenic Rat. The complexity of the human system and the limitations associated with undertaking invasive clinical studies has contributed in large measure to the confusion regarding the underlying causes of bone loss in HIV-1 infection and led us to exploit an animal model, the HIV-1 transgenic (Tg) rat, a model that is not confounded by lifestyle factors and effects of ART, to investigate the effects of HIV-1 on bone turnover.

Constitutive expression of HIV-1 viral proteins directed by a replication defective HIV-1 viral genome, integrated into the rat DNA, leads to a syndrome in these animals that significantly resembles the immunologic and clinical abnormalities observed in human AIDS [167]. Using this model we documented for the first time a severe defect in skeletal homeostasis that led to a significant decline in BMD and in bone volume. These alterations in skeletal mass were consistent with significantly elevated osteoclast numbers and bone resorption, a consequence of a significant decline in B-cell OPG production, compounded by a significant increase in B-cell production of RANKL. Production of RANKL is indeed an established property of activated B cells

[168, 169] and of B-cell precursors [170]. This imbalance in the RANKL/OPG ratio was favorable to osteoclastic bone resorption and was likely further exacerbated by a dramatic increase in the number of osteoclast precursors [171].

These data link the disruptive impact of HIV infection on B-cell homeostasis to direct changes in bone turnover. In the context of humans, these alterations in the immunoskeletal interface are likely compounded by patient specific lifestyle factors and AIDS-associated pathologies thus contributing to the extremely high rates of bone disease exhibited by this population. Clinical studies to ratify these changes in humans are currently underway.

6.3. HIV, ART, and Inflammatory Bone Loss. While lymphocytes appear to play an important role in favor of the preservation of bone mass under physiological conditions, activated T and B cells, characteristic of inflammatory processes, are potent destroyers of bone and may cause skeletal degeneration in a wide range of pathological contexts.

Paradoxically, although HIV-1 infection leads to profound immunodeficiency, an inflammatory undercurrent is recognized to coexist in AIDS patients [22, 172] and is a strong predictor of disease progression [173]. Although the etiology is poorly defined, chronic immune activation is thought to result, in part, from persistent residual HIV-1 replication, chronic coinfections, and HIV-induced gastrointestinal mucosal damage that leads to internalization of high concentrations of bacterial metabolites and components including lipopolysaccharide (LPS), a bacterial cell wall protein that is potently immunogenic and leads to activation of both the innate and adaptive immune systems [173, 174]. LPS-induced inflammatory responses have long been recognized to stimulate production of RANKL, IL-1, and TNFα [175]. This inflammatory state in HIV-infected patients persists indefinitely even in the context of ART and may contribute to drive up bone resorption in AIDS patients even in the setting of effective viral suppression.

While ART has dramatically extended lifespan, troublesome metabolic complications including osteoporosis and elevated fracture prevalence are now undermining the quality of life of patients living on chronic ART [19]. Although HIV-1 infection and AIDS all contribute to severe skeletal deterioration, ART itself has long been recognized to independently contribute to bone loss [143] although the responsible mechanisms remain to be established. Resolving the contributions of HIV infection and AIDS, traditional osteoporosis risk factors, lifestyle factors, and ART to skeletal decline have been challenging [145, 147, 176]. In addition, because ART is used clinically as a combinatorial coformulation of multiple drug classes including protease inhibitors (PIs), nucleoside reverse transcriptase inhibitors (NRTIs), nonnucleoside reverse transcriptase inhibitors (NNRTIs), integrase inhibitors (IIs), and entry (fusion) inhibitors, with yet others in development, ascribing specific effects to specific drug classes has been difficult. This is further complicated by the fact that for each class of drug multiple variants exist that differ in chemical structure making for a very wide range of different formulations in different patients and between different studies.

Attempts to circumvent these confounders have involved *in vitro* or *in vivo* animal studies of ART; however the data has often been difficult to reconcile with clinical observations. PIs such as the ubiquitously used ritonavir have long been associated with bone loss in patients [176–181]; however when mice were treated with ritonavir in the absence of viral infection bone mass was found to be significantly improved rather than worsened [182]. Mechanistically, ritonavir was reported to inhibit osteoclast differentiation and abrogated bone resorption by disrupting the osteoclast cytoskeleton. Furthermore, ritonavir blunted parathyroid-hormone- (PTH-) induced osteoclastogenesis in mice and *in vitro* was found to suppress RANKL-induced NF-κB and Akt activation, signaling pathways critical to osteoclast formation and function. By contrast in the same study indinavir, a PI of different chemical structure, was inert and exhibited none of the effects observed for ritonavir [182].

By contrast, in another study ritonavir and saquinavir (but not indinavir and nelfinavir) were reported to promote T-cell production of RANKL following exposure to soluble HIV-1 envelope glycoprotein gp120 *in vitro* [183].

NRTIs have also been associated with bone loss in humans [176, 177, 184]. Zidovudine (AZT) the first drug approved for treatment of HIV-1-infection is of the NRTI class and although seldom prescribed now has in fact been found to promote bone loss in mice and to stimulate osteoclast formation *in vitro* along with two other NRTIs Didanosine (DDI) and Lamivudine (3TC) [185, 186].

Although there is presently no agreement on the mechanisms of ART-induced bone loss *in vivo*, accumulating evidence suggests that to some degree all classes of ART have a negative influence on bone turnover [187, 188] and the magnitude of bone loss is greatest within the first 2 years of therapy [150, 189, 190].

Because all ART regimens act to rejuvenate immune function through a repopulation of T cells (and B cells), a process that begins immediately following ART-initiation, but often continues for up to two years [191], current research in our laboratory is investigating whether ART-induced bone loss is, in part, a consequence of immune reignition leading to a transitory inflammatory bone loss. The recovery of T cells (and B cells) in the setting of ART is complex and likely differs between patients, involving peripheral expansion of existing T-cell pools in some, and/or IL-7 mediated thymic reactivation in others [191, 192]. T-cell and B-cell homeostatic expansion is a process involving lymphocyte activation and proliferation, conditions propitious for production of inflammatory and osteoclastogenic cytokines including TNFα and RANKL. These mechanisms may significantly resemble the bone loss associated with animal models of postmenopausal osteoporosis (described later in detail) which too involve IL-7-driven thymic-dependent differentiation of bone-marrow-derived progenitors and thymic-independent peripheral expansion of mature T cells [193].

While bone loss in the context of HIV infection and ART is ultimately likely to be explained by a combination of multiple factors that likely differ significantly between different individual patients, the recent appreciation for how immune function controls basal bone turnover and the role of inflammation in driving bone loss is likely to provide a new perspective on skeletal degeneration in AIDS patients and ultimately lead to new therapies to combat bone loss, through modulation of the immunoskeletal interface.

6.4. Lymphocytes and Alveolar Bone Loss in Periodontal Infection. Periodontal infection is a major cause of tooth loss in adults and is characterized by inflammation of the supporting tissues of the teeth, resulting in resorption of alveolar bone as well as loss of the soft tissue attachment to the tooth [194].

B cells have been reported to limit bone resorption in periodontitis as evidenced by *in vivo* animal studies involving T-cell deficient nude rats or rats treated with anti-B cell antibody. Periodontal bone loss was assessed following inoculation with *Actinomyces viscosus* or *Bacteroides gingivalis* and revealed that anti-B-cell-antibody-treated rats had significantly less periodontal bone support, whereas no difference was found between normal, nude, and thymus-grafted rats. The study concluded that while permanent T lymphocyte deficiency did not interfere with periodontal disease development, acute moderate reduction in B cells predisposed the animals for aggravation of alveolar bone loss [195]. One explanation for this outcome is that B cells are necessary to control the growth of periodontal bacteria and indeed in this study 95% of the inoculated rats raised serum IgG or IgM antibody against one or more of the microorganisms to which they were exposed [195]. However, another possibility is that B-cell OPG production ameliorates alveolar bone loss. Interestingly, it has been reported that B cells activated in the presence of helper T cells (Th)1 cytokines were found to inhibit osteoclastogenesis while B cells activated in the presence of Th2 cytokines increased osteoclastogenesis [196].

Although T cells did not appear to play an important role in supporting periodontal bone loss in the Klausen et al. study [195], other investigations have indeed implicated T cells in periodontal bone loss [197]. In fact, periodontal tissues from human patients with periodontal infection have been reported to express significantly higher levels of RANKL protein and significantly lower levels of OPG. In this study RANKL was associated with lymphocytes and macrophages, the latter not being a typical source of RANKL, while OPG protein was associated with endothelial cells [198].

In another study unfractionated peripheral blood mononuclear cells from periodontal patients revealed a high degree of spontaneous T-cell-dependent osteoclast formation compared to controls and were consistent with overexpression of RANKL and TNFα by T cells. Furthermore, anti-RANKL and anti-TNFα antibodies significantly inhibited osteoclastogenesis suggesting that T cells support spontaneous osteoclastogenesis in periodontal disease via RANKL and TNFα overexpression [199].

Furthermore, high levels of serum IL-7 associated with peripheral blood B cells from periodontal patients have been suggested to be responsible for T-cell-dependent osteoclastogenesis [200]. Indeed we have reported that IL-7 is a potent inducer of RANKL production by human peripheral blood derived T cells [125] (discussed later in detail). Furthermore, bone loss may be exacerbated by TNF-related apoptosis-inducing ligand (TRAIL) production suppressing osteoblast formation [201].

In another study, double-color confocal microscopy revealed that less than 20% of B cells and T cells were found to express RANKL in healthy gingival tissues, while in diseased gingival tissues, more than 50% and 90% of T cells and B cells, respectively, expressed RANKL. As RANKL production by nonlymphoid cells was not observed, this study concluded that B and T lymphocytes are the primary sources of RANKL in the bone resorptive lesion of periodontal disease [169].

Taken together both T cells and B cells have been implicated in alveolar bone loss in periodontitis, likely due to enhanced RANKL production, as a consequence of immune activation and potentially exacerbated by diminished OPG production by B cells and secretion of inflammatory cytokines such as IL-6, IL-7, and TNFα.

6.5. Lymphocytes and Osteoclastic Bone Loss in Rheumatoid Arthritis. Rheumatoid arthritis is another inflammatory disease; however in contrast to periodontitis where inflammation is driven by bacterial infection, rheumatoid arthritis stems from an autoimmune condition leading to immune-mediated deterioration of cartilage and bone in the affected joints [202]. This is the result of a state of chronic inflammation that develops in the synovial membrane of affected joints and afflicts approximately 2 percent of the adult population causing chronic pain and fatigue, crippling, and loss of daily function and can cause permanent disability and increased mortality [203]. Rheumatoid arthritis not only causes destruction of cartilage but also disrupts systemic control of bone remodeling causing a systemic bone loss [204]. A major characteristic of rheumatoid arthritis is a dense lymphoid infiltration into the synovial membrane with high concentrations of activated T and B cells that drives not only initiation of the inflammatory state but is also in large measure responsible for the bone loss associated with rheumatoid arthritis [203, 205–208]. In rheumatoid arthritis activated T and B cells are potent inducers of osteoclastic bone resorption through direct RANKL secretion as well as through production of TNFα, a cytokine of key importance in the etiology of rheumatoid arthritis. In fact, transgenic overexpression of TNFα in mice leads to a robust inflammatory state characterized by bone and joint destruction that closely mimics that of human rheumatoid arthritis [209, 210]. TNFα ablation, by contrast, prevents both inflammation and bone loss in TNFα transgenic mice [82], and pharmacological TNFα inhibitors, such as TNFα receptor decoy receptors, are effective agents for amelioration of rheumatoid arthritis in human patients [84, 211–214].

Although bone erosions are ameliorated by TNFα inhibitors, it remains unclear whether this is a direct consequence of the beneficial action of these pharmaceuticals on TNFα-mediated inflammation (upstream of bone turnover) or whether there is a direct beneficial effect on bone formation and/or resorption or a combination of both mechanisms. Given studies by others and us in animal models, reduction of TNFα is expected to boost bone formation while simultaneously reducing bone resorption [90, 98, 113].

Interestingly, high levels of IL-7 have also been reported in rheumatoid arthritis and may contribute to the cycle of inflammation and/or bone loss [215–220]. Indeed, injections of IL-7 in arthritic mice cause expansion of T and B cells and increased levels of proinflammatory mediators and intensify arthritis severity and joint destruction. These actions were accompanied by increased Th1 and Th17 activity and suggest that IL-7 could be an important mediator in arthritic conditions and that targeting IL-7 or its receptor may represent a novel therapeutic strategy [221]. In contrast to IL-7 administration, antibody neutralization of the IL-7 receptor significantly reduced clinical arthritis severity in association with reduced radiographic joint damage [221].

Th17 cells are another major subset of T-helper cells and named for their expression of the cytokine IL-17 and have long been suggested to play a role in rheumatoid arthritis [222]. Levels of IL-17 in synovial fluids are reported to be significantly higher in rheumatoid arthritis patients than osteoarthritis patients, and anti-IL-17 antibody was shown to significantly inhibit osteoclast formation induced by culture media derived from rheumatoid arthritis synovial tissues. Furthermore, treatment of cocultures of mouse hemopoietic cells with primary osteoblasts stimulated with IL 17 induced osteoclast differentiation, which was completely inhibited by OPG. Expression of RANKL by osteoblasts in response to IL-17 was further confirmed *in vitro* suggesting that IL-17-induced osteoclastic bone loss is a consequence of RANKL expression by osteoblasts [223].

In another study IL-17 adenoviral overexpression in the knee joint of type II collagen-immunized mice (a murine model of rheumatoid arthritis) promoted osteoclastic bone erosions in cortical, subchondral, and trabecular bone along with expression of RANKL and its receptor RANK in the synovial infiltrate and at sites of focal bone erosions. IL-17 not only enhanced RANKL expression but also strongly upregulated the RANKL/OPG ratio in the synovium, while systemic OPG treatment prevented joint damage induced by local IL-17 overexpression. These findings suggest T cell IL-17 to be an important inducer of RANKL expression stimulating osteoclastogenesis and bone erosion in arthritis [224].

Consistent with these assertions antibody neutralization of IL-17 in a murine model of rheumatoid arthritis, the TNFα transgenic mouse, using IL-17 neutralizing antibody while only having minor effects on TNFα-induced inflammation, effectively reduced local and systemic bone loss by blocking osteoclast differentiation *in vivo*. These protective effects on bone erosions were consistent with a shift to bone-protective T-cell responses such as enhanced Th2 differentiation, IL-4 and IL-12 expressions, and increased regulatory T-cell (Treg) numbers. The data highlight IL-17 as a putative therapeutic target for ameliorating bone destruction associated with T-cell activation in rheumatoid arthritis [225].

7. Role of the Immunoskeletal Interface in Estrogen Deficiency-Induced Bone Loss

A cause-effect relationship between estrogen deficiency and postmenopausal osteoporosis has existed for over 70 years. Loss of estrogen at the time of the menopause results in an accelerated phase of bone loss impacting predominantly cancellous (trabecular) bone that declines rapidly over a 4–8-year period. Thereafter, this is replaced by a second slow phase of bone loss in which the rate of cancellous bone loss is reduced, but the rate of cortical bone loss is unchanged or increased. This bone loss continues indefinitely, mediated in large measure by the development of a state of secondary hyperparathyroidism [226].

One of the most surprising aspects to emerge in the past 15 years is the profound contribution of the immune system to bone loss in estrogen deficiency [15, 17, 227]. For more than a decade we have investigated the cascade of inflammatory cytokines that regulate the immune system and bone turnover in a murine model of estrogen deficiency, the ovariectomized mouse [15, 17, 43, 70, 77, 137, 193, 228–235]. Some of the key findings from these studies are presented in the following.

7.1. B Cells in Ovariectomy-Induced Bone Loss. The role of B cells in the bone loss associated with estrogen deficiency remains contentious. Almost 2 decades ago it was observed that ovariectomy in mice leads to a surge in B lymphopoiesis [236] and that estrogen administration can suppress B lymphopoiesis [237]. These studies lead to the suggestion that cells of the B lineage may contribute to ovariectomy-induced bone loss, and in 1997 a landmark paper demonstrated that the lymphopoietic cytokine IL-7 caused a potent rise in B lymphopoiesis when injected into mice, an event that was paralleled by a significant loss of BMD [238].

Interestingly, immature B cell populations expressing the marker B220 have been suggested to transdifferentiate along the osteoclast pathway *in vitro* [239] providing a potential enhanced source of osteoclast precursors and an explanation for a role of B-lineage cells in ovariectomy-induced bone loss. Although the potential for B220 cells to function as osteoclast precursors *in vitro* has been independently verified by us and others [240, 241], the role of such cells *in vivo* remains unclear.

After the discovery of RANKL as the key osteoclastogenic cytokine, expression of this factor by B-lineage cells ($B220^+$ cells, which in the bone marrow represent multiple populations of early B-cell precursors, immature B cells, and mature B cells) has been reported to be more abundant in ovariectomized mice than in sham-operated mice [170]. RANKL from B cells isolated from the bone marrow of estrogen deficient postmenopausal women have been demonstrated to secrete RANKL [242], providing a plausible mechanism for a role of B cells in estrogen deficiency bone loss.

In an attempt to demonstrate a cause-effect relationship between B-lymphopoiesis and bone loss in estrogen deficiency we performed ovariectomy on B-cell KO mice and examined bone loss by DEXA and microcomputed tomography (μCT). Surprisingly, after compensating for differences in basal bone mass between WT and B cell KO controls, ovariectomized B cell KO mice lost an identical percentage of bone mass to that of WT controls, excluding a role of mature B cells in bone loss associated with this model, although this KO retains early B-cell precursors that might contribute to the process [243].

Recently, however, to overcome the confounder of altered bone turnover in B-cell KO mice, Onal et al. made use of a state-of-the-art conditional B-cell RANKL KO mouse, to reevaluate the role of mature B cells in ovariectomy-induced bone loss. This high sensitivity model did indeed reveal a small contribution of mature B cells to ovariectomy-induced bone loss as mice lacking RANKL in B lymphocytes were partially protected from the increase in osteoclast numbers and bone loss caused by ovariectomy in cancellous bone, although not in cortical bone, in the conditional KO mice [122].

7.2. The Role of T Cells and IL-7 in Ovariectomy-Induced Bone Loss. A surprising finding over the last decade and a half has been the identification of a central role for T cells in the osteoclastic bone loss associated with ovariectomy in mice and recent translational data from clinical studies providing tantalizing support for a role of T cells in human postmenopausal bone loss.

In an attempt to further dissect the IL-7-induced bone loss reported by Miyaura et al., and ascribed to B cells [238], we examined the action of IL-7 in fractionated peripheral blood cells *in vitro* and made the surprising discovery that IL-7 potently promoted *in vitro* osteoclast formation but only in the presence of T cells. We further demonstrated that IL-7 stimulates the production of RANKL by T cells and that OPG could significantly, although not completely, repress IL-7-induced osteoclastogenesis [125]. Indeed, IL-7 is an established master regulator of T-cell homeostasis [244]; however these were the first studies to demonstrate that IL-7 is an inducer of T-cell RANKL production. Importantly, we were able to further demonstrate that ovariectomy enhances the production of IL-7 *in vivo* and that antibody directed neutralization of IL-7 prevented ovariectomy-induced bone loss in mice. In addition, IL-7 neutralization augmented bone formation suggesting that IL-7 was an osteoblast inhibitor and indeed IL-7 injection into mice inhibited bone formation *in vivo* suggesting that IL-7 may uncouple bone formation from bone resorption, exacerbating ovariectomy-induced bone loss [70].

Additional studies in mice revealed that IL-7-administration induces bone loss by a mechanism that involves production of RANKL, but also involved TNFα *ex vivo* [240]. In fact, *in vivo* IL-7 has multiple complex actions that impact almost every step in T-cell maturation, development, and function [244], and consistent with this concept we further demonstrated that in ovariectomy, IL-7 stimulated both thymic-dependent differentiation of bone-marrow-derived progenitors and thymic-independent, peripheral expansion of mature T cells. Almost 50% of the bone loss observed was through thymic-dependent effects of IL-7 as thymectomy decreases by half, the bone loss and stimulation of T lymphopoiesis induced by estrogen deficiency [193, 245]. The role of the thymus in postmenopausal osteoporosis in humans is presently unclear, given that at advanced age significant thymic atrophy has almost always taken place. However, studies in aged mice and rats have revealed that thymic regeneration may indeed occur, in part, in response to estrogen deficiency [246], and aged women have increased numbers of circulating recent thymic emigrants, an index of thymic output, relative to aged men [247].

How IL-7 is regulated is still unclear; however one study has reported that liver-derived insulin-like growth factor 1 (IGF-1) is permissive for ovariectomy-induced trabecular bone loss by modulation of the number of T cells and the expression of IL-7. In these studies IGF-1 KO mice were shown to be protected from ovariectomy-induced bone loss and T-cell expansion suggesting an action upstream of IL-7 [248].

Not all studies have reported a role for IL-7 in ovariectomy-induced bone loss. In fact, in contrast to the osteoclastogenic effects of IL-7 mediated through the immune system, it has been reported that IL-7 directly inhibits osteoclast formation *in vitro* [241]. In these studies IL-7 suppressed RANKL and M-CSF-induced osteoclast formation in murine bone marrow cultures derived from WT mice but not IL-7 receptor null mice. However, bone marrow from IL-7 receptor null mice generated significantly lower numbers of osteoclasts when treated with RANKL, vitamin D, or PTH showing complex effects of IL-7 [241]. The reasons for the different responses *in vitro* and *in vivo* are unclear, but may relate in part to the fact that IL-7-induced osteoclastogenesis *in vivo* occurs largely by a mechanism involving the stimulation of T-cell activation and expansion and production of RANKL and TNFα, while *in vitro* in the context of high doses of RANKL these effects are masked and a direct antiosteoclastogenic effect appears to be the dominant activity. Indeed, a similar effect is observed by IFNγ (discussed later in detail).

We have also reported that IL-7 is inhibitory to osteoblast differentiation [70] and may suppress the production of osteoclastogenic cytokines by these cells in coculture systems involving PTH and vitamin D-induced RANKL production.

In another model system, however, it was reported that IL-7 KO mice had increased osteoclasts and decreased trabecular bone volume compared with WT mice and lost similar amounts of trabecular bone following ovariectomy to that of WT animals. Interestingly, IL-7 KO mice were protected from cortical but not trabecular bone lost after ovariectomy [249]. Additional studies by the same group involving a model in which IL-7 was transgenically overexpressed using a 2.3-kb rat collagen 1a1 promoter to drive the expression of human IL-7 specifically in osteoblasts found increased trabecular bone volume *in vivo* by μCT and decreased osteoclast formation in vitro. Surprisingly this bone phenotype was only evident in female mice. The authors hypothesized that overexpression of IL-7 in the bone marrow microenvironment may change the distribution and/or the differentiation of osteoclast progenitors by disturbing the balance of lineage development *in situ* [250].

In contrast to these studies a global IL-7 overexpressing transgenic mouse in which the IL-7 transgene was under control of an estrogen alpha promoter was reported to have a bone marrow cavity that was considerably expanded and with cortical bone showing focal osteolysis [251]. More recently in-depth analysis of this animal further revealed a specific phenotype characterized by an age-related loss of trabecular bone in both axial and long bones. Osteopenia was the result of an increased number of active osteoclasts on the surface of trabecular bone. The overexpression of IL-7 also created an osteoclastogenic bone marrow microenvironment that promoted the commitment of precursors towards the osteoclast lineage [252].

The conflicting reports for IL-7 actions by multiple independent groups of investigators reveal a complex action of this cytokine on bone homeostasis that remains to be fully understood.

Interestingly, bone disease occurs in over 70%–80% of patients with the B-cell cancer multiple myeloma and represents a significant source of morbidity and mortality [253]. Human myeloma cells have been reported to stimulate RANKL production by T cells, by a mechanism involving IL-7 and/or IL-6 [254]. This group has further shown a role for IL-7 in the suppressed osteoblast formation and differentiation induced by multiple myeloma cells from human patients [255]. Other studies have further investigated the mechanism for suppression of bone formation in multiple myeloma and report that increased levels of the transcriptional repressor growth factor independent 1 (Gfi1), a novel transcriptional repressor of the critical osteoblast transcription factor Runx2, may play an important role. Interestingly, Gfi1 induction was blocked by anti-TNFα and anti-IL-7 antibodies [256].

Taken together the data suggest that as in ovariectomy and rheumatoid arthritis IL-7 may play a critical role in the enhanced bone resorption and suppressed bone formation associated with multiple myeloma.

7.3. The Role of T-Cell TNF Production in Ovariectomy-Induced Bone Loss. TNFα has long been recognized as an important cytokine in postmenopausal osteoporosis [26, 42, 74, 75, 257]; however a surprising recent discovery was that T cells are the likely source of this cytokine. Support of a role for T-cell production of TNFα in ovariectomy-induced bone loss came from studies by our group demonstrating that ovariectomy-induced a significant expansion of TNFα-producing T cells in WT mice but failed to do so in T-cell deficient nude mice. The data suggested that ovariectomy caused an expansion of TNFα secreting T-cells, although without altering production of TNFα per cell. The critical role of TNFα production in ovariectomy-induced bone loss was further demonstrated in a study in which ovariectomy failed to induce bone loss in TNFα KO mice and mice deficient in the p55 (type I) TNFα receptor. By contrast, p75 (type II) TNFα receptor ablation failed to prevent ovariectomy-induced bone loss. Finally, adoptive transfer of T cells from TNFα KO mice into T-cell deficient mice revealed a key role for T-cell-specific TNFα production in the mechanism of ovariectomy-induced bone loss [228].

Interestingly, a recent study suggests that expansion of senescent CD4âĄžCD28$^-$ T cells may be the responsible TNFα secreting T-cell population involved in ovariectomy-induced bone loss as estrogen deficiency led to increased prevalence of TNFα secreting CD4$^+$CD28$^-$ T cells and even that could be reversed using the isoflavonoid daidzein [258].

The mechanism by which TNFα from T cells promotes osteoclast formation is not entirely clear, however it is established that TNFα amplifies the activity of endogenous RANKL as well as stimulating RANKL production by osteoblasts and their precursors [68, 259]. Interestingly, like B cells, T cells derived from estrogen deficient women have been demonstrated to express increased levels of RANKL [242] however a direct specific role for T-cell-derived RANKL in the mouse ovariectomy model has not been demonstrated. In fact, a recent study using a conditional RANKL KO mouse has demonstrated that ablation of RANKL in T cells failed to prevent or attenuate ovariectomy-induced bone loss [122]. These data suggest that although T cells have the capacity to secrete RANKL, it is predominantly TNFα that accounts for ovariectomy-induced bone loss.

Recent studies from our group show that the T-cell costimulatory molecule CD40L not only functions in the regulation of B-cell OPG production, but further mediates expansion of osteoblast precursors, promotes osteoblast proliferation, and differentiation and regulates osteoblast precursor production of M-CSF, RANKL, and OPG. Ovariectomy thus failed to promote bone loss and increase bone resorption in mice depleted of T cells or lacking CD40L, suggesting that cross-talk between T cells and osteoblast precursor mediated by CD40L plays a pivotal role in the disregulation of osteoblastogenesis and osteoclastogenesis induced by ovariectomy [235]. The data further suggest that RANKL production by osteoblasts may be the target of T-cell-derived TNFα.

Interestingly, a recent study further suggests that TNFα production from T cells promotes an increase in sclerostin, a potent Wnt-pathway antagonist and antiosteoblastic factor, that may contribute to the relatively reduced bone formation associated with estrogen deficiency. While sclerostin expression in WT mice was stimulated by ovariectomy and reversed by estrogen treatment as well as by pharmacological TNFα neutralization, T-cell deficient nude mice showed no response to ovariectomy [260].

8. IFNγ, a Key Mediator of Ovariectomy-Induced Bone Loss and T-Cell TNFα Production

Taken together the accumulated evidence suggests that estrogen deficiency leads to overexpression of IL-7 that culminates in T-cell activation and production of osteoclastogenic cytokines, predominantly TNFα. How T cells are activated in estrogen deficiency, however, turns out to be complex. CD4$^+$ T cell activation requires two distinct signals, the first signal of which is generated by engagement of the T-cell receptor (TCR) on CD4$^+$ helper T cells with major histocompatibility complex (MHC) class II (MHCII) bearing antigens on the surface of professional antigen presenting cells (APCs) including B cells, dendritic cells, and macrophages. This signal renders T cells inactive or anergic unless a second "costimulatory" signal is transmitted through association of the CD28 receptor on T cells, with B7 molecules (B7-1 (CD80) and B7-2 (CD86)), expressed on professional APCs. Once both signals have been received, the T cell becomes activated, undergoes clonal expansion, and produces characteristic cytokines depending on its ultimate differentiation program [261].

IL-7 is known to increase the sensitivity of T cells to otherwise weak antigenic stimuli, amplifying the antigenic response and driving up T-cell activation. IL-7 production thus acts to increase the magnitude of T-cell responses to otherwise weak antigens that are normally tolerogenic and that do not usually promote significant immune activation. IL-7 further increases immune activation by promoting production of IFNγ, a classic Th1 T-cell cytokine. IFNγ is a potent inducer of macrophage class II transactivator (CIITA) protein [262] a key transcription factor that upregulates MHCII expression on macrophages promoting antigenic responses.

Attesting to the importance of IFNγ in ovariectomy-induced bone loss we have further demonstrated that ovariectomy upregulates IFNγ that induces CIITA, increasing antigen presentation by macrophages, enhancing T-cell activation, and prolonging the lifespan of active T cells. As a consequence ovariectomy fails to induce bone loss in IFNγ receptor null mice. Attesting to the importance of antigen presentation in this system mice possessing a transgenic T-cell receptor that is responsive only to ovalbumin, a protein not endogenously present in mice, are protected from ovariectomy-induced bone loss, but undergo bone loss in response to estrogen deficiency following administration of ovalbumin [229].

The fact that ovariectomy was muted in the face of an inactive T-cell receptor strongly suggests that antigen presentation is a necessary component of ovariectomy-induced bone loss; however an intriguing question arises as to the nature of the antigen or antigens involved and whether a unique antigen is generated during estrogen deficiency that drives T-cell activation. In fact, because ovalbumin was found to support bone loss during estrogen deficiency the data would suggest that a specific type of antigen is not required and that any antigen capable of activating T cells is able to support bone resorption [229]. In addition, the capacity of IL-7 to reduce T-cell sensitivity to weak prevailing antigens coupled with the IFNγ-induced MHCII expression likely all converges to upregulate basal antigen presentation responses to endogenous foreign and self-antigens.

An interesting concept in immunology is that T-cell survival in the periphery is dependent on self-peptides that serve to maintain the longevity of mature T cells. This weak antigenic "tickling" does not induce T-cell activation or proliferation but simply helps to maintain the peripheral pool. In conditions where total T cell numbers are reduced, these self-ligands become overtly stimulatory and cause naive T cells to proliferate and undergo homeostatic expansion [263]. An intriguing possibility is that estrogen deficiency may promote T-cell expansion by a similar mechanism reliant on these physiological weak self-peptides that normally function in maintenance of T-cell homeostasis. An alternative explanation is that ovariectomy simply increases the sensitivity of T cells to foreign antigens including bacterial metabolites and cell membranes (LPSs), peptide products of digestion that are routinely absorbed in the gut and antigens inhaled into the lungs. Together, these foreign and self-antigens all conspire to sustain a weak basal antigenic activity that is necessary for the maintenance of T-cell peripheral pools [263–265].

Future studies remain to be conducted to definitively determine the types of antigens responsible for ovariectomy-induced bone loss.

Interestingly, IFNγ has further been reported to possess potent direct inhibitory actions on osteoclast formation by impeding the RANKL-RANK signaling pathway and inducing degradation of the RANK adapter protein, TRAF6 preventing RANKL-induced activation of NF-κB and JNK [266]. Consistent with these studies IFNγ suppresses RANKL-induced cathepsin K expression in differentiating osteoclast precursors [267].

Given the need for IFNγ activity in promoting ovariectomy-induced bone loss *in vivo*, the data suggest that the direct inhibitory actions of IFNγ may compete with the proosteoclastogenic indirect actions. This was further investigated in T-cell null mice where systemic administration of IFNγ was found to cause bone loss in T-cell replete but not T-cell deficient mice. Thus under conditions of estrogen deficiency the net balance of IFNγ action was biased toward bone resorption in this study [232]. In another study administration of IFNγ *in vivo* was also reported to lead to bone loss and fails to ameliorate cyclosporin A-induced osteopenia [268]. Interestingly, in a study focusing largely on the effect of IFNγ on bone formation, IFNγ receptor KO mice were reported to reflect an osteoporotic phonotype due to reduced bone formation and elevated bone resorption [269].

The data suggesting antiosteoporotic actions of IFNγ conflict, however, with a number of clinical studies that have used IFNγ administration to treat excessive bone formation by upregulating bone resorption in conditions of osteopetrosis [270–272].

These different outcomes again reflect how subtle changes in experiment conditions may lead to very different results. While the actions of IFNγ appear to be contradictory between studies, it has been reported that early exposure to RANKL can prime osteoclast precursors to form in the presence of high levels of IFNγ using mechanisms independent of the signaling molecules signal transducers and activators of transcription (STAT)1 and TRAF6 [273], thus providing an explanation for how chronic IFNγ stimulation *in vivo* may overcome the inhibitory effects on osteoclast formation under inflammatory states.

9. TGFβ, a Potent Inhibitor of Immune Activation and Ovariectomy-Induced Bone Loss

As discussed previously the role of TGFβ in bone biology is extremely complex with both stimulatory and inhibitory effects on both osteoclastogenesis and osteoblastogenesis reported. Interestingly, in the context of estrogen deficiency and immune activation, TGFβ appears to play an upstream protective role and represents a central mechanism by which estrogen protects the body against inflammatory bone loss.

We have shown that ovariectomy diminishes expression of TGFβ in the bone microenvironment, while transgenic mice overexpressing a dominant-negative TGFβ type II receptor, specifically in T cells, were completely insensitive to the bone-sparing effect of estrogen and as in the case of control WT mice ovariectomy led to production of IFNγ, T-cell activation, and T-cell TNFα production. Furthermore, overexpression of TGFβ *in vivo* using a somatic gene therapy technique was found to prevent ovariectomy-induced bone loss. These findings suggest that stimulation of TGFβ production in the bone marrow is a critical "upstream" mechanism by which estrogen prevents bone loss [137]. The reduction in TGFβ signaling, associated with estrogen deficiency, may further serve to stimulate IL-7 production, thus intensifying the inflammatory response and driving up bone resorption [17].

The critical role of the immune system in ovariectomy-induced bone loss has been further validated in an independent study where estrogen deficiency failed to induce osteoporosis in immunocompromised bg-nu/nu-xid mice, a strain deficient in T, B, and NK cells [274].

In another study, however, ovariectomy was not found to alter the percentage of T lymphocytes in the bone marrow and spleen, and in fact small decreases were observed. In a comparison of bone mass in 3 strains of immunocompromised mice (T-cell deficient nude and TCRα KO mice and double T-cell and B-cell deficient recombination activating gene (RAG)2 KO mice) bone loss with ovariectomy was consistently observed in WT mice but was variably present in immunocompromised mice as measured by DEXA. In contrast, μCT and histomorphometry showed similar trabecular bone loss after ovariectomy in all strains but found protection from cortical bone loss in nude and TCRα KO mice, but not in RAG2 KO mice [275]. The reason for the difference in outcomes between this study and that of others remains unclear.

10. TGFβ and Regulatory T Cells (Tregs) in Bone Homeostasis

Tregs also known as suppressor T cells are a potent immunomodulatory T-cell subset that are critical for the prevention of spontaneous autoimmune disease by moderating inflammatory T-cell responses. Tregs further function to restore immune homeostasis after inflammatory responses in order to limit inflammation and prevent chronic inflammatory diseases [276].

Kim et al. found that Tregs inhibit osteoclast differentiation from peripheral blood mononuclear cells in a cytokine-dependent and cell-to-cell contact-independent manner and proposed that TGFβ and IL-4 cytokine secreted by Th2 cells may be the key cytokines responsible for the suppressive function of Tregs [277]. Another recent study has implicated Tregs in the mechanism by which estrogen suppresses osteoclast differentiation and bone resorption through Treg production of IL-10 and TGFβ1 [278].

Another mechanism by which Tregs maintain control of immune function is by secretion of Cytotoxic T-Lymphocyte Antigen 4 (CTLA4), an inhibitor that binds to CD80 and CD86 coreceptors on APC and blocking their association with CD28 on T cells, thus dulling inflammatory responses [279]. We have previously reported that one mechanism by which estrogen deficiency induces bone loss is by upregulating CD80 on dendritic cells. As an antagonist of CD80/CD28 costimulation we found that a pharmacological derivative of CTLA4, CTLA4-Ig, was able to prevent ovariectomy-induced bone loss by downmodulating the inflammatory cascade leading to T-cell activation and TNFα production and downmodulating osteoclastogenesis and bone resorption in mice *in vivo* [233].

Interestingly, Tregs have also been shown to directly inhibit osteoclast formation by CD11b monocytes treated with M-CSF and RANKL, as well as to suppress resorption of pits *in vitro* by mature osteoclasts. An important finding was that the key Treg cytokines TGFβ, IL-4 and IL-10 were not essential to this inhibitory effect on osteoclastogenesis; however, direct antiosteoclastogenic effects of CTLA4 mediated on purified osteoclast precursors were documented. The data suggest that in addition to an anti-inflammatory role of CTLA4, this receptor may directly suppress osteoclastogenesis by binding to CD80/CD86 on mononuclear osteoclast precursors [280, 281].

11. The Th17 T-Cell Subset and Bone Loss in Estrogen Deficiency

Th17 cells are another subset of T-helper cells and named for their expression of the cytokine IL-17. To study the role of IL-17 in ovariectomy-induced bone loss Goswami et al. ovariectomized IL-17 receptor KO mice and quantified bone turnover. Surprisingly, the IL-17 receptor KO mice were found to be markedly more susceptible to ovariectomy-induced bone loss than sham controls. Although no changes in Th1, Th2, or Th17 cytokines were detected in serum, constitutively elevated leptin, a factor that regulates metabolism and satiety, but also bone metabolism, was further increased following ovariectomy and suggested as a putative mechanism to account for exaggerated bone loss [282].

In contrast to the IL-17 receptor KO, Tyagi et al. induced a functional block of IL-17 using neutralizing monoclonal antibody and found a complete prevention of ovariectomy-induced bone loss. Ovariectomy was further observed to lead to a significant expansion in Th17 $CD4^+$ T cells and a dramatic elevation in the serum concentration of IL-17, events suppressed by administration of exogenous estrogen to mice. *In vitro*, IL-17 treatment was found to upregulate the expression of the receptor RANK on osteoclast precursors and to upregulate expression of TNFα, IL-6, and RANKL by osteoblasts. These effects were potently downmodulated by addition of estrogen to the cultures. These findings suggest that estrogen deficiency leads to increased differentiation of Th17 cells and induces bone loss by increasing proosteoclastogenic cytokines including TNFα and RANKL from osteoblasts [283].

12. Reactive Oxygen Species (ROS) and Immune Activation in Ovariectomy-Induced Bone Loss

Recently, increases in reactive oxygen species (ROS) have been implicated in the upstream actions of estrogen deficiency, aging and the bone loss associated with diabetes [233, 284, 285]. ROS have significant direct effects on the generation and survival of osteoclasts, osteoblasts, and osteocytes [284]. An important mediator of ROS in osteoblast progenitors is the ROS-activated FoxO transcription factors that converge on the bone anabolic Wnt signaling pathway, decoying β-catenin from binding to target genes necessary for osteoblast differentiation and decreasing osteoblastogenesis [284]. Ovariectomy not only alters the generation of ROS, but the antioxidant defense capacity of the cell is altered increasing sensitivity to the direct stimulatory effects of ROS on osteoclast formation and activity ([286, 287], Lean, 2004 #3124).

However, ROS also mediate potent actions on the immune system and have the capacity to indirectly promote osteoclastogenesis by altering the immunoskeletal interface. Superoxide promotes maturation of human dendritic cells and is reported to upregulate the costimulatory molecules CD80 and CD86 [288]. Indeed, we have further found that ROS induced by estrogen deficiency in mice upregulates CD80 on mouse dendritic cells [233]. Because CD80 is a key ratification signal for T-cell activation through its counterpart CD28 on the T cell [289], upregulation of CD80 facilitates antigen-dependent T-cell activation and hence promotes production of TNFα by T cells. Accordingly, bone loss is prevented by treatment of ovariectomized mice with either antioxidants or CTLA4-Ig, an inhibitor of CD80/CD28 costimulation [233].

13. Human Postmenopausal Osteoporosis and the Immunoskeletal Interphase

As the vast majority of studies have thus far been conducted using animal models of postmenopausal osteoporosis, these outcomes remain to be ratified in humans. In a number of cases animal studies have generated conflicting data, and consequently given the complexity and lack of uniformity among humans there are multiple complex outcomes that may be predicted.

One of the most interesting studies in humans addresses the production of RANKL by bone marrow cells in early postmenopausal women. In this study surface RANKL expression was quantified by two-color flow cytometry on isolated bone marrow mononuclear cells derived from premenopausal women, early postmenopausal women, and age-matched, estrogen-treated postmenopausal women. The surface concentration of RANKL per cell was increased in postmenopausal women compared to premenopausal women and estrogen-treated postmenopausal women by two- to threefold for MSCs, T cells, B cells, and total RANKL-expressing cells [242]. This study suggests that RANKL production by T cells and B cells may contribute to bone loss during estrogen deficiency in humans. Studies of human and animal lymphocytes do indeed suggest that both T and B cells have the innate capacity to secrete RANKL however a defined role for T-cell generated RANKL in ovariectomy-induced bone loss has not been demonstrated. In fact, the animal studies reported previously suggest that TNFα production by T cells is more important to the mechanism of ovariectomy-induced bone loss in mice.

Few human studies have been conducted to assess the role of T cells in postmenopausal osteoporosis but one recent clinical study reported that women with postmenopausal osteoporosis exhibit an increased T-cell activity and elevated production of TNFα and RANKL production compared to healthy postmenopausal controls [290]. These data provide enticing support to a role of T cells in the etiology of postmenopausal bone loss in humans as suggested by the animal models.

IFNγ is a cytokine with complex action *in vitro* and in animal models with both stimulatory [229, 232, 273] and inhibitory effects [266, 267, 269] being reported.

In humans the weight of evidence is in favor of a net pro-osteoclastogenic activity as clinical studies have employed IFNγ to treat excessive bone formation by stimulating bone resorption in osteopetrosis [270–272].

Detailed clinical studies are now needed to establish the role of the immunoskeletal interface in human disease and the role of the inflammatory state in postmenopausal osteoporosis.

14. The Role of T Cells in the Bone Loss Associated with Hyperparathyroidism

Hyperparathyroidism is a condition whereby enhanced levels PTH lead to accelerated bone resorption and bone loss. High-turnover bone disease caused by secondary hyperparathyroidism is common in end-stage renal disease [291] and may contribute to bone loss in the slow phase of bone loss in postmenopausal women and in senile osteoporosis in aged men [226].

Primary hyperparathyroidism is associated with accelerated bone loss, osteopenia, and increased bone turnover and is an independent risk factor for fractures [292]. In animal models continuous infusion of PTH (cPTH) mimics primary and secondary hyperparathyroidism leading to osteoclastic bone resorption and bone loss. Paradoxically, when PTH is administered in an intermittent fashion (iPTH), mimicked in animals by a single daily injection, this pulsatile delivery of PTH leads to a relatively weak induction of bone resorption that is overcompensated for by a robust stimulation of bone formation leading to a net gain of bone mass [293]. In humans this anabolic effect of PTH has been exploited as a therapeutic strategy to improve bone mass in postmenopausal osteoporosis and other osteoporotic conditions [294].

Hyperparathyroidism and cPTH treatment increase bone turnover in trabecular and cortical bone, as evidenced by elevations in histomorphometric and biochemical markers of resorption and formation although mild hyperparathyroidism and cPTH injection in young mice may actually cause a modest increase in cancellous bone [292]. This bone loss is mediated, in part, through enhanced production of M-CSF [295] and RANKL by BMSC and osteoblasts, coupled with a decline in OPG production [296].

Over a decade ago an interesting report emerged describing the absence of a catabolic response to PTH in athymic T-cell deficient mice that underwent xenotransplantation of parathyroid gland fragments obtained from patients with primary or secondary hyperparathyroidism, and parathyroid cells maintained in culture from patients with secondary hyperparathyroidism. Despite extremely high plasma iPTH levels, hypercalcemia or hypophosphatemia was not observed, and no difference in active bone resorption surface or number of osteoclasts was seen by bone histomorphometry. The authors hypothesized that the characteristic deficit of T-cell function and of cytokine and growth factor production may protect nude mice with chronic hypersecretion of human PTH from hypercalcemia and bone lesions [297].

These data appeared to conflict however with an older study in which T-cell deficient nude mice were infused with human parathyroid hormone-related protein (PTHrP), a physiological ligand that binds to the same PTH receptor and has the same net biological activity as PTH. In this study serum calcium was significantly increased in nude mice infused with PTHrP compared with control nude mice, and static bone histomorphometry revealed increased osteoclast area, number of osteoclasts, and osteoclast perimeter in trabecular bone of lumbar vertebrae, as well as increasing bone formation in nude mice [298].

The reason for the discrepancies in response is unclear, however nude mice are a "leaky" phenotype that are known to recover T cells as they age due to extrathymic maturation. Furthermore, these animals have complex metabolism with delayed onset of puberty and rapidly lose fertility potentially resulting from changes in the estrogen responsiveness of tissues [275, 299, 300]. We have further reported that nude mice have increased BMD 4 weeks after birth but rapidly lose BMD relative to WT mice as they age, due to an imbalance in the RANKL/OPG ratio, a consequence of diminished B-cell OPG production [140].

Recently, we revisited the issue of T-cell-dependent PTH activity and confirmed that T cells play an essential permissive role in hyperparathyroidism as cPTH failed to induce osteoclast formation, bone resorption, and cortical bone loss in nude mice lacking T cells. We further demonstrated that T cells provide proliferative and survival cues to stromal cells and sensitize stromal cells to PTH through CD40L on activated T cells. Consequently, deletion of T cells or CD40L blunted the bone catabolic activity of PTH by decreasing bone marrow stromal cell number, RANKL/OPG production, and osteoclastogenic activity. To overcome some of the limitations of genetic T-cell KO models antibody-mediated deletion of T cells was further employed as an alternative model and further supported a need for T cells to mediate PTH-induced bone loss [301].

To investigate the role of direct PTH signaling in T cells during PTH-induced bone loss we used a mouse in which the PTH receptor had been conditionally silenced specifically in T cells using Cre/Lox technology. Using this strain a direct effect of PTH on T cells was shown to be necessary to support PTH-induced bone loss. Mechanistically, and similar to conditions of ovariectomy, PTH activation of the T-cell PTH receptor was shown to stimulate T-cell production of TNFα, suggesting a cause-effect relationship between this cytokine and cPTH-induced bone loss. To prove this the capacity of T cells to produce TNFα was conditionally ablated by reconstitution of T-cell deficient mice with T cells from TNFα KO mice, by adoptive transfer. The chimeric mouse with all sources of TNFα intact, except for that derived from T cells, was significantly protected from bone loss following PTH administration relative to T-cell deficient mice reconstituted with WT T cells [292].

Because CD40L expression is a feature of activated T cells, in a follow-up study we further demonstrated a role for antigen presentation in cPTH-induced bone loss and reported that inhibition of antigen presentation, through silencing of either class I or class II MHC-TCR interactions, prevented cortical bone loss induced by cPTH treatment *in vivo*. Finally, the costimulation inhibitor CTLA4-Ig was found to prevent iPTH-induced bone loss in WT mice demonstrating a need for normal APC activity to support iPTH-induced bone resorption [302].

Taken together the data suggest that T cells are essential participants in the bone loss associated with PTH and function in part by promoting T-cell production of TNFα and in part by sensitizing stromal cells to PTH through CD40/CD40L interactions.

15. The Role of T Cells in the Bone Anabolic Effect of PTH

Interestingly, T cells are not only pertinent to the bone loss associated with hyperparathyroidism, but also appear to be key mediators of the bone anabolic activity associated with iPTH administration.

Although T cells have long been implicated in the bone loss associated with hyperparathyroidism, there is no specific link between the anabolic activity of iPTH and T cells. Anabolic PTH is presently the only FDA approved anabolic therapy for fracture prevention in postmenopausal women [303]. Anabolic PTH improves bone mass and strength by promoting bone formation by increasing the number [304], activity, and longevity of osteoblasts through activation of preexisting quiescent bone lining cells [305], increased osteoblast proliferation [293, 306], and differentiation [293, 304, 306] and activation of survival signaling through attenuation of preosteoblast and osteoblast apoptosis [307–309].

An important mode of PTH action on bone formation involves regulation of the anabolic Wnt pathway in osteoclasts and their precursors culminating in the nuclear translocation of β-catenin. Wnt signaling is antagonized at the level of ligand binding to the Wnt receptors low-density lipoprotein receptor-related protein (LRP)5 and 6 by sclerostin, a protein synthesized in the bone microenvironment, in large measure by osteocytes [310]. Indeed a key mechanism of PTH activity is the downregulation of sclerostin leading to increased osteoblast sensitivity to prevailing Wnt ligands [311].

Interestingly, a key question that remains unclear is the nature and source of the Wnt ligands that support osteoblastogenesis in response to PTH.

T cells have long been recognized as a source of Wnt10b [312, 313], and we consequently investigated T cells as a source of this Wnt ligand under conditions of anabolic PTH treatment in mice. In fact, iPTH was found to significantly increase the production of Wnt10b by bone marrow $CD8^+$ T cells leading to activation of canonical Wnt signaling in preosteoblasts. Demonstrating a key role of T cells in anabolic PTH action T cell null mice displayed diminished Wnt signaling in preosteoblasts and blunted osteoblastic commitment, proliferation, differentiation, and lifespan. These actions culminated in a diminished anabolic response in trabecular bone and a failure to increase bone strength. Furthermore, mice conditionally lacking Wnt10b production specifically in their T cells failed to induce an anabolic response to iPTH [314].

Further studies involving conditional silencing of the PTH receptor specifically in T cells were found to blunt the capacity of iPTH to induce T-cell production of Wnt10b, thus abrogating activation of Wnt signaling in osteoblasts, expansion of the osteoblastic pool, and increased BMD and trabecular bone volume in response to iPTH. These data thus revealed a direct action of PTH on the T cell leading to Wnto10b production [315].

Taken together that data demonstrated a key permissive role for T cells in the mechanism by which iPTH increases bone strength, suggesting that T-cell osteoblast crosstalk pathways may provide pharmacological targets for bone anabolism [314].

16. Conclusions

Over the past 2 decades phenomenal progress has been made in understanding how the immune system impacts and regulates the skeleton in physiological and pathological conditions through the immunoskeletal interface. Although most of the lessons learned have been in animal models and although the outcomes between studies have not always been consistent, tantalizing data from human studies has begun to translate and ratify some aspects of these findings in humans.

The existence of the immunoskeletal interface has wide repercussions for a range or disease conditions including inflection (periodontitis and HIV) and inflammation (rheumatoid arthritis, Crones disease, inflammaging, and estrogen deficiency, a condition that significantly resembles an inflammatory state).

Although bone loss is characteristic of aging, the immune system also undergoes significant changes during aging and immunosenescence is recognized as a major outcome. Contraction of T-cell receptor diversity leads to a diminished capacity of T cells to respond to pathogenic stimuli, and accumulation of autoreactive T cells that predispose to increased incidence of autoimmune disease is common. One of the most consistent characteristics of the aging immune system is the accumulation of $CD28^-$ T cells that fail to respond productively to antigen presentation [316, 317]. An important question that remains to be answered is how these changes in the aging immune system impact the immunoskeletal interface and alter basal bone turnover, bone turnover associated with estrogen deficiency, and anabolic and catabolic bone turnover mediated by PTH.

A better understanding of these concepts may ultimately lead to novel approaches to the treatment of skeletal disease in multiple contexts involving, in part, modulators of immune function to treat downstream bone alterations. Indeed, the field of rheumatoid arthritis has been aggressive in adopting immunomodulatory biologic agents including TNFα inhibitors, T-cell costimulation suppressors, and B-cell depleting antibodies [213, 214, 318] to ameliorate inflammatory disease. Future therapeutic approaches may be able to incorporate some of these agents and pathways in some cases into new antiosteoporotic applications. The role of the NF-κB pathway in bone formation and resorption as well as in inflammation further lends itself to exploitation for amelioration of bone disease.

Despite the progress made we have likely only scratched the "tip of the iceberg" concerning the functioning of the immunoskeletal interface in basal and pathological bone turnover, and many important discoveries likely await future elucidation.

Acknowledgments

M. N. Weitzmann gratefully acknowledges research support by Grants from the Biomedical Laboratory Research and Development Service of the VA Office of Research and Development (5I01BX000105), the National Institute of Arthritis and Musculoskeletal and Skin Diseases (NIAMS) of the National Institutes of Health under Award nos. R01AR059364 and R01AR056090 and by the National Institute on Aging (NIA) under Award nos. R01AG040013. The content is solely the responsibility of the author and does not necessarily represent the official views of the National Institutes of Health.

References

[1] S. Weiner and W. Traub, "Bone structure: from angstroms to microns," *The FASEB Journal*, vol. 6, no. 3, pp. 879–885, 1992.

[2] T. A. Franz-Odendaal, "Induction and patterning of intramembranous bone," *Frontiers in Bioscience*, vol. 16, no. 7, pp. 2734–2746, 2011.

[3] S. C. Manolagas, "Birth and death of bone cells: basic regulatory mechanisms and implications for the pathogenesis and treatment of osteoporosis," *Endocrine Reviews*, vol. 21, no. 2, pp. 115–137, 2000.

[4] S. C. Manolagas and R. L. Jilka, "Mechanisms of disease: bone marrow, cytokines, and bone remodeling—emerging insights

into the pathophysiology of osteoporosis," *The New England Journal of Medicine*, vol. 332, no. 5, pp. 305–311, 1995.

[5] S. Khosla, S. Amin, and E. Orwoll, "Osteoporosis in men," *Endocrine Reviews*, vol. 29, no. 4, pp. 441–464, 2008.

[6] J. A. Eisman, E. R. Bogoch, R. Dell et al., "Making the first fracture the last fracture: ASBMR task force report on secondary fracture prevention," *Journal of Bone and Mineral Research*, vol. 27, no. 10, pp. 2039–2046, 2012.

[7] O. Johnell and J. A. Kanis, "An estimate of the worldwide prevalence and disability associated with osteoporotic fractures," *Osteoporosis International*, vol. 17, no. 12, pp. 1726–1733, 2006.

[8] C. J. Todd, C. J. Freeman, C. Camilleri-Ferrante et al., "Differences in mortality after fracture of hip: the East Anglian audit," *British Medical Journal*, vol. 310, no. 6984, pp. 904–908, 1995.

[9] D. M. Black, L. Palermo, M. C. Nevitt et al., "Comparison of methods for defining prevalent vertebral deformities: the study of osteoporotic fractures," *Journal of Bone and Mineral Research*, vol. 10, no. 6, pp. 890–902, 1995.

[10] "Prevention and management of osteoporosis," *World Health Organization Technical Report Series*, vol. 921, pp. 1–164, 2003.

[11] J. R. Lewis, S. K. Z. Hassan, R. T. Wenn, and C. G. Moran, "Mortality and serum urea and electrolytes on admission for hip fracture patients," *Injury*, vol. 37, no. 8, pp. 698–704, 2006.

[12] A. Brainsky, H. Glick, E. Lydick et al., "The economic cost of hip fractures in community-dwelling older adults: a prospective study," *Journal of the American Geriatrics Society*, vol. 45, no. 3, pp. 281–287, 1997.

[13] R. Burge, B. Dawson-Hughes, D. H. Solomon, J. B. Wong, A. King, and A. Tosteson, "Incidence and economic burden of osteoporosis-related fractures in the United States, 2005–2025," *Journal of Bone and Mineral Research*, vol. 22, no. 3, pp. 465–475, 2007.

[14] M. C. Horowitz and J. A. Lorenzo, "The origins of osteoclasts," *Current Opinion in Rheumatology*, vol. 16, no. 4, pp. 464–468, 2004.

[15] M. N. Weitzmann and R. Pacifici, "The role of T lymphocytes in bone metabolism," *Immunological Reviews*, vol. 208, pp. 154–168, 2005.

[16] H. Takayanagi, "Mechanistic insight into osteoclast differentiation in osteoimmunology," *Journal of Molecular Medicine*, vol. 83, no. 3, pp. 170–179, 2005.

[17] M. N. Weitzmann and R. Pacifici, "Estrogen deficiency and bone loss: an inflammatory tale," *Journal of Clinical Investigation*, vol. 116, no. 5, pp. 1186–1194, 2006.

[18] J. Lorenzo, M. Horowitz, and Y. Choi, "Osteoimmunology: interactions of the bone and immune system," *Endocrine Reviews*, vol. 29, no. 4, pp. 403–440, 2008.

[19] I. Ofotokun and M. N. Weitzmann, "HIV-1 infection and antiretroviral therapies: risk factors for osteoporosis and bone fracture," *Current Opinion in Endocrinology, Diabetes and Obesity*, vol. 17, no. 6, pp. 523–529, 2010.

[20] A. Leibbrandt and J. M. Penninger, "Novel functions of RANK(L) signaling in the immune system," *Advances in Experimental Medicine and Biology*, vol. 658, pp. 77–94, 2010.

[21] I. Ofotokun and M. N. Weitzmann, "HIV and bone metabolism," *Discovery Medicine*, vol. 11, pp. 385–393, 2011.

[22] I. Ofotokun, E. McIntosh, and M. N. Weitzmann, "HIV: inflammation and bone," *Current HIV/AIDS Reports*, vol. 9, pp. 16–25, 2012.

[23] R. Pacifici, "Role of T cells in ovariectomy induced bone loss—revisited," *Journal of Bone and Mineral Research*, vol. 27, pp. 231–239, 2012.

[24] R. Baron, L. Neff, W. Brown, D. Louvard, and P. J. Courtoy, "Selective internalization of the apical plasma membrane and rapid redistribution of lysosomal enzymes and mannose 6-phosphate receptors during osteoclast inactivation by calcitonin," *Journal of Cell Science*, vol. 97, no. 3, pp. 439–447, 1990.

[25] S. L. Teitelbaum, "Bone resorption by osteoclasts," *Science*, vol. 289, no. 5484, pp. 1504–1508, 2000.

[26] R. Pacifici, C. Brown, E. Puscheck et al., "Effect of surgical menopause and estrogen replacement on cytokine release from human blood mononuclear cells," *Proceedings of the National Academy of Sciences of the United States of America*, vol. 88, no. 12, pp. 5134–5138, 1991.

[27] S. C. Manolagas, T. Bellido, and R. L. Jilka, "New insights into the cellular, biochemical, and molecular basis of postmenopausal and senile osteoporosis: roles of IL-6 and gp130," *International Journal of Immunopharmacology*, vol. 17, no. 2, pp. 109–116, 1995.

[28] N. Takahashi, T. Akatsu, N. Udagawa et al., "Osteoblastic cells are involved in osteoclast formation," *Endocrinology*, vol. 123, no. 5, pp. 2600–2602, 1988.

[29] W. S. Simonet, D. L. Lacey, C. R. Dunstan et al., "Osteoprotegerin: a novel secreted protein involved in the regulation of bone density," *Cell*, vol. 89, no. 2, pp. 309–319, 1997.

[30] E. Tsuda, M. Goto, S. I. Mochizuki et al., "Isolation of a novel cytokine from human fibroblasts that specifically inhibits osteoclastogenesis," *Biochemical and Biophysical Research Communications*, vol. 234, no. 1, pp. 137–142, 1997.

[31] D. L. Lacey, E. Timms, H. L. Tan et al., "Osteoprotegerin ligand is a cytokine that regulates osteoclast differentiation and activation," *Cell*, vol. 93, no. 2, pp. 165–176, 1998.

[32] K. Matsuzaki, N. Udagawa, N. Takahashi et al., "Osteoclast differentiation factor (ODF) induces osteoclast-like cell formation in human peripheral blood mononuclear cell cultures," *Biochemical and Biophysical Research Communications*, vol. 246, no. 1, pp. 199–204, 1998.

[33] D. M. Anderson, E. Maraskovsky, W. L. Billingsley et al., "A homologue of the TNF receptor and its ligand enhance T-cell growth and dendritic-cell function," *Nature*, vol. 390, no. 6656, pp. 175–179, 1997.

[34] B. R. Wong, R. Josien, S. Y. Lee et al., "TRANCE (Tumor necrosis factor [TNF]-related Activation-induced Cytokine), a new TNF family member predominantly expressed in t cells, is a dendritic cell-specific survival factor," *The Journal of Experimental Medicine*, vol. 186, no. 12, pp. 2075–2080, 1997.

[35] H. Hsu, D. L. Lacey, C. R. Dunstan et al., "Tumor necrosis factor receptor family member RANK mediates osteoclast differentiation and activation induced by osteoprotegerin ligand," *Proceedings of the National Academy of Sciences of the United States of America*, vol. 96, no. 7, pp. 3540–3545, 1999.

[36] S. Khosla, "Minireview: the OPG/RANKL/RANK system," *Endocrinology*, vol. 142, no. 12, pp. 5050–5055, 2001.

[37] T. Suda, N. Takahashi, N. Udagawa, E. Jimi, M. T. Gillespie, and T. J. Martin, "Modulation of osteoclast differentiation and function by the new members of the tumor necrosis factor receptor and ligand families," *Endocrine Reviews*, vol. 20, no. 3, pp. 345–357, 1999.

[38] H. J. Choi, Y. R. Park, M. Nepal et al., "Inhibition of osteoclastogenic differentiation by Ikarisoside A in RAW 264.7 cells via JNK and NF-κB signaling pathways," *European Journal of Pharmacology*, vol. 636, no. 1–3, pp. 28–35, 2010.

[39] T. Maruyama, H. Fukushima, K. Nakao et al., "Processing of the NF-κB2 precursor p100 to p52 is critical for RANKL-induced osteoclast differentiation," *Journal of Bone and Mineral Research*, vol. 25, no. 5, pp. 1058–1067, 2010.

[40] T. Ogasawara, M. Katagiri, A. Yamamoto et al., "Osteoclast differentiation by RANKL requires NF-κB-mediated downregulation of cyclin-dependent kinase 6 (Cdk6)," *Journal of Bone and Mineral Research*, vol. 19, no. 7, pp. 1128–1136, 2004.

[41] S. Vaira, M. Alhawagri, I. Anwisye, H. Kitaura, R. Faccio, and D. V. Novack, "RelA/p65 promotes osteoclast differentiation by blocking a RANKL-induced apoptotic JNK pathway in mice," *Journal of Clinical Investigation*, vol. 118, no. 6, pp. 2088–2097, 2008.

[42] S. Srivastava, M. N. Weitzmann, S. Cenci, F. P. Ross, S. Adler, and R. Pacifici, "Estrogen decreases TNF gene expression by blocking JNK activity and the resulting production of c-Jun and JunD," *Journal of Clinical Investigation*, vol. 104, no. 4, pp. 503–513, 1999.

[43] S. Srivastava, G. Toraldo, M. N. Weitzmann, S. Cenci, F. P. Ross, and R. Pacifici, "Estrogen decreases osteoclast formation by down-regulating receptor activator of NF-κB ligand (RANKL)-induced JNK activation," *Journal of Biological Chemistry*, vol. 276, no. 12, pp. 8836–8840, 2001.

[44] H. Hirotani, N. A. Tuohy, J. T. Woo, P. H. Stern, and N. A. Clipstone, "The calcineurin/nuclear factor of activated T cells signaling pathway regulates osteoclastogenesis in RAW264.7 cells," *Journal of Biological Chemistry*, vol. 279, no. 14, pp. 13984–13992, 2004.

[45] K. Matsuo, D. L. Galson, C. Zhao et al., "Nuclear factor of activated T-cells (NFAT) rescues osteoclastogenesis in precursors lacking c-Fos," *Journal of Biological Chemistry*, vol. 279, no. 25, pp. 26475–26480, 2004.

[46] H. Takayanagi, "The role of NFAT in osteoclast formation," *Annals of the New York Academy of Sciences*, vol. 1116, pp. 227–237, 2007.

[47] M. H. Helfrich, C. W. Thesingh, R. H. P. Mieremet, and A. S. van Iperen-van Gent, "Osteoclast generation from human fetal bone marrow in cocultures with murine fetal long bones. A model for *in vitro* study of human osteoclast formation and function," *Cell and Tissue Research*, vol. 249, no. 1, pp. 125–136, 1987.

[48] T. Inaoka, G. Bilbe, O. Ishibashi, K. I. Tezuka, M. Kumegawa, and T. Kokubo, "Molecular cloning of human cDNA for cathepsin K: novel cysteine proteinase predominantly expressed in bone," *Biochemical and Biophysical Research Communications*, vol. 206, no. 1, pp. 89–96, 1995.

[49] B. F. Boyce, T. Yoneda, C. Lowe, P. Soriano, and G. R. Mundy, "Requirement of pp60(c-src) expression for osteoclasts to form ruffled borders and resorb bone in mice," *Journal of Clinical Investigation*, vol. 90, no. 4, pp. 1622–1627, 1992.

[50] T. A. Hentunen, S. H. Jackson, H. Chung et al., "Characterization of immortalized osteoclast precursors developed from mice transgenic for both bcl-X(L) and simian virus 40 large T antigen," *Endocrinology*, vol. 140, no. 7, pp. 2954–2961, 1999.

[51] J. Clover, R. A. Dodds, and M. Gowen, "Integrin subunit expression by human osteoblasts and osteoclasts *in situ* and in culture," *Journal of Cell Science*, vol. 103, no. 1, pp. 267–271, 1992.

[52] S. L. Teitelbaum, "The osteoclast and its unique cytoskeleton," *Annals of the New York Academy of Sciences*, vol. 1240, pp. 14–17, 2011.

[53] M. J. Oursler, L. V. Bell, B. Clevinger, and P. Osdoby, "Identification of osteoclast-specific monoclonal antibodies," *Journal of Cell Biology*, vol. 100, no. 5, pp. 1592–1600, 1985.

[54] Y. Y. Kong, H. Yoshida, I. Sarosi et al., "OPGL is a key regulator of osteoclastogenesis, lymphocyte development and lymph-node organogenesis," *Nature*, vol. 397, no. 6717, pp. 315–323, 1999.

[55] N. Bucay, I. Sarosi, C. R. Dunstan et al., "Osteoprotegerin-deficient mice develop early onset osteoporosis and arterial calcification," *Genes and Development*, vol. 12, no. 9, pp. 1260–1268, 1998.

[56] H. Min, S. Morony, I. Sarosi et al., "Osteoprotegerin reverses osteoporosis by inhibiting endosteal osteoclasts and prevents vascular calcification by blocking a process resembling osteoclastogenesis," *The Journal of Experimental Medicine*, vol. 192, no. 4, pp. 463–474, 2000.

[57] A. E. Hughes, S. H. Ralston, J. Marken et al., "Mutations in TNFRSF11A, affecting the signal peptide of RANK, cause familial expansile osteolysis," *Nature Genetics*, vol. 24, no. 1, pp. 45–48, 2000.

[58] M. P. Whyte, S. E. Obrecht, P. M. Finnegan et al., "Osteoprotegerin deficiency and juvenile Paget's disease," *The New England Journal of Medicine*, vol. 347, no. 3, pp. 175–184, 2002.

[59] M. P. Whyte, P. N. Singhellakis, M. B. Petersen, M. Davies, W. G. Totty, and S. Mumm, "Juvenile Paget's disease: the second reported, oldest patient is homozygous for the TNFRSF11B "Balkan" mutation (966_969delTGACinsCTT), which elevates circulating immunoreactive osteoprotegerin levels," *Journal of Bone and Mineral Research*, vol. 22, no. 6, pp. 938–946, 2007.

[60] M. P. Whyte and S. Mumm, "Heritable disorders of the RANKL/OPG/RANK signaling pathway," *Journal of Musculoskeletal Neuronal Interactions*, vol. 4, no. 3, pp. 254–267, 2004.

[61] M. P. Whyte, W. G. Totty, D. V. Novack, X. Zhang, D. Wenkert, and S. Mumm, "Camurati-engelmann disease: unique variant featuring a novel mutation in TGFβ1 encoding transforming growth factor beta 1 and a missense change in TNFSF11 encoding RANK ligand," *Journal of Bone and Mineral Research*, vol. 26, no. 5, pp. 920–933, 2011.

[62] B. Bolon, C. Carter, M. Daris et al., "Adenoviral delivery of osteoprotegerin ameliorates bone resorption in a mouse ovariectomy model of osteoporosis," *Molecular Therapy*, vol. 3, no. 2, pp. 197–205, 2001.

[63] C. Capparelli, S. Morony, K. Warmington et al., "Sustained antiresorptive effects after a single treatment with human recombinant osteoprotegerin (OPG): a pharmacodynamic and pharmacokinetic analysis in rats," *Journal of Bone and Mineral Research*, vol. 18, no. 5, pp. 852–858, 2003.

[64] M. S. Ominsky, P. J. Kostenuik, P. Cranmer, S. Y. Smith, and J. E. Atkinson, "The RANKL inhibitor OPG-Fc increases cortical and trabecular bone mass in young gonad-intact cynomolgus monkeys," *Osteoporosis International*, vol. 18, no. 8, pp. 1073–1082, 2007.

[65] P. J. Bekker, D. Holloway, A. Nakanishi, M. Arrighi, P. T. Leese, and C. R. Dunstan, "The effect of a single dose of osteoprotegerin in postmenopausal women," *Journal of Bone and Mineral Research*, vol. 16, no. 2, pp. 348–360, 2001.

[66] M. R. McClung, E. M. Lewiecki, S. B. Cohen et al., "Denosumab in postmenopausal women with low bone mineral density," *The New England Journal of Medicine*, vol. 354, no. 8, pp. 821–831, 2006.

[67] S. R. Cummings, J. S. Martin, M. R. McClung et al., "Denosumab for prevention of fractures in postmenopausal women with osteoporosis," *The New England Journal of Medicine*, vol. 361, no. 8, pp. 756–765, 2009.

[68] L. C. Hofbauer, D. L. Lacey, C. R. Dunstan, T. C. Spelsberg, B. L. Riggs, and S. Khosla, "Interleukin-1β and tumor necrosis factor-κ, but not interleukin-6, stimulate osteoprotegerin ligand gene expression in human osteoblastic cells," *Bone*, vol. 25, no. 3, pp. 255–259, 1999.

[69] S. Wei, H. Kitaura, P. Zhou, F. Patrick Ross, and S. L. Teitelbaum, "IL-1 mediates TNF-induced osteoclastogenesis," *Journal of Clinical Investigation*, vol. 115, no. 2, pp. 282–290, 2005.

[70] M. N. Weitzmann, C. Roggia, G. Toraldo, L. Weitzmann, and R. Pacifici, "Increased production of IL-7 uncouples bone formation from bone resorption during estrogen deficiency," *Journal of Clinical Investigation*, vol. 110, no. 11, pp. 1643–1650, 2002.

[71] F. Arai, T. Miyamoto, O. Ohneda et al., "Commitment and differentiation of osteoclast precursor cells by the sequential expression of c-Fms and receptor activator of nuclear factor κB (RANK) receptors," *The Journal of Experimental Medicine*, vol. 190, no. 12, pp. 1741–1754, 1999.

[72] R. Pacifici, J. L. Vannice, L. Rifas, and R. B. Kimble, "Monocytic secretion of interleukin-1 receptor antagonist in normal and osteoporotic women: effects of menopause and estrogen/progesterone therapy," *Journal of Clinical Endocrinology and Metabolism*, vol. 77, no. 5, pp. 1135–1141, 1993.

[73] R. B. Kimble, J. L. Vannice, D. C. Bloedow et al., "Interleukin-1 receptor antagonist decreases bone loss and bone resorption in ovariectomized rats," *Journal of Clinical Investigation*, vol. 93, no. 5, pp. 1959–1967, 1994.

[74] R. Kitazawa, R. B. Kimble, J. L. Vannice, V. T. Kung, and R. Pacifici, "Interleukin-1 receptor antagonist and tumor necrosis factor binding protein decrease osteoclast formation and bone resorption in ovariectomized mice," *Journal of Clinical Investigation*, vol. 94, no. 6, pp. 2397–2406, 1994.

[75] R. B. Kimble, A. B. Matayoshi, J. L. Vannice, V. T. Kung, C. Williams, and R. Pacifici, "Simultaneous block of interleukin-1 and tumor necrosis factor is required to completely prevent bone loss in the early postovariectomy period," *Endocrinology*, vol. 136, no. 7, pp. 3054–3061, 1995.

[76] R. B. Kimble, S. Srivastava, F. Patrick Ross, A. Matayoshi, and R. Pacifici, "Estrogen deficiency increases the ability of stromal cells to support murine osteoclastogenesis via an interleukin-1- and tumor necrosis factor-mediated stimulation of macrophage colony-stimulating factor production," *Journal of Biological Chemistry*, vol. 271, no. 46, pp. 28890–28897, 1996.

[77] S. Cenci, M. N. Weitzmann, C. Roggia et al., "Estrogen deficiency induces bone loss by enhancing T-cell production of TNF-α," *Journal of Clinical Investigation*, vol. 106, no. 10, pp. 1229–1237, 2000.

[78] J. Lam, S. Takeshita, J. E. Barker, O. Kanagawa, F. P. Ross, and S. L. Teitelbaum, "TNF-α induces osteoclastogenesis by direct stimulation of macrophages exposed to permissive levels of RANK ligand," *Journal of Clinical Investigation*, vol. 106, no. 12, pp. 1481–1488, 2000.

[79] K. Fuller, C. Murphy, B. Kirstein, S. W. Fox, and T. J. Chambers, "TNFα potently activates osteoclasts, through a direct action independent of and strongly synergistic with RANKL," *Endocrinology*, vol. 143, no. 3, pp. 1108–1118, 2002.

[80] Y. H. Zhang, A. Heulsmann, M. M. Tondravi, A. Mukherjee, and Y. Abu-Amer, "Tumor necrosis factor-α (TNF) stimulates RANKL-induced osteoclastogenesis via coupling of TNF type 1 receptor and RANK signaling pathways," *Journal of Biological Chemistry*, vol. 276, no. 1, pp. 563–568, 2001.

[81] K. Kobayashi, N. Takahashi, E. Jimi et al., "Tumor necrosis factor α stimulates osteoclast differentiation by a mechanism independent of the ODF/RANKL-RANK interaction," *The Journal of Experimental Medicine*, vol. 191, no. 2, pp. 275–285, 2000.

[82] K. Redlich, B. Görtz, S. Hayer et al., "Repair of local bone erosions and reversal of systemic bone loss upon therapy with anti-tumor necrosis factor in combination with osteoprotegerin or parathyroid hormone in tumor necrosis factor-mediated arthritis," *American Journal of Pathology*, vol. 164, no. 2, pp. 543–555, 2004.

[83] N. Saidenberg-Kermanac'H, A. Corrado, D. Lemeiter, M. C. deVernejoul, M. C. Boissier, and M. E. Cohen-Solal, "TNF-α antibodies and osteoprotegerin decrease systemic bone loss associated with inflammation through distinct mechanisms in collagen-induced arthritis," *Bone*, vol. 35, no. 5, pp. 1200–1207, 2004.

[84] A. M. Reimold, "New indications for treatment of chronic inflammation by TNF-α blockade," *American Journal of the Medical Sciences*, vol. 325, no. 2, pp. 75–92, 2003.

[85] B. F. Boyce, L. Xing, G. Franzoso, and U. Siebenlist, "Required and nonessential functions of nuclear factor-kappa B in bone cells," *Bone*, vol. 25, no. 1, pp. 137–139, 1999.

[86] T. J. Hall, M. Schaeublin, H. Jeker, K. Fuller, and T. J. Chambers, "The role of reactive oxygen intermediates in osteoclastic bone resorption," *Biochemical and Biophysical Research Communications*, vol. 207, no. 1, pp. 280–287, 1995.

[87] S. Vaira, T. Johnson, A. C. Hirbe et al., "RelB is the NF-κB subunit downstream of NIK responsible for osteoclast differentiation," *Proceedings of the National Academy of Sciences of the United States of America*, vol. 105, no. 10, pp. 3897–3902, 2008.

[88] J. Liu, S. Wang, P. Zhang, N. Said-Al-Naief, S. M. Michalek, and X. Feng, "Molecular mechanism of the bifunctional role of lipopolysaccharide in osteoclastogenesis," *Journal of Biological Chemistry*, vol. 284, no. 18, pp. 12512–12523, 2009.

[89] V. Iotsova, J. Caamaño, J. Loy, Y. Yang, A. Lewin, and R. Bravo, "Osteopetrosis in mice lacking NF-κB1 and NF-κB2," *Nature Medicine*, vol. 3, no. 11, pp. 1285–1289, 1997.

[90] K. Strait, Y. Li, D. L. Dillehay, and M. N. Weitzmann, "Suppression of NF-κB activation blocks osteoclastic bone resorption during estrogen deficiency," *International Journal of Molecular Medicine*, vol. 21, no. 4, pp. 521–525, 2008.

[91] R. Feng, G. Anderson, G. Xiao et al., "SDX-308, a nonsteroidal anti-inflammatory agent, inhibits NF-κB activity, resulting in strong inhibition of osteoclast formation/activity and multiple myeloma cell growth," *Blood*, vol. 109, no. 5, pp. 2130–2138, 2007.

[92] J. C. Clohisy, T. Hirayama, E. Frazier, S. K. Han, and Y. Abu-Amer, "NF-κB signaling blockade abolishes implant particle-induced osteoclastogenesis," *Journal of Orthopaedic Research*, vol. 22, no. 1, pp. 13–20, 2004.

[93] S. Dai, T. Hirayama, S. Abbas, and Y. Abu-Amer, "The IκB kinase (IKK) inhibitor, NEMO-binding domain peptide, blocks osteoclastogenesis and bone erosion in inflammatory arthritis," *Journal of Biological Chemistry*, vol. 279, no. 36, pp. 37219–37222, 2004.

[94] X. Lu, P. Farmer, J. Rubin, and M. S. Nanes, "Integration of the NfκB p65 subunit into the vitamin D receptor transcriptional complex: identification of p65 domains that inhibit 1,25-dihydroxyvitamin D3-stimulated transcription," *Journal of Cellular Biochemistry*, vol. 92, no. 4, pp. 833–848, 2004.

[95] L. Gilbert, X. He, P. Farmer et al., "Inhibition of osteoblast differentiation by tumor necrosis factor-α," *Endocrinology*, vol. 141, no. 11, pp. 3956–3964, 2000.

[96] M. S. Nanes, "Tumor necrosis factor-κ: molecular and cellular mechanisms in skeletal pathology," *Gene*, vol. 321, no. 1-2, pp. 1–15, 2003.

[97] E. C. Wahl, J. Aronson, L. Liu et al., "Restoration of regenerative osteoblastogenesis in aged mice: modulation of TNF," *Journal of Bone and Mineral Research*, vol. 25, no. 1, pp. 114–123, 2010.

[98] Y. Li, A. Li, K. Strait, H. Zhang, M. S. Nanes, and M. N. Weitzmann, "Endogenous TNFα lowers maximum peak bone mass and inhibits osteoblastic smad activation through NF-κB," *Journal of Bone and Mineral Research*, vol. 22, no. 5, pp. 646–655, 2007.

[99] M. Wan and X. Cao, "BMP signaling in skeletal development," *Biochemical and Biophysical Research Communications*, vol. 328, no. 3, pp. 651–657, 2005.

[100] E. J. Moerman, K. Teng, D. A. Lipschitz, and B. Lecka-Czernik, "Aging activates adipogenic and suppresses osteogenic programs in mesenchymal marrow stroma/stem cells: the role of PPAR-γ2 transcription factor and TGF-β/BMP signaling pathways," *Aging Cell*, vol. 3, no. 6, pp. 379–389, 2004.

[101] F. Zhang, T. Qiu, X. Wu et al., "Sustained BMP signaling in osteoblasts stimulates bone formation by promoting angiogenesis and osteoblast differentiation," *Journal of Bone and Mineral Research*, vol. 24, no. 7, pp. 1224–1233, 2009.

[102] S. D. Boden, "The ABCs of BMPs," *Orthop Nurs*, vol. 24, pp. 49–52, 2005.

[103] K. Janssens, P. Ten Dijke, S. Janssens, and W. Van Hul, "Transforming growth factor-β1 to the bone," *Endocrine Reviews*, vol. 26, no. 6, pp. 743–774, 2005.

[104] Y. Tang, X. Wu, W. Lei et al., "TGF-β1-induced migration of bone mesenchymal stem cells couples bone resorption with formation," *Nature Medicine*, vol. 15, no. 7, pp. 757–765, 2009.

[105] N. Selvamurugan, S. Kwok, T. Alliston, M. Reiss, and N. C. Partridge, "Transforming growth factor-β1 regulation of collagenase-3 expression in osteoblastic cells by cross-talk between the Smad and MAPK signaling pathways and their components, Smad2 and Runx2," *Journal of Biological Chemistry*, vol. 279, no. 18, pp. 19327–19334, 2004.

[106] S. Spinella-Jaegle, S. Roman-Roman, C. Faucheu et al., "Opposite effects of bone morphogenetic protein-2 and transforming growth factor-β1 on osteoblast differentiation," *Bone*, vol. 29, no. 4, pp. 323–330, 2001.

[107] J. Gebken, A. Feydt, J. Brinckmann, H. Notbohm, P. K. Müller, and B. Bätge, "Ligand-induced downregulation of receptors for TGF-β in human osteoblast-like cells from adult donors," *Journal of Endocrinology*, vol. 161, no. 3, pp. 503–510, 1999.

[108] Y. Takeuchi, M. Suzawa, T. Kikuchi, E. Nishida, T. Fujita, and T. Matsumoto, "Differentiation and transforming growth factor-β receptor down-regulation by collagen-$\alpha 2\beta 1$ integrin interaction is mediated by focal adhesion kinase and its downstream signals in murine osteoblastic cells," *Journal of Biological Chemistry*, vol. 272, no. 46, pp. 29309–29316, 1997.

[109] R. A. Eliseev, E. M. Schwarz, M. J. Zuscik, R. J. O'Keefe, H. Drissi, and R. N. Rosier, "Smad7 mediates inhibition of Saos2 osteosarcoma cell differentiation by NFκB," *Experimental Cell Research*, vol. 312, no. 1, pp. 40–50, 2006.

[110] R. Guo, M. Yamashita, Q. Zhang et al., "Ubiquitin ligase Smurf1 mediates tumor necrosis factor-induced systemic bone loss by promoting proteasomal degradation of bone morphogenetic signaling proteins," *Journal of Biological Chemistry*, vol. 283, no. 34, pp. 23084–23092, 2008.

[111] T. Mukai, F. Otsuka, H. Otani et al., "TNF-α inhibits BMP-induced osteoblast differentiation through activating SAPK/JNK signaling," *Biochemical and Biophysical Research Communications*, vol. 356, no. 4, pp. 1004–1010, 2007.

[112] M. Yamaguchi and M. N. Weitzmann, "The estrogen 17β-estradiol and phytoestrogen genistein mediate differential effects on osteoblastic NF-κB activity," *International Journal of Molecular Medicine*, vol. 23, no. 2, pp. 297–301, 2009.

[113] J. Chang, Z. Wang, E. Tang et al., "Inhibition of osteoblastic bone formation by nuclear factor-κB," *Nature Medicine*, vol. 15, no. 6, pp. 682–689, 2009.

[114] M. Yamaguchi and M. N. Weitzmann, "Vitamin K2 stimulates osteoblastogenesis and suppresses osteoclastogenesis by suppressing NF-κB activation," *International Journal of Molecular Medicine*, vol. 27, no. 1, pp. 3–14, 2011.

[115] M. Yamaguchi, J. L. Arbiser, and M. N. Weitzmann, "Honokiol stimulates osteoblastogenesis by suppressing NF-κB activation," *International Journal of Molecular Medicine*, vol. 28, pp. 1049–1053, 2011.

[116] M. Yamaguchi and M. N. Weitzmann, "Zinc stimulates osteoblastogenesis and suppresses osteoclastogenesis by antagonizing NF-κB activation," *Molecular and Cellular Biochemistry*, vol. 355, pp. 179–186, 2011.

[117] M. Yamaguchi and M. N. Weitzmann, "The bone anabolic carotenoids p-hydroxycinnamic acid and β-cryptoxanthin antagonize NF-κB activation in MC3T3 preosteoblasts," *Molecular Medicine Reports*, vol. 2, no. 4, pp. 641–644, 2009.

[118] M. Yamaguchi and M. N. Weitzmann, "The bone anabolic carotenoid p-hydroxycinnamic acid promotes osteoblast mineralization and suppresses osteoclast differentiation by antagonizing NF-κB activation," *International Journal of Molecular Medicine*, vol. 30, no. 3, pp. 708–712, 2012.

[119] J. Xiong, M. Onal, R. L. Jilka, R. S. Weinstein, S. C. Manolagas, and C. A. O'Brien, "Matrix-embedded cells control osteoclast formation," *Nature Medicine*, vol. 17, pp. 1235–1241, 2011.

[120] D. A. Corral, M. Amling, M. Priemel et al., "Dissociation between bone resorption and bone formation in osteopenic transgenic mice," *Proceedings of the National Academy of Sciences of the United States of America*, vol. 95, no. 23, pp. 13835–13840, 1998.

[121] M. C. Horowitz, A. L. M. Bothwell, D. G. T. Hesslein, D. L. Pflugh, and D. G. Schatz, "B cells and osteoblast and osteoclast development," *Immunological Reviews*, vol. 208, pp. 141–153, 2005.

[122] M. Onal, J. Xiong, X. Chen et al., "Receptor activator of nuclear factor kappaB ligand (RANKL) protein expression by B lymphocytes contributes to ovariectomy-induced bone loss," *The Journal of Biological Chemistry*, vol. 287, pp. 29851–29860, 2012.

[123] T. Nakashima, M. Hayashi, T. Fukunaga et al., "Evidence for osteocyte regulation of bone homeostasis through RANKL expression," *Nature Medicine*, vol. 17, pp. 1231–1234, 2011.

[124] M. N. Weitzmann, S. Cenci, L. Rifas, J. Haug, J. Dipersio, and R. Pacifici, "T cell activation induces human osteoclast formation via receptor activator of nuclear factor κB ligand-dependent and -independent mechanisms," *Journal of Bone and Mineral Research*, vol. 16, no. 2, pp. 328–337, 2001.

[125] M. N. Weitzmann, S. Cenci, L. Rifas, C. Brown, and R. Pacifici, "Interleukin-7 stimulates osteoclast formation by up-regulating

the T-cell production of soluble osteoclastogenic cytokines," *Blood*, vol. 96, no. 5, pp. 1873–1878, 2000.

[126] L. Rifas and M. N. Weitzmann, "A novel T cell cytokine, secreted osteoclastogenic factor of activated T cells, induces osteoclast formation in a RANKL-independent manner," *Arthritis and Rheumatism*, vol. 60, no. 11, pp. 3324–3335, 2009.

[127] L. Rifas, R. Civitelli, and L. V. Avioli, "Activated T cells stimulate IL-6 production by human osteoblasts via soluble factors and cell contact," *Journal of Bone and Mineral Research*, vol. 12, p. S436, 1998.

[128] J. R. Edwards, S. G. Sun, R. Locklin et al., "LIGHT (TNFSF14), a novel mediator of bone resorption, is elevated in rheumatoid arthritis," *Arthritis and Rheumatism*, vol. 54, no. 5, pp. 1451–1462, 2006.

[129] D. M. Shinar and G. A. Rodan, "Biphasic effects of transforming growth factor-β on the production of osteoclast-like cells in mouse bone marrow cultures: the role of prostaglandins in the generation of these cells," *Endocrinology*, vol. 126, no. 6, pp. 3153–3158, 1990.

[130] R. J. Sells Galvin, C. L. Gatlin, J. W. Horn, and T. R. Fuson, "TGF-β enhances osteoclast differentiation in hematopoietic cell cultures stimulated with RANKL and M-CSF," *Biochemical and Biophysical Research Communications*, vol. 265, no. 1, pp. 233–239, 1999.

[131] N. J. Horwood, V. Kartsogiannis, J. M. W. Quinn, E. Romas, T. J. Martin, and M. T. Gillespie, "Activated T lymphocytes support osteoclast formation *in vitro*," *Biochemical and Biophysical Research Communications*, vol. 265, no. 1, pp. 144–150, 1999.

[132] C. Chenu, J. Pfeilschifter, G. R. Mundy, and G. D. Roodman, "Transforming growth factor β inhibits formation of osteoclast-like cells in long-term human marrow cultures," *Proceedings of the National Academy of Sciences of the United States of America*, vol. 85, no. 15, pp. 5683–5687, 1988.

[133] D. E. Hughes, A. Dai, J. C. Tiffee, H. H. Li, G. R. Munoy, and B. F. Boyce, "Estrogen promotes apoptosis of murine osteoclasts mediated by TGF-β," *Nature Medicine*, vol. 2, no. 10, pp. 1132–1135, 1996.

[134] M. N. Weitzmann, S. Cenci, J. Haug, C. Brown, J. DiPersio, and R. Pacifici, "B lymphocytes inhibit human osteoclastogenesis by secretion of TGFbeta," *Journal of Cellular Biochemistry*, vol. 78, pp. 318–324, 2000.

[135] H. Takai, M. Kanematsu, K. Yano et al., "Transforming growth factor-β stimulates the production of osteoprotegerin/osteoclastogenesis inhibitory factor by bone marrow stromal cells," *Journal of Biological Chemistry*, vol. 273, no. 42, pp. 27091–27096, 1998.

[136] J. M. W. Quinn, K. Itoh, N. Udagawa et al., "Transforming growth factor β affects osteoclast differentiation via direct and indirect actions," *Journal of Bone and Mineral Research*, vol. 16, no. 10, pp. 1787–1794, 2001.

[137] Y. Gao, W. P. Qian, K. Dark et al., "Estrogen prevents bone loss through transforming growth factor β signaling in T cells," *Proceedings of the National Academy of Sciences of the United States of America*, vol. 101, no. 47, pp. 16618–16623, 2004.

[138] I. Itonaga, A. Sabokbar, S. G. Sun et al., "Transforming growth factor-β induces osteoclast formation in the absence of RANKL," *Bone*, vol. 34, no. 1, pp. 57–64, 2004.

[139] T. J. Yun, P. M. Chaudhary, G. L. Shu et al., "OPG/FDCR-1, a TNF receptor family member, is expressed in lymphoid cells and is up-regulated by ligating CD40," *Journal of Immunology*, vol. 161, no. 11, pp. 6113–6121, 1998.

[140] Y. Li, G. Toraldo, A. Li et al., "B cells and T cells are critical for the preservation of bone homeostasis and attainment of peak bone mass *in vivo*," *Blood*, vol. 109, no. 9, pp. 3839–3848, 2007.

[141] D. Grcevic, S. K. Lee, A. Marusic, and J. A. Lorenzo, "Depletion of CD4 and CD8 T lymphocytes in mice *in vivo* enhances 1,25-dihydroxyvitamin D_3-stimulated osteoclast-like cell formation *in vitro* by a mechanism that is dependent on prostaglandin synthesis," *Journal of Immunology*, vol. 165, no. 8, pp. 4231–4238, 2000.

[142] E. Lopez-Granados, S. T. Temmerman, L. Wu et al., "Osteopenia in X-linked hyper-IgM syndrome reveals a regulatory role for CD40 ligand in osteoclastogenesis," *Proceedings of the National Academy of Sciences of the United States of America*, vol. 104, no. 12, pp. 5056–5061, 2007.

[143] P. Tebas, W. G. Powderly, S. Claxton et al., "Accelerated bone mineral loss in HIV-infected patients receiving potent antiretroviral therapy," *AIDS*, vol. 14, no. 4, pp. F63–F67, 2000.

[144] K. Mondy and P. Tebas, "Emerging bone problems in patients infected with human immunodeficiency virus," *Clinical Infectious Diseases*, vol. 36, no. 2, pp. S101–S105, 2003.

[145] K. Mondy, K. Yarasheski, W. G. Powderly et al., "Longitudinal evolution of bone mineral density and bone markers in human immunodeficiency virus-infected individuals," *Clinical Infectious Diseases*, vol. 36, no. 4, pp. 482–490, 2003.

[146] J. S. Huang, S. J. Wilkie, M. P. Sullivan, and S. Grinspoon, "Reduced bone density in androgen-deficient women with acquired immune deficiency syndrome wasting," *Journal of Clinical Endocrinology and Metabolism*, vol. 86, no. 8, pp. 3533–3539, 2001.

[147] M. J. Bolland and A. Grey, "HIV and low bone density: responsible party, or guilty by association?" *IBMS BoneKEy*, vol. 8, pp. 7–15, 2011.

[148] S. E. Dolan, J. S. Huang, K. M. Killilea, M. P. Sullivan, N. Aliabadi, and S. Grinspoon, "Reduced bone density in HIV-infected women," *AIDS*, vol. 18, no. 3, pp. 475–483, 2004.

[149] J. Thomas and S. M. Doherty, "HIV infection—a risk factor for osteoporosis," *Journal of Acquired Immune Deficiency Syndromes*, vol. 33, no. 3, pp. 281–291, 2003.

[150] G. A. McComsey, P. Tebas, E. Shane et al., "Bone disease in HIV infection: a practical review and recommendations for HIV care providers," *Clinical Infectious Diseases*, vol. 51, no. 8, pp. 937–946, 2010.

[151] T. T. Brown and R. B. Qaqish, "Antiretroviral therapy and the prevalence of osteopenia and osteoporosis: a meta-analytic review," *AIDS*, vol. 20, no. 17, pp. 2165–2174, 2006.

[152] S. L. Hui, C. W. Slemenda, and C. C. Johnston, "Age and bone mass as predictors of fracture in a prospective study," *Journal of Clinical Investigation*, vol. 81, no. 6, pp. 1804–1809, 1988.

[153] World Health Organization, "Assessment of fracture risk and its application to screening for postmenopausal osteoporosis. Report of a WHO Study Group," *World Health Organization Technical Report Series*, vol. 843, pp. 1–129, 1994.

[154] S. H. Abbasi-Jahromi, A. Matayoshi, R. Kimble, A. Dimarogonas, and R. Pacifici, "Bone quality factor analysis: a new noninvasive technique for the measurement of bone density and bone strength," *Journal of Bone and Mineral Research*, vol. 11, no. 5, pp. 594–599, 1996.

[155] V. Amorosa and P. Tebas, "Bone disease and HIV infection," *Clinical Infectious Diseases*, vol. 42, no. 1, pp. 108–114, 2006.

[156] G. Guaraldi, P. Ventura, M. Albuzza et al., "Pathological fractures in AIDS patients with osteopenia and osteoporosis

induced by antiretroviral therapy," *AIDS*, vol. 15, no. 1, pp. 137–138, 2001.

[157] V. A. Triant, T. T. Brown, H. Lee, and S. K. Grinspoon, "Fracture prevalence among human immunodeficiency virus (HIV)-infected versus non-HIV-infected patients in a large U.S. healthcare system," *Journal of Clinical Endocrinology and Metabolism*, vol. 93, no. 9, pp. 3499–3504, 2008.

[158] J. H. Arnsten, R. Freeman, A. A. Howard, M. Floris-Moore, Y. Lo, and R. S. Klein, "Decreased bone mineral density and increased fracture risk in aging men with or at risk for HIV infection," *AIDS*, vol. 21, no. 5, pp. 617–623, 2007.

[159] J. Prior, D. Burdge, E. Maan et al., "Fragility fractures and bone mineral density in HIV positive women: a case-control population-based study," *Osteoporosis International*, vol. 18, no. 10, pp. 1345–1353, 2007.

[160] J. A. Womack, J. L. Goulet, C. Gibert et al., "Increased risk of fragility fractures among HIV infected compared to uninfected male veterans," *PLoS ONE*, vol. 6, no. 2, Article ID e17217, 2011.

[161] B. Young, C. N. Dao, K. Buchacz, R. Baker, and J. T. Brooks, "Increased rates of bone fracture among HIV-infected persons in the HIV outpatient study (HOPS) compared with the US general population, 2000-2006," *Clinical Infectious Diseases*, vol. 52, no. 8, pp. 1061–1068, 2011.

[162] M. T. Yin, Q. Shi, D. R. Hoover et al., "Fracture incidence in HIV-infected women: results from the Women's Interagency HIV Study," *AIDS*, vol. 24, no. 17, pp. 2679–2686, 2010.

[163] S. Desai and A. Landay, "Early immune senescence in HIV disease," *Current HIV/AIDS Reports*, vol. 7, no. 1, pp. 4–10, 2010.

[164] A. De Milito, "B lymphocyte dysfunctions in HIV infection," *Current HIV Research*, vol. 2, no. 1, pp. 11–21, 2004.

[165] S. Moir, J. Ho, A. Malaspina et al., "Evidence for HIV-associated B cell exhaustion in a dysfunctional memory B cell compartment in HIV-infected viremic individuals," *The Journal of Experimental Medicine*, vol. 205, no. 8, pp. 1797–1805, 2008.

[166] M. Morrow, A. Valentin, R. Little, R. Yarchoan, and G. N. Pavlakis, "A splenic marginal zone-like peripheral blood $CD27^{+}B220^{-}$ B cell population is preferentially depleted in HIV type 1-infected individuals," *AIDS Research and Human Retroviruses*, vol. 24, no. 4, pp. 621–633, 2008.

[167] W. Reid, M. Sadowska, F. Denaro et al., "An HIV-1 transgenic rat that develops HIV-related pathology and immunologic dysfunction," *Proceedings of the National Academy of Sciences of the United States of America*, vol. 98, no. 16, pp. 9271–9276, 2001.

[168] N. Manabe, H. Kawaguchi, H. Chikuda et al., "Connection between B lymphocyte and osteoclast differentiation pathways," *Journal of Immunology*, vol. 167, no. 5, pp. 2625–2631, 2001.

[169] T. Kawai, T. Matsuyama, Y. Hosokawa et al., "B and T lymphocytes are the primary sources of RANKL in the bone resorptive lesion of periodontal disease," *American Journal of Pathology*, vol. 169, no. 3, pp. 987–998, 2006.

[170] M. Kanematsu, T. Sato, H. Takai, K. Watanabe, K. Ikeda, and Y. Yamada, "Prostaglandin E2 induces expression of receptor activator of nuclear factor-κB ligand/osteoprotegrin ligand on pre-B cells: implications for accelerated osteoclastogenesis in estrogen deficiency," *Journal of Bone and Mineral Research*, vol. 15, no. 7, pp. 1321–1329, 2000.

[171] T. Vikulina, X. Fan, M. Yamaguchi et al., "Alterations in the immuno-skeletal interface drive bone destruction in HIV-1 transgenic rats," *Proceedings of the National Academy of Sciences of the United States of America*, vol. 107, no. 31, pp. 13848–13853, 2010.

[172] S. G. Deeks, "HIV infection, inflammation, immunosenescence, and aging," *Annual Review of Medicine*, vol. 62, pp. 141–155, 2011.

[173] S. G. Deeks, "Immune dysfunction, inflammation, and accelerated aging in patients on antiretroviral therapy," *Topics in HIV Medicine*, vol. 17, no. 4, pp. 118–123, 2009.

[174] J. M. Brenchley, D. A. Price, T. W. Schacker et al., "Microbial translocation is a cause of systemic immune activation in chronic HIV infection," *Nature Medicine*, vol. 12, no. 12, pp. 1365–1371, 2006.

[175] W. Zou and Z. Bar-Shavit, "Dual modulation of osteoclast differentiation by lipopolysaccharide," *Journal of Bone and Mineral Research*, vol. 17, no. 7, pp. 1211–1218, 2002.

[176] C. Duvivier, S. Kolta, L. Assoumou et al., "Greater decrease in bone mineral density with protease inhibitor regimens compared with nonnucleoside reverse transcriptase inhibitor regimens in HIV-1 infected naive patients," *AIDS*, vol. 23, no. 7, pp. 817–824, 2009.

[177] A. B. Hansen, N. Obel, H. Nielsen, C. Pedersen, and J. Gerstoft, "Bone mineral density changes in protease inhibitor-sparing vs. nucleoside reverse transcriptase inhibitor-sparing highly active antiretroviral therapy: data from a randomized trial," *HIV Medicine*, vol. 12, no. 3, pp. 157–165, 2011.

[178] K. Briot, S. Kolta, P. Flandre et al., "Prospective one-year bone loss in treatment-naïve HIV+ men and women on single or multiple drug HIV therapies," *Bone*, vol. 48, pp. 1133–1139, 2011.

[179] M. G. A. van Vonderen, P. Lips, M. A. van Agtmael et al., "First line zidovudine/lamivudine/lopinavir/ritonavir leads to greater bone loss compared to nevirapine/lopinavir/ritonavir," *AIDS*, vol. 23, no. 11, pp. 1367–1376, 2009.

[180] P. Rivas, M. Górgolas, R. García-Delgado, M. Díaz-Curiel, A. Goyenechea, and M. L. Fernández-Guerrero, "Evolution of bone mineral density in AIDS patients on treatment with zidovudine/lamivudine plus abacavir or lopinavir/ritonavir," *HIV Medicine*, vol. 9, no. 2, pp. 89–95, 2008.

[181] J. Fernández-Rivera, R. García, F. Lozano et al., "Relationship between low bone mineral density and highly active antiretroviral therapy including protease inhibitors in HIV-infected patients," *HIV Clinical Trials*, vol. 4, no. 5, pp. 337–346, 2003.

[182] M. W. H. Wang, S. Wei, R. Faccio et al., "The HIV protease inhibitor ritonavir blocks osteoclastogenesis and function by impairing RANKL-induced signaling," *Journal of Clinical Investigation*, vol. 114, no. 2, pp. 206–213, 2004.

[183] J. M. Fakruddin and J. Laurence, "HIV envelope gp120-mediated regulation of osteoclastogenesis via receptor activator of nuclear factor κB ligand (RANKL) secretion and its modulation by certain HIV protease inhibitors through interferon-γ/RANKL cross-talk," *Journal of Biological Chemistry*, vol. 278, no. 48, pp. 48251–48258, 2003.

[184] D. P. Wanner, A. Tyndall, and U. A. Walker, "Tenofovir-induced osteomalacia," *Clinical and Experimental Rheumatology*, vol. 27, no. 6, pp. 1001–1003, 2009.

[185] G. Pan, X. Wu, M. A. McKenna, X. Feng, T. R. Nagy, and J. M. McDonald, "AZT enhances osteoclastogenesis and bone loss," *AIDS Research and Human Retroviruses*, vol. 20, no. 6, pp. 608–620, 2004.

[186] G. Pan, M. Kilby, and J. M. McDonald, "Modulation of osteoclastogenesis induced by nucleoside reverse transcriptase inhibitors," *AIDS Research and Human Retroviruses*, vol. 22, no. 11, pp. 1131–1141, 2006.

[187] T. T. Brown, G. A. McComsey, M. S. King, R. B. Qaqish, B. M. Bernstein, and B. A. Da Silva, "Loss of bone mineral

density after antiretroviral therapy initiation, independent of antiretroviral regimen," *Journal of Acquired Immune Deficiency Syndromes*, vol. 51, no. 5, pp. 554-561, 2009.

[188] D. Bruera, N. Luna, D. O. David, L. M. Bergoglio, and J. Zamudio, "Decreased bone mineral density in HIV-infected patients is independent of antiretroviral therapy," *AIDS*, vol. 17, no. 13, pp. 1917–1923, 2003.

[189] J. E. Gallant, S. Staszewski, A. L. Pozniak et al., "Efficacy and safety of tenofovir DF vs stavudine in combination therapy in antiretroviral-naive patients: a 3-year randomized trial," *Journal of the American Medical Association*, vol. 292, no. 2, pp. 191–201, 2004.

[190] H. J. Stellbrink, C. Orkin, J. R. Arribas et al., "Comparison of changes in bone density and turnover with abacavir-lamivudine versus tenofovir-emtricitabine in HIV-infected adults: 48-week results from the ASSERT study," *Clinical Infectious Diseases*, vol. 51, no. 8, pp. 963–972, 2010.

[191] J. M. Franco, A. Rubio, M. Martínez-Moya et al., "T-cell repopulation and thymic volume in HIV-1-infected adult patients after highly active antiretroviral therapy," *Blood*, vol. 99, no. 10, pp. 3702–3706, 2002.

[192] R. C. Kalayjian, J. Spritzler, M. Pu et al., "Distinct mechanisms of T cell reconstitution can be identified by estimating thymic volume in adult HIV-1 disease," *Journal of Infectious Diseases*, vol. 192, no. 9, pp. 1577–1587, 2005.

[193] M. R. Ryan, R. Shepherd, J. K. Leavey et al., "An IL-7-dependent rebound in thymic T cell output contributes to the bone loss induced by estrogen deficiency," *Proceedings of the National Academy of Sciences of the United States of America*, vol. 102, no. 46, pp. 16735–16740, 2005.

[194] J. Wactawski-Wende, S. G. Grossi, M. Trevisan et al., "The role of osteopenia in oral bone loss and periodontal disease," *Journal of Periodontology*, vol. 67, no. 10, pp. 1076–1084, 1996.

[195] B. Klausen, H. P. Hougen, and N. E. Fiehn, "Increased periodontal bone loss in temporarily B lymphocyte-deficient rats," *Journal of Periodontal Research*, vol. 24, no. 6, pp. 384–390, 1989.

[196] Y. Choi and J. J. Kim, "B cells activated in the presence of Th1 cytokines inhibit osteoclastogenesis," *Experimental and Molecular Medicine*, vol. 35, no. 5, pp. 385–392, 2003.

[197] M. A. Taubman and T. Kawai, "Involvement of T-lymphocytes in periodontal disease and in direct and indirect induction of bone resorption," *Critical Reviews in Oral Biology and Medicine*, vol. 12, no. 2, pp. 125–135, 2001.

[198] T. Crotti, M. D. Smith, R. Hirsch et al., "Receptor activator NF κB ligand (RANKL) and osteoprotegerin (OPG) protein expression in periodontitis," *Journal of Periodontal Research*, vol. 38, no. 4, pp. 380–387, 2003.

[199] G. Brunetti, S. Colucci, P. Pignataro et al., "T cells support osteoclastogenesis in an *in vitro* model derived from human periodontitis patients," *Journal of Periodontology*, vol. 76, no. 10, pp. 1675–1680, 2005.

[200] S. Colucci, G. Mori, G. Brunetti et al., "Interleukin-7 production by B lymphocytes affects the T cell-dependent osteoclast formation in an *in vitro* model derived from human periodontitis patients," *International Journal of Immunopathology and Pharmacology*, vol. 18, no. 3, pp. 13–19, 2005.

[201] G. Mori, G. Brunetti, S. Collucci et al., "Osteoblast apoptosis in periodontal disease: role of TNF-related apoptosis-inducing ligand," *International Journal of Immunopathology and Pharmacology*, vol. 22, no. 1, pp. 95–103, 2009.

[202] M. Feldmann, F. M. Brennan, and R. N. Maini, "Rheumatoid arthritis," *Cell*, vol. 85, no. 3, pp. 307–310, 1996.

[203] J. C. W. Edwards, L. Szczepański, J. Szechiński et al., "Efficacy of B-cell-targeted therapy with rituximab in patients with rheumatoid arthritis," *The New England Journal of Medicine*, vol. 350, no. 25, pp. 2572–2581, 2004.

[204] G. Schett and J. P. David, "The multiple faces of autoimmune-mediated bone loss," *Nature Reviews Endocrinology*, vol. 6, no. 12, pp. 698–706, 2010.

[205] C. Fournier, "Where do T cells stand in rheumatoid arthritis?" *Joint Bone Spine*, vol. 72, no. 6, pp. 527–532, 2005.

[206] Y. Y. Kong, U. Felge, I. Sarosi et al., "Activated T cells regulate bone loss and joint destruction in adjuvant arthritis through osteoprotegerin ligand," *Nature*, vol. 402, no. 6759, pp. 304–309, 1999.

[207] X. He, A. H. Kang, and J. M. Stuart, "Anti-human type II collagen $CD19^+$ B cells are present in patients with rheumatoid arthritis and healthy individuals," *Journal of Rheumatology*, vol. 28, no. 10, pp. 2168–2175, 2001.

[208] K. Yanaba, Y. Hamaguchi, G. M. Venturi, D. A. Steeber, S. Clair, and T. F. Tedder, "B cell depletion delays collagen-induced arthritis in mice: arthritis induction requires synergy between humoral and cell-mediated immunity," *Journal of Immunology*, vol. 179, no. 2, pp. 1369–1380, 2007.

[209] P. Li and E. M. Schwarz, "The TNF-α transgenic mouse model of inflammatory arthritis," *Springer Seminars in Immunopathology*, vol. 25, no. 1, pp. 19–33, 2003.

[210] G. Schett, K. Redlich, S. Hayer et al., "Osteoprotegerin protects against generalized bone loss in tumor necrosis factor-transgenic mice," *Arthritis and Rheumatism*, vol. 48, no. 7, pp. 2042–2051, 2003.

[211] R. Fleischmann, I. Iqbal, P. Nandeshwar, and A. Quiceno, "Safety and efficacy of disease-modifying anti-rheumatic agents: focus on the benefits and risks of etanercept," *Drug Safety*, vol. 25, no. 3, pp. 173–197, 2002.

[212] J. K. Jenkins and K. J. Hardy, "Biological modifier therapy for the treatment of rheumatoid arthritis," *American Journal of the Medical Sciences*, vol. 323, no. 4, pp. 197–205, 2002.

[213] A. M. Reimold, "TNFalpha as therapeutic target: new drugs, more applications," *Current Drug Targets: Inflammation & Allergy*, vol. 1, pp. 377–392, 2002.

[214] N. T. Ilowite, "Update on biologics in juvenile idiopathic arthritis," *Current Opinion in Rheumatology*, vol. 20, no. 5, pp. 613–618, 2008.

[215] M. Natsumeda, K. Nishiya, and Z. Ota, "Stimulation by interleukin-7 of mononuclear cells in peripheral blood, synovial fluid and synovial tissue from patients with rheumatoid arthritis," *Acta Medica Okayama*, vol. 47, no. 6, pp. 391–397, 1993.

[216] F. De Benedetti, M. Massa, P. Pignatti, M. Kelley, C. R. Faltynek, and A. Martini, "Elevated circulating interleukin-7 levels in patients with systemic juvenile rheumatoid arthritis," *Journal of Rheumatology*, vol. 22, no. 8, pp. 1581–1585, 1995.

[217] L. Leistad, M. Østensen, and A. Faxvaag, "Detection of cytokine mRNA in human, articular cartilage from patients with rheumatoid arthritis and osteoarthritis by reverse transcriptase-polymerase chain reaction," *Scandinavian Journal of Rheumatology*, vol. 27, no. 1, pp. 61–67, 1998.

[218] S. Harada, M. Yamamura, H. Okamoto et al., "Production of interleukin-7 and interleukin-15 by fibroblast-like synoviocytes from patients with rheumatoid arthritis," *Arthritis & Rheumatism*, vol. 42, pp. 1508–1516, 1999.

[219] S. Colucci, G. Brunetti, F. P. Cantatore et al., "Lymphocytes and synovial fluid fibroblasts support osteoclastogenesis through

RANKL, TNFα, and IL-7 in an *in vitro* model derived from human psoriatic arthritis," *Journal of Pathology*, vol. 212, no. 1, pp. 47–55, 2007.

[220] S. M. Churchman and F. Ponchel, "Interleukin-7 in rheumatoid arthritis," *Rheumatology*, vol. 47, no. 6, pp. 753–759, 2008.

[221] S. A. Y. Hartgring, C. R. Willis, D. Alcorn et al., "Blockade of the interleukin-7 receptor inhibits collagen-induced arthritis and is associated with reduction of T cell activity and proinflammatory mediators," *Arthritis and Rheumatism*, vol. 62, no. 9, pp. 2716–2725, 2010.

[222] E. Lubberts, "IL-17/Th17 targeting: on the road to prevent chronic destructive arthritis?" *Cytokine*, vol. 41, no. 2, pp. 84–91, 2008.

[223] S. Kotake, N. Udagawa, N. Takahashi et al., "IL-17 in synovial fluids from patients with rheumatoid arthritis is a potent stimulator of osteoclastogenesis," *Journal of Clinical Investigation*, vol. 103, no. 9, pp. 1345–1352, 1999.

[224] E. Lubberts, L. Van den Bersselaar, B. Oppers-Walgreen et al., "IL-17 promotes bone erosion in murine collagen-induced arthritis through loss of the receptor activator of NF-κB ligand/osteoprotegerin balancel," *Journal of Immunology*, vol. 170, no. 5, pp. 2655–2662, 2003.

[225] K. Zwerina, M. Koenders, A. Hueber et al., "Anti IL-17A therapy inhibits bone loss in TNF-α-mediated murine arthritis by modulation of the T-cell balance," *European Journal of Immunology*, vol. 42, no. 2, pp. 413–423, 2012.

[226] B. L. Riggs, S. Khosla, and L. J. Melton, "Sex steroids and the construction and conservation of the adult skeleton," *Endocrine Reviews*, vol. 23, no. 3, pp. 279–302, 2002.

[227] J. A. Clowes, B. L. Riggs, and S. Khosla, "The role of the immune system in the pathophysiology of osteoporosis," *Immunological Reviews*, vol. 208, pp. 207–227, 2005.

[228] C. Roggia, Y. Gao, S. Cenci et al., "Up-regulation of TNF-producing T cells in the bone marrow: a key mechanism by which estrogen deficiency induces bone loss *in vivo*," *Proceedings of the National Academy of Sciences of the United States of America*, vol. 98, no. 24, pp. 13960–13965, 2001.

[229] S. Cenci, G. Toraldo, M. N. Weitzmann et al., "Estrogen deficiency induces bone loss by increasing T cell proliferation and lifespan through IFN-γ-induced class II transactivator," *Proceedings of the National Academy of Sciences of the United States of America*, vol. 100, no. 18, pp. 10405–10410, 2003.

[230] M. N. Weitzmann and R. Pacifici, "Role of the immune system in postmenopausal bone loss," *Current Osteoporosis Reports*, vol. 3, no. 3, pp. 92–97, 2005.

[231] M. N. Weitzmann and R. Pacifici, "Estrogen regulation of immune cell bone interactions," *Annals of the New York Academy of Sciences*, vol. 1068, no. 1, pp. 256–274, 2006.

[232] Y. Gao, F. Grassi, M. R. Ryan et al., "IFN-γ stimulates osteoclast formation and bone loss *in vivo* via antigen-driven T cell activation," *Journal of Clinical Investigation*, vol. 117, no. 1, pp. 122–132, 2007.

[233] F. Grassi, G. Tell, M. Robbie-Ryan et al., "Oxidative stress causes bone loss in estrogen-deficient mice through enhanced bone marrow dendritic cell activation," *Proceedings of the National Academy of Sciences of the United States of America*, vol. 104, no. 38, pp. 15087–15092, 2007.

[234] M. N. Weitzmann and R. Pacifici, "T cells: unexpected players in the bone loss induced by estrogen deficiency and in basal bone homeostasis," *Annals of the New York Academy of Sciences*, vol. 1116, pp. 360–375, 2007.

[235] J. Y. Li, H. Tawfeek, B. Bedi et al., "Ovariectomy disregulates osteoblast and osteoclast formation through the T-cell receptor CD40 ligand," *Proceedings of the National Academy of Sciences of the United States of America*, vol. 108, no. 2, pp. 768–773, 2011.

[236] T. Masuzawa, C. Miyaura, Y. Onoe et al., "Estrogen deficiency stimulates B lymphopoiesis in mouse bone marrow," *Journal of Clinical Investigation*, vol. 94, no. 3, pp. 1090–1097, 1994.

[237] M. C. Erlandsson, C. A. Jonsson, U. Islander, C. Ohlsson, and H. Carlsten, "Oestrogen receptor specificity in oestradiol-mediated effects on B lymphopoiesis and immunoglobulin production in male mice," *Immunology*, vol. 108, no. 3, pp. 346–351, 2003.

[238] C. Miyaura, Y. Onoe, M. Inada et al., "Increased B-lymphopoiesis by interleukin 7 induces bone loss in mice with intact ovarian function: similarity to estrogen deficiency," *Proceedings of the National Academy of Sciences of the United States of America*, vol. 94, no. 17, pp. 9360–9365, 1997.

[239] T. Sato, T. Shibata, K. Ikeda, and K. Watanabe, "Generation of bone-resorbing osteoclasts from $B220^+$ cells: its role in accelerated osteoclastogenesis due to estrogen deficiency," *Journal of Bone and Mineral Research*, vol. 16, no. 12, pp. 2215–2221, 2001.

[240] G. Toraldo, C. Roggia, W. P. Qian, R. Pacific, and M. N. Weitzmann, "IL-7 induces bone loss *in vivo* by induction of receptor activator of nuclear factor κB ligand and tumor necrosis factor α from T cells," *Proceedings of the National Academy of Sciences of the United States of America*, vol. 100, no. 1, pp. 125–130, 2003.

[241] S. K. Lee, J. F. Kalinowski, S. L. Jastrzebski, L. Puddington, and J. A. Lorenzo, "Interleukin-7 is a direct inhibitor of *in vitro* osteoclastogenesis," *Endocrinology*, vol. 144, no. 8, pp. 3524–3531, 2003.

[242] G. Eghbali-Fatourechi, S. Khosla, A. Sanyal, W. J. Boyle, D. L. Lacey, and B. L. Riggs, "Role of RANK ligand in mediating increased bone resorption in early postmenopausal women," *Journal of Clinical Investigation*, vol. 111, no. 8, pp. 1221–1230, 2003.

[243] Y. Li, A. Li, X. Yang, and M. N. Weitzmann, "Ovariectomy-induced bone loss occurs independently of B cells," *Journal of Cellular Biochemistry*, vol. 100, no. 6, pp. 1370–1375, 2007.

[244] T. J. Fry and C. L. Mackall, "Interleukin-7: master regulator of peripheral T-cell homeostasis?" *Trends in Immunology*, vol. 22, no. 10, pp. 564–571, 2001.

[245] M. Robbie-Ryan, R. Pacifici, and M. N. Weitzmann, "IL-7 drives T cell-mediated bone loss following ovariectomy," *Annals of the New York Academy of Sciences*, vol. 1068, no. 1, pp. 348–351, 2006.

[246] M. Utsuyama and K. Hirokawa, "Hypertrophy of the thymus and restoration of immune functions in mice and rats by gonadectomy," *Mechanisms of Ageing and Development*, vol. 47, no. 3, pp. 175–185, 1989.

[247] J. Pido-Lopez, N. Imami, and R. Aspinall, "Both age and gender affect thymic output: more recent thymic migrants in females than males as they age," *Clinical and Experimental Immunology*, vol. 125, no. 3, pp. 409–413, 2001.

[248] M. K. Lindberg, J. Svensson, K. Venken et al., "Liver-derived IGF-I is permissive for ovariectomy-induced trabecular bone loss," *Bone*, vol. 38, no. 1, pp. 85–92, 2006.

[249] S. K. Lee, J. F. Kalinowski, C. Jacquin, D. J. Adams, G. Gronowicz, and J. A. Lorenzo, "Interleukin-7 influences osteoclast function *in vivo* but is not a critical factor in ovariectomy-induced bone loss," *Journal of Bone and Mineral Research*, vol. 21, no. 5, pp. 695–702, 2006.

[250] H. L. Aguila, S. H. Mun, J. Kalinowski, D. J. Adams, J. A. Lorenzo, and S. K. Lee, "Osteoblast-specific overexpression of human interleukin-7 rescues the bone mass phenotype of interleukin-7-deficient female mice," *Journal of Bone and Mineral Research*, vol. 27, pp. 1030–1042, 2012.

[251] H. O. Valenzona, R. Pointer, R. Ceredig, and D. G. Osmond, "Prelymphomatous B cell hyperplasia in the bone marrow of interleukin-7 transgenic mice: precursor B cell dynamics, microenvironmental organization and osteolysis," *Experimental Hematology*, vol. 24, no. 13, pp. 1521–1529, 1996.

[252] D. Salopek, D. Grčević, V. Katavić, N. Kovačić, I. K. Lukić, and A. Marušić, "Increased bone resorption and osteopenia are a part of the lymphoproliferative phenotype of mice with systemic over-expression of interleukin-7 gene driven by MHC class II promoter," *Immunology Letters*, vol. 121, no. 2, pp. 134–139, 2008.

[253] A. Huston and G. D. Roodman, "Role of the microenvironment in multiple myeloma bone disease," *Future Oncology*, vol. 2, no. 3, pp. 371–378, 2006.

[254] N. Giuliani, S. Colla, R. Sala et al., "Human myeloma cells stimulate the receptor activator of nuclear factor-κB ligand (RANKL) in T lymphocytes: a potential role in multiple myeloma bone disease," *Blood*, vol. 100, no. 13, pp. 4615–4621, 2002.

[255] N. Giuliani, S. Colla, F. Morandi et al., "Myeloma cells block RUNX2/CBFA1 activity in human bone marrow osteoblast progenitors and inhibit osteoblast formation and differentiation," *Blood*, vol. 106, no. 7, pp. 2472–2483, 2005.

[256] S. D'Souza, D. del Prete, S. Jin et al., "Gfi1 expressed in bone marrow stromal cells is a novel osteoblast suppressor in patients with multiple myeloma bone disease," *Blood*, vol. 118, no. 26, pp. 6871–6880, 2011.

[257] R. B. Kimble, S. Bain, and R. Pacifici, "The functional block of TNF but not of IL-6 prevents bone loss in ovariectomized mice," *Journal of Bone and Mineral Research*, vol. 12, no. 6, pp. 935–941, 1997.

[258] A. M. Tyagi, K. Srivastava, K. Sharan, D. Yadav, R. Maurya, and D. Singh, "Daidzein prevents the increase in $CD4^+CD28null$ T cells and B lymphopoesis in ovariectomized mice: a key mechanism for anti-osteoclastogenic effect," *PLoS ONE*, vol. 6, no. 6, Article ID e21216, 2011.

[259] F. Gori, L. C. Hofbauer, C. R. Dunstan, T. C. Spelsberg, S. Khosla, and B. Lawrence Riggs, "The expression of osteoprotegerin and RANK ligand and the support of osteoclast formation by stromal-osteoblast lineage cells is developmentally regulated," *Endocrinology*, vol. 141, no. 12, pp. 4768–4776, 2000.

[260] B. J. Kim, S. J. Bae, S. Y. Lee et al., "TNF-α mediates the stimulation of sclerostin expression in an estrogen-deficient condition," *Biochemical and Biophysical Research Communications*, vol. 424, no. 1, pp. 170–175, 2012.

[261] M. H. Sayegh, "Finally, CTLA4Ig graduates to the clinic," *Journal of Clinical Investigation*, vol. 103, no. 9, pp. 1223–1225, 1999.

[262] A. Muhlethaler-Mottet, W. D. Berardino, L. A. Otten, and B. Mach, "Activation of the MHC class II transactivator CIITA by interferon-γ requires cooperative interaction between Stat1 and USF-1," *Immunity*, vol. 8, no. 2, pp. 157–166, 1998.

[263] B. Ernst, D. S. Lee, J. M. Chang, J. Sprent, and C. D. Surh, "The peptide ligands mediating positive selection in the thymus control T cell survival and homeostatic proliferation in the periphery," *Immunity*, vol. 11, no. 2, pp. 173–181, 1999.

[264] C. Tanchot, F. A. Lemonnier, B. Pérarnau, A. A. Freitas, and B. Rocha, "Differential requirements for survival and proliferation of CD8 naive or memory T cells," *Science*, vol. 276, no. 5321, pp. 2057–2062, 1997.

[265] C. D. Surh and J. Sprent, "Homeostasis of naive and memory T cells," *Immunity*, vol. 29, no. 6, pp. 848–862, 2008.

[266] H. Takayanagi, K. Ogasawara, S. Hida et al., "T-cell-mediated regulation of osteoclastogenesis by signalling cross-talk between RANKL and IFN-γ," *Nature*, vol. 408, no. 6812, pp. 600–605, 2000.

[267] M. Pang, A. F. Martinez, J. Jacobs, W. Balkan, and B. R. Troen, "RANK ligand and interferon gamma differentially regulate cathepsin gene expression in pre-osteoclastic cells," *Biochemical and Biophysical Research Communications*, vol. 328, no. 3, pp. 756–763, 2005.

[268] G. N. Mann, T. W. Jacobs, F. J. Buchinsky et al., "Interferon-γ causes loss of bone volume *in vivo* and fails to ameliorate cyclosporin A-induced osteopenia," *Endocrinology*, vol. 135, no. 3, pp. 1077–1083, 1994.

[269] G. Duque, D. C. Huang, N. Dion et al., "Interferon-γ plays a role in bone formation *in vivo* and rescues osteoporosis in ovariectomized mice," *Journal of Bone and Mineral Research*, vol. 26, no. 7, pp. 1472–1483, 2011.

[270] R. M. Rodriguiz, L. L. Key, and W. L. Ries, "Combination macrophage-colony stimulating factor and interferon-γ administration ameliorates the osteopetrotic condition in microphthalmic (mi/mi) mice," *Pediatric Research*, vol. 33, no. 4, pp. 384–389, 1993.

[271] L. L. Key, R. M. Rodriguiz, S. M. Willi et al., "Long-term treatment of osteopetrosis with recombinant human interferon gamma," *The New England Journal of Medicine*, vol. 332, no. 24, pp. 1594–1599, 1995.

[272] P. R. Madyastha, S. U. Yang, W. L. Ries, and L. L. Key Jr., "IFN-γ enhances osteoclast generation cultures of peripheral blood from osteopetrotic patients and normalizes superoxide production," *Journal of Interferon and Cytokine Research*, vol. 20, no. 7, pp. 645–652, 2000.

[273] W. Huang, R. J. O'Keefe, and E. M. Schwarz, "Exposure to receptor-activator of NFκB ligand renders pre-osteoclasts resistant to IFN-γ by inducing terminal differentiation," *Arthritis Research & Therapy*, vol. 5, no. 1, pp. R49–59, 2003.

[274] T. Yamaza, Y. Miura, Y. Bi et al., "Pharmacologic stem cell based intervention as a new approach to osteoporosis treatment in rodents," *PLoS ONE*, vol. 3, no. 7, Article ID e2615, 2008.

[275] S. K. Lee, Y. Kadono, F. Okada et al., "T lymphocyte-deficient mice lose trabecular bone mass with ovariectomy," *Journal of Bone and Mineral Research*, vol. 21, no. 11, pp. 1704–1712, 2006.

[276] W. A. Goodman, K. D. Cooper, and T. S. McCormick, "Regulation generation: the suppressive functions of human regulatory T cells," *Critical Reviews in Immunology*, vol. 32, no. 1, pp. 65–79, 2012.

[277] Y. G. Kim, C. K. Lee, S. S. Nah, S. H. Mun, B. Yoo, and H. B. Moon, "Human $CD4^+CD25^+$ regulatory T cells inhibit the differentiation of osteoclasts from peripheral blood mononuclear cells," *Biochemical and Biophysical Research Communications*, vol. 357, no. 4, pp. 1046–1052, 2007.

[278] C. Y. Luo, L. Wang, C. Sun, and D. J. Li, "Estrogen enhances the functions of $CD4^+CD25^+Foxp3^+$ regulatory T cells that suppress osteoclast differentiation and bone resorption *in vitro*," *Cellular and Molecular Immunology*, vol. 8, no. 1, pp. 50–58, 2011.

[279] K. Wing, T. Yamaguchi, and S. Sakaguchi, "Cell-autonomous and -non-autonomous roles of CTLA-4 in immune regulation," *Trends in Immunology*, vol. 32, pp. 428–433, 2011.

[280] M. M. Zaiss, R. Axmann, J. Zwerina et al., "Treg cells suppress osteoclast formation: a new link between the immune system and bone," *Arthritis and Rheumatism*, vol. 56, no. 12, pp. 4104–4112, 2007.

[281] R. Axmann, S. Herman, M. Zaiss et al., "CTLA-4 directly inhibits osteoclast formation," *Annals of the Rheumatic Diseases*, vol. 67, no. 11, pp. 1603–1609, 2008.

[282] J. Goswami, N. Hernández-Santos, L. A. Zuniga, and S. L. Gaffen, "A bone-protective role for IL-17 receptor signaling in ovariectomy-induced bone loss," *European Journal of Immunology*, vol. 39, no. 10, pp. 2831–2839, 2009.

[283] A. M. Tyagi, K. Srivastava, M. N. Mansoori, R. Trivedi, N. Chattopadhyay, and D. Singh, "Estrogen deficiency induces the differentiation of IL-17 secreting Th17 cells: a new candidate in the pathogenesis of osteoporosis," *PLoS ONE*, vol. 7, Article ID e44552, 2012.

[284] S. C. Manolagas, "From estrogen-centric to aging and oxidative stress: a revised perspective of the pathogenesis of osteoporosis," *Endocrine Reviews*, vol. 31, no. 3, pp. 266–300, 2010.

[285] S. C. Manolagas and M. Almeida, "Gone with the Wnts: β-catenin, T-cell factor, forkhead box O, and oxidative stress in age-dependent diseases of bone, lipid, and glucose metabolism," *Molecular Endocrinology*, vol. 21, no. 11, pp. 2605–2614, 2007.

[286] J. M. Lean, J. T. Davies, K. Fuller et al., "A crucial role for thiol antioxidants in estrogen-deficiency bone loss," *Journal of Clinical Investigation*, vol. 112, no. 6, pp. 915–923, 2003.

[287] J. M. Lean, C. J. Jagger, B. Kirstein, K. Fuller, and T. J. Chambers, "Hydrogen peroxide is essential for estrogen-deficiency bone loss and osteoclast formation," *Endocrinology*, vol. 146, no. 2, pp. 728–735, 2005.

[288] S. Kantengwa, L. Jornot, C. Devenoges, and L. P. Nicod, "Superoxide anions induce the maturation of human dendritic cells," *American Journal of Respiratory and Critical Care Medicine*, vol. 167, no. 3, pp. 431–437, 2003.

[289] E. Bjorgo and K. Tasken, "Novel mechanism of signaling by CD28," *Immunology Letters*, vol. 129, pp. 1–6, 2010.

[290] P. D'Amelio, A. Grimaldi, S. Di Bella et al., "Estrogen deficiency increases osteoclastogenesis up-regulating T cells activity: a key mechanism in osteoporosis," *Bone*, vol. 43, no. 1, pp. 92–100, 2008.

[291] J. S. Lindberg and S. M. Moe, "Nephrology-specific issues in women's health osteoporosis in end-stage renal disease," *Seminars in Nephrology*, vol. 19, no. 2, pp. 115–122, 1999.

[292] H. Tawfeek, B. Bedi, J. Y. Li et al., "Disruption of PTH receptor 1 in t cells protects against PTH-induced bone loss," *PLoS ONE*, vol. 5, no. 8, Article ID e12290, 2010.

[293] S. Nishida, A. Yamaguchi, T. Tanizawa et al., "Increased bone formation by intermittent parathyroid hormone administration is due to the stimulation of proliferation and differentiation of osteoprogenitor cells in bone marrow," *Bone*, vol. 15, no. 6, pp. 717–723, 1994.

[294] A. B. Hodsman, D. C. Bauer, D. W. Dempster et al., "Parathyroid hormone and teriparatide for the treatment of osteoporosis: a review of the evidence and suggested guidelines for its use," *Endocrine Reviews*, vol. 26, no. 5, pp. 688–703, 2005.

[295] E. C. Weir, C. W. G. M. Lowik, I. Paliwal, and K. L. Insogna, "Colony stimulating factor-1 plays a role in osteoclast formation and function in bone resorption induced by parathyroid hormone and parathyroid hormone-related protein," *Journal of Bone and Mineral Research*, vol. 11, no. 10, pp. 1474–1481, 1996.

[296] Y. L. Ma, R. L. Cain, D. L. Halladay et al., "Catabolic effects of continuous human PTH (1-38) *in vivo* is associated with sustained stimulation of RANKL and inhibition of osteoprotegerin and gene-associated bone formation," *Endocrinology*, vol. 142, no. 9, pp. 4047–4054, 2001.

[297] B. G. Hory, M. C. Roussanne, S. Rostand, A. Bourdeau, T. B. Drüeke, and J. Gogusev, "Absence of response to human parathyroid hormone in athymic mice grafted with human parathyroid adenoma, hyperplasia or parathyroid cells maintained in culture," *Journal of Endocrinological Investigation*, vol. 23, no. 5, pp. 273–279, 2000.

[298] T. J. Rosol, C. C. Capen, and R. L. Horst, "Effects of infusion of human parathyroid hormone-related protein-(1-40) in nude mice: histomorphometric and biochemical investigations," *Journal of Bone and Mineral Research*, vol. 3, no. 6, pp. 699–706, 1988.

[299] H. E. Alten and P. Groscurth, "The postnatal development of the ovary in the "nude" mouse," *Anatomy and Embryology*, vol. 148, no. 1, pp. 35–46, 1975.

[300] H. Nagasawa and R. Yanai, "Mammary growth and function and pituitary prolactin secretion in female nude mice," *Acta Endocrinologica*, vol. 86, no. 4, pp. 794–802, 1977.

[301] Y. Gao, X. Wu, M. Terauchi et al., "T cells potentiate PTH-induced cortical bone loss through CD40L signaling," *Cell Metabolism*, vol. 8, no. 2, pp. 132–145, 2008.

[302] B. Bedi, J. Y. Li, F. Grassi, H. Tawfeek, M. N. Weitzmann, and R. Pacifici, "Inhibition of antigen presentation and T cell costimulation blocks PTH-induced bone loss," *Annals of the New York Academy of Sciences*, vol. 1192, pp. 215–221, 2010.

[303] R. M. Neer, C. D. Arnaud, J. R. Zanchetta et al., "Effect of parathyroid hormone (1-34) on fractures and bone mineral density in postmenopausal women with osteoporosis," *The New England Journal of Medicine*, vol. 344, no. 19, pp. 1434–1441, 2001.

[304] I. U. Schmidt, H. Dobnig, and R. T. Turner, "Intermittent parathyroid hormone treatment increases osteoblast number, steady state messenger ribonucleic acid levels for osteocalcin, and bone formation in tibial metaphysis of hypophysectomized female rats," *Endocrinology*, vol. 136, no. 11, pp. 5127–5134, 1995.

[305] H. Dobnig and R. T. Turner, "Evidence that intermittent treatment with parathyroid hormone increases bone formation in adult rats by activation of bone lining cells," *Endocrinology*, vol. 136, no. 8, pp. 3632–3638, 1995.

[306] G. J. Pettway, J. A. Meganck, A. J. Koh, E. T. Keller, S. A. Goldstein, and L. K. McCauley, "Parathyroid hormone mediates bone growth through the regulation of osteoblast proliferation and differentiation," *Bone*, vol. 42, no. 4, pp. 806–818, 2008.

[307] R. L. Jilka, "Molecular and cellular mechanisms of the anabolic effect of intermittent PTH," *Bone*, vol. 40, no. 6, pp. 1434–1446, 2007.

[308] R. L. Jilka, R. S. Weinstein, T. Bellido, P. Roberson, A. M. Parfitt, and S. C. Manolagas, "Increased bone formation byprevention of osteoblast apoptosis with parathyroid hormone," *Journal of Clinical Investigation*, vol. 104, no. 4, pp. 439–446, 1999.

[309] T. Bellido, A. A. Ali, L. I. Plotkin et al., "Proteasomal degradation of Runx2 shortens parathyroid hormone-induced anti-apoptotic signaling in osteoblasts: a putative explanation for why intermittent administration is needed for bone anabolism," *Journal of Biological Chemistry*, vol. 278, no. 50, pp. 50259–50272, 2003.

[310] P. V. N. Bodine and B. S. Komm, "Wnt signaling and osteoblastogenesis," *Reviews in Endocrine & Metabolic Disorders*, vol. 7, no. 1-2, pp. 33–39, 2006.

[311] T. Bellido, A. A. Ali, I. Gubrij et al., "Chronic elevation of parathyroid hormone in mice reduces expression of sclerostin by osteocytes: a novel mechanism for hormonal control of osteoblastogenesis," *Endocrinology*, vol. 146, no. 11, pp. 4577–4583, 2005.

[312] G. Hardiman, S. Albright, J. I. Tsunoda, T. McClanahan, and F. Lee, "The mouse Wnt-10B gene isolated from helper T cells is widely expressed and a possible oncogene in BR6 mouse mammary tumorigenesis," *Gene*, vol. 172, no. 2, pp. 199–205, 1996.

[313] Y. Ouji, M. Yoshikawa, A. Shiroi, and S. Ishizaka, "Wnt-10b secreted from lymphocytes promotes differentiation of skin epithelial cells," *Biochemical and Biophysical Research Communications*, vol. 342, no. 4, pp. 1063–1069, 2006.

[314] M. Terauchi, J. Y. Li, B. Bedi et al., "T lymphocytes amplify the anabolic activity of parathyroid hormone through Wnt10b signaling," *Cell Metabolism*, vol. 10, no. 3, pp. 229–240, 2009.

[315] B. Bedi, J. Y. Li, H. Tawfeek et al., "Silencing of parathyroid hormone (PTH) receptor 1 in T cells blunts the bone anabolic activity of PTH," *Proceedings of the National Academy of Sciences of the United States of America*, vol. 109, no. 12, pp. E725–E733, 2012.

[316] J. J. Goronzy and C. M. Weyand, "T-cell senescence and contraction of T-cell repertoire diversity—catalysts of autoimmunity and chronic inflammation," *Arthritis Research and Therapy*, vol. 5, no. 5, pp. 225–234, 2003.

[317] A. N. Vallejo, M. Schirmer, C. M. Weyand, and J. J. Goronzy, "Clonality and longevity of $CD4^{+}$CD28(null) T cells are associated with defects in apoptotic pathways," *Journal of Immunology*, vol. 165, no. 11, pp. 6301–6307, 2000.

[318] M. H. Weisman, "What are the risks of biologic therapy in rheumatoid arthritis? An update on safety," *Journal of Rheumatology*, vol. 29, no. 65, pp. 33–38, 2002.

3

Mechanisms for Covalent Immobilization of Horseradish Peroxidase on Ion-Beam-Treated Polyethylene

Alexey V. Kondyurin, Pourandokht Naseri, Jennifer M. R. Tilley, Neil J. Nosworthy, Marcela M. M. Bilek, and David R. McKenzie

Applied and Plasma Physics, School of Physics, University of Sydney, A28, Sydney, NSW 2006, Australia

Correspondence should be addressed to Alexey V. Kondyurin; a.kondyurin@physics.usyd.edu.au

Academic Editors: E. A. Abou Neel, S. S. Banerjee, and P. Ferruti

The surface of polyethylene was modified by plasma immersion ion implantation. Structure changes including carbonization and oxidation were observed. High surface energy of the modified polyethylene was attributed to the presence of free radicals on the surface. The surface energy decay with storage time after treatment was explained by a decay of the free radical concentration while the concentration of oxygen-containing groups increased with storage time. Horseradish peroxidase was covalently attached onto the modified surface by the reaction with free radicals. Appropriate blocking agents can block this reaction. All aminoacid residues can take part in the covalent attachment process, providing a universal mechanism of attachment for all proteins. The native conformation of attached protein is retained due to hydrophilic interactions in the interface region. The enzymatic activity of covalently attached protein remained high. The long-term activity of the modified layer to attach protein is explained by stabilisation of unpaired electrons in sp^2 carbon structures. A high concentration of free radicals can give multiple covalent bonds to the protein molecule and destroy the native conformation and with it the catalytic activity. The universal mechanism of protein attachment to free radicals could be extended to various methods of radiation damage of polymers.

1. Introduction

The attachment of proteins to polymer surfaces provides a means of modifying the response of an organism to the surface and is therefore an important step for improving the biocompatibility and functionality of medical implant table devices [1]. In medicine, the immune response can cause adverse reactions to implanted prosthetics or during operations in which blood is exposed to the surfaces of medical devices such as heart-lung machines. In biosensors, attached proteins may be used to detect the presence of molecules in the environment. The attached protein must be strongly bound to the surface to prevent it being washed off under operational conditions including a high rate of flow of liquid across the surface [2]. Additionally the surface must allow the protein to preserve its bioactivity [3].

Given the rigorous protocols that must be undertaken to obtain approvals for the use of new polymer materials in medical applications, it is preferable to modify the surface of an existing polymer than to develop an entirely new polymer material. The preparation of polymer surfaces for protein binding can be done using a number of chemical and physical modifications, such as the attachment of linker molecules to provide covalent binding through specific active groups [4, 5] plasma treatment [6–12] UV treatment [13–16], and ion beam implantation [17–20].

Despite its importance in applications, the attachment mechanism of proteins on polymer surfaces is not yet well understood [21–27]. The uncertainty of the mechanism could make the behaviour of the surface unpredictable in a given application. In a limited number of applications, the physical adsorption on a polymer surface is acceptable. However, in some applications, the stronger attachment provided by covalent bonding is desirable and linker groups have been employed to achieve this [28]. The mechanism of attachment provided by linker groups is usually assumed to be covalent bonding via the chemistry that is expected for the active group of the linker and the protein, based on a general knowledge of polymer and protein chemistry. However, without clear experimental evidence of the reaction products and without analysis of the reaction conditions, it should not be assumed that the expected chemistry has in fact occurred. The linker binding method has disadvantages as it restricts significantly the range of available substrates, restricting its use in biomedical applications, which usually need to satisfy specific requirements. Biomechanical properties, low toxicity, biostability, and suitability for sterilization are all important and may dictate the choice of substrate. Also, the linker method is not suitable for all proteins since a suitable group is required in the external protein surface and the linker chemistry could affect conformation.

The methods of achieving protein binding based on radiation damage in polymers (plasma treatment, UV light, and ion beam implantation) can provide strong binding, possibly covalent binding, to polymer surfaces and has been achieved without the use of specific linker groups [29–35]. These methods appear to be widely applicable to many polymer surfaces and to many proteins. The mechanism of binding has been assumed to be through physical intermolecular interactions, morphology of the surface, reactive groups, including oxygen containing groups, or radical containing groups, but there is at present, no direct evidence as to the actual mechanism.

When a polymer is subjected to modification by an ion beam, energy transfer from the impacting ions to the target atoms occurs, generating broken bonds, ionisation and electronic and vibrational excitation of the macromolecules. A large number of investigations of different kinds of polymers under ion beam impact have been reported and overviewed [36–38]. The ion beam implantation for improvement of protein attachment on polyethylene [39], polytetrafluorethylene [40], polystyrene [41], and Nylon [42] has been reported. Strong bonding between the modified polymer surface and active enzyme molecules including horseradish peroxidase (HRP), soybean peroxidase, catalase, and tropoelastin was observed together with the preservation of the enzyme's catalytic activity.

The proposed mechanisms of protein attachment that have been proposed for binding to modified polymers are in contradiction with each other and do not explain observations. For example, an appearance of oxygen containing groups in polymer surface after radiation damage causes an increase in surface energy, especially its polar part [10, 36–38, 43–48]. If the mechanism is of protein binding is assumed to be via physical adsorption, protein attachment should be stronger on nonpolar surfaces [49, 50]. Therefore, the modified surface should be less attractive to protein, a result that is not supported by experimental results [29–34]. The increase of protein attachment after modification has been associated with an increase of the effective surface area, but in a number of investigations of polymers after radiation modification the surface morphology does not change or the surface becomes even smoother [51, 52]. The appearance of oxygen containing groups has been proposed as the reason for strong protein attachment [53], but polymers with oxygen containing groups in macromolecules do not provide strong attachment of proteins without modification [54]. The present investigation aims to determine the actual mechanism of protein attachment realised one example of polymer surface modification—ion beam implantation achieved by plasma immersion ion implantation (PIII). In particular, we investigate whether the covalent bounding is constrained by the surface energy, surface chemistry, or morphology. To achieve this, we will investigate the correlation of covalent binding with the presence of oxygen-containing groups, surface roughness, and surface energy determined with contact angle.

We apply PIII modification to low-density polyethylene (LDPE) and ultrahigh molecular weight polyethylene (UHMWPE) and attach HRP [55], a widely used enzyme, with available biological, crystallographic, and spectroscopic data. The polyethylene polymers are used in applications such as medical devices, including human body prosthetics, where protein attachment plays important role. Polyethylene when untreated is a representative hydrocarbon polymer with a high hydrophobicity. The modification of polyethylene by ion beam implantation [56–72] has been investigated.

2. Experiment

Polyethylene (PE) film of low density (LDPE) and ultrahigh molecular weight (UHMWPE) was purchased from Goodfellow. PE strips of 2×5 cm^2 area and 0.200, 0.020, and 0.075 mm thickness were washed with ethanol and dried minimum one day before using.

Horseradish Peroxidase (HRP) cat.no.P6782 and all other chemicals were purchased from Sigma. The nitrogen gas used for PIII was 99.99% pure.

Plasma immersion ion implantation was carried out in an inductively coupled radiofrequency plasma powered at 13.56 MHz. The plasma power was 100 W with reverse power of 12 W when matched. The plasma density during treatment was monitored by a Langmuir probe with rf-block from Hiden Analytical Ltd. The base pressure was 10^{-6} Torr ($\sim10^{-4}$ Pa). The pressure of nitrogen during implantation was $2\cdot10^{-3}$ Torr ($4.4\cdot10^{-2}$ Pa) and the pressure of argon during implantation was $3.3\cdot10^{-4}$ Torr ($7.3\cdot10^{-3}$ Pa). This difference of pressure provided the same plasma density for nitrogen and argon plasma. Acceleration of ions from the plasma was achieved by the application of high voltage (20 kV) bias pulses of 20 μs duration to the sample holder at a frequency of 50 Hz. The thickness of modified layer of polyethylene is 70 nm, as it was calculated in [37, 38].

The samples were mounted on a stainless steel holder, with a stainless steel mesh, electrically connected to the holder of 150 mm diameter, placed 45 mm in front of the sample surface. In experiments with chemical vacuum chamber, the sample holder of 25 mm diameter without mesh was used.

The ion fluence was calculated from the number of high voltage pulses multiplied by the fluence corresponding to one pulse. The fluence of one high voltage pulse was determined by comparing UV transmission spectra from polyethylene films implanted under conditions used here to samples implanted with known fluences in previous PIII and ion beam treatment experiments [38].

The fluence rate for wide sample holder with mesh was 10^{13} ions/cm^2 per second and for small sample holder without mesh was $4 \cdot 10^{13}$ ions/cm^2 per second of PIII treatment time. The samples were treated for durations of 20–800 secs, corresponding to implantation ion fluences of $(0.5–10) \cdot 10^{15}$ ions/cm^2.

For chemical posttreatment without contact with air, the chemical vacuum chamber connected to the plasma chamber was used. Chemical chamber was closed from plasma chamber during plasma treatment (Figure 1). Protein solution or acrylic acid solution in metal bath was placed into chemical chamber, pumped up to vapour pressure of the solution (20 Torr). Then the chamber was vented by nitrogen up to atmospheric pressure (750 Torr). This cycle of pumping and venting of chemical chamber was repeated 5 times to remove the atmospheric oxygen from the chemical chamber up to $2.4 \cdot 10^{-7}$% or $2 \cdot 10^{-6}$ Torr (estimation). Then the bath with solution was removed into bottom part and closed from main volume of the chemical chamber. Then the chemical chamber was pumped up to pressure of plasma chamber.

The sample was moulded on metal holder with diameter of 25 mm, placed into plasma chamber, and treated. After PIII treatment the sample was taken by mechanical arm and moved into chemical chamber at residual pressure of 10^{-4}-10^{-5} Torr. Then the plasma chamber was closed from chemical chamber. The chemical chamber was filled by nitrogen up to pressure of 20 Torr and the bath with solution was opened and moved up to the chemical chamber. The sample was immersed into the bath with solution. After exposure in solution the chamber was opened and the sample was used for an analysis.

The wettability of PE was measured using the sessile drop method. Kruss contact angle equipment DS10 was employed to measure the contact angles. Deionised water and Diiodomethane were dropped on the sample and the angle between edge of drop and the surface was measured. Surface energy and its components (polar and dispersive parts) were calculated using the Rabel model with regression method.

Optical microphotographs of the polyethylene surface were made with microscope Axioskop, Carl Zeiss Jena attached with CCD camera KS-100-3.0. Zeiss software was used for image treatment. The 3D images of sample surface were obtained using an atomic force microscope (AFM) Rasterscope C-21 (DME, Denmark) with software Dual Scope/Rasterscope SPM 1.3.2. The measurements were done in FZR, Germany.

After PIII treatment, the PE samples were incubated in HRP solution (50 μg/mL in 10 mM sodium phosphate buffer pH 7) overnight at 23°C. In kinetics study, the time of incubation varied. After incubation, PE samples were washed six times (20 minutes each wash) in buffer (10 mM sodium phosphate buffer pH 7). Samples for FTIR ATR spectral analysis were washed in de-ionised water for 10 seconds to remove buffer salts from the PE surface.

HRP activity was measured by two methods. In the first method, the PE sample (13 mm × 15 mm) was clamped between two stainless steel plates separated by an O-ring (inner diameter 8 mm, outer diameter 11 mm) which sealed to the plasma-treated surface. The top plate contained a 5 mm diameter hole. TMB assay was added to the polymer surface. After 30 seconds 25 μL was removed and added to 50 μL of 2 M HCl followed by 25 μL of unreacted TMB to make the volume up to 100 μL. Optical density was then measured at a wavelength of 450 nm using a DU 530 Beckman spectrophotometer.

In the second method, the PE quadrant sample of 1 cm^2 was placed on bottom of UV spectrophotometer cuvette. The micromixer with 10 mm length and 0.5 mm diameter mixer bar and electrical micromotor was placed on the top of the cuvette. Speed rate of mixer was 100 rpm. The cuvette was placed in spectrophotometer and TMB solution was added to the cuvette. The spectrophotometer recorded optical density at 635 nm wavelength in kinetics mode.

The protein solution of 1 ng/mL concentration was prepared by dilution of concentrated solution for analysis of catalytic activity of protein corresponding to monolayer of protein. Such low concentration can give error because of protein attachment on walls of the glass and polymer volumes used for dilution. The BSA sealing of the surfaces of volumes at dilution was used against the protein attachment.

FTIR-ATR spectra from the PE samples were recorded using a Digilab FTS7000 FTIR spectrometer fitted with an ATR accessory (Harrick, USA) with trapezium Germanium crystal and incidence angle of 45°. To obtain sufficient signal/noise ratio and resolution of spectral bands, we used 500 scans and a resolution of 1 cm^{-1}. Differences, obtained by subtraction, between spectra of samples before and after PIII treatment were used to detect changes associated with the surface treatment. All spectral analysis was done using GRAMS software.

FTIR ATR spectra of polyethylene were recorded in situ after PIII treatment. The plasma chamber was connected with spectral chemical chamber (Figure 1). The infrared beam from spectrometer passed through KRS-6 window into spectral chamber with ATR accessory. After ATR accessory, the beam returns to spectrometer through the KRS-6 window to detector. The spectral chamber was under the same vacuum during measurements as the plasma chamber. The polyethylene sample was placed on high voltage electrode in plasma chamber and treated there. The treated polyethylene sample was replaced by mechanical arm from high voltage electrode of plasma chamber to ATR crystal in spectral chamber without breaking of vacuum. Therefore, the sample was not exposed by air between PIII treatment and FTIR ATR spectra recording. The ATR crystal of 2 mm diameter had hemispherical geometry. Because of focused infrared beam, the angle of beam incident was different and the conditions of attenuated total reflection were not fulfilled for all beam angles. It provided high sensitivity of the analysis, but quantitative measurements were not possible. For comparison, the same ATR attachment was used at presence of air in the spectral chamber and the treated polyethylene sample was exposed on air after PIII treatment.

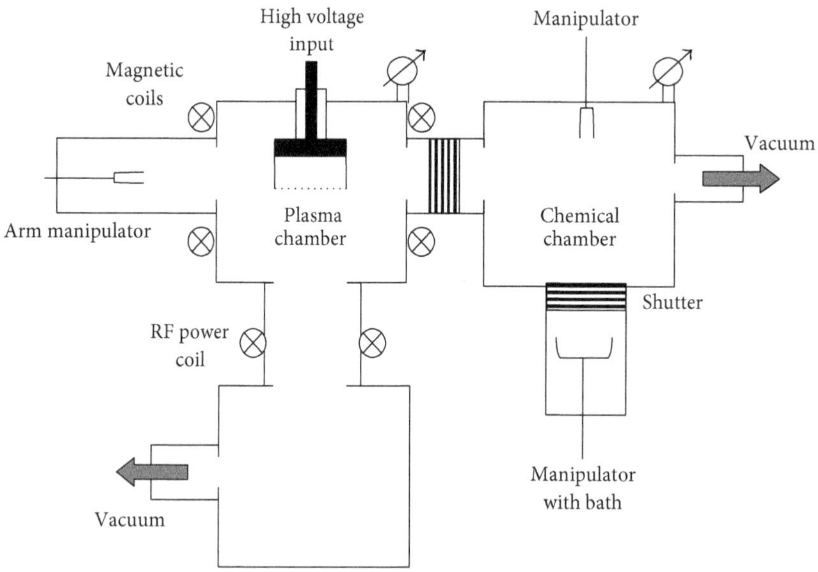

FIGURE 1: Plasma immersion ion implantation chamber with attached chemical chamber for posttreatment of polymer sample after PIII treatment. The sample is treated in "plasma chamber" by plasma and ion beam, which is extracted from plasma under high voltage. The high energy ions are bombarding the sample through the mesh. After treatment, the sample is moving with the arm manipulator into "chemical chamber," where the top manipulator grabs the sample and put to the bath with solution. The manipulator with bath can be replaced with ATR crystal when FTIR ATR spectra of PIII-treated sample can be recorded under vacuum. All manipulations can be done under vacuum or inert gas.

Micro-Raman spectra were recorded in a backscattering mode excited by Nd:YAG laser irradiation (2ω, wavelength = 532.14 nm) on a diffraction double-monochromator spectrometer (HR800, Jobin Yvon) with the LabRam 010 system (Lastek, Adelaide, SA, Australia). An optical microscope was used for focusing the exciting laser beam and for collecting the Raman scattered light. An objective of 100 units was used. The sample surface position alignment during the Raman signal acquisition was adjusted according to an image projected onto a screen from a microscope-mounted charged coupling device camera. The intensity of the laser beam was adjusted to avoid overheating of the samples. A spectral resolution of 4 cm^{-1} was used. The number of scans was selected from the range of 100–4000 to provide a sufficient signal/noise ratio for the spectra. LabRam software was used for spectral analysis.

XPS measurements were done with a spectrometer (Specs, Berlin, Germany) equipped with an Al X-ray source with a monochromator operated at 200 W, a hemispherical analyzer, and a line delay detector with nine channels. Survey spectra were acquired for binding energies in the range of 0–1200 eV at a pass energy of 30 eV. C_{1s}, O_{1s}, and N_{1s} region spectra were acquired at a pass energy of 23 eV with 10 scans to obtain a higher spectral resolution and to lower the noise level. S_{2p} region spectra were acquired at a pass energy of 30 eV with 50 scans and a 0.5-s dwelling time to obtain even lower noise levels. CASA software was used for spectral analysis.

3. Results and Discussion

3.1. Structure Changes in Polyethylene Surface Layer Resulting from PIII Treatment. The effect of ion bombardment during PIII was readily observed as a darkening of the treated polyethylene. The dark colour corresponds to carbonization of the surface layer of polyethylene and increases with ion fluence. The dark colour remains after washing of the modified polyethylene surface with water, buffer and the organic solvents toluene, ethanol, and acetone. The carbonization was studied by Raman and UV-vis spectroscopy.

The micro-Raman spectrum of the modified surface layer shows peaks which are interpreted as vibrational modes of pure carbon structures and do not show any lines attributed to vibrations of polyethylene macromolecules (Figure 2). The spot of the focused laser beam in the Raman spectrometer is about 10 μm, larger than the thickness of the modified layer of polyethylene (70 nm). The intensity of the carbon lines is significantly higher than the intensity of the polyethylene lines because of a resonance Raman effect which is observed because the laser wavelength is resonantly absorbed by the electrons in the carbon structures. The spectrum is fitted by individual Gauss functions with maxima at 1587 cm^{-1} and 1350 cm^{-1}. These lines are interpreted as E_{2g} vibrations ("G" peak at 1587 cm^{-1}) and A_{1g} vibrations ("D" peak at 1350 cm^{-1}) of graphitic structures [73, 74]. Using known correlations of the ratio of Raman peak intensities $I(D)/I(G)$ and the D and G peak positions with the characteristic size

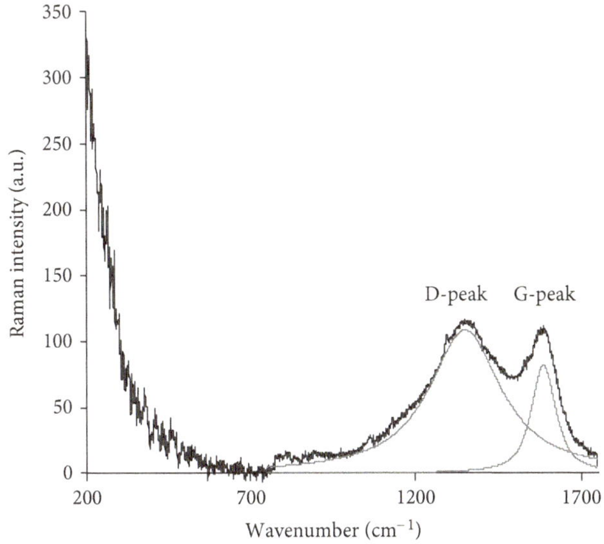

FIGURE 2: Micro-Raman spectrum of polyethylene treated by PIII with nitrogen ions of 20 keV energy and 10^{16} ions/cm^2 fluence. The spectrum is fitted with mixed Lorentz+Gauss functions at 1350 and 1587 cm^{-1} positions corresponding to the "D" and "G" peaks of carbon structures, respectively.

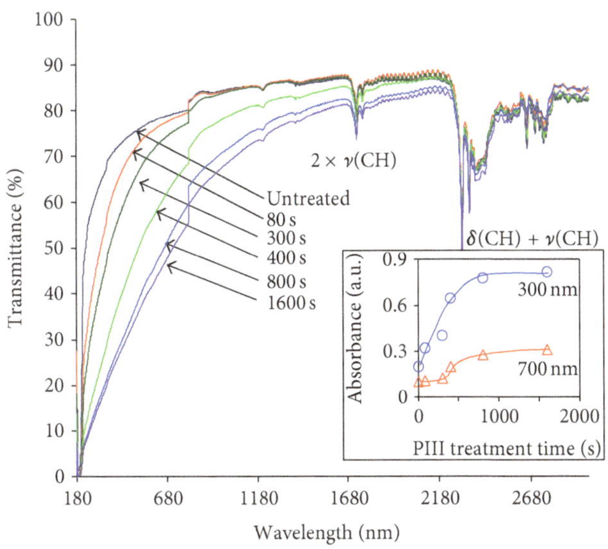

FIGURE 3: UV-Vis transmission spectra of polyethylene film after PIII treatment to a range of fluences of nitrogen ions with 20 keV energy. The time of PIII treatment is shown on the graph. The absorbance at short wavelength (300 nm) grows quicker with PIII treatment time, than the absorbance at long wavelength (700 nm).

of graphitic structural domains [75], the carbonised layer is found to consist of graphitic islands of a characteristic size of 1 nm.

Quantitative analysis of the extent of carbonization can be extracted from the UV-Vis spectra of the polyethylene film. Untreated polyethylene has an absorption at short wavelengths of less than 250 nm. The UV-vis transmission spectra of PIII-treated polyethylene films shows a broad absorption (Figure 3) with a shoulder that progressively shifts to the red and increases in intensity as the fluence of ions increases.

These changes of absorbance can be viewed from two different standpoints. The absorbance is caused by unsaturated carbon structures including condensed aromatic rings and polyene groups. An increase in size of the conjugated regions of unsaturated carbon structures causes a red shift in their absorption Therefore, the observed red shift and increase of intensity of the absorption shows that there is a progressive increase of the unsaturated group concentration and an in the size of conjugated structures with increasing fluence of PIII treatment. For example, the shoulder of absorbance for polyethylene after 1600 sec of PIII treatment is observed at 2.5 μm wavelength, corresponding to large islands consisting of conjugated aromatic rings arranged in graphite-like structures—nanographite islands. Using the Woodward-Fieser rule [76, 77], the absorbance at 2.5 nm wavelength corresponds to graphitic island containing about 40 conjugated aromatic rings, that would have characteristic size of about 1.5 nm. This value is comparable with the 1 nm size of graphite islands estimated from the Raman spectra.

The shift of the absorbance corresponds to decrease of the gap between energy bands corresponding to valence electrons and conduction electrons. The well-known Tauc formula can be used to calculate the energy gap in ion beam implanted polymers, as shown in [38]. With increasing PIII fluence the energy gap narrows from 3 eV for untreated polyethylene to 0.6 eV for polyethylene treated for 1600 sec.

The appearance of unpaired electrons associated with free radicals in modified polyethylene is observed in electron spin resonance (ESR) spectra as shown in Figure 4. The untreated polyethylene film contains a low concentration of unpaired electrons. Free radicals in as received polymer can be generated by environmental factors such as light, temperature, and oxygen species (ozone, peroxide and excited oxygen molecules) as well as trapped residual free radicals remaining after the polymerisation process. The ESR intensity of the untreated sample shown in Figure 4 corresponds to the natural concentration of free radicals in the bulk sample of 50 μm thickness.

The principal contribution to the ESR spectrum of the treated sample is attributed to the thin modified surface layer of 70 nm thickness. Allowing for the difference in thickness of the polyethylene film (50 μm) and the modified layer (70 nm), the observed increase in the ESR signal for the PIII-treated sample of 160 times corresponds to a factor of 10^5 times greater free radical concentration in the PIII-treated surface layer compared to the untreated material. The intensity of the ESR spectrum decreases slowly with storage time of the sample at room temperature, showing that the unpaired electrons recombine as a result of free radical reactions.

The g-factor (0.0028) of ESR signal of PIII-treated polyethylene is close to the g-factor of free electrons (0.0025) and corresponds to the g-factor unpaired free electrons delocalised on graphite structures [78–82]. Original position of such electrons can be on edges of graphite structures.

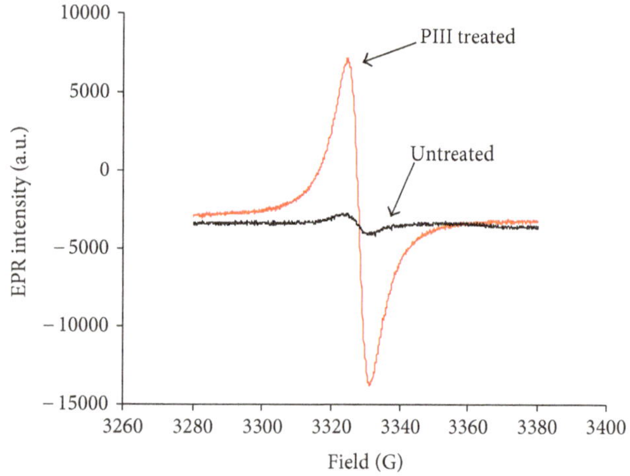

FIGURE 4: ESR spectra of LDPE film before and after PIII treatment. PIII treatment was done with 20 keV energy nitrogen ions to an ion fluence of 2×10^{16} ions/cm^2. The spectrum of the treated polyethylene surface was recorded after 30 minutes of exposure to air at room temperature.

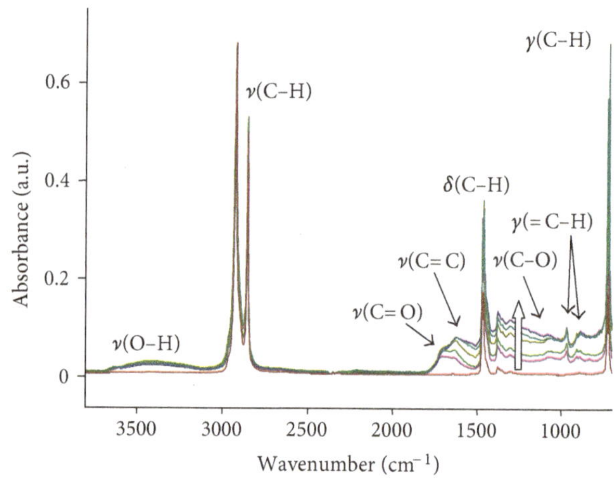

FIGURE 5: FTIR ATR spectra of LDPE after PIII treatment. Thick array shows fluence increase of PIII treatment: from untreated to 10^{15}, 2×10^{15}, 5×10^{15}, 10^{16}, 2×10^{16} ions/cm^2. The spectra were recorded after stabilization during 2 weeks storage time after PIII treatment. The intensity of unsaturated and oxygen-containing group lines increases with fluence of PIII.

Usually, the unpaired electrons have short life time under room temperature conditions due to high activity. In the case of PIII-treated polyethylene, the saving of the free radicals is due to delocalisation of unpaired electron on π-electrons of graphite structure so, that free radical does not have a possibility to be terminated by hydrogen, oxygen, or other active particles placed near the graphite islands. The aromatic ring π-electrons stabilise these unpaired electrons.

The FTIR ATR spectra of treated polyethylene show significant changes in the surface layer after PIII treatment (Figure 5). The broad continuous band from 1700 to 700 cm^{-1}, interpreted as vibrations in disordered carbonised layers, appears after PIII treatment. The intensity of this band grows with the duration of the PIII treatment. Vibrational modes of this carbonised layer have very broad frequency distribution. The vibrational states corresponding to individual carbon structures are not resolved.

Some narrow vibration lines related to new structures are observed in the spectra of treated samples. These lines in the region of 1750–1600 cm^{-1} correspond to ν(C=O) vibrations in carbonyl, carboxyl, aldehyde, lactone, and ester groups, and ν(C=C) vibrations in unsaturated hydrocarbons fragments and aromatic rings. Narrow peaks at 921, 907, and 887 cm^{-1} corresponding to vinyl, vinylidene, and vinylene groups, respectively are observed. The broad line in the region 3600–3200 cm^{-1} corresponds to ν(OH) vibrations of hydroxyl, carboxyl, and peroxide groups.

All these spectral changes caused by the PIII treatment are observed as additional features superimposed on the intense vibrational spectra of unmodified polyethylene macromolecules, which consist of asymmetrical and symmetrical stretch vibrations ν(C–H) at 2917 and 2860 cm^{-1}, bending vibrations in $-CH_2-$ groups δ(C–H) at 1462 cm^{-1} and in $-CH_3$ branch end groups at 1375 cm^{-1}, and out-of-plane vibrations γ(C–H) at 720/730 cm^{-1} doublet. The

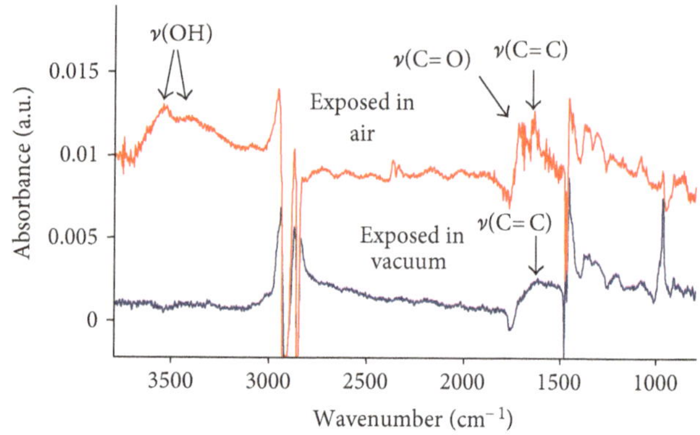

FIGURE 6: Differential FTIR ATR spectra of PIII-treated UHMWPE sample exposed to air and exposed to vacuum after treatment. The PIII treatment time is 200 sec for both samples. The sample without air contact does not have oxygen-containing groups in the surface layer. The spectra were recorded on single reflection hemispherical ATR Germanium crystal.

intensity of the lines related to unmodified polyethylene macromolecules is higher than the intensity of lines of the newly introduced groups. The difference in intensity corresponds to the ratio of the modified layer thickness (70 nm) and to the depth of the FTIR ATR analysis (700–400 nm, depending on wavenumber).

The appearance of lines corresponding to oxygen containing groups (C=O and OH) shows that the oxidation of the PIII-modified layer occurs after exposure of the treated polyethylene samples to air. Residual oxygen in the plasma chamber is expected to have a partial pressure of not more than 10^{-5} torr. Therefore, the oxygen incorporation into modified polyethylene structure could be expected to occur at a rate 10^{-7} time less in plasma chamber than in air.

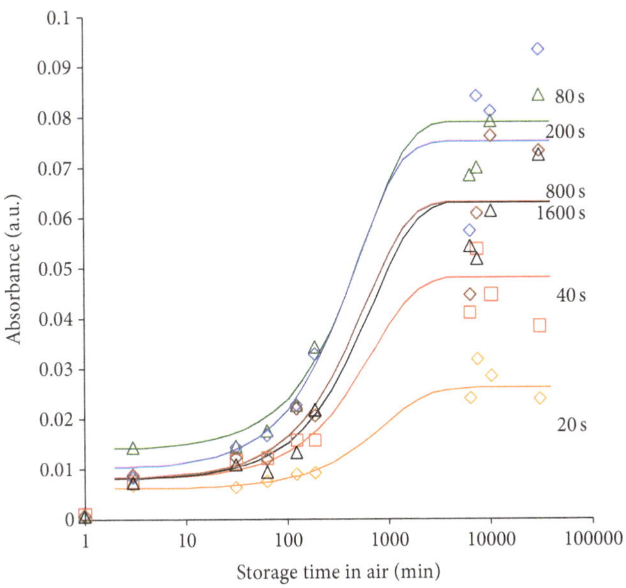

FIGURE 7: The ATR-FTIR absorbance intensity due to the 1712 cm^{-1} carbonyl line ν(C=O) normalized to the 2917 cm^{-1} line of $\nu(CH_2)$ stretch vibrations of UHMWPE as a function of storage time after PIII treatment for various times of PIII treatment.

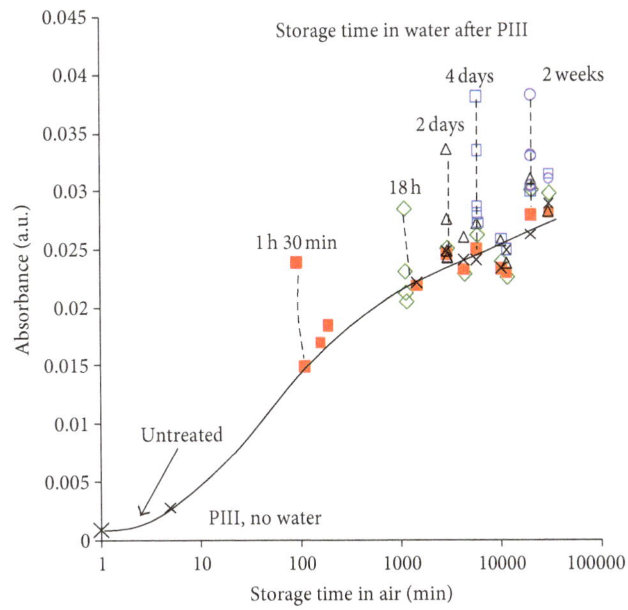

FIGURE 8: Normalized absorbance intensity due to hydroxyl groups (3400 cm^{-1}) in FTIR ATR spectra of UHMWPE as a function of time of storage after PIII treatment. The time of storage under water is shown annotated in the figure. When the sample is taken from water, the adsorbed water in gives a contribution in the intensity of ν(OH) line. After 30–40 mins the water evaporates.

Figure 6 shows the ATR-IR spectrum of the nonoxidized PIII-treated surface observed in situ before contact of the sample with air. These spectra show that the modified layer of polyethylene does not contain any oxygen containing groups When the sample is exposed to air after treatment, the spectra of the same sample shows the ν(C=O) and ν(OH) lines of oxygen-containing groups. We conclude that oxygen containing groups appear in the surface layer as result of reaction with air, not with residual oxygen in the plasma chamber.

The intensity of the oxygen containing group lines increases with time after modification. For example, the dependence of the absorption due to carbonyl group vibrations at 1712 cm^{-1} on storage time after PIII is presented in Figure 7. The normalized absorbance of the ν(C=O) line increases with time of storage in air. This means that the concentration of carbonyl groups in the surface layer grows with time. The saturation level of the carbonyl group concentration depends on the ion fluence (PIII time). The maximal concentration is observed for median times of PIII treatment (80 sec), corresponding to an ion fluence of 10^{15} ions/cm^2. The same effect was observed for PIII-treated polystyrene when oxidation was maximal at such an ion fluence, which provides the highest level of macromolecule destruction but not a fully carbonised surface layer [43]. This means that oxidation primarily results from the interaction of free radicals created by damage to the macromolecular chains with atmospheric oxygen. The appearance of carbonised structure decreases the level of oxidation due to stabilization of free radicals on π-electron clouds as discussed above.

The oxidation process is facilitated by exposure to oxygen but not on exposure to water. The storage kinetics of PIII-treated polyethylene stored under water show the same concentration curve of oxygen-containing groups as for modified polyethylene sample stored in air. Storage under water does not cause any increase in OH; for example, the dependence of ν(OH) line absorbance at 3400 cm^{-1} wavenumber is presented in Figure 8. The samples were treated by PIII and immediately placed in μQ-water. The air exposure time between venting of the PIII chamber by air and placing in water was 2-3 minutes. This is a relatively short time in comparison with the kinetics of the process of some days. The oxidation under water occurred due to the oxygen dissolved in water. The samples were kept under water before spectrum measurement. Removed from water sample was kept on air and measured by spectra. After complete evaporation of water from the surface layer of polyethylene (up to 3 hours), the ν(OH) absorbance points lay on the same curve as for oxidation kinetics on air. The position of maximum and shape of the line is similar for the samples stored in air and under water. This means that storage under water does not change the oxidation kinetics and that the presence of water during oxidation does not play a role. The same similarity of the oxidation kinetics is observed using ν(C=O) vibration line.

The changes of chemical structure have been observed by XPS spectra. The spectra of untreated polyethylene has singlet C_{1s} line and low intensive O_{1s} line (0.1% from carbon line intensity) showing the oxidation of polyethylene surface under environmental factors such as light, atmospheric oxygen, and cosmic rays (Figure 9). After PIII treatment, the spectrum shows C_{1s}, O_{1s}, and N_{1s} multiplet lines. The fitting of these lines gives separate peaks of new bonds such as

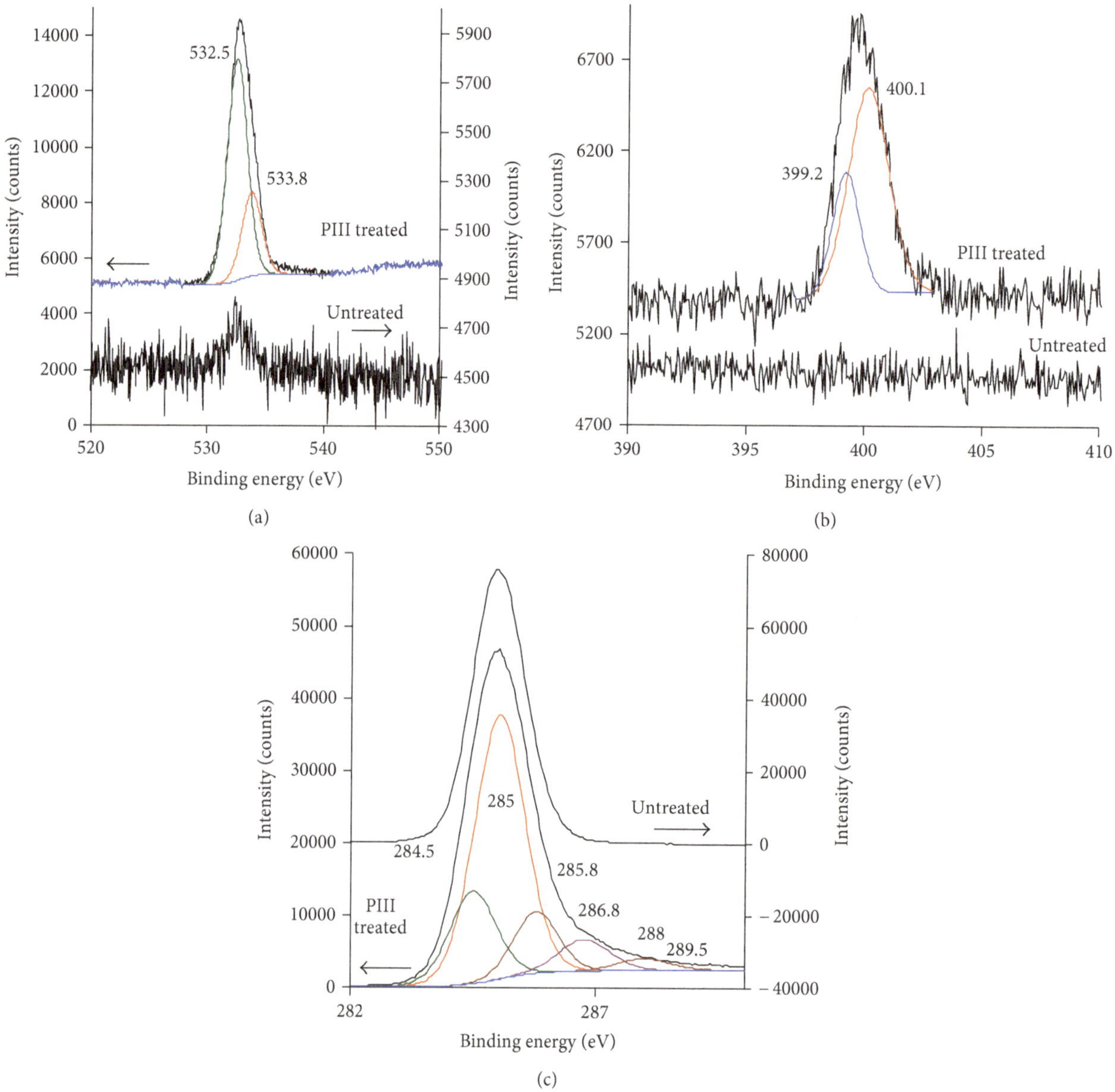

FIGURE 9: (a) O_{1s} line of XPS fitted spectra of UHMWPE before and after PIII treatment with Ar ions of 20 keV energy and 10^{16} ions/cm^2 fluence. Untreated polyethylene has 532.5 eV low intensity line of oxygen in C=O bond. The PIII-treated polyethylene has two O_{1s} lines: 532.5 eV of C=O and N=O bonds and 533.8 eV of C–O and N–O bonds. (b) N_{1s} line of XPS fitted spectra of UHMWPE before and after PIII treatment with Ar ions of 20 keV energy and 10^{16} ions/cm^2 fluence. The untreated polyethylene does not contain nitrogen. The PIII-treated polyethylene has two N_{1s} lines: 399.2 eV of C=N and N=O bonds and 400.1 eV of C–N and N–O bonds. (c) C_{1s} line of XPS fitted spectra of UHMWPE before and after PIII treatment with Ar ions of 20 keV energy and 10^{16} ions/cm^2 fluence. The untreated polyethylene has singlet C_{1s} line at 285 eV. The PIII-treated polyethylene has a number of C_{1s} lines: 284.5 eV and 285 eV of hydrocarbon bonds, and 285.8, 286.8, 288, and 289.5 eV of carbon in various oxygen and nitrogen bonds.

C–O, C=O, C–N, C=N, N–O, and N=O. The appearance of oxygen (Figure 9(a)) in high concentration (10% of total elements) is consistent with the new oxygen containing groups observed by FTIR spectra of PIII-treated polyethylene and with previous results [43]. The nitrogen in polyethylene after PIII with nitrogen ions can be explained with capturing of implanted nitrogen ions in modified layer. The nitrogen (2% of total elements) in polyethylene after PIII with argon ions (Figure 9(b)) can be only explained by reactions of modified polyethylene with atmospheric nitrogen after exposure of the treated samples in air.

The structure transformations in polyethylene surface layer during and after PIII can be explained by free radical reactions. There is extensive literature discussing free radical reactions in polyethylene resulting from different kinds of radiations including ion beam implantation, UV, VUV, electron beam, gamma-irradiation, X-ray irradiation [83–85]. Examples of reaction induced by ions (i) are shown in

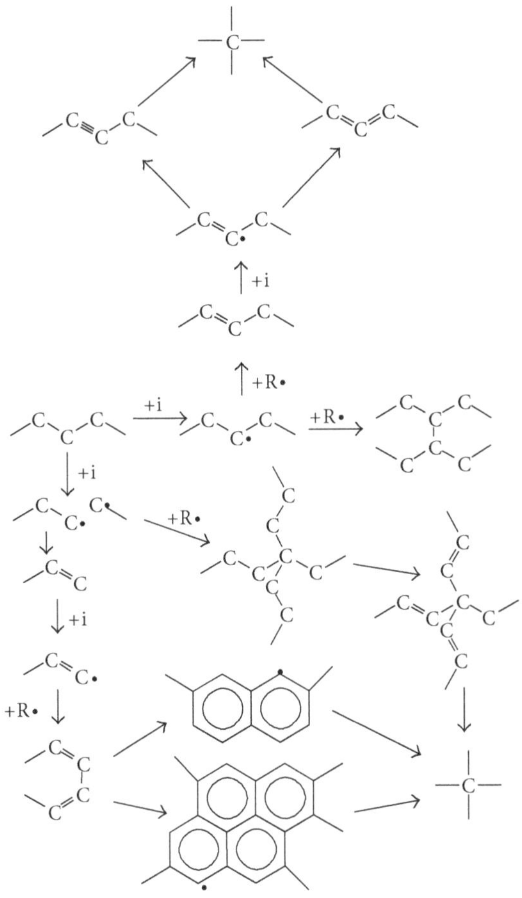

Scheme 1

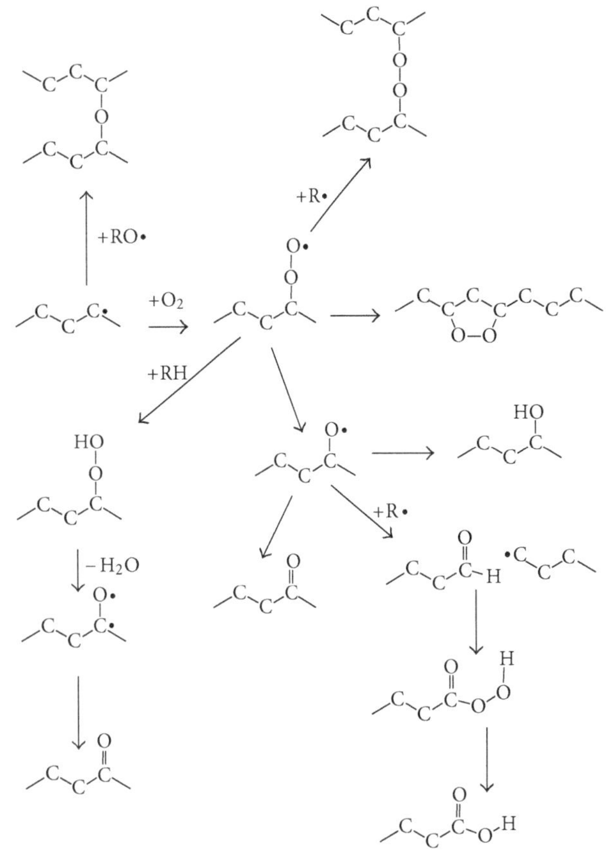

Scheme 2

(Scheme 1). Many of these reactions involve free radicals ($R^{\bullet}$) created by ions.

The scheme shows that initial polyethylene structure becomes enriched in double bond groups, condensed aromatic rings, crosslinks and amorphous carbon. At very high fluences the structure is transformed into highly crosslinked amorphous carbon.

After exposure of the treated surface to the atmosphere, oxidation reactions may follow, such those shown in (Scheme 2).

The stable oxygen-containing groups such as carbonyl, carboxyl, aldehyde, hydroxyl, ester, ether are created.

After exposure of the treated surface to the atmosphere, the reactions of atmospheric nitrogen with multiradicals may follow, such those shown in (Scheme 3).

Carbon structures containing sp^2 and sp^3 hybridisations, oxygen-containing groups and unsaturated carbon-carbon bonds in macromolecules are observed in FTIR and Raman spectra as shown above. Some free radicals remain active in the modified surface layer even for long storage times after the PIII treatment. The chemical structure of the modified polyethylene surface explains its reactivity in many different kind of chemical reactions.

The surface of polyethylene after PIII becomes textured with corrugations as observed using optical microscopy and using AFM in scanning mode (Figure 10). The lateral wave period is $2.3 \pm 0.2\,\mu$m and the peak to peak amplitude of the wave is about $0.35 \pm 0.05\,\mu$m. Assuming the corrugations are sinusoidal, the effective surface area of the polyethylene increases by 1.2 ± 0.1 times after PIII. The reason for the corrugations structure may be internal stresses caused by carbonisation of the surface layer, dehydration processes and crosslinking. All of these processes decrease the volume of the modified layer. The direction of the corrugations may be influenced by residual stresses generated during the rolling of the polyethylene films. In our experiment, the modified layer is 70 nm, much less than the unmodified PE layer, so that relaxation of the internal stresses is accommodated in the modified layer.

3.2. Surface Energy of PIII Modified Polyethylene. The untreated polyethylene surface is hydrophobic with a wetting angle of a water drop on untreated polyethylene surface of higher than 90° degrees. Immediately after PIII treatment, the water contact angle becomes very low, near 24° degrees that is, very hydrophilic (Figure 11). The same sharp changes of wetting angle are observed for formamide, methyleneiodide and glycerol drops. The total surface energy increases from 24 to 67 MJ/m^2 (Figure 12). The contributions of the polar and dispersive parts of the total surface energy are different. The polar part of the surface energy increases significantly from

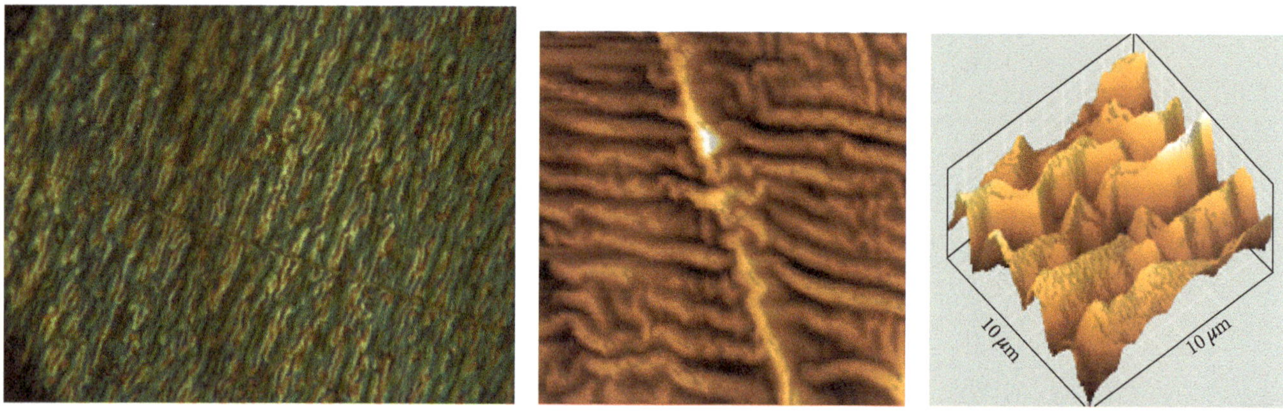

(a) (b)

Figure 10: (a) Optical microphotos (size of 120 μm × 92 μm) of polyethylene after PIII treatment. The wave structure appears after PIII treatment while untreated film is smooth. (b) AFM image of polyethylene surface after PIII. The lateral scale is 30 μm (left image) and 10 μm (right image). Vertical scale is 1 μm. The average wave's period is 2.3 μm.

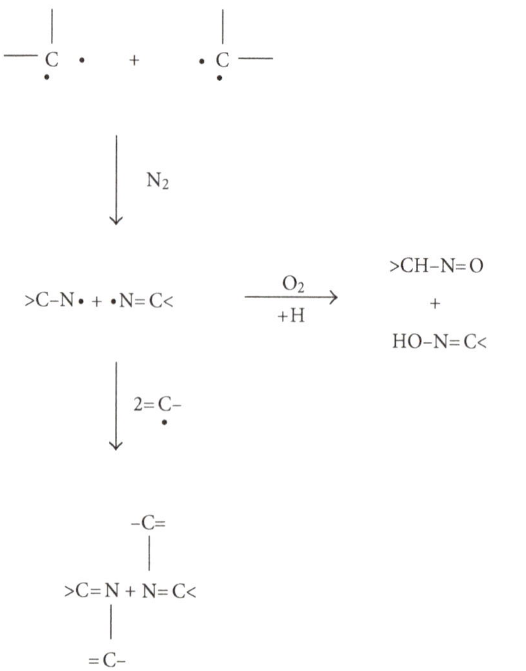

Scheme 3

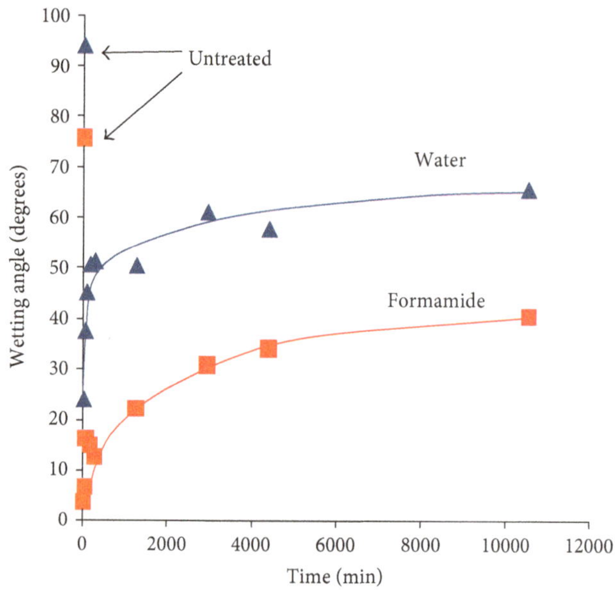

Figure 11: Water and formamide wetting angles of LDPE with time after PIII treatment. Marked signs correspond to untreated LDPE surface. Most recover of contact angle occurs shortly after PIII. However, the contact angle never comes back to initial.

4 MJ/m^2 to 44 MJ/m^2. The dispersive part does not change much from 20 MJ/m^2 to 22 MJ/m^2.

The wetting angle and the surface energy of PIII-modified polyethylene are not stable with time of storing after treatment. The water contact angle increases to 60–70° degrees after 2 weeks of storing time on air. The total energy decreases to 44 MJ/m^2, the polar part of the surface energy decreases to 14 MJ/m^2. The dispersive part of the surface energy increases slightly to 30 MJ/m^2.

The increase in surface energy is caused by chemical transformations in the modified polyethylene surface, in particular, the appearance of high energy polar groups. The same increase is observed after plasma treatment, UV light, electron and γ-irradiation [10, 14, 46]. The decrease in surface energy observed after storage of the modified material may have the same origin as similar surface energy decreases observed after plasma polymerisation or plasma treatment of polymer surfaces [86, 87].

The surface energy decrease and recovery of hydrophobicity with time in the plasma treated polymers has been attributed to the reptation or diffusion of the surface polymer chains and the rotation of high energy surface functional groups back into the polymer bulk [47]. Surface energy is thereby reduced and hydrophobicity increased. However, for

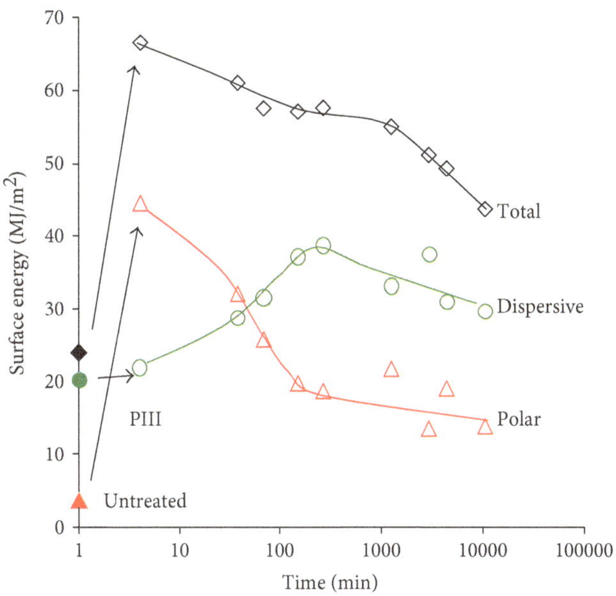

FIGURE 12: Total surface energy and its parts (polar and dispersic) of LDPE with time after PIII treatment. Full signs correspond to untreated LDPE surface. Empty signs correspond to PIII-treated LDPE surface. Continuous lines correspond to (1) and (2).

a PIII-treated surface layer the diffusion of polymer chains as in the reptation picture should be hindered by the dense crosslinking associated with highly carbonised structures appearing after high fluence modification.

The explanation of rotation of high energy surface functional groups at the polymer surface in polar media like water is not observed in our case of PIII-treated polyethylene. Although the contact angle reduce from 60–70° degrees to 51° by immersion in water, our FTIR data (Figure 8) shows that this is associated by uptake of water rather than the rotation of high energy groups. The concentration of –OH groups clearly increases upon contact with water and then gradually decreases again. The water molecules remain in PIII-modified layer longer time than required to evaporate drop of water from the surface. This is possibly connected with absorption of water molecules on oxygen containing groups and free radicals, which would cause a slow diffusion of the water molecules from the modified surface layer. After complete removing the water molecules as evidence by the reduction of the OH line intensity, the water contact angle increases again to 56°. Therefore, the recovery of high wettability under exposure in water can be explained by diffused water in the modified layer and the low contact angle after immersion is due to strong contribution of water-water interactions in the surface layer.

Another possible explanation for hydrophobic recovery may be via the adsorption of adventitious carbon and hydrocarbons on the activated surface during atmospheric exposure [48]. The changes in wettability in this study were repeatable despite the variable nature of the uncontrolled laboratory atmosphere and the FTIR-ATR spectra did not show any significant growth in lines attributed to adsorbed hydrocarbons on the surface. Besides that, the decay of the water wetting angle is the same in air and in vacuum under 10^{-5} Torr pressure. In the last case, an adsorption of adventitious carbon and hydrocarbons on the activated surface is excluded or decreased. Therefore, the adsorption mechanism of the decay can be excluded.

We believe that the changes in surface energy observed with storage time after modification are associated with chemical changes in the surface of the modified polyethylene. The character and kinetics of these transformations is complex and depend on a number of reactions characterized by different rates of reaction. The macrokinetics may be applied to simulate these transformations. These relaxation processes may be fitted using exponential functions that correspond to first-order reactions. Exponential functions were fitted to the total and polar component of the surface energy and agreement between experimental data and the theoretical curve was found (Figure 12). The fitted curve is a biexponential function of the form

$$\sigma = \sigma_1 \cdot \exp\left(-\frac{t}{t_1}\right) + \sigma_2 \cdot \exp\left(-\frac{t}{t_2}\right) + \sigma_\infty, \quad (1)$$

where t_1 and t_2 are the characteristic times of the decay, σ_∞ is the surface energy of the modified polyethylene after infinite storage time, and the $(\sum \sigma_i + \sigma_\infty)$ value is the surface energy of modified polyethylene immediately after PIII treatment. After fitting of experimental points, the equations for polar and dispersive parts of the surface energy are given by the following:

$$\begin{aligned}\sigma_{\text{dispersive}} &= 7.5 \cdot \exp\left(-\frac{t}{5000}\right) \\ &\quad - 18 \cdot \exp\left(-\frac{t}{60}\right) + 31\ \left(\text{MJ/m}^2\right), \\ \sigma_{\text{dispersive}} &= 15 \cdot \exp\left(-\frac{t}{60000}\right) \\ &\quad + 27 \cdot \exp\left(-\frac{t}{50}\right) + 4\ \left(\text{MJ/m}^2\right),\end{aligned} \quad (2)$$

where t is in minutes. The characteristic time shows that the wettability of the modified polyethylene is stabilized 3-4 days after PIII treatment. The total surface energy immediately following PIII treatment is 67 MJ/m^2 with polar component of 46 MJ/m^2. The surface energy after infinite storage time (35 MJ/m^2 with a 4 MJ/m^2 polar component) is not the same as the value for the untreated polyethylene surface (23.8 MJ/m^2 with a 3.7 MJ/m^2 polar component). The change in surface energy is determined mostly by the polar component. The dispersive component of the surface energy remains in the range of 20–30 MJ/m^2 for untreated and for modified polyethylene surfaces.

The total surface energy immediately following PIII treatment (67 MJ/m^2) is much higher than normally reported for an equilibrium property of a polymer which show total surface energies not exceeding 45–50 MJ/m^2 [88]. There are two possible sources for the high surface energy: newly introduced oxygen containing polar groups and free radicals. An examination of the literature shows that surface energies as high as 67 MJ/m^2 cannot be explained by a coverage of the new polar groups that we observe. The surface energies reported for carbonyl containing group all have surface energy below 50 MJ/m^2 [88], for example, polymethylmethacrylate with high concentration of C=O groups in the backbone (49 MJ/m^2), polycarbonate with aromatic rings and carbonyl groups in the backbone (46.7 MJ/m^2), and polyetherester ketone PEEK with ether, ester and, aromatic ring groups in the backbone (46 MJ/m^2). In the case of hydrogenated and oxidized surfaces of diamond and graphite, surface energies of 47 MJ/m^2 and 65.8 MJ/m^2, respectively have been reported [89]. A low surface energy is observed for fullerenes which do not have unpaired electrons at the surfaces (48.1 MJ/m^2) [90] and carbon nitrides (51.9–41.9 MJ/m^2) [91].

The surface energy of carbon structures like graphite and diamond is sensitive to a presence of dangling bonds at the surfaces. The surface energy of carbon structures terminated with unpaired electrons is reported to be in range of 4000 MJ/m^2 to 1000 MJ/m^2 [92, 93]. This high surface energy arises from the presence of free radicals in the surface layer. We do not expect such a high coverage of the surface of our modified polyethylene by free electrons associated with free radical groups; however, the high surface energy does indicate that the PIII treatment results in the generation of a significant number of free radicals at the freshly treated polymer surface. The presence and disappearance of free radicals on the modified polyethylene surfaces changes the polar component of the surface energy, not the dispersive component, as expected of the strong polar electrostatic interactions of free uncoupled electrons.

Therefore, we propose that most of the changes of wettability and surface energy of the PIII-modified polyethylene are produced by free radicals in the top layer that is in contact with the wetting liquid. Residual differences in surface energy for untreated and PIII-modified polyethylene after long storage times are connected with stable groups that appear after the completion of the free radical reactions.

The presented above results show that the PIII-treated surface has been changed dramatically. The surface becomes richer with polar intermolecular interactions; the chemical groups such as hydroxyl, carbonyl, carboxyl, aldehyde, ester, ether, carbon unsaturated groups, aromatic condensed structures and the number of free radicals change chemical activity of the surface layer; changes in morphology of the surface give higher effective surface area.

3.3. Improved Attachment of Protein on PIII-Treated Surfaces. The untreated polyethylene surface during incubation in buffer solution with HRP attaches protein molecules. The FTIR ATR spectrum of an incubated polyethylene surface after subtraction of the spectrum of polyethylene incubated in buffer solution without protein shows the presence of characteristic lines 3300 cm^{-1} of Amide A, 1650 cm^{-1} of Amide I and 1540 cm^{-1} of Amide II related to strongly absorbing vibrational modes of the protein molecules (Figure 13). The spectrum of PIII-modified polyethylene incubated in protein solution shows the same lines. However, the protein lines in the spectra of the PIII-treated surface are more intense than in the spectra of untreated polyethylene sample. We have developed a normalisation procedure for a quantitative measure of the amount of attached protein using all three Amide lines.

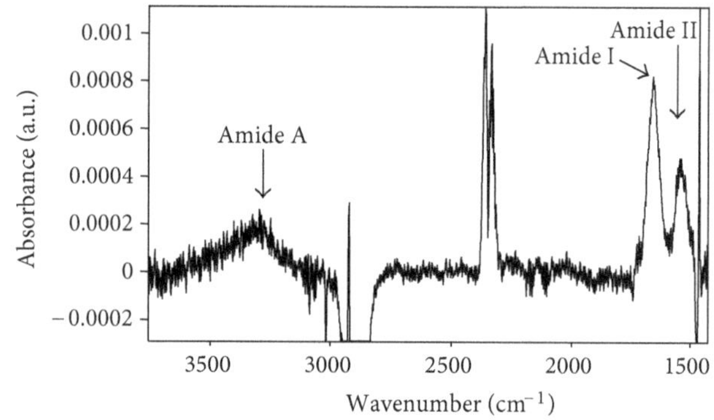

Figure 13: FTIR ATR spectra of attached HRP protein on LDPE. The spectra of LDPE is subtracted. Three main lines Amide A, I and II of protein are clear visible. The centre peak is CO_2 gas in FTIR spectrometer. The regions of polyethylene lines (2980–2820 cm^{-1} and 1480–1450 cm^{-1}) are noisy after subtraction.

The intensity of the protein lines is significantly lower than that of the vibrational lines of the underlying polyethylene. This is consistent with the protein layer being thinner than the penetration depth of the infrared beam. Therefore, the intensity of polyethylene lines can be used as an internal normalization standard for the protein spectrum. According to Bouger-Lambert-Beer law, an absorbance (A) for infrared transmission spectra is given

$$A = \varepsilon \cdot C \cdot h, \tag{3}$$

where C is a concentration of the absorbing groups, h is thickness of the layer, and ε is extinction coefficient, the structure effect can be analyzed by changes of the concentration C of the groups. In the case of ATR spectra, the depth penetration of the infrared beam into a sample immediately adjacent to the crystal is

$$h = \frac{\lambda}{\sqrt{n_{21}^2 - \cos^2(\theta)}}, \tag{4}$$

where h is the depth penetration of the infrared beam into the sample, n_{21} is a ratio of refractive indexes of ATR crystal and the sample, Lambda is the wavelength of infrared beam. An effective amount of attached protein P can be calculated using

$$P = \frac{\sum_i k_i \cdot (A(\text{Amide}_i)/A(\text{CH}_2))}{3}, \tag{5}$$

where $A(\text{Amide}_i)$ is the absorbance of i Amide line, $A(CH_2)$ is the absorbance of $-CH_2-$ stretch vibration line

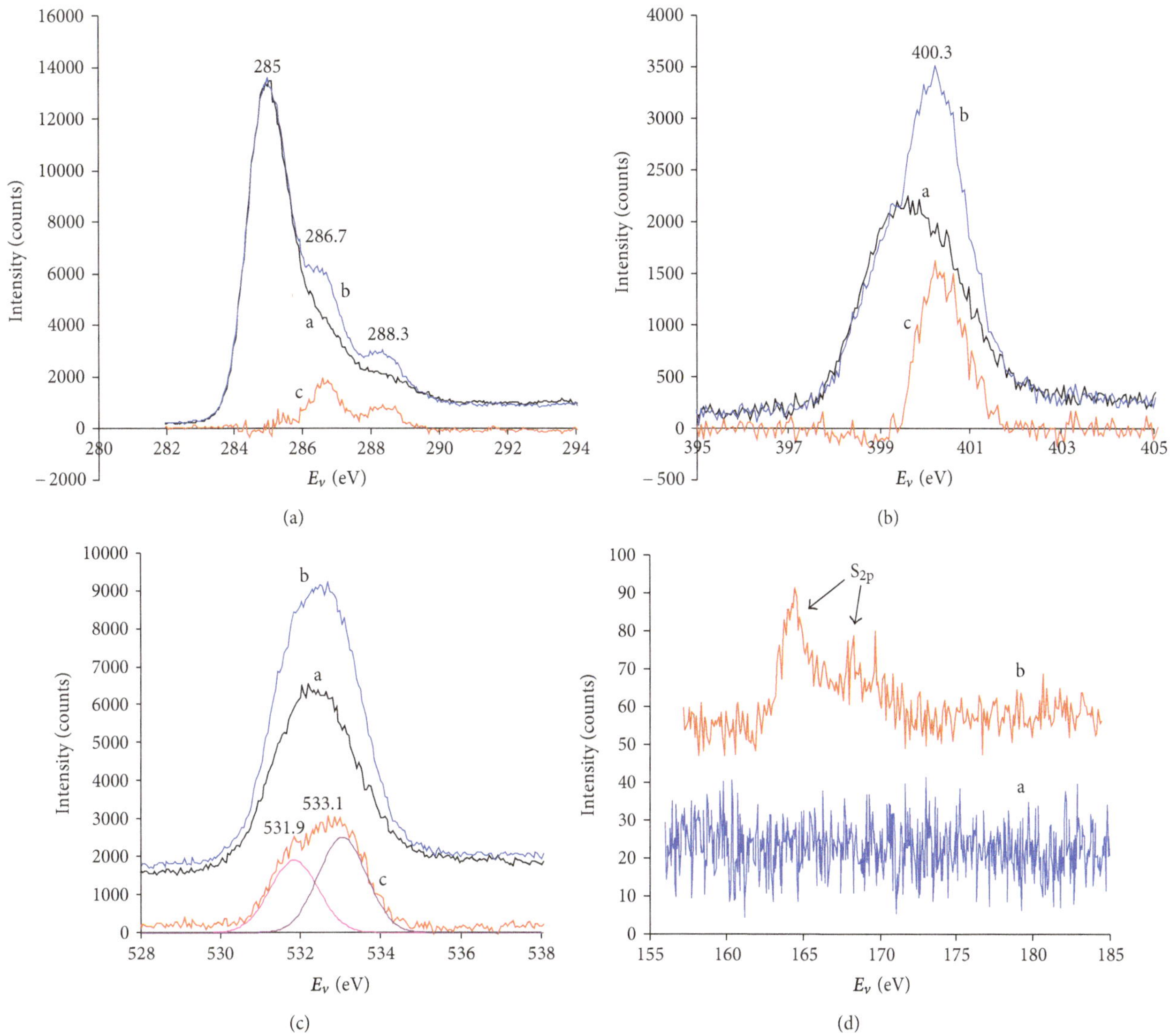

FIGURE 14: (a) XPS C_{1s} line of N+ PIII-treated UHMWPE without (a) and with (b) attached HRP protein and difference between these two spectra (c). (b) XPS N_{1s} line of N+ PIII-treated UHMWPE without (a) and with (b) attached HRP protein and difference between these two spectra (c). (c) XPS O_{1s} line of N+ PIII-treated UHMWPE without (a) and with (b) attached HRP protein and difference between these two spectra (c) with two fitted individual peaks. (d) XPS S_{2p} lines of N+ PIII-treated UHMWPE without (a) and with (b) attached HRP protein.

at 2917 cm^{-1} or the bending vibration line at 1462 cm^{-1}, k_i is normalising coefficient as ratio of Amide-i/Amide I extinction coefficients multiplied by the ratio of penetration depth of the infrared beam at the Amide-i wavenumber and the Amide I wavenumber. The amount of attached protein on PIII-modified polyethylene is approximately doubled in comparison with untreated polyethylene. The same difference was observed in our previous experiments with polystyrene [41], Teflon [40] and Nylon [42].

The presence of protein is also observed by XPS spectra. XPS spectra of PIII-treated polyethylene surfaces with and without attached HRP protein are presented in Figures 14(a)–14(d). The samples after incubation in protein solution were rinsed with μQ-water, dried and placed in the vacuum chamber of the XPS spectrometer. The XPS spectra were recorded in C_{1s}, O_{1s}, N_{1s}, and S_{2p} regions. The HRP protein monolayer is not expected to be higher than 7–9 nm; therefore the X-ray beam will penetrate through the protein layer and enter the polymer surface even when the polymer is completely covered by a protein layer. Therefore, the spectra show the protein layer peaks as well as the polymer surface peaks in different proportions. Subtraction of the XPS spectra of the polymer surface will give spectra of the protein layer only.

The C_{1s} carbon peak of the PIII-treated polyethylene surface (Figure 14(a)) is a multiplet due to the presence of oxygen-containing and nitrogen-containing groups. The C_{1s} peak at 285 eV has a long tail on the high energy side of the main peak. The spectrum of PIII-treated polyethylene with attached HRP shows clearly visible shoulders at 286.7 and 288.3 eV. The fitting analysis of this tail is problematic, because of high variability of the different oxygen-containing and nitrogen-containing groups in the PIII-treated surface layer. However, the subtraction procedure can give separated protein spectrum with 286.7 and 288.3 eV peaks attributed to C–N and C=O groups accordingly. The same peaks are observed in XPS spectra of HRP prepared as a thick layer on a silicon wafer substrate.

The XPS spectra of untreated polyethylene do not show a nitrogen (N_{1s}) line while PIII-treated polyethylene contains a small amount of nitrogen and shows a nitrogen peak (Figure 14(b)). The presence of such a nitrogen peak could be explained by reaction of free radicals with implanted nitrogen and nitrogen absorbed from the air after PIII treatment. The attachment of HRP protein gives an additional peak at 400.3 eV on the top of the N_{1s} peak of PIII treated polyethylene. The subtraction reveals the protein N_{1s} peak as shown in Figure 14(b).

The oxygen O_{1s} peak appears in XPS spectra of polyethylene only after PIII treatment as the result of oxidation of the surface layer in air. The peak consists of two individual peaks for oxygen in C–O and C=O bonds (Figure 14(c)). The presence of HRP protein on the surface increases the intensity of the O_{1s} peak as HRP contains oxygen. The subtracted spectra also show peaks at 531.85 and 533.05 eV attributed to oxygen in C–O and C=O bonds of HRP respectively.

The presence of sulphur-containing amino acids Cysteine and Methylcysteine in HRP protein gives rise to the S_{2p} peak in the XPS spectra of PIII-treated polyethylene with attached HRP (Figure 14(d)). The HRP protein contains 10 Cysteine and 7 Methylcysteine residues that contribute 17 sulphur atoms to one HRP molecule. The structure of the HRP molecule allows the amount of sulphur to be calculated at 0.54 atomic %. The XPS spectrum of HRP molecule on PIII-treated polyethylene surface shows 0.16 atomic % of sulphur calculated from the relative ratio of the S_{2p} peak intensity to the sum of C_{1s}, O_{1s}, and N_{1s} peak intensities. This is consistent result, because the X-ray beam of XPS spectrometer penetrates deeper into the sample than the maximum available thickness of HRP monolayer (the longest dimension of the HRP molecule is 7 nm). The XPS spectra of the sample without HRP attachment does not show S_{2p} peak higher than the noise level (±0.04%).

The amount of attached HRP protein is difficult to determine from the intensity of the elemental C_{1s}, O_{1s}, and N_{1s} peaks. The protein peaks overlap the same peaks of the PIII-treated polyethylene. The penetration depth of XPS analysis is close to the thickness of the protein layer and the subtracted spectra cannot be used to consistently subtract the polyethylene peaks. The S_{2p} region can be used for analysis as there is no sulphur in the polyethylene, however the concentration of sulphur atoms and corresponding intensity of S_{2p} peak is low in the protein and gives quantitative measurements of limited accuracy. Following these results, we used XPS for qualitative analysis of protein on the surface as only additional support for the FTIR results.

3.4. Conformation of Attached Protein. Knowledge of the conformation of an attached protein is important to understand the activity of the protein molecule and its functionality in a biological system. Attached HRP protein on untreated hydrocarbon polymeric materials does not preserve its native conformation [94]. We have investigated the conformation of attached protein on PIII-treated polyethylene using the Amide I line in FTIR ATR spectroscopy.

The spectra of HRP in the Amide I region were analysed for bulk HRP protein dried on Germanium crystal, and for attached HRP protein on PIII-treated polyethylene surfaces. The bulk layer was selected as a control because the interactions of the protein molecules with any substrate are absent. The spectrum in the Amide I and II regions for the protein on PIII-treated polyethylene is similar to the spectrum in the same regions for a bulk layer on a Ge crystal. The position of the maximum, the width and shape of lines remain the same when the protein is covalently attached.

The detailed analysis was done by fitting the Amide I region using individual peaks. These individual peaks characterise the presence of different structures in the protein molecule: α-helices, β-sheets and random chains. The individual conformation of a protein is characterised by unique number of concentrations of such structures. The change of conformation results in a change in the relative concentrations of these structures.

For a first approximation to determine the number and positions of individual peaks, the 2nd derivative of the measured spectrum and a deconvolution of it using Fourier transformation were evaluated and interpreted with the aid of the literature [95–97]. A simple unconstrained fitting procedure to extract the multiple components was unsatisfactory as the position and width of the components were not well determined. The fitting procedure was therefore carried out by constraining the width and positions of the individual peaks to a narrow range. The results of fitting are presented in Figure 15. The 1683 cm^{-1} and 1676 cm^{-1} lines are interpreted as vibrations in regions with β-turns, the 1661 and 1649 cm^{-1} lines are attributed to vibrations in α-helices, the line at 1636 cm^{-1} is attributed to random structures and the line at 1623 cm^{-1} is interpreted as vibrations in β-sheets. Using (5), the relative concentrations of the protein chain structures were calculated from the intensity of the individual peaks.

Following the fitting results, the HRP protein in the bulk dry layer consists of 49% of α-helices, 23% β-turns, 17% of random structures, and 11% of β-sheets. This structure is in agreement with the reference data of 50% of α-helices of HRP in crystal form determined from X-ray diffraction [98] and 30–40% of α-helices of HRP in PBS buffer solution [97]. The intensity of the spectra of the attached layer is significantly lower than in bulk protein layer, but the noise level is still low enough to get useful fitting results. The attached protein on an untreated surface has 45% of α-helices, 19% β-turns, 14% random structures and 17% β-sheets. The conformation of attached protein on the PIII-treated surface was found to consist of 43% α-helices, 23% β-turns, 14% random structures, and 12% β-sheets. These values are close to the values of HRP protein in the bulk layer. Therefore, we conclude that the conformation of HRP protein in a covalently attached

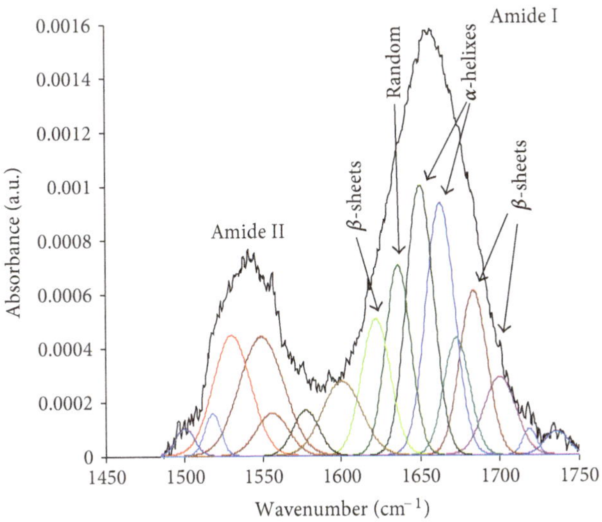

FIGURE 15: Fitting results of Amide I and II region in FTIR ATR spectra of dry attached HRP on PIII-treated polyethylene.

monolayer on the PIII-treated polyethylene surface remains similar to that in a bulk layer.

3.5. Catalytic Activity of the Attached Protein. The attached protein is active in catalysing the decomposition reaction of peroxide. The activity is provided by interaction of a porphyrin ring with a calcium ion as its active centre with the peroxide molecule. When the conformation of protein has been changed, the activity of the protein is lost. Therefore, the analysis of the protein activity can be used as a simple test for the presence of HRP in its native conformation.

The activity of HRP can be tested with TMB and ABTS assays. The assay molecules are changed by reaction with oxygen ions, which come from the catalytically decomposed hydrogen peroxide. The changes in assay molecules are quantified using the colour of the solution as determined by an optical density in UV-vis spectroscopy. The rate of the decomposition reaction depends on the concentration of active protein molecules in solution. The optical density of the test solution can therefore be used as a measurement of protein activity. In the case of a high concentration of peroxide, the rate of the reaction follows the first-[order dependence on the concentration of the protein molecules:

$$dC = P \cdot dt, \tag{6}$$

where C is the concentration of coloured assay product molecules, P is the concentration of active protein attached on the surface.

The optical densities of TMB solutions, in which untreated and PIII-treated polyethylene with attached protein are immersed, are presented in Figure 16(a). The amount of free protein in solution was monitored and found to be small so that all changes in assay colour are caused by surface attached protein. The zero catalytic activity of the polyethylene before and after modification without attached protein was also confirmed.

For comparison of the activity of molecules in solution with those attached on surfaces, the activity of protein in solution was tested with the same assay. The concentration in solution was prepared by dilution of a known amount of protein corresponding to the 80 ng/cm^2 of protein on the surface at complete coverage [41]. During the dilution procedure, the walls of all glass containers were blocked by BSA to prevent loss of the protein due to attachment of the HRP on the glass walls.

The curve of the kinetics for the assay reaction of attached protein on untreated polyethylene is a factor of 2 lower than for attached protein on PIII-treated polyethylene. Therefore, the amount of active protein on the PIII-treated surface is a factor of 2 higher than for protein on the untreated surface. This difference corresponds to the difference in total amount of protein attached on the surface as confirmed by FTIR ATR spectra.

The kinetics curve of diluted protein in solution is higher than for attached protein on PIII-treated surfaces. Because the HRP forms a monolayer on the polymer surface, the amount of active protein is close to the amount of total protein attached on the modified surface within experimental error. The difference between the activity of diluted protein in solution and protein attached on the surface can be explained by steric hindrance of the assay molecules in accessing the active centre of the protein. The presence of the polymer surface on one side and the dense packing of protein molecules on the surface both contribute to the steric hindrance. The influence of the density of packing on activity is shown in Figure 16(b) as a plot of protein activity as a function of the amount of protein attached as measured by FTIR ATR. The saturation in the curve shows this steric hindrance effect on the assay.

3.6. Stability of Attached Protein. Attached protein can be removed from untreated polyethylene surface with sufficient time of washing in buffer solution only. The kinetics of washing is presented in Figure 17 and is determined by the probability of breaking of the intermolecular interactions between the protein and the surface. The activity of the attached protein is proportional to the amount of protein.

Attached protein from an untreated polyethylene surface can be more quickly removed by washing in detergents. The detergents sodium dodecylsulfate (SDS), Triton X100, and Tween 20 were used for washing. These detergents are accepted as effective detergents to wash proteins away from different surfaces [99, 100]. Due to presence of polar and non-polar chemical groups in detergent molecule, these detergents provide a number of strong interactions with the protein and break the intermolecular interactions between the protein molecules and the polyethylene surface. Once the interactions are broken, the protein molecule is washed away. This process on an untreated polyethylene surface is observed by the disappearance of the protein peaks in FTIR spectra and the loss of activity of protein after washing in detergents.

Since part of the protein attached on a PIII-treated polyethylene can be washed in buffer, this portion of the protein is not bonded covalently. However, some of the

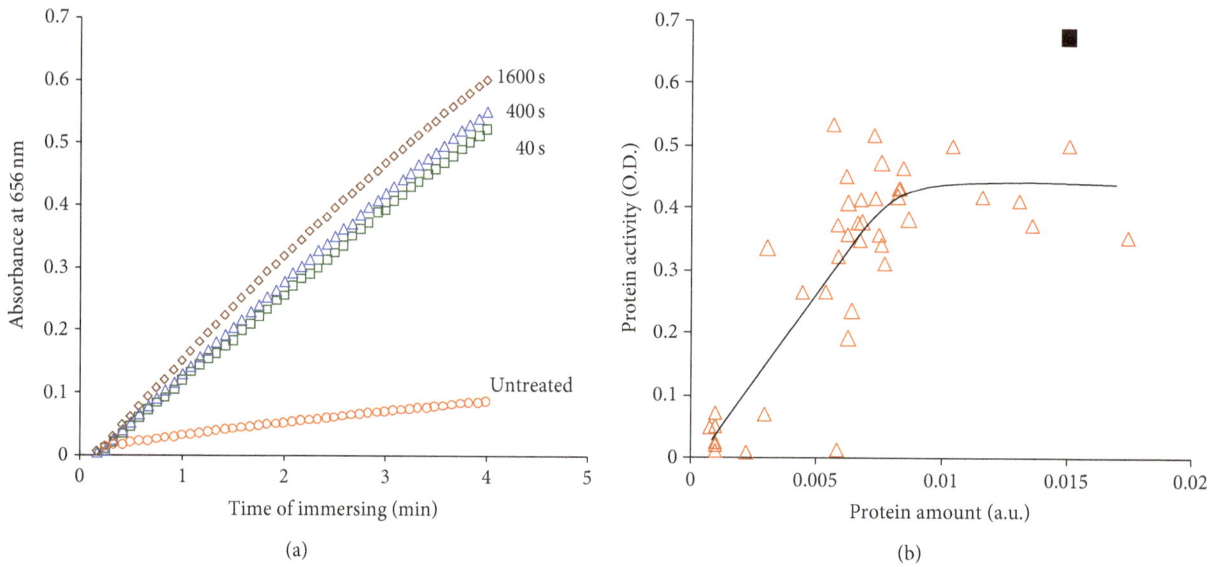

FIGURE 16: (a) Absorbance of TMB solution in dependence on the immersing time of UHMWPE surface with attached HRP. The curves of various PIII treatment time and the curve for untreated polyethylene are marked. (b) Catalytic activity of attached HRP on PIII-treated polyethylene in dependence of protein amount determined by FTIR ATR spectra. Full square is activity of HRP in solution with the concentration proportional to a complete monolayer of the protein on the surface.

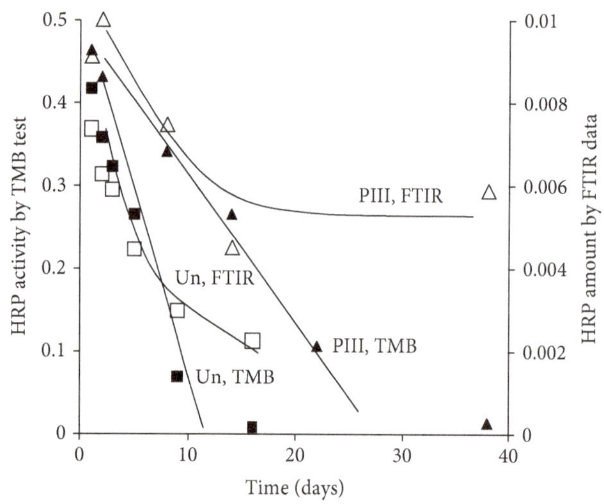

FIGURE 17: HRP activity (by TMB test data) and amount of HRP (by FTIR data) on untreated (Un) and PIII-treated (PIII) UHMWPE surface with storing time in buffer solution at room temperature after protein attachment.

protein remains attached on a PIII-treated polyethylene surface even after a long time of washing. The same amount of protein remains on PIII-treated protein after washing in SDS, Triton X100, and Tween 20 detergents. These protein molecules cannot be washed away because of strong interactions between protein molecule and PIII-modified surface. Such strong interactions cannot be provided by physical intermolecular interactions, but can be explained by the formation of chemical bonds between protein molecules and the surface. These chemical bonds cannot be broken with these detergents even after long washing times.

It has been shown previously that the attachment of proteins depends on the pH its environment (buffer) [54, 101]. The pH effect on attachment of HRP was tested experimentally. The protein from buffer solution with various values of pH was attached on untreated and PIII-treated polyethylene surface. The amount of attached protein was measured by FTIR ATR spectroscopy and was found not to depend on the pH of the buffer for both untreated and treated polyethylene as shown in Figure 18(a). The amount of covalently attached protein after washing in SDS detergent was also measured by FTIR ATR spectroscopy and found not to depend on the pH of the soaking solution over the range pH6 to pH8.

In general, the addition of ionic compounds into a buffer changes the ionic force of the buffer and can change the absorption of protein onto a surface immersed in the buffer [54, 101, 102]. The influence of adding NaCl on HRP protein attachment was tested experimentally. The protein from solution with different concentrations of NaCl was attached on untreated and PIII-treated polyethylene surfaces. The amount of attached and covalently bonded protein does not depend on the salt concentration in the range 0 to 1 mMol, as shown by FTIR ATR spectroscopy (Figure 18(b)). The same result was observed for various concentrations of $Mg(OH)_2$ additive in HRP solution.

The concentration dependence of the amount of HRP attached on treated and untreated polyethylene in buffer after overnight incubation is shown in (Figure 18(c)). In the low concentration region (up to 10 mg/mL), the amount of attached protein on untreated polyethylene increases with protein concentration. This can be explained by an increasing

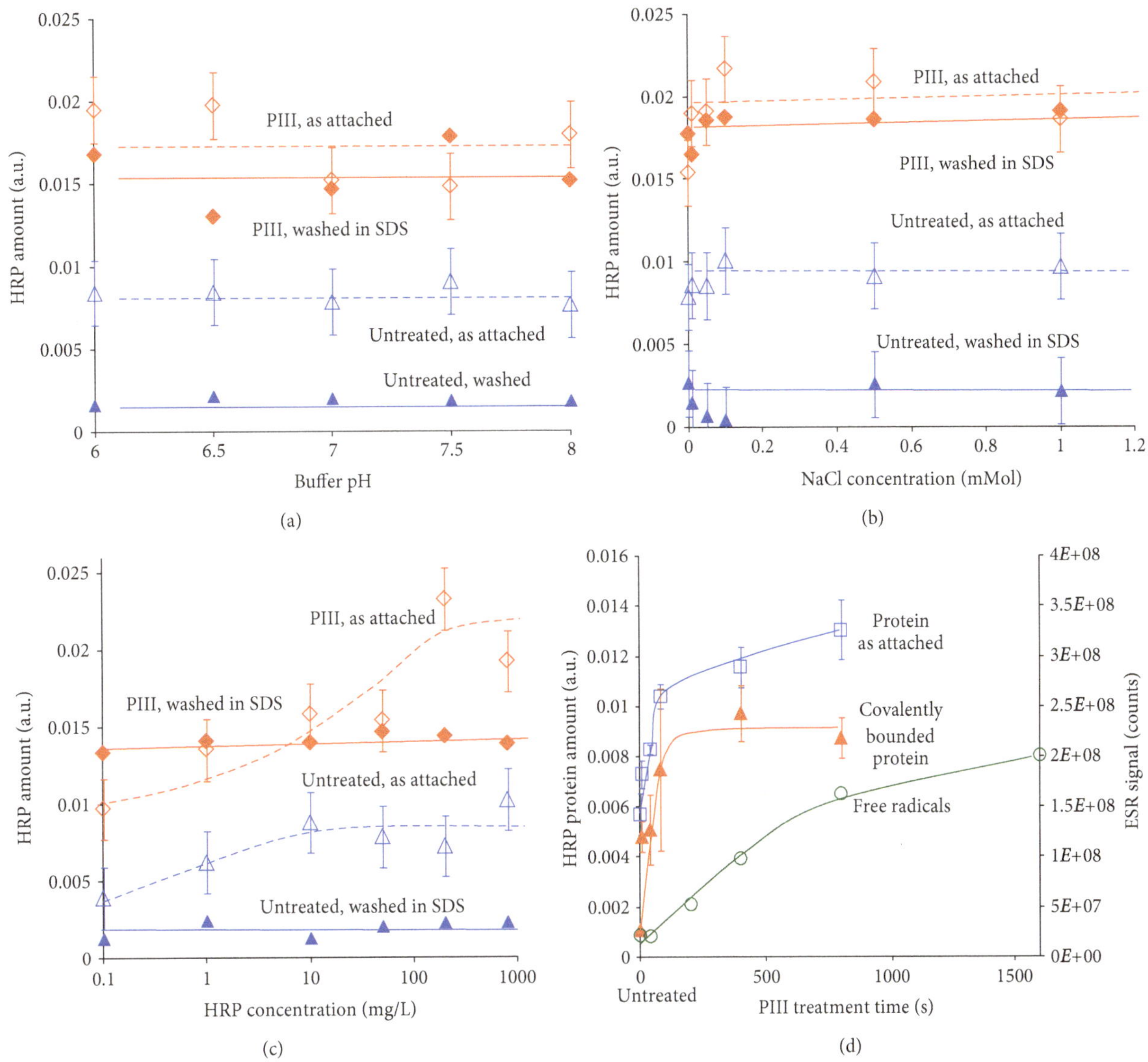

FIGURE 18: (a) Amount of attached HRP protein on untreated (blue) and PIII-treated (red) polyethylene in dependence on pH of HRP solution before (empty signs) and after washing in SDS detergent during 1 hour at 70°C (full signs). The amount of attached protein does not depend on pH of buffer solution. (b) Amount of attached HRP protein on untreated (blue) and PIII-treated (red) polyethylene in dependence on salt NaCl concentration of HRP solution before (empty signs) and after washing in SDS detergent during 1 hour at 70°C (full signs). The amount of attached protein does not depend on salt concentration. (c) Amount of attached HRP protein on untreated (blue) and PIII-treated (red) polyethylene in dependence on concentration of HRP solution before (empty signs) and after washing in SDS detergent during 1 hour at 70°C (full signs). (d) Amount of attached HRP protein on polyethylene in dependence on PIII treatment time before (empty signs) and after washing in SDS detergent (full signs). The saturation of protein amount with PIII treatment time is observed for total protein amount and for amount of covalently attached protein. Low amount of free radicals is enough to achieve the saturation stage of protein attachment.

probability of protein contact with the polyethylene surface. In the region of high concentrations (from 10 mg/mL of protein), the amount of attached protein on untreated polyethylene does not depend on the protein concentration in solution. The amount of protein attached on PIII-treated surface is higher than attached on untreated polyethylene for all applied concentrations and does not depend on the concentration of the protein in solution.

After washing in detergent, the amount of protein attached on untreated polyethylene was significantly decreased and remains constant for all applied concentrations of protein in solution. The amount of protein attached on PIII-treated polyethylene does not change (in error bar diapason) after washing in detergent for protein solutions with low concentration (up to 10 mg/L). For solutions with higher concentration (from 10 mg/L), some protein attached on the PIII-modified surface was washed away. However, the amount of covalently bounded protein on PIII-treated surface remains independent of the concentration of protein solution. Therefore, the attachment of protein on untreated and PIII-treated surfaces behaves differently.

The catalytic activity of the HRP is connected with its specific conformation. The influence of conformation change (unfolding) on the attachment process was analysed by unfolding the HRP prior to attachment. The unfolding of the HRP was done with boiling in buffer solution for 30 minutes after which all activity was destroyed. After that the protein was attached on PIII-treated and untreated polyethylene surfaces. The amount of the attached and covalently attached inactive protein was found to be similar as for active protein. Therefore, the conformation of HRP protein does not play role in the attachment process on either untreated or PIII-treated polyethylene surface.

The amount of attached protein of PIII-treatment increases with time and shows saturation (Figure 18(d)). The amount of covalently attached protein increases with the time of PIII treatment and also shows saturation. The concentration of free radicals increases in the same range of PIII treatment times. A perfect correlation between the amount of attached protein and the measured free radical concentration is not observed because the measured free radical concentration includes radicals in the bulk of the polyethylene. Only surface free radicals are effective in the attachment process. This difference in roles of the two types of radicals has the effect of a saturation in the protein amount earlier than the saturation of the free radical concentration. The saturation of the amount of protein covalently attached is achieved after about 10^{15} ions/cm^2 fluence of ion beam.

The ability to attach a protein with chemical bonds to PIII-treated polyethylene remains after long time. To investigate the aging effect of PIII treatment, the polyethylene samples were treated and stored under laboratory conditions (in a closed dark container, stabilized at a temperature of 23°C and at 70% relative humidity) for two years. The amount of attached protein on freshly prepared PIII surface is slightly higher than on the aged PIII-treated surface (Table 1). The amount of covalently bonded protein on a 2-year-old PIII-treated polyethylene surface and on a freshly treated surface is the same within error bars. Together with protein attachment, the ATR FTIR spectra and the surface energy of PIII-treated samples do not show significant changes during two years of storage after a stabilization in first month after PIII treatment. Therefore, the surface remains active to covalent attachment of protein after at least two years of storage.

Table 1: Amount of attached HRP protein (determined from FTIR ATR using (5)) on UHMWPE treated by PIII with 20 keV energy Nitrogen ions at 10^{16} ions/cm^2 fluence.

Substrate	As attached	Washed in SDS
Untreated	0.0093 ± 0.0014	0.0005 ± 0.0007
PIII treated, new	0.0171 ± 0.0001	0.0095 ± 0.0001
PIII treated, after 2 years	0.0136 ± 0.0004	0.0085 ± 0.0021

3.7. *Functionalization of the Polyethylene Surface and Protein Attachment/Influence of Oxygen Containing Groups on Covalent Attachment of Protein.*

In this section, we analyse previous explanations of the attachment of protein on surfaces that have been treated by ions, electrons, or ionising radiation. If the attachment of protein on a PIII-treated surface is provided by chemical bonds, which are formed between protein molecules and surface active groups during incubation of the treated polymer in a protein solution, the surface activity can be simulated by artificially introducing active groups into the surface layer during synthesis of the polymer film. The conditions of incubation are not specific as described above; therefore, the reaction (or reactions) must be realised easy. It means that the groups of modified layer must be active enough to take part in chemical reaction with protein under normal conditions of soaking. The untreated polyethylene does not provide the chemical bonds, the active groups in the surface of polyethylene appear after modification, therefore the analysis of new groups appeared after PIII can be used for creation of simulated active surface layer to protein attachment.

To investigate the groups responsible for protein attachment, the modified polyethylene surface was simulated by introducing selected chemically active groups. It is well documented that oxygen containing groups such as carbonyl, carboxyl, aldehyde, and hydroxyl can provide chemical bonds with protein molecules [54]. As described above, the PIII-modified layer of polyethylene contains a number of oxygen containing groups that appear as the result of free radical reactions with atmospheric oxygen after exposure of the treated samples in air. The presence of such active groups is considered in the literature as a reason for the strong adhesion of modified polyethylene surfaces to epoxy and polyurethane adhesives. The reactions responsible are between epoxy and isocyanate groups of the adhesive with carboxyl and hydroxyl groups of the modified polyethylene [71] in the interface region. Similar reactions can be expected to be responsible for the covalent protein attachment.

The presence of hydroxyl, carboxyl, and aldehyde groups on the polyethylene surface after PIII would give rise to a potential for a reaction between the amine group of Lysine and these oxygen containing groups:

$$\begin{gathered}\text{R–OH} + \text{H}_2\text{N-Protein} \longrightarrow \text{R–NH-Protein} + \text{H}_2\text{O}\\ \text{R–COOH} + \text{H}_2\text{N-Protein} \longrightarrow \text{R–CO–NH-Protein} + \text{H}_2\text{O}\\ \text{R–COH} + \text{H}_2\text{N-Protein} \longrightarrow \text{R–CH=N-Protein} + \text{H}_2\text{O}\end{gathered} \tag{7}$$

These reactions are used to bind HRP to specific compounds in a number of biotechnological tools [3, 5, 54, 95, 102].

The reaction of carboxyl group is more probable due to higher activity of carboxyl group with amine than the activity of hydroxyl or aldehyde groups with amine. The carboxyl groups can be introduced in a polymer surface by means of copolymerisation reactions without any need for radiation damage to the polyethylene. To prove the concept of using carboxyl-amine reactions for protein immobilisation, we intentionally introduced active carboxyl groups into polyethylene.

The copolymer of ethylene and methacrilyc acid with 17 wt% concentration of methacrylic acid monomer was used as a model surface. The MMA concentration corresponds to the theoretical density of 1 carboxyl group per 14 methylene groups in the copolymer. The samples were moulded between hot plates covered by Teflon film from granules of copolymer. After moulding, the surface of the copolymer was treated with ethanol, acetone, and water. The concentration of residual Teflon macromolecules on the copolymer surface after moulding was monitored by ATR-FTIR spectra and found to be undetectable. The ratio of the $\nu(C{=}O) = 1690\,cm^{-1}$ from the carboxyl group and the $\nu(CH_2) = 2917\,cm^{-1}$ lines of the polyethylene absorbance was found to depend on solvent treatment (ethanol, acetone, and water) after moulding. The hydrophilic solvent causes slightly higher concentration of carboxyl groups in the surface layer observed as a higher intensity of $\nu(C{=}O)$ line than freshly moulded or after hydrophobic solvent treatment (Table 2). However, even after treatment with the hydrophobic solvent toluene, the surface layer of the moulded film still contains carboxyl groups, although somewhat reduced in concentration. The activity of carboxyl groups was confirmed by a test reaction with sodium hydroxide which causes the appearance of a sodium carboxylate line at $1574\,cm^{-1}$. Therefore, the carboxyl groups on the surface of the moulded film are active. The surface of polyethylene with introduced carboxyl groups becomes slightly hydrophilic, the water contact angle decreasing from 90° for the as received polyethylene to 88° for the copolymer.

The activated polyethylene samples were soaked in protein solution as described above and tested by FTIR ATR spectra and protein activity. The amount of attached HRP molecules on the surface with carboxyl groups is lower than on untreated polyethylene surface. After washing with detergents, the amount of HRP molecules decreased below the level for untreated polyethylene. Therefore, the presence of active carboxylic groups in a copolymer does not provide a covalent attachment of HRP.

The minimisation of the influence of oxygen-containing groups in PIII-treated samples could be realised in an experiment in which a protein is attached on the surface that has never had contact with air after the PIII treatment. In a realisation of this experiment, the protein solution was placed in a vacuum chamber termed the "chemical vacuum chamber," separate but connected to, the plasma treatment chamber and this chamber was pumped down to about 20 Torr pressure when water starts to boil. The chemical chamber was then vented with nitrogen up to atmospheric pressure. The procedure of pumping and venting was repeated 5 times. Then the container with protein solution was closed and the chemical vacuum chamber was pumped down to 10^{-3} mTorr.

The PIII-treated sample of polyethylene was moved from the plasma chamber into the chemical chamber under a vacuum of 10^{-3} mTorr by means of an arm manipulator. Then the chemical chamber was isolated from the plasma chamber, vented with pure nitrogen up to either a partial vacuum (20 mTorr) or 760 Torr and the container with protein solution was opened into the chemical chamber. The sample was immersed in the protein solution and soaked there overnight. After that, the chamber was vented and opened to air and a washing procedure to remove loosely bound protein was applied. Due to the exclusion of oxygen from the freshly treated PIII-treated sample until protein was applied, the oxygen-containing group concentration is expected to be significantly less than in the normal process in which samples are exposed to air after PIII treatment (see Section 3.1) and the concentration of free radicals is expected to be higher.

The amount of attached protein in partial vacuum (20 mTorr of nitrogen) and in nitrogen atmosphere (760 Torr) was found to be as high as for a PIII-treated sample exposed to air as usual. The attached protein remains on these surfaces after all detergent washing, showing that it is covalently bound.

These experiments confirm the copolymer experiments described above and confirm that the presence of carboxyl groups on the surface is not responsible for protein attachment and cannot cause covalent bonding of protein by means of carboxyl groups on the surface reacting with an amine group of the protein.

The activity of other groups such as aldehyde, hydroxide, lactone, carbonyl and others is less than for carboxyl, and the reactions of these groups with amine groups of amino acid residuals has a smaller probability. For example, the attachment of HRP molecules on PMMA with a high concentration of ester groups, on polyamide with high concentration of amide groups, on PEEK with high concentration of ester and carbonyl groups, is lower or the same as for untreated polyethylene [42, 103]. The effect of carbon-carbon unsaturated groups on protein attachment can be studied with polystyrene which contains aromatic rings. As shown above, the attachment of protein on untreated polystyrene is low [41]. A full analysis of the active groups present in a selection of representative polymers is shown in Table 3.

Therefore, the presence of active oxygen containing and unsaturated groups in the surface layer cannot cause high attachment of the protein as well as covalent bonding of protein and the appearance of such groups in the surface layer of PIII-modified polyethylene is not the reason of high attachment of protein and covalent bonding of protein molecules to the surface (Table 3).

The surface of PIII-modified polyethylene contains free radicals with a high concentration. The free radicals disappear over time due to their high activity in accepting any mobile atom or molecule capable of reacting with it from the environment. Free radicals have the ability to migrate along macromolecules and between macromolecular chains from the surface layer into the bulk. At the same time, free radicals are stabilized by the presence of condensed aromatic rings due to the delocalisation of electrons on pi orbitals in aromatic structures. Also free radicals are also stabilized by the presence of nitroxyl groups and thiazyl groups. The stabilization of free radicals is increased by steric hindrance effects. This applies when the free radical belongs to a group, which is surrounded by neighbouring groups in such a way that any other molecule cannot come close to the free radical.

All these mechanisms are discussed in the literature [83–85]. In our experiments on several polymers, the ESR signal of free radicals remains for a long time (months) after PIII treatment.

Active free radicals are present on the surface of polymers after PIII treatment. This was proved in previous experiments on ion beam modified PTFE [104], when the free radicals from modified PTFE caused crosslinking reaction in thick layer of a resin placed on the PTFE surface. The free radicals reactions on modified polymer surface have been proposed as a mechanism for protein attachment [105].

Free radicals can take part in the chemical reactions with protein molecules and provide the formation of chemical bonds between the modified surface layer of a polymer and an attached protein. However, a synthesis of initial polymer macromolecules with active free radicals in the surface layer appears not to be possible.

FTIR analysis of the quantity of HRP showed that the amount of protein attached to a sample exposed only to vacuum is the same as for air-exposed sample (Table 4). However, the activity of protein is less in a sample exposed in vacuum, than for the air-exposed sample. The deconvolution of the Amide I line shows that the conformation is different for protein attached to a surface in air and in vacuum (Figure 19). The intensity of 1638 cm^{-1} line, attributed to disordered chains, is higher for the vacuum attached protein. In addition, the spectrum to spectrum deviation for different samples is stronger for samples that had protein attached in vacuum. Such a strong deviation implies that the protein conformation is random. Such random conformation variations suggest that the conformation is subject to change by a random factor such as a high concentration of free radicals randomly distributed on the surface. A high concentration of free radicals will lead to more than one covalent bond forming between the molecule and the surface. This multiple bond formation will have the effect of causing both the random conformation changes and the loss of protein activity through excessive unfolding.

In summary, there is a significant body of evidence that free radicals are responsible for the formation of the observed covalent bonds between protein and a PIII-modified surface.

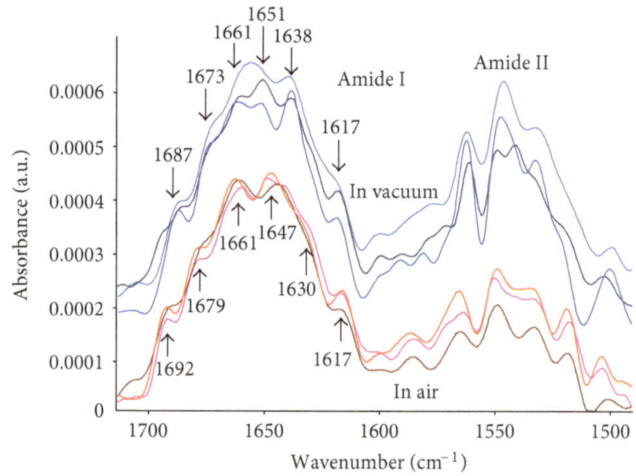

FIGURE 19: Self-deconvoluted FTIR ATR spectra of HRP attached on PIII-treated LDPE exposed to air (three bottom spectra) and vacuum (three top spectra) for three different samples of each treatment. The spectrum to spectrum deviation for different samples is stronger for samples that had protein attached in vacuum (top spectra).

3.8. Blocking of Covalent Attachment to PIII-Treated Surfaces. If free radicals are responsible for covalent attachment, it should be possible to block the activity of free radicals selectively by using specific blocking agents that are applied after the PIII treatment and before the protein attachment.

It was found that covalent attachment of protein on PIII-treated polyethylene can be blocked by the application of specific low molecular weight components. In experiment, the PIII modified polyethylene surface was treated by Styrene, Hexene, polytetrahydrofuran (PTHF), Ethylenediamine, Benzyl mercaptan, and 2,2,6,6-Tetramethylpiperidine 1-oxyl (TEMPO) in different solvents (toluene, acetone, and ethanol). After treatment, the polyethylene samples were washed with pure solvents to remove non-bonded blocking molecules. The presence of the applied blocking agents on the polyethylene surface was monitored by FTIR ATR spectra using specific group lines of the attached molecules. The control experiment with initial polyethylene showed that the blocking molecules do not stick to the unmodified surface and the washing procedure is sufficient to remove all unbounded blocking molecules. All blocking agents are observed as attached to the PIII-treated surface. After blocking, the protein was attached on the treated polyethylene surface as described above. The amount of attached protein before and after SDS detergent washing by FTIR ATR spectra is shown in Table 5.

The amount of attached protein depends on the details of the intermolecular interactions between protein molecules and the blocked surface, which in turn depends on the blocking agent. The adsorption of hydrocarbon compounds (hexene and styrene) on a PIII-modified surface does not change the amount of attached protein very much. The presence of polar groups in the blocking molecule (e.g., ethylenediamine, polytetrahydrofurane, and TEMPO) decreases the amount of the attached protein. This trend is in accordance with known data on a protein attachment on hydrophobic surfaces [49].

The amount of covalently attached protein, as tested by SDS washing, is the same on adsorbed hexene and styrene layers as it is on the unblocked PIII-treated surface. The amount of covalently attached protein decreases on surfaces blocked with ethylenediamine and PTHF. The lowest amount of covalently bonded protein is observed on the surfaces blocked with adsorbed TEMPO and Benzyl mercaptan.

None of the blocking molecules tested are expected to have a specific chemical activity to the protein once attached on the surface and the chemical attachment of the protein molecules to the blocked surface is therefore not expected. Blocking agents that contain free radicals may show a different behaviour on a surface that contains free radicals. Hexene and styrene molecules contain carbon double bonds

TABLE 2: Amount of HRP attached protein (see (5)) on untreated and PIII-treated UHMWPE and on copolymer of polyethylene and methancrylic acid (co-PE-MMA) before and after washing in detergents. The HRP protein attachment was done on PIII-treated sample in air, in nitrogen at low pressure (30 Torr), and high pressure (760 Torr). Carbonyl group relative concentration is measured by intensity ratio of 1691 cm^{-1} line and 1462 cm^{-1} line in FTIR ATR spectra. The average error bar for the protein amount is 0.0010.

Sample description	Amount of attached after incubation	Amount after SDS	Amount after Triton	Amount after Tween 20	C=O concentration before attachment
Untreated	0.0087	0.0041	0.0018	0.0023	~0
PIII, in air	0.0198	0.0143	0.0142	0.0167	0.14
PIII, in N_2, 30 Torr	0.0182	0.0161	0.0106	0.0100	~0
PIII, in N_2, 760 Torr	0.0255	0.0147	0.0186	0.0180	~0
co-PE-MMA, pressed	0.0086	0	0.0033	0.0024	0.46
co-PE-MMA, pressed and ethanol washed	0.0057	0	0.0014	0.0029	0.53

TABLE 3: Chemical groups and polymer representatives available for covalent attachment of protein.

Active chemical group	Polymer representative	Is a protein covalently attached?
Methylene, $-CH_2-$	Polyethylene	No
Double carbon bond, -C=C-	Polystyrene	No
Hydroxyl, -OH	Polyvinyl alcohol	No
Ether, C–O	Polyethylene terephtalate	No
Carbonyl, C=O	Polyethylene terephtalate	No
Aldehyde, CH=O	Polyacrolein	No
Carboxyl, -COOH	Polymethacrylic acid	No
Free radical, R•	No known example	?
Combination of all these groups	PIII treatment of polyethylene	Yes

TABLE 4: Amount (see (5)) and catalytic activity of HRP protein on PIII-modified LDPE attached in air and in vacuum.

	Attachment on air	Attachment in vacuum
Protein amount as attached	0.020 ± 0.001	0.023 ± 0.001
Activity of protein	0.54 ± 0.06	0.45 ± 0.02

which open in the presence of free radicals to give a possibility of polymerisation to form a polyhexene or polystyrene layer

$$\text{R–CH=CH}_2 + {}^{\bullet}\text{R}' \longrightarrow \text{R–CHR}'\text{–CH}_2{}^{\bullet} \quad (8)$$

The final radical on the right hand side can be used for the next reaction with a new molecule of styrene or hexene or the radical could be kept and used for the protein attachment. Also, one layer of polystyrene or polyhexene macromolecules synthesised on the surface is able to transfer a free radical along the macromolecule to the new surface above the attached layer

$$\text{R–CH}^{\bullet}\text{–CH}_2\text{–R}' \longrightarrow \text{R–CH}_2\text{–CH}^{\bullet}\text{–R}' \quad (9)$$

Following this scheme, the hexene and styrene cannot block the covalent attachment of the protein, in agreement with experimental observation.

Ethylenediamine and PTHF contain oxygen or nitrogen in backbone chain of the molecule. In the presence of free radicals, these molecules can be attached by the hydrocarbon part of the molecule to the surface, but the oxygen and nitrogen atoms in these molecules are likely to be separated from the parent molecule in the presence of a free radical and the free radical cannot be kept in the blocking molecule

$$\text{R–CH}^{\bullet}\text{–CH}_2\text{–O–R}' \longrightarrow \text{R–CH=CH}_2 + {}^{\bullet}\text{O–R}' \quad (10)$$

Therefore, these molecules cannot transfer a free radical through the layer. Therefore, after attachment of these molecules, the protein attachment becomes impossible. These two molecules (Ethylenediamine and PTHF) can partially block the surface against the protein attachment, which is observed in experiment.

The highest blocking ability is observed for TEMPO and benzyl mercaptan molecules. TEMPO contains a free radical stabilized by aromatic ring conjugated with nitroxyl group, but the activity of the free radical in TEMPO is high enough to cause free radical reactions in chemical processing. Therefore, the attachment of TEMPO to PIII-modified surface is expected to be a reaction between two free radicals—one from TEMPO and one from the surface

$$\text{R}^{\bullet} + {}^{\bullet}\text{O–R}' \longrightarrow \text{R–O–R}' \quad (11)$$

After attachment of TEMPO the PIII-modified surface does not have free radicals and the protein attachment is blocked completely. The same reason is with benzyl mercaptan molecules, where S–H group is very active to free radicals

$$2\text{R}^{\bullet} + \text{HS–R}' \longrightarrow \text{R–H} + \text{R–S–R}' \quad (12)$$

Table 5: Amount of attached HRP protein (see (5)) on PIII-treated UHMWPE with various blocking agents of the surface. Detergent SDS was applied for analysis of covalently attached protein. The average error bar for the protein amount is 0.0010.

Blocking agent	Formula	As attached	After SDS washing
No blocking		0.0164	0.0113
Hexene	$CH_3(CH_2)_3CH{=}CH_2$	0.0162	0.0090
Styrene	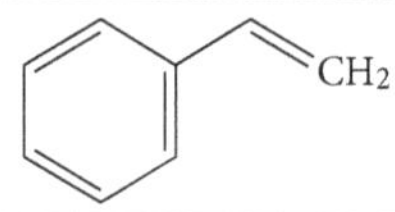	0.0156	0.0098
Ethylenediamine	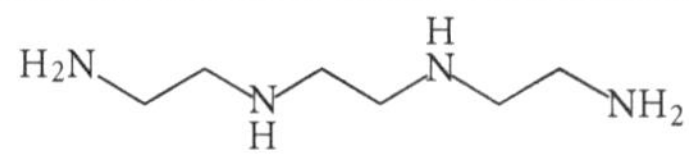	0.0122	0.0049
Polytetrahydrofuran (PTHF)	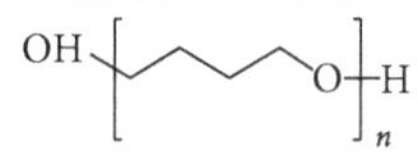	0.0102	0.0060
TEMPO	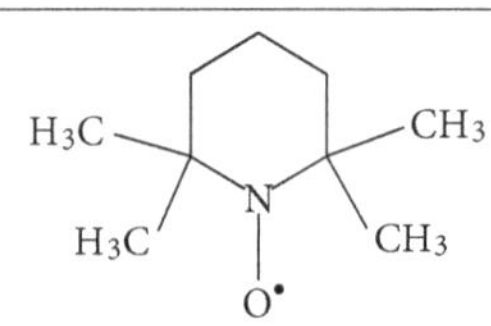	0.0119	0.0015
Benzyl mercaptan	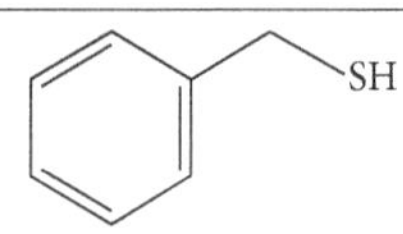	0.0078	0.0018

As a result, the free radicals on the surface react with benzyl mercaptan and TEMPO that renders the modified polyethylene surface to be inactive for protein attachment.

Therefore, the reactions of specific blockers support the free radical mechanism for the covalent binding of protein to PIII-modified surfaces.

3.9. Attachment of Polyamino Acids. This study was undertaken to determine which chemical groups in a protein take part in the covalent bonding to a PIII-modified surface via a free radical. Free radicals are able to react with a wide range of molecules. From this point of view, it is likely that all amino acid residues in a protein molecule can take part in covalent bonding with a PIII-treated surface. One chemical bond is enough to give a covalent attachment of protein molecule. To confirm that the covalent binding is possible via many different types of amino acid residues, we attached a number of different polyamino acids on PIII-treated polyethylene. In this way, we simulated by attachment of selected amino acid residues when they are present in a protein molecule.

The activity of polyethylene surface after ion beam implantation to free alanine and leucine was observed earlier [106]. But due to their low molecular mass, it is possible that individual amino acids could diffuse into the bulk. To confirm that the reaction is on the surface, we used polyamino acids of high molecular mass to exclude diffusion into the bulk. In 20 of the most common amino acids, there are 7 different chemically active groups present in the side chains (methyl, aromatic ring, hydroxyl, amine, mercapto, carboxyl, and pyridine). Therefore, the activity of 20 amino acids can be simulated by attachment of 7 different polyamino acids, each having one of the 7 different side chain groups.

The attachment of polyamino acids was carried out on untreated and PIII-treated polyethylene and tested with FTIR ATR spectroscopy. The molecular mass of polyamino acids was selected as to be as close as possible to the molecular mass of HRP. All polyamino acids were attached from aqueous buffer solution, except Poly-l-tryptophan which has limited solubility in aqueous solution and was attached from acetone solution. The SDS washing procedure to test for covalent attachment was the same as for protein attachment except for Poly-l-tryptophan, which was washed with pure solvent only. The results of attachment experiments are presented in Table 6.

As can be seen from Table 6, not all polyamino acids are well attached. This means that the end groups (base and acid) and the amide backbone groups presented in all amino acids can be excluded from consideration as active binding groups, and the binding must take place via a side group.

An amount of attached Poly-l-histidine and Poly-l-lysine is high both before and after SDS washing. This is similar to the behaviour observed for HRP on the PIII-treated polyethylene. Poly-l-glycine is a hydrophobic polyamino acid and the amount of Poly-l-glycine present both before and after washing is lower than the amount of attached Poly-l-histidine and Poly-l-lysine. This expected since the PIII-treated polyethylene is mildly hydrophilic. However, some Poly-l-glycine molecules remain after detergent washing on the PIII-treated surface, showing that covalent bonding takes place.

Table 6: Amount of polyamino acids (see (5)) on PIII-treated polyethylene immediately after incubation (as attached) and after SDS washing (except for Poly-l-tryptophan, Poly-L-arginine, Poly-DL-alanine, and Poly-L-isoleucine as described in the text). The average error bar for the polyamino acid amount is 0.0005.

Aminoacid	Polyaminoacid	Side-chain groups	As attached	After detergent washing
Glycine	Poly-L-glycine (in buffer)	$-CH_2-$	0.0092	0.0025
Alanine	Poly-DL-alanine (in acetone)	$-CH_3$	0.0074	0.0074
Isoleucine	Poly-L-isoleucine (in acetone)		0.016	0.016
Similar to:				
Leucine				
Valine				
Proline				
Lysine	Poly-l-lysine (in buffer)	$-CH_2-$	0.0077	0.0073
Arginine	Poly-L-arginine (in DMFA)	$-NH_2$	0.014	0.014
Histidine	Poly-l-histidine (in buffer)	-NH-	0.016	0.013
		=N-		
		-CH=		
Tryptophan	Poly-l-tryptophan (in acetone)	-NH-	0.0171	0.0087
		-CH=		
Tyrosine	Poly-l-tyrosine (in buffer)	-OH	0.0022	0.0002
Threonine	Poly-L-threonine (in acetone)	-CH=	0.011	0.011
Glutamic acid	Poly-l-glutamic acid (in buffer)	$-CH_2-$	0.0002	0.0002
		-COOH		
Similar to:				
Aspartic acid				
Methionine	Poly-L-methionine (in acetone)	$-CH_2-$	0.025	0.025
		-SH		
Similar to: cystein				

Poly-l-tryptophan, Poly-L-methionine, Poly-L-threonine, Poly-L-isoleucine, and Poly-DL-alanine were attached from acetone solution. In this case, the physical interactions between the surface and these molecules are quite different from those that would apply in aqueous solution due to presence of acetone molecules. However the attachment is provided by chemical bonds on PIII-treated surface should be the same, independent of the environment. The chemical bonding will be covalent since no physical interactions will be strong enough to withstand washing in pure acetone.

Poly-l-glutamic acid has a low attachment ability on the PIII-treated surface. The PIII-treated polyethylene has acid groups on the surface as discussed in Section 3.1. In buffer solution, the acid groups are converted to ionic form and prevent close contact of the surface with acidic molecules from solution. Therefore, it is likely that Poly-l-glutamic acid molecules cannot come close enough to the surface to allow a chemical reaction with free radicals.

Poly-l-tyrosine was attached from a basic solution due to its low solubility in a pH neutral solution. Because of the presence of carboxyl acid groups on the surface and sodium ions in solution, the Poly-l-tyrosine molecules have the same problem as Poly-l-glutamic acid to achieve a sufficiently close interaction with the surface to achieve any kind of chemical interaction. This could be the reason why Poly-l-tyrosine shows low attachment ability on the PIII-treated surface. Note, however, that Poly-l-tyrosine shows high attachment ability on the untreated polyethylene surface where ionic interactions near the surface do not play a major role. Besides, Poly-L-threonine is strongly attached from acetone solution.

A mercapto group reaction with PIII-treated polyethylene surface was observed at poly-L-Methionine attachment. Methionine and Cystein –SH groups are expected to be involved in chemical reaction with free radicals of PIII-modified surface.

In summary, all polyamino acids are potentially capable of attachment to the PIII-treated surface. The low attachment that was observed in specific cases we explain by specific ionic interactions in the layer of buffer near the surface. Such a universal behaviour of amino acids residues with the PIII-modified surface is provided by the presence of active free radicals. However, in a protein molecule, the ability of an individual amino acid residue to take part in chemical bonding with the PIII-treated surface depends also on the conformation of the protein and on the orientation of the protein molecule relative to the surface.

The universal character of protein attachment to free radicals could be extended to various methods of radiation damage of polymers, if it can be demonstrated that these methods provide a sufficient concentration of active free radicals on or near the surface. In that case the mechanism of protein attachment described in this work could be applied

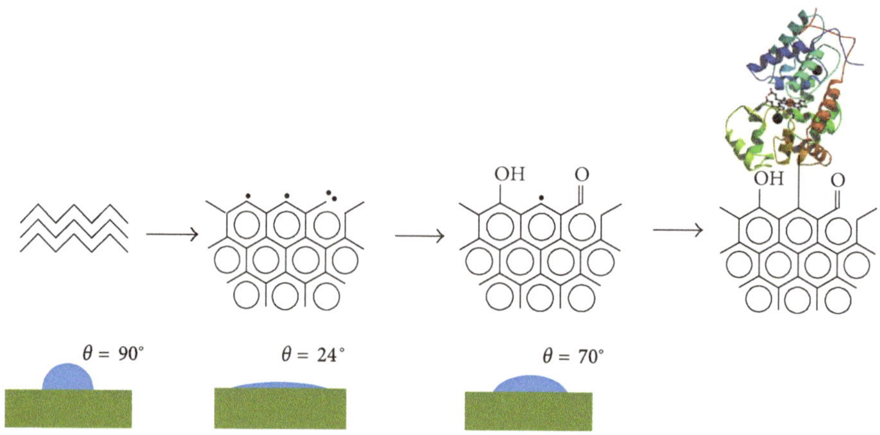

FIGURE 20: Stages of protein attachment: untreated polyethylene with high contact angle; PIII-treated polyethylene with high concentration of free radicals and low contact angle; aged PIII modified polyethylene with oxygen-containing groups and residual free radicals stabilised on π-electrons; protein is bounded to residual free radicals.

to damage by glow discharge plasma, UV light irradiation, electron beam modification, X-ray modification, γ-irradiation, and mechanodestruction (polishing and scratching) of carbon-containing polymers as well carbon deposition methods that create carbon structures (such as graphite clusters, carbon nanotubes and graphene) with stabilised free radicals. The stages of PIII treatment of polyethylene and protein attachment are presented in Figure 20.

4. Conclusion

Plasma immersion ion implantation is a type of ion beam implantation and produces structural changes in a thin surface layer of polyethylene. These changes include the following:

(i) a carbonisation process in which unsaturated groups containing double bonds, conjugated double bonds, aromatic rings, condensed aromatic rings in increasing numbers that eventually form graphitic islands;

(ii) appearance of active free radicals and free radicals that show long-term stability;

(iii) appearance of oxygen-containing groups such as carboxyl, carbonyl, aldehyde, and hydroxyl groups after exposure of the treated sample to air;

(iv) appearance of nitrogen-containing groups during implantation and after exposure of the treated sample to air;

(v) an increase in surface energy that coincides with the appearance of free radicals and decreases with storage time as the free radicals decay and oxygen-containing groups appear;

(vi) a wavelike morphology of the surface.

The amount of protein attached on a PIII-treated surface is up to 2 times higher than on an untreated surface. The attachment on the PIII-treated surface is through the formation of covalent bonds between the protein molecule and the modified surface, while the attachment on the untreated surface is through physical intermolecular interactions.

The covalent bonds between the protein molecule and the modified surface are formed by a reaction with active free radicals, which are preserved in conjugated structures due to delocalisation of unpaired free electrons. The blocking of the modified surface with selected molecules eliminates free radicals or prevents their migration, in turn preventing the covalent attachment of protein.

The protein molecule has a number of active amino acid residues available for bonding to free radicals at the surface. This means that the PIII-treated surface can provide a covalent attachment for all kinds of proteins provided that the protein molecule is able to come close enough to establish a chemical bond. The universal character of protein attachment to free radicals could be extended to various methods of radiation damage of polymers, if it can be demonstrated that these methods provide a sufficient concentration of active free radicals on or near the surface.

The native conformation of attached protein is retained on a PIII-treated surface due to hydrophilic interactions at the interface. However, a high concentration of free radicals on the surface can give rise to multiple covalent bonds with the protein molecule that destroy the native conformation with a consequent loss of catalytic activity. Therefore, the retention of protein conformation (and activity) requires an optimisation of the free radical concentration on the surface.

Acknowledgments

Authors would like to acknowledge the contribution of Helen Smith and Robert Thompson, who took part in experiments with polyamino acids and proteins.

References

[1] A. Schmid, J. S. Dordick, B. Hauer, A. Kiener, M. Wubbolts, and B. Witholt, "Industrial biocatalysis today and tomorrow," *Nature*, vol. 409, no. 6817, pp. 258–268, 2001.

[2] R. M. Ottenbrite, Ed., *Frontiers in Biomedical Polymer Applications*, Technomic Publishing Company, Lancaster, UK, 1998.

[3] B. J. Ryan, N. Carolan, and C. Fagain, "Horseradish and soybean peroxidases: comparable tools for alternative niches?" *Trends in Biotechnology*, vol. 24, no. 8, pp. 355–363, 2006.

[4] S. P. Shukla and S. Devi, "Covalent coupling of peroxidase to a copolymer of acrylamide (AAm)-2-hydroxyethyl methaacrylate (HEMA) and its use in phenol oxidation," *Process Biochemistry*, vol. 40, no. 1, pp. 147–154, 2005.

[5] K. F. Fernandes, C. S. Lima, H. Pinho, and C. H. Collins, "Immobilization of horseradish peroxidase onto polyaniline polymers," *Process Biochemistry*, vol. 38, no. 9, pp. 1379–1384, 2003.

[6] J. D. Whittle, N. A. Bullett, R. D. Short, C. W. I. Douglas, A. P. Hollander, and J. Davies, "Adsorption of vitronectin, collagen and immunoglobulin-G to plasma polymer surfaces by enzyme linked immunosorbent assay (ELISA)," *Journal of Materials Chemistry*, vol. 12, no. 9, pp. 2726–2732, 2002.

[7] J. L. Bohnert, B. C. Fowler, T. A. Horbett, and A. S. Hoffman, "Plasma gas discharge deposited fluorocarbon polymers exhibit reduced elutability of adsorbed albumin and fibrinogen," *Journal of Biomaterials Science*, vol. 1, no. 4, pp. 279–297, 1990.

[8] A. Dekker, K. Reitsma, T. Beugeling, A. Bantjes, J. Feijen, and W. G. van Aken, "Adhesion of endothelial cells and adsorption of serum proteins on gas plasma-treated polytetrafluoroethylene," *Biomaterials*, vol. 12, no. 2, pp. 130–138, 1991.

[9] T. Chandy, G. S. Das, R. F. Wilson, and G. H. R. Rao, "Use of plasma glow for surface-engineering biomolecules to enhance bloodcompatibility of Dacron and PTFE vascular prosthesis," *Biomaterials*, vol. 21, no. 7, pp. 699–712, 2000.

[10] F. Poncin-Epaillard and G. Legeay, "Surface engineering of biomaterials with plasma techniques," *Journal of Biomaterials Science*, vol. 14, no. 10, pp. 1005–1028, 2003.

[11] U. König, M. Nitschke, A. Menning et al., "Plasma modification of polytetrafluoroethylene for immobilization of the fibrinolytic protein urokinase," *Surface and Coatings Technology*, vol. 116–119, pp. 1011–1015, 1999.

[12] P. K. Chu, J. Y. Chena, L. P. Wang, and N. Huang, "Plasma-surface modification of biomaterials," *Materials Science and Engineering R*, vol. 36, pp. 143–206, 2002.

[13] M. M. Browne, G. V. Lubarsky, M. R. Davidson, and R. H. Bradley, "Protein adsorption onto polystyrene surfaces studied by XPS and AFM," *Surface Science*, vol. 553, no. 1–3, pp. 155–167, 2004.

[14] V. N. Vasilets, A. V. Kuznetsov, and V. I. Sevastianov, "Vacuum ultraviolet treatment of polyethylene to change surface properties and characteristics of protein adsorption," *Journal of Biomedical Materials Research A*, vol. 69, no. 3, pp. 428–435, 2004.

[15] K. Yanagisawa, T. N. Murakami, Y. Tokuoka, A. Ochiai, M. Takahashi, and N. Kawashima, "Immobilization and enzymatic activity of glucose oxidase on polystyrene surface modified with ozone aeration and UV irradiation in distilled water and/or aqueous ammonia solution," *Colloids and Surfaces B*, vol. 48, no. 1, pp. 67–71, 2006.

[16] G. V. Lubarsky, M. M. Browne, S. A. Mitchell, M. R. Davidson, and R. H. Bradley, "The influence of electrostatic forces on protein adsorption," *Colloids and Surfaces B*, vol. 44, no. 1, pp. 56–63, 2005.

[17] M. Manso, A. Valsesia, M. Lejeune, D. Gilliland, G. Ceccone, and F. Rossi, "Tailoring surface properties of biomedical polymers by implantation of Ar and He ions," *Acta Biomaterialia*, vol. 1, no. 4, pp. 431–440, 2005.

[18] M. Manso, C. R. Navas, D. Gilliland, P. G. Ruiz, and F. Rossi, "Cellular response to oxygen containing biomedical polymers modified by Ar and He implantation," *Acta Biomaterialia*, vol. 3, no. 5, pp. 735–743, 2007.

[19] L. Bačáková, V. Švorčík, V. Rybka et al., "Adhesion and proliferation of cultured human aortic smooth muscle cells on polystyrene implanted with N^+, F^+ and Ar^+ ions: correlation with polymer surface polarity and carbonization," *Biomaterials*, vol. 17, no. 11, pp. 1121–1126, 1996.

[20] K. Rockova-Hlavackova, V. Svorcik, L. Bacakova, B. Dvorankova, J. Heitz, and V. Hnatowicz, "Bio-compatibility of ion beam-modified and RGD-grafted polyethylene," *Nuclear Instruments and Methods in Physics Research B*, vol. 225, pp. 275–282, 2004.

[21] M. Bellion, L. Santen, H. Mantz et al., "Protein adsorption on tailored substrates: long-range forces and conformational changes," *Journal of Physics Condensed Matter*, vol. 20, no. 40, Article ID 404226, 2008.

[22] A. Ladiwala, F. Xia, Q. Luo, C. M. Breneman, and S. M. Cramer, "Investigation of protein retention and selectivity in HIC systems using quantitative structure retention relationship models," *Biotechnology and Bioengineering*, vol. 93, no. 5, pp. 836–850, 2006.

[23] P. M. Biesheuvel, F. A. M. Leermakers, and M. A. C. Stuart, "Self-consistent field theory of protein adsorption in a non-Gaussian polyelectrolyte brush," *Physical Review E*, vol. 73, no. 1, Article ID 011802, 2006.

[24] H. Noh and E. A. Vogler, "Volumetric interpretation of protein adsorption: mass and energy balance for albumin adsorption to particulate adsorbents with incrementally increasing hydrophilicity," *Biomaterials*, vol. 27, no. 34, pp. 5801–5812, 2006.

[25] N. Barnthip, P. Parhi, A. Golas, and E. A. Vogler, "Volumetric interpretation of protein adsorption: kinetics of protein-adsorption competition from binary solution," *Biomaterials*, vol. 30, no. 33, pp. 6495–6513, 2009.

[26] I. Szleifer, "Protein adsorption on surfaces with grafted polymers: a theoretical approach," *Biophysical Journal*, vol. 72, no. 2 I, pp. 595–612, 1997.

[27] F. Fang, J. Satulovsky, and I. Szleifer, "Kinetics of protein adsorption and desorption on surfaces with grafted polymers," *Biophysical Journal*, vol. 89, no. 3, pp. 1516–1533, 2005.

[28] J. Black and G. Hastings, Eds., *Handbook of Biomaterial Properties*, Chapman and Hall, London, UK, 1998.

[29] J. C. Lin and S. L. Cooper, "Surface characterization and ex vivo blood compatibility study of plasma modified small diameter tubing: effect of sulphur dioxide and hexamethyl disiloxane plasmas," *Biomaterials*, vol. 16, no. 13, pp. 1017–1023, 1995.

[30] A. V. Kondyurin, M. F. Maitz, and I. V. Kondyurina, "Cell growth on plasma immersion ion implanted polymer surfaces, abstract," in *Proceedings of the E-MRS European Materials Conference*, MRS, Warsaw, Poland, September 2004.

[31] R. M. France and R. D. Short, "Plasma treatment of polymers effects of energy transfer from an argon plasma on the surface chemistry of poly(styrene), low density poly(ethylene), poly(propylene) and poly(ethylene terephthalate)," *Journal of the Chemical Society*, vol. 93, no. 17, pp. 3173–3178, 1997.

[32] E. Selli, G. Mazzone, C. Oliva et al., "Characterisation of poly(ethylene terephthalate) and cotton fibres after cold SF6 plasma treatment," *Journal of Materials Chemistry*, vol. 11, no. 8, pp. 1985–1991, 2001.

[33] S. W. Lee, J. W. Hong, M. Y. Wye, J. H. Kim, H. J. Kang, and Y. S. Lee, "Surface modification and adhesion improvement of PTFE film by ion beam irradiation," *Nuclear Instruments and Methods in Physics Research B*, vol. 219-220, no. 1-4, pp. 963–967, 2004.

[34] P. Wang, K. L. Tan, E. T. Kang, and K. G. Neoh, "Surface functionalization of low density polyethylene films with grafted poly(ethylene glycol) derivatives," *Journal of Materials Chemistry*, vol. 11, no. 12, pp. 2951–2957, 2001.

[35] J. P. Chen, D. Kiaei, and A. S. Hoffman, "Activity of horseradish peroxide adsorbed on radio frequency glow discharge-treated polymers," *Journal of biomaterials science*, vol. 5, no. 1-2, pp. 167–182, 1993.

[36] D. Fink, *Fundamentals of Ion-Irradiated Polymers*, Springer, Berlin, Germany, 2004.

[37] V. B. Odzhaev, I. P. Kozlov, V. N. Popok, and D. B. Sviridov, *Ion Implantation of Polymers*, Belorussian State University, Minsk, Belarus, 1998.

[38] A. Kondyurin and M. Bilek, *Ion Beam Treatment of Polymers*, Elsevier, Oxford, UK, 2007.

[39] N. J. Nosworthy, J. P. Y. Ho, A. Kondyurin, D. R. McKenzie, and M. M. M. Bilek, "The attachment of catalase and poly-l-lysine to plasma immersion ion implantation-treated polyethylene," *Acta Biomaterialia*, vol. 3, no. 5, pp. 695–704, 2007.

[40] A. Kondyurin, N. J. Nosworthy, and M. M. M. Bilek, "Attachment of horseradish peroxidase to polytetrafluorethylene (teflon) after plasma immersion ion implantation," *Acta Biomaterialia*, vol. 4, no. 5, pp. 1218–1225, 2008.

[41] B. K. Gan, A. Kondyurin, and M. M. M. Bilek, "Comparison of protein surface attachment on untreated and plasma immersion ion implantation treated polystyrene: protein Islands and carpet," *Langmuir*, vol. 23, no. 5, pp. 2741–2746, 2007.

[42] A. Kondyurin, N. J. Nosworthy, M. M. M. Bilek, R. Jones, and P. J. Pigram, "Surface attachment of horseradish peroxidase to nylon modified by plasma-immersion ion implantation," *Journal of Applied Polymer Science*, vol. 120, no. 5, pp. 2891–2903, 2011.

[43] A. Kondyurin, P. Naseri, K. Fisher, D. R. McKenzie, and M. M. M. Bilek, "Mechanisms for surface energy changes observed in plasma immersion ion implanted polyethylene: the roles of free radicals and oxygen-containing groups," *Polymer Degradation and Stability*, vol. 94, no. 4, pp. 638–646, 2009.

[44] A. Kondyurin, V. Karmanov, and R. Guenzel, "Plasma immersion ion implantation of polyethylene," *Vacuum*, vol. 64, no. 2, pp. 105–111, 2001.

[45] N. Gavrilov, D. Yakusheva, and A. Kondyurin, "Structure of polyethylene after pulse ion beam treatment," *Journal of Applied Polymer Science*, vol. 69, no. 6, pp. 1071–1077, 1998.

[46] A. M. Abdul-Kader, A. Turos, R. M. Radwan, and A. M. Kelany, "Surface free energy of ultra-high molecular weight polyethylene modified by electron and gamma irradiation," *Applied Surface Science*, vol. 255, no. 17, pp. 7786–7790, 2009.

[47] H. Yasuda, *Plasma Polymerization*, Academic, New York, NY, USA, 1985.

[48] V. I. Povstugar, V. I. Kodolov, and S. S. Mikhailova, *Composition and Properties of Surface of Polymer Materials*, Khimiya, Moscow, Russia, 1988.

[49] D. Kiaei, A. S. Hoffman, and T. A. Horbett, "Tight binding of albumin to glow discharge treated polymers," *Journal of Biomaterials Science*, vol. 4, no. 1, pp. 35–44, 1992.

[50] Y. Ikada, "Blood-compatible polymers," in *Polymers in Medicine. Advances in Polymer Science*, pp. 103–140, Springer, Berlin, Germany, 1984.

[51] R. L. Clough, "High-energy radiation and polymers: a review of commercial processes and emerging applications," *Nuclear Instruments and Methods in Physics Research B*, vol. 185, no. 1–4, pp. 8–33, 2001.

[52] A. Valenza, A. M. Visco, L. Torrisi, and N. Campo, "Characterization of ultra-high-molecular-weight polyethylene (UHMWPE) modified by ion implantation," *Polymer*, vol. 45, no. 5, pp. 1707–1715, 2004.

[53] M. Bosetti, L. Zanardi, P. Bracco, L. Costa, and M. Cannas, "In vitro evaluation of the inflammatory activity of ultra-high molecular weight polyethylene," *Biomaterials*, vol. 24, no. 8, pp. 1419–1426, 2003.

[54] F. Rusmini, Z. Zhong, and J. Feijen, "Protein immobilization strategies for protein biochips," *Biomacromolecules*, vol. 8, no. 6, pp. 1775–1789, 2007.

[55] N. C. Veitch, "Horseradish peroxidase: a modern view of a classic enzyme," *Phytochemistry*, vol. 65, no. 3, pp. 249–259, 2004.

[56] L. Calcagno, G. Compagnini, and G. Foti, "Structural modification of polymer films by ion irradiation," *Nuclear Instruments and Methods in Physics Research B*, vol. 65, no. 1–4, pp. 413–422, 1992.

[57] M. B. Lewis and E. H. Lee, "Chemical G-values of ion-irradiated polymers," *Nuclear Instruments and Methods in Physics Research B*, vol. 69, no. 2-3, pp. 341–348, 1992.

[58] V. Hnatowicz, J. Vacík, J. Červená et al., "Doping of ion implanted polyethylene with metallocarborane," *Nuclear Instruments and Methods in Physics Research B*, vol. 105, no. 1–4, pp. 241–244, 1995.

[59] V. N. Popok, V. B. Odzhaev, I. P. Kozlov, I. I. Azarko, I. A. Karpovich, and D. V. Sviridov, "Ion beam effects in polymer films: structure evolution of the implanted layer," *Nuclear Instruments and Methods in Physics Research B*, vol. 129, no. 1, pp. 60–64, 1997.

[60] V. Švorčík, E. Arenholz, V. Hnatowicz, V. Rybka, R. Öchsner, and H. Ryssel D, "AFM surface investigation of polyethylene modified by ion bombardment," *Nuclear Instruments and Methods in Physics Research B*, vol. 142, no. 3, pp. 349–354, 1998.

[61] V. Švorčík, V. Rybka, J. Vacík, V. Hnatowicz, R. Öchsner, and H. Ryssel, "Li^+ grafting of ion irradiated polyethylene," *Nuclear Instruments and Methods in Physics Research B*, vol. 149, no. 3, pp. 331–335, 1999.

[62] A. Tóth, T. Bell, I. Bertóti, M. Mohai, and B. Zelei, "Surface modification of polyethylene by low keV ion beams," *Nuclear Instruments and Methods in Physics Research B*, vol. 148, no. 1–4, pp. 1131–1135, 1999.

[63] V. B. Odzhaev, V. N. Popok, E. I. Kozlova, O. N. Jankovskij, and I. A. Karpovich, "Electrical properties of polyethylene modified by ion implantation and diffusion," *Nuclear Instruments and Methods in Physics Research B*, vol. 166, pp. 655–659, 2000.

[64] V. N. Popok, I. I. Azarko, V. B. Odzhaev, A. Tóth, and R. I. Khaibullin, "High fluence ion beam modification of polymer surfaces: EPR and XPS studies," *Nuclear Instruments and Methods in Physics Research B*, vol. 178, no. 1–4, pp. 305–310, 2001.

[65] T. Oka, H. Kanbe, F. Yatagai, and Y. Hama, "Changes in the chemical structure and the mechanical properties of single-site polyethylene induced by ion-beam irradiation," *Nuclear Instruments and Methods in Physics Research B*, vol. 208, no. 1–4, pp. 181–184, 2003.

[66] J. Davenas and P. Thévenard, "Models of the hydrogen release from polymers under ion beam irradiation," *Nuclear Instruments and Methods in Physics Research B*, vol. 208, no. 1–4, pp. 170–175, 2003.

[67] A. Lacoste and J. Pelletier, "Processing considerations with plasma-based ion implantation of polymers: theoretical aspects, limitations, and experimental results," *Nuclear Instruments and Methods in Physics Research B*, vol. 208, no. 1–4, pp. 260–266, 2003.

[68] K. Prosková, V. Svorcík, V. Rybka, and V. Hnatowicz, "Selected degradation reactions in polyethylene irradiated with Ar^+ and Xe^+ ions," *Radiation Physics and Chemistry*, vol. 58, no. 2, pp. 153–156, 2000.

[69] M. Veres, M. Füle, S. Tóth et al., "Raman scattering of ultra-high molecular weight polyethylene treated by plasma-based ion implantation," *Thin Solid Films*, vol. 482, no. 1-2, pp. 211–215, 2005.

[70] A. Kondyurin, R. Khaybullin, N. Gavrilov, and V. Popok, "Pulse and continuous ion beam treatment of polyethylene," *Vacuum*, vol. 68, no. 4, pp. 341–347, 2002.

[71] G. A. Mesyats, Y. S. Klyachkin, N. V. Gavrilov, N. V. Mizgulin, R. M. Yakushev, and A. V. Kondyurin, "Ion beam modification of polyethylene and adhesion to epoxy adhesive," *Vacuum*, vol. 47, no. 9, pp. 1085–1087, 1996.

[72] A. Kondyurin, E. Pecheva, and L. Pramatarova, "Calcium phosphate formation on plasma immersion ion implanted low density polyethylene and polytetrafluorethylene surfaces," *Journal of Materials Science*, vol. 19, no. 3, pp. 1145–1153, 2008.

[73] C. Mapelli, C. Castiglioni, G. Zerbi, and K. Müllen, "Common force field for graphite and polycyclic aromatic hydrocarbons," *Physical Review B*, vol. 60, no. 18, pp. 12710–12725, 1999.

[74] P. C. Painter, M. M. Coleman, and J. L. Koenig, *The Theory of Vibrational Spectroscopy and Its Application to Polymeric Materials*, Wiley, New York, NY, USA, 1982.

[75] A. C. Ferrari and J. Robertson, "Interpretation of Raman spectra of disordered and amorphous carbon," *Physical Review B*, vol. 61, no. 20, pp. 14095–14107, 2000.

[76] R. B. Woodward, "Structure and the absorption spectra of α,β-unsaturated ketones," *Journal of the American Chemical Society*, vol. 63, no. 4, pp. 1123–1126, 1941.

[77] L. F. Fieser, M. Fieser, and S. Rajagopalan, "Absorption spectroscopy and the structures of the diosterols," *Journal of Organic Chemistry*, vol. 13, no. 6, pp. 800–806, 1948.

[78] R. J. Gambino and J. A. Thompson, "Spin resonance spectroscopy of amorphous carbon films," *Solid State Communications*, vol. 34, no. 1, pp. 15–18, 1980.

[79] K. Fabisiak, S. Orzeszko, F. Rozpoch, and J. Szatkowski, "RF Plasma deposited amorphous carbon films electronic and optical properties," *Journal of Non-Crystalline Solids*, vol. 99, no. 1, pp. 12–22, 1988.

[80] G. Fusco, A. Tagliaferro, W. I. Milne, and J. Robertson, "Paramagnetic centres in tetrahedral amorphous carbon," *Diamond and Related Materials*, vol. 6, no. 5–7, pp. 783–786, 1997.

[81] R. C. Barklie, "Characterisation of defects in amorphous carbon by electron paramagnetic resonance," *Diamond and Related Materials*, vol. 10, no. 2, pp. 174–181, 2001.

[82] G. A. Viana, R. G. Lacerda, F. L. Freire, and F. C. Marques, "ESR investigation of graphite-like amorphous carbon films revealing itinerant states as the ones responsible for the signal," *Journal of Non-Crystalline Solids*, vol. 354, no. 19–25, pp. 2135–2137, 2008.

[83] J. F. Rabek, *Polymer Photodegradation: Mechanisms and Experimental Methods*, Chapman and Hall, London, UK, 1995.

[84] N. M. Emanuel and A. L. Buchachenko, *Chemical Physics of Molecular Decomposition and Ageing of Polymers*, Nauka, Moscow, Russia, 1988.

[85] N. Grassie and G. Scott, *Polymer Degradation & Stabilisation*, Cambridge University Press, Cambridge, UK, 1985.

[86] H. Steinhauser and G. Ellinghorst, "Corona treatment of isotactic polypropylene in nitrogen and carbondioxide," *Die Angewandte Makromolekulare Chemie*, vol. 120, no. 1, pp. 177–191, 1984.

[87] H. Yasuda, *Luminous Chemical Vapor Deposition and Interface Engineering*, Marcel Dekker, New York, NY, USA, 2005.

[88] M. F. Herman, Ed., *Encyclopedia of Polymer Science and Technology*, John Wiley, New York, NY, USA, 3rd edition, 2004.

[89] L. Ostrovskaya, V. Perevertailo, V. Ralchenko, A. Dementjev, and O. Loginova, "Wettability and surface energy of oxidized and hydrogen plasma-treated diamond films," *Diamond and Related Materials*, vol. 11, no. 3–6, pp. 845–850, 2002.

[90] Y. Tajima, T. Matsuura, Y. Numata, D. Yamazaki, H. Kawamura, and H. Osedo, "Surface free energy and wettability determination of various fullerene derivative films on amorphous carbon wafer," *Japanese Journal of Applied Physics*, vol. 47, no. 7, pp. 5730–5733, 2008.

[91] P. Y. Tessier, L. Pichon, P. Villechaise et al., "Carbon nitride thin films as protective coatings for biomaterials: synthesis, mechanical and biocompatibility characterizations," *Diamond and Related Materials*, vol. 12, no. 3–7, pp. 1066–1069, 2003.

[92] E. Papirer, E. Brendle, F. Ozil, and H. Balard, "Comparison of the surface properties of graphite, carbon black and fullerene samples, measured by inverse gas chromatography," *Carbon*, vol. 37, no. 8, pp. 1265–1274, 1999.

[93] T. W. Ebbesen, Ed., *Carbon Nanotubes. Preparation and Properties*, CRC Press, London, UK, 1996.

[94] D. B. Berkowitz and D. W. Webert, "The inactivation of horseradish peroxidase by a polystyrene surface," *Journal of Immunological Methods*, vol. 47, no. 1, pp. 121–124, 1981.

[95] W. Al-Azzam, E. A. Pastrana, Y. Ferrer, Q. Huang, R. Schweitzer-Stenner, and K. Griebenow, "Structure of poly(ethylene glycol)-modified horseradish peroxidase in organic solvents: infrared amide I spectral changes upon protein dehydration are largely caused by protein structural changes and not by water removal per se," *Biophysical Journal*, vol. 83, no. 6, pp. 3637–3651, 2002.

[96] Y. Maeda, M. Fujihara, and I. Ikeda, "Spectroscopic study on structure of horseradish peroxidase in water and dimethyl sulfoxide mixture," *Biopolymers*, vol. 67, no. 2, pp. 107–112, 2002.

[97] I. E. Holzbaur, A. M. English, and A. A. Ismail, "FTTR study of the thermal denaturation of horseradish and cytochrome *c* peroxidases in D_2O," *Biochemistry*, vol. 35, no. 17, pp. 5488–5494, 1996.

[98] G. I. Berglund, G. H. Carlsson, A. T. Smith, H. Szöke, A. Henriksen, and J. Hajdu, "The catalytic pathway of horseradish peroxidase at high resolution," *Nature*, vol. 417, pp. 463–468, 2002.

[99] D. V. Bax, D. R. McKenzie, A. S. Weiss, and M. M. M. Bilek, "The linker-free covalent attachment of collagen to plasma

immersion ion implantation treated polytetrafluoroethylene and subsequent cell-binding activity," *Biomaterials*, vol. 31, no. 9, pp. 2526–2534, 2010.

[100] D. V. Bax, D. R. McKenzie, A. S. Weiss, and M. M. M. Bilek, "Linker-free covalent attachment of the extracellular matrix protein tropoelastin to a polymer surface for directed cell spreading," *Acta Biomaterialia*, vol. 5, no. 9, pp. 3371–3381, 2009.

[101] T. W. Perkins, D. S. Mak, T. W. Root, and E. N. Lightfoot, "Protein retention in hydrophobic interaction chromatography: modeling variation with buffer ionic strength and column hydrophobicity," *Journal of Chromatography A*, vol. 766, no. 1-2, pp. 1–14, 1997.

[102] G. Greene, H. Radhakrishna, and R. Tannenbaum, "Protein binding properties of surface-modified porous polyethylene membranes," *Biomaterials*, vol. 26, no. 30, pp. 5972–5982, 2005.

[103] A. Kondyurin and M. Bilek, "Etching and structure changes in PMMA coating under argon plasma immersion ion implantation," *Nuclear Instruments and Methods in Physics Research B*, vol. 269, no. 12, pp. 1361–1369, 2011.

[104] G. Mesyats, Y. Klyachkin, N. Gavrilov, and A. Kondyurin, "Adhesion of polytetrafluorethylene modified by an ion beam," *Vacuum*, vol. 52, no. 3, pp. 285–289, 1999.

[105] A. Kondyurin and M. Maitz, "Surface modification of ePTFE and implants using the same," US patent 2007/0050007 A1, 2007.

[106] V. Švorčík, V. Hnatowicz, P. Stopka et al., "Amino acids grafting of Ar^+ ions modified PE," *Radiation Physics and Chemistry*, vol. 60, no. 1-2, pp. 89–93, 2001.

4

Large-Scale Survey of Unselected Automated Visual Fields in a Major Reading Center: Patterns and Data Analysis

Lilly Zborowski-Naveh,[1,2] Rita Ehrlich,[3] Moshe Luski,[1,3,4] Dov Weinberger,[1,3,4] Mona Boaz,[5] and Dan D. Gaton[1,3,4]

[1] *Deptartment of Ophthalmology, MOR Institute for Medical Data, 51108 Bnei Brak, Israel*
[2] *Department of Ophthalmology, Wolfson Medical Center, 58100 Holon, Israel*
[3] *Department of Ophthalmology, Rabin Medical Center, Beilinson Hospital, 49100 Petach Tikva, Israel*
[4] *Sackler Faculty of Medicine, Tel Aviv University, 69978 Tel Aviv, Israel*
[5] *Department of Epidemiology, Wolfson Medical Center, 58100 Holon, Israel*

Correspondence should be addressed to Dan D. Gaton; gaton@post.tau.ac.il

Academic Editors: R. Kröger and H. Noma

A prospective, randomized study was conducted to survey a large number of automated perimetry examinations in a central reading institute, obtaining practical information on unselected referred patients and their clinician "consumers". Visual field records of 1041 patients were obtained, each evaluated by one of three glaucoma specialists. Statistical analysis was applied on demographics, physician characteristics, test reliability and visual field scores. Reliability was scored on a scale of 1 (excellent) to 5 (uninterpretable). Data from earlier examinations of these patients was also analyzed. The large majority of patients (70.4%) were referred due to glaucoma, ocular hypertension or suspected glaucoma. Most of the patients had threshold strategies: FastPac 24-2 or 30-2 (88.9%), Full Threshold (0.7%), and 10-2 (0.5%). In only 7 patients was short-wavelength automated perimetry (SWAP) performed. The Swedish Interactive Testing Algorithm (SITA) was applied in 1.0% of cases. More than half (56.8%) of the population had a reliability score of 1, and 22.7% had a score of 2, indicating a valid result for 79.4% of patients, providing clinically useful information. Linear regression analyses indicated that the Mean Defect was a better predictor of the visual field score than the Corrected Pattern Standard Deviation (CPSD), for the entire group and for each visual field score subgroup.

1. Introduction

Visual field evaluation is critical in glaucoma and neuro-ophthalmic diagnosis and followup. All the major studies of the last decade or so including EMGT [1], AGIS [2], OHTS [3], and CIGTS [4] have used visual field criteria to establish eligibility and for followup. Each of those studies created their own scoring system and their criteria for defining progression. In all cases the reliability requirements were high, and the patients needed to be available for fairly frequent exams.

In the real world of clinical practice our patients are often less than perfect candidates, they may not return exactly on schedule for their exams, and the community-based ophthalmologists may not all be "up to speed" on perimetry interpretation. The study scoring systems are not always available or practical for everyday clinical use.

In our country, most visual field examinations are referred to diagnostic centers. The Mor Institute provides comprehensive state-of-the-art diagnostic services to 500,000 patients per year. It receives referrals from about 150 ophthalmologists nationwide and performs more than 10,000 perimetry examinations annually. One of three glaucoma specialists reads the printouts and returns a written evaluation to the referring physician.

We sought to utilize this large group of unselected patients' examinations to gain insight into real everyday practice and to determine how to improve test results and patient care as well as physician practice patterns.

TABLE 1: Visual field scoring system.

Score	Degree of damage	Description
1	No damage	Normal visual field
2	Mild damage	Enlarged blind spot, slight nasal or temporal depression, mild peripheral constriction, and mild diffuse or nonspecific changes
3	Moderate damage	Changes in one quadrant or moderate nasal depression, relative central, or cecocentral scotomas
4	Advanced damage	Changes in two quadrants above or below the midline or advanced nasal depression. Deep central or cecocentral depression
5	Severe damage	Significant defects above and below the midline
6	End stage	Tubular field with or without a temporal island

To the best of our knowledge, no similar survey of this scale has been reported to date.

2. Materials and Methods

The present prospective study included all automated perimetry examinations conducted at the Mor Institute during one month (August 2002). The participating technicians were experienced and have been trained to both monitor fixation and encourage the patients during testing. The printouts were read by three of the authors (L. Zborowski-Naveh, M. Lusky, and D. D. Gaton). The readers evaluated the printout as usual and sent a letter with the results to the referring physician. They then completed the survey questionnaire. The right eye or the only eye of each patient was included in the survey.

The survey queried four categories of information: patient-related characteristics (age, gender, and referring diagnosis); physician-related characteristics (test algorithm and test target size requested); test results (reliability score, reasons for loss of reliability, visual field score, mean deviation, and corrected pattern standard deviation); and longitudinal data, where applicable (number of previous examinations, change in reliability score, and change in visual field score).

Reliability was scored on a scale of 1 (excellent) to 5 (uninterpretable). The reader assigned a score on the basis of four parameters: fixation loss; false-positive errors; false-negative errors; white scotomas. For any field with a reliability score greater than 1, the reason was cited as any of the above, alone or in combination.

A linear visual field scoring system was designed to correspond to practical clinical usage. The criteria for score assignment are provided in Table 1.

2.1. Data Analysis. Data were analyzed with the SPSS for Windows, version 15.0.1 (SPSS Inc., Chicago, IL, USA). For continuous variables (age and visual field score), descriptive statistics were calculated and reported as mean ± standard deviation. Categorical variables (specific diagnosis and patient gender) were described using frequency distributions. Continuous variables were compared by reader and by age group using one-way analysis of variance (ANOVA). Continuous variables were compared by diagnostic group (glaucoma versus ocular hypertension) and gender using t-test for independent samples. Associations between continuous variables and age were analyzed with Pearson's correlation coefficients. Previous test results were compared to present results using t-test for paired samples. All tests were two-sided and considered significant at $P < 0.05$.

TABLE 2: Distribution of referring diagnoses by mean age.

Diagnosis	N (%)	Mean age (years)
Glaucoma	337 (32.4)	68.8
OHT/suspected glaucoma	395 (38)	63.2
Retinal pathology (except myopia)	29 (4.0)	61.5
Neurologic/headache	160 (15.4)	47.9
Myopia	8 (0.8)	46.4
Cataract	2 (0.2)	83.1

$^*P < 0.001$.
OHT: Ocular hypertension.

3. Results

During the study period, 1041 visual field records were obtained.

3.1. Patient-Related Data. Mean age of the surveyed population was 61.87 (±17.10) years (range 6–93). Only 18.2% were younger than 50 years; 70.8% were aged 50 to 79 years, and 11.9% were aged 80 years or more.

Significant differences were noted in the proportion and age of men and women referred for testing. Women comprised 56.6% of the survey population and were of mean age 59.95 (±17.42) years. Men comprised 43.4% of the population and were of mean age 64.32 (±16.38) years. There were more women than men in each decade of life except the ninth ($P = .047$).

The distribution of referring diagnoses by number of patients and mean age is shown in Table 2. The large majority of patients (70.4%) were referred for reasons related to glaucoma; known glaucoma, ocular hypertension (OHT), or suspected glaucoma. There was a significant difference in mean patient age among the diagnostic groups ($P < 0.001$), with the youngest patients referred mainly for neurology/headache and myopia. Clinically, the most significant variation was the 5-year difference between the glaucoma and the OHT/suspected glaucoma groups ($P < 0.001$). Forty-two of the 395 patients (10.6%) with OHT/suspected glaucoma

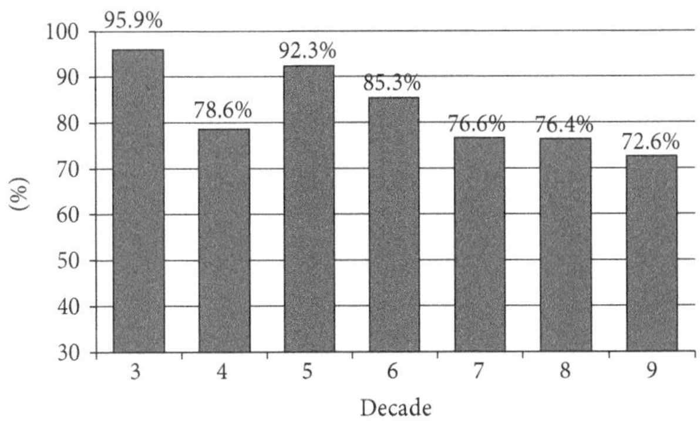

FIGURE 1: Percent of patients in each decade of life with a reliability score of 1 or 2.

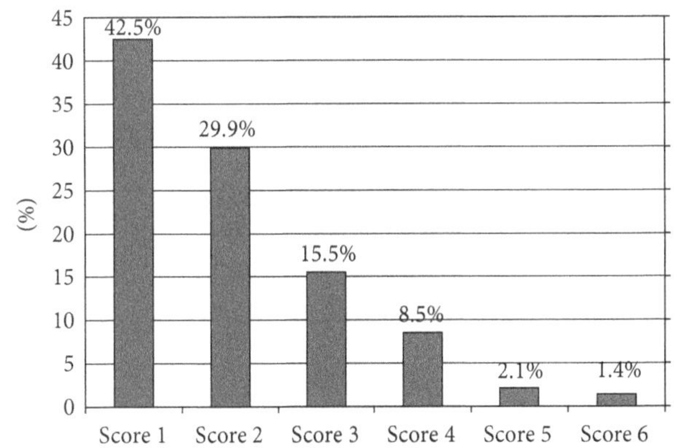

FIGURE 2: Distribution of visual field scores.

were aged 50 years or less and an additional 5 were aged 51 to 55 years.

3.2. Physician-Related Data. The referring physician specified the test algorithm to be used. Most of the patients were tested with threshold strategies: FastPac 24-2 or 30-2 (88.9%), full threshold (0.7%), and 10-2 programs (0.5%). The 3-zone 120-point screening program was specified by 6.7% of physicians, and the macula program with red and white targets, by 1.1%. In only 7 patients short-wavelength (blue-yellow) automated perimetry (SWAP) was performed; 6 of them had OHT/suspected glaucoma and were aged 55 years or less. The Swedish interactive testing algorithm (SITA) was applied in 1.0% of cases.

3.3. Test Results

3.3.1. Reliability. The mean reliability score was 1.68. There was a small but statistically significant difference in mean score between men (1.71) and women (1.66) ($P < 0.001$).

The tests of more than half (56.8%) the survey population had a reliability score of 1, and 22.7% had a score of 2, indicating a valid result for 79.4% of patients. An additional 15.8% had a reliability score of 3 which can at times still provide clinically useful information.

TABLE 3: Mean visual field scores of the 3 readers.

Reader	N	Mean score*
1	348	1.9827 ± 1.2875
2	347	2.0870 ± 1.1042
3	346	1.9681 ± 1.0711

*$P \leq 0.340$.

TABLE 4: Mean visual field score by diagnosis.

Diagnosis	N	Mean visual field score
Myopia	8	2.38
Retinal-vascular	17	2.29
Glaucoma	333	2.28*
Neurologic/headache	158	2.17
Macular changes	12	1.92
OHT/suspected glaucoma	392	1.92*
Hydroxychloroquine	12	1.58

*$P < 0.001$.
OHT: ocular hypertension.

Reliability was correlated with patient age. When children were excluded, we found a steady decrease in the proportion of "excellent" reliability test scores (score 1 by age group), from 91.7% for patients in the third decade to 47.1% for patients in the ninth decade ($P < 0.001$). The decrease in reliability with age was sustained when we grouped patients with test scores 1 or 2 together. Nevertheless, even in the over-80-year group, 72.6% of patients had a valid test result (Figure 1).

The most common reason cited by the readers for low test reliability was loss of fixation (90.3% of cases), followed by false-negatives (25%) and false-positives (7.0%).

3.3.2. Visual Field Score. Each field was assigned a damage score, and each of the glaucoma specialists (L. Zborowski-Naveh, M. Lusky, and D. D. Gaton) read about one-third of the fields. No statistically significant difference was found among the mean scores of the 3 readers (Table 3). The mean score for the entire group was 2.01. The distribution of visual field scores is shown in Figure 2.

Table 4 summarizes the mean visual field scores by diagnosis. The myopia group (which was also the youngest) had the highest score, and the hydroxychloroquine group the lowest. Although the difference in mean score between the glaucoma group (2.28) and OHT/suspected glaucoma group (1.92) was not large, it was statistically significant ($P < 0.001$).

3.3.3. Correlation of Visual Field and Reliability Scores. The visual field score was positively correlated to the reliability score ($r = 0.36$): the lower the reliability, the greater the chance of a defective visual field.

3.3.4. Mean Deviation (MD). The mean MD for the 935 size III threshold tests was −3.30 dB (±3.57 dB). The mean MD in the group of patients aged 40 years or less was −3.68 ± 4.4 dB. However, from the fifth through the ninth decade, there was a steady decrease in MD, from −2.3 dB to −4.24 dB ($P < 0.001$).

3.3.5. Corrected Pattern Standard Deviation (CPSD). The mean CPSD for the 935 size III threshold tests was 1.94 dB. A nonsignificant trend toward an increase in CPSD with age was observed.

There was a significant correlation of the MD with the CPSD ($r = .27$, $P < 0.001$), and of both the MD and the CPSD with the visual field score ($r = .55$, $P < 0.001$ and $.54$, $P < 0.001$, resp.). Linear regression analyses indicated, however, that the MD was a better predictor of the visual field score than the CPSD, for the entire group and for each visual field score subgroup.

3.4. Longitudinal Data. A previous visual field test was available for comparison for 608 of the 1041 patients (58.1%) (Table 5). Analysis of the number of patients in whom the disease progressed yielded a significant difference between the glaucoma and the OHT/suspected glaucoma groups (25% versus 15.8%, resp., $P < 0.012$).

In 505 of the 608 cases, the previous or the first in a series of visual field exams was available. The current mean reliability score for this subgroup was 1.75. The mean reliability score assigned to the earlier visual field test was 1.63. This difference was not statistically significant, suggesting the absence of a "learning effect" for reliability.

Table 5: Rates of progression/stability when previous fields were available.

	Entire group	Glaucoma	OHT/Suspected glaucuoma
	N (%)	*N* (%)	*N* (%)
Stable	463 (76.5)	176 (71)	184 (82.8)
Progressed	116 (19.2)	62 (25)*	35 (15.8)*
Improved	22 (3.6)	10 (4)	3 (1.4)
Indeterminate	7 (0.7)		

*$P < 0.012$.
OHT: ocular hypertension.

4. Discussion

This survey is unique in the literature of perimetry in that it included a very large population of entirely unselected cases. Our purpose was to extract useful clinical information that could be applied to daily practice. All other studies were either limited to small groups without pathology [5] or selected study groups with exclusion of unreliable fields [1–7].

The finding that glaucoma was the main reason for the test (70%) was expected. The progressive increase of the MD with age has also been described in the literature [5]. Other results were less obvious.

4.1. Demographics. Female patients accounted for 56.6% of the whole population; however, this rate is only slightly higher than the proportion of women in the general population (53.9% for those 45 years old or more) [8]. The mean age of the women was significantly lower than that of the men (59.95 and 64.32 years, resp.), which may reflect an actual gender-related difference in the age distribution of patients with these pathologies. Some of the earlier population-based studies of the incidence or prevalence of glaucoma [9–11] did not show any gender- or age-related difference, whereas others reported a higher prevalence in men [12–14]. Only in the Hispanic population in the United States [15] was a higher prevalence noted in women.

Our finding may also be explained by a bias in diagnostic referrals or a difference in utilization of primary health care services. The possibility that the difference is a result of chance cannot be entirely discounted either. This question merits further study.

The older mean age (by more than 5 years) of the glaucoma group than the OHT/suspected glaucoma group, combined with the significantly higher visual field damage score in the patients with glaucoma, supports the notion that glaucoma is preceded either by OHT or by suspicious disc changes.

4.2. Algorithm Requested. The low rate of requests for the SITA program (1%) suggests a certain degree of conservatism among our referring physicians and highlights an important area in which educational activities may be applied.

The SWAP program was used in only 7 patients, although we identified 47 patients with OHT or suspected glaucoma who were 55 years old or less at the time of examination. SWAP testing can detect visual field damage earlier than standard white on white perimetry, [16] and it is particularly suitable for younger patients because of their low incidence of nuclear sclerosis. Yet it was not applied in most of the patients in our population who might have benefited from it, maybe due to lack of clinician awareness at the time of patient recruitment to the study.

4.3. Reliability and Visual Field. About 80% of our random, unselected population were able to cooperate well enough for the clinician to obtain a reliable field (Figure 1). Test reliability in an additional 15% was rated intermediate, that is, sufficient for the clinician to obtain partially useful, if not entirely accurate, information. Even the group of patients in the ninth decade of life had a 72.6% rate of valid field results. These data suggest that clinicians should not hesitate to test the elderly with automated perimetry.

The ocular hypertension treatment study (OHTS) [3] reported better reliability results than ours with 79% of patients having reliable fields by strict criteria and 97% by slightly more liberal criteria, corresponding roughly to our level 1 and 2. Although the trend in our study was similar, the difference in reliability was probably attributable to the more restricted patient population in the OHTS.

Like in the OHTS, the most common reason for loss of reliability in our study was fixation loss. Accordingly, reliability correlated with the visual field score. These findings suggest a confounding effect of reliability on test results. Therefore, focusing efforts on improving fixation of the examinees will result in better reliability and "cleaner" test results.

Patients with advanced field loss may find it difficult to maintain fixation, and even slight movements at the margins of deep scotomas can easily produce false-negative results. This might explain some of the shared variability in reliability and damage. In addition, a true decrease in reliability can be the cause of a falsely poor result, producing a confounding effect. Therefore, it is important to improve reliability for each examination, especially in patients with advanced field loss.

Previous studies have described a learning effect of repeated visual field testing on test results, even when the initial reliability was good [17–19]. Our data, however, do not support a specific learning effect. In general, reliability or lack thereof persisted from the first test to the later one. We do not suggest that repeated attempts should not be made to improve test reliability, only that these attempts may not always succeed as intended. Learning effects may be stronger if the examinations are closely spaced in time. Further analysis of the time elapsing between repeated examinations should be made in future studies.

The MD and the CPSD both correlated with the visual field score, but the MD was a better predictor. This is contrary to our expectations of a lower predictive value of the MD, given its greater sensitivity to lens changes or refractive errors than the CPSD [10, 20], at least at the level of early to moderate field damage.

4.4. Implications for Physicians. This study was not designed to evaluate the criteria of the community physicians for requesting perimetry. However, the fact that 42.5% of the fields were normal might suggest that the "threshold" for referral was fairly low and that a healthy degree of suspicion was being maintained.

In our survey, the referring physician assigned the diagnosis; consequently, there was no standardization of the diagnostic criteria or diagnostic confirmation. Nevertheless, we found a clear and significant difference in the mean visual field score between the glaucoma group (2.28) and the OHT/suspected glaucoma group (1.92), in addition to a significantly higher rate of deterioration in the glaucoma group (25% versus 15.8%). The findings were not necessarily confirmed by repeated fields, but the statistics of progression could imply that more aggressive treatment of glaucoma in the community is needed. This is consistent with the results of the Advanced Glaucoma Intervention Study (AGIS) [21] and others [13, 22], which demonstrated a benefit for consistently lower pressure in preventing further field loss in patients with glaucoma.

5. Summary

In summary, we describe the results of a large-scale survey of unselected patients undergoing automated perimetry. We were able to gain significant insight into reliability according to patient age and, perhaps, the behavior of disease progression in this group of patients as well as into visual field scores according to referring clinical diagnosis. In addition, the actual practice patterns of a large and representative group of ophthalmologists were delineated.

We were able to gain insight into the patterns of physician referral and learn where to focus additional education for better utilization of perimetry options. Most patients are capable of giving a test result reliable enough to be clinically useful even in the elderly age bracket. The need for more aggressive treatment of glaucoma patients is implied in the proportion of cases with progression.

References

[1] M. C. Leske, A. Heijl, L. Hyman, and B. Bengtsson, "Early manifest glaucoma trial: design and baseline data," *Ophthalmology*, vol. 106, no. 11, pp. 2144–2153, 1999.

[2] D. E. Gaasterland, F. Ederer, E. K. Sullivan, J. Caprioli, and M. N. Cyrlin, "Advanced glaucoma intervention study: 2. Visual field test scoring and reliability," *Ophthalmology*, vol. 101, no. 8, pp. 1445–1455, 1994.

[3] C. A. Johnson, J. L. Keltner, K. E. Cello et al., "Baseline visual field characteristics in the ocular hypertension treatment study," *Ophthalmology*, vol. 109, no. 3, pp. 432–437, 2002.

[4] D. C. Musch, P. R. Lichter, K. E. Guire, and C. L. Standardi, "The collaborative initial glaucoma treatment study: study design, methods, and baseline characteristics of enrolled patients," *Ophthalmology*, vol. 106, no. 4, pp. 653–662, 1999.

[5] A. Heijl, G. Lindgren, and J. Olsson, "Perimetric threshold variability and age," *Archives of Ophthalmology*, vol. 106, no. 4, pp. 450–452, 1988.

[6] A. Heijl, M. C. Leske, B. Bengtsson et al., "Measuring visual field progression in the early manifest glaucoma trial," *Acta Ophthalmologica Scandinavica*, vol. 81, no. 3, pp. 286–293, 2003.

[7] M. O. Gordon and M. A. Kass, "The ocular hypertension treatment study. Design and baseline description of the participants," *Archives of Ophthalmology*, vol. 117, no. 5, pp. 573–583, 1999.

[8] Israel Bureau of Statistics, 2004.

[9] J. M. Tielsch, A. Sommer, J. Katz, R. M. Royall, H. A. Quigley, and J. Javitt, "Racial variations in the prevalence of primary open-angle glaucoma: the Baltimore eye survey," *Journal of the American Medical Association*, vol. 266, no. 3, pp. 369–374, 1991.

[10] B. E. K. Klein, R. Klein, W. E. Sponsel et al., "Prevalence of glaucoma: the Beaver Dam Eye Study," *Ophthalmology*, vol. 99, no. 10, pp. 1499–1504, 1992.

[11] P. Mitchell, W. Smith, K. Attebo, and P. R. Healey, "Prevalence of open-angle glaucoma in Australia: the blue mountains eye study," *Ophthalmology*, vol. 103, no. 10, pp. 1661–1669, 1996.

[12] L. Hyman, S. Y. Wu, A. M. S. Connell et al., "Prevalence and causes of visual impairment in the Barbados Eye Study," *Ophthalmology*, vol. 108, no. 10, pp. 1751–1756, 2001.

[13] H. A. Kahn, H. M. Leibowitz, J. P. Ganley et al., "The Framingham eye study. I. Outline and major prevalence findings," *American Journal of Epidemiology*, vol. 106, no. 1, pp. 17–32, 1977.

[14] I. Dielemans, J. R. Vingerling, R. C. W. Wolfs, A. Hofman, D. E. Grobbee, and P. T. de Jong, "The prevalence of primary open-angle glaucoma in a population-based study in The Netherlands. The Rotterdam Study," *Ophthalmology*, vol. 101, no. 11, pp. 1851–1855, 1994.

[15] J. Rodriguez, R. Sanchez, B. Munoz et al., "Causes of blindness and visual impairment in a population-based sample of U.S. Hispanics," *Ophthalmology*, vol. 109, no. 4, pp. 737–743, 2002.

[16] M. F. Delgado, N. T. A. Nguyen, T. A. Cox et al., "Automated perimetry: a report by the American Academy of Ophthalmology," *Ophthalmology*, vol. 109, no. 12, pp. 2362–2374, 2002.

[17] A. Heijl and B. Bengtsson, "The effect of perimetric experience in patients with glaucoma," *Archives of Ophthalmology*, vol. 114, no. 1, pp. 19–22, 1996.

[18] H. Matsuo, G. Tomita, Y. Suzuki, and M. Araie, "Learning effect and measurement variability in frequency-doubling technology perimetry in chronic open-angle glaucoma," *Journal of Glaucoma*, vol. 11, no. 6, pp. 467–473, 2002.

[19] M. Iester, P. Capris, A. Pandolfo, M. Zingirian, and C. E. Traverso, "Learning effect, short-term fluctuation, and long-term fluctuation in frequency doubling technique," *American Journal of Ophthalmology*, vol. 130, no. 2, pp. 160–164, 2000.

[20] B. Koucheki, K. Nouri-Mahdavi, G. Patel, D. Gaasterland, and J. Caprioli, "Visual field changes after cataract extraction: the AGIS experience," *American Journal of Ophthalmology*, vol. 138, no. 6, pp. 1022–1028, 2004.

[21] D. E. Gaasterland, F. Ederer, A. Beck et al., "The Advanced Glaucoma Intervention Study (AGIS): 7. The relationship between control of intraocular pressure and visual field deterioration," *American Journal of Ophthalmology*, vol. 130, no. 4, pp. 429–440, 2000.

[22] I. Goldberg, "Relationship between intraocular pressure and preservation of visual field in glaucoma," *Survey of Ophthalmology*, vol. 48, supplement 1, pp. S3–S7, 2003.

5

Hepatitis C Virus, Cryoglobulinemia, and Kidney: Novel Evidence

Fabrizio Fabrizi

Division of Nephrology and Dialysis, Maggiore Hospital and IRCCS Foundation, Pad. Croff, Via Commenda 15, 20122 Milano, Italy

Correspondence should be addressed to Fabrizio Fabrizi; fabrizi@policlinico.mi.it

Academic Editors: I. Shoji and W. Vogel

Hepatitis C virus infection can lead to chronic active hepatitis, cirrhosis, and liver failure; however, it is also associated with a wide range of extra-hepatic complications. HCV is associated with a large spectrum of histopathological lesions in both native and transplanted kidneys, and it is increasingly recognized as an instigator of B cell lympho-proliferative disorders including mixed cryoglobulinemia. Mixed cyoglobulinemia is a systemic vasculitis primarily mediated by immune complexes; it is characterized by variable organ involvement including skin lesions, chronic hepatitis, glomerulonephritis, peripheral neuropathy, and arthralgias. The most frequent HCV-associated nephropathy is type I membranoproliferative glomerulonephritis, usually in the context of type II mixed cryoglobulinemia. Various approaches have been tried for the treatment of HCV-related glomerulonephritis, including immunosuppressive therapy (corticosteroids and cytotoxic agents), plasma exchange and antiviral agents. Data on the antiviral treatment of HCV-associated glomerulonephritis are not abundant but encouraging results have been provided. Immunosuppressive therapy is particularly recommended for cryoglobulinemic kidney disease. Recent evidence has been accumulated on rituximab therapy for HCV-related cryoglobulinemic glomerulonephritis exists but several questions related to its use remain unclear. Distinct approaches should be considered for the treatment of HCV-associated cryoglobulinemic glomerulonephritis according to the level of proteinuria and kidney failure.

1. Introduction

Cryoglobulinemia is a pathologic condition in which the blood contains immunoglobulins that have the property of reversible precipitation from human serum cooled to 4°C. The discovery in the human serum of proteins which reversibly precipitate in the cold was made in 1933 [1]. In 1947, Lerner and Watson found that these proteins were γ-globulins and introduced the term cryoglobulins (cold precipitable serum globulins) [2]. A detailed nosographic placement to the cryoglobulinemic disease within the vast family of systemic vasculitis was made by Meltzer et al. who first described the clinical syndrome of essential mixed cryoglobulinemia (EMC), characterized by purpura, weakness, arthralgias, and, in some patients, organ involvement [3]. On the grounds of immunochemical studies, Brouet et al. identified 3 types of cryoglobulins [4]. In type I, the cryoprecipitable immunoglobulin is a single monoclonal Ig. Types II and III cryoglobulinemias are both mixed types (MC), composed of at least two immunoglobulins. In both of them, a polyclonal immunoglobulin G (IgG) is bound to another Ig which is an antiglobulin and acts as a rheumatoid factor (RF). The main difference between two types of MCs is that in type II, the RF usually of the IgM class is monoclonal, whereas in type III, it is polyclonal. Both components of MCs, IgG, and IgM RF are necessary for precipitation in the cold, whereas the individual components do not have this property. Patients are considered to have a significant cryoglobulin level when it is >0.05 g/L on two determinations. Some laboratories characterize cryoglobulinemia using immunofixation or immunoelectrophoresis, and quantify the cryoglobulin level by determining the cryocrit, as the percentage of the total volume. The use of immunoblotting for immunochemical characterization is a sensitive and specific method allowing a full identification in 98% [5]. When a cryoglobulin is suspected, serum should be kept warm, and tests should be carried out at 37°C. Serum cryoglobulins may also interfere with spurious quantitation of plasma proteins and erythrocyte sedimentation rate, pseudoleucocytosis, pseudothrombocytosis, or pseudomacrocytosis.

Mixed cryoglobulinemia represent 60% to 75% of all cryoglobulinemias and are found in connective tissue diseases, infectious, or lymphoproliferative disorders, that is, secondary MC. Since the identification of hepatitis C virus

Table 1: Extrahepatic manifestations of HCV infection.

Source	
Kidney	Membranoproliferative GN, membranous nephropathy, focal segmental sclerosis, fibrillary GN, immunotactoid nephropathy, IgA nephropathy, tubulointerstitial nephritis, thrombotic microangiopathy
Skin	Purpura, ulcers; lichen planus; porphyria cutanea tarda
Lung	Alveolitis; pulmonary fibrosis
Joints	Arthralgias; nonerosive arthritis
Thyroid	Autoimmune thyroiditis; hypothyroidism; thyroid cancer
Bone marrow	Monoclonal gammopathies; B-cell lymphoma
Nerves	Peripheral neuropathy; mononeuritis
Muscles	Polymyositis
Glands	Xerostomia; xeroftalmia

[6, 7], many authors have recognized it as the cause of 80% to 90% of MC [8, 9]. HCV is primarily associated with type II MC (which typically has an IgM*k* RF with antiidiotypic activity), and to a lesser extent, with type III MC [10–12]. In the absence of identified etiologic factor (<5% of all MC), cryoglobulinemic vasculitis is defined as essential or idiopathic. This paper aims to describe, main characteristics of HCV-related cryoglobulinemia with a special focus on kidney involvement.

1.1. Epidemiology. Beside chronic liver disease, relevant extrahepatic manifestations of HCV include cryoglobulinemia, lymphoproliferative disorders, and renal diseases (Table 1). Several investigators have given evidence of the association between HCV and glomerular disease in both native [5] and transplanted kidneys [13–15]. A variety of kidney diseases have been associated with HCV. The kidney manifestations of HCV are uncommon, and the available information on their frequency is mostly based on small studies. El-Serag et al. [16] identified 34,204 hospitalized male veterans with HCV (cases) in the US and 136,816 randomly selected patients without HCV (controls) between 1992 and 1999. A significantly greater proportion of HCV-infected patients had porphyria cutanea tarda (0.77% versus 0.06%, $P < 0.0001$), vitiligo (0.17% versus 0.10%, $P = 0.0002$), lichen planus (0.30% versus 0.13%, $P < 0.0001$), and cryoglobulinemia (0.57% versus 0.05%, $P < 0.0001$). There was a greater proportion of membranoproliferative glomeulonerphritis among patients with HCV (0.36% versus 0.05%, $P < 0.0001$), but not membranous glomerulopathy (0.33% versus 0.19%, $P = 0.86$).

During the last decade, some surveys extracted from large clinical databases have suggested an impact of HCV on incidence (and prevalence) of kidney disease [17–23]. Hepatitis C coinfection was also linked with a significant increase in the risk of HIV-related kidney disease [24, 25]. Patients with HCV might be more likely to have diabetes, obesity, or human immunodeficiency virus, these conditions being independently associated with kidney disease. Chronic HCV is associated with mixed cryoglobulinemia and membranoproliferative glomerulonephritis, and these, in turn, can lead to kidney function impairment [26]. It remains unclear whether and to what extent HCV affects renal function in the whole population. In contrast, four cross-sectional surveys have shown a significant link between HCV and proteinuria in apparent healthy individuals, and the pooled risk of proteinuria in patients with HIV-HCV compared those without HCV coinfection was consistently increased [17, 22, 27, 28].

Multivariate regression models showed that anti-HCV positive rate was significantly associated with proteinuria independently of common metabolic factors, such as diabetes mellitus, arterial hypertension, obesity, and dyslipidemia [28]. Type I MPGN associated with type II MC remains the most common form of kidney disease associated with HCV. Less frequently described kidney lesions are MPGN without cryoglobulinemia and membranous nephropathy. Occasional cases of focal segmental glomerulosclerosis, fibrillary or immunotactoid glomerulopathies, and thrombotic microangiopathy have also been reported [5]. In addition, vasculitis and interstitial nephritis have been associated with HCV. More recent information has been accumulated on the association between HCV and glomerular disease in liver- [29, 30] or kidney/liver [31] transplanted population. The natural history of these HCV-associated nephropathies is characterized by remission and relapsing phases; however, the long-term outcome is not well known.

1.2. Pathophysiology of Mixed Cryoglobulinemia Vasculitis. Cryoglobulinemia vasculitis is a systemic vasculitis, that mainly affects the small and, less frequently, medium sized arteries and veins. It is characterized by the deposition of immune complexes containing rheumatoid factor, IgG, HCV RNA, and complement on endothelial surfaces, eliciting vascular inflammation. Mixed cryoglobulinemia is also characterized by the proliferation of B-cell clones producing pathogenic IgM with RF activity. MC represents an example of immune complex vasculitis. Intravascular cryoglobulin precipitation is induced by cold temperature and may involve primarily the skin, the peripheral nerve, and the kidney. A leukocytoclastic reaction is commonly involved in vessel damage of the cutaneous vasculitis. In patients with peripheral neuropathy, nerve pathological analysis often highlights moderate to severe axonal damages (axonal degeneration, differential fascicular loss of axons, signs of demyelinization) associated with a small-size vessel vasculitis (arterioles, venules, and capillaries) and an inflammatory infiltrate composed only of monocytes and T lymphocytes, without necrotizing angiitis [32]. Morphological features observed on kidney biopsies of patients with renal involvement are characterized by an important monocyte infiltrate with double contours of the basement membrane, large eosinophilic and amorphous intraluminal thrombi, evocative of membranoproliferative glomerulonephritis (MPGN). Immunofluorescence study shows intraglomerular subendothelial deposits of IgG, IgM (identical to those of the cryoprecipitates), and complement components. In addition, vasculitis of small renal arteries is present in one-third of patients. Extracapillary crescents are rarely observed. In contrast to cutaneous vasculitis [33], HCV RNA has not been prominently detected in immune complexes in renal lesions and has not been detected in the peripheral neuropathy lesions.

These findings suggest that various pathophysiological processes are involved in different target organs. The prevalent pathogenetic mechanism of HCV-associated cryoglobulinemic glomerulonephritis is represented by the deposition in the glomerulus of a monoclonal IgM RF with particular affinity for the glomerular matrix, an RF produced by permanent clones of B lymphocytes activated by the virus. Cumulative data suggest that HCV particles may be bound directly or indirectly to B-cells, but HCV rarely infects B-cells [34–36]. Marukian et al. [37] have shown that B-cells lack necessary entry receptors and cannot support replication of HCV. In a minority of cases, immune complexes composed of HCV antigens and anti-HCV IgG antibody might deposit in the glomerular structures, in the absence of a concomitant type II MC with a monoclonal IgM RF, indicating an immune complex glomerulonephritis similar to that observed in patients infected with hepatitis B virus. Such a mechanism could explain the noncryoglobulinemic GN rarely observed by others in patients with chronic HCV [38].

1.3. The Role of HCV Itself in Mixed Cryoglobulinemia. Various pieces of evidence support the aetiological role of HCV in mixed cryoglobulinemia. A high proportion of patients with MC and chronic liver disease have serologic evidence of HCV infection [39]. A high prevalence of HCV RNA was detected in the great majority (up to 90%) of patients with type II essential MC [40–42]. An increased concentration (up to 10-fold) of IgG anti-HCV antibody in the cryoprecipitate was measured [41]. The majority of the known HCV antigens (core, E1, E2, NS34, NS4, and NS5) and their corresponding antibodies are described in both cryoprecipitate and vascular lesions in tissue sections [43]. HCV RNA was found in the cryoprecipitate of patients with type II MC concentrated up to 1,000 times the respective levels in supernatants [41, 42].

Hepatitis C virus exerts a chronic stimulus on the immune system, which may lead to the proliferation of B-cell clones producing IgM with RF activity. Charles and Dustin [44] have suggested that specific HCV proteins are necessary for clonal B-cell expansion. High concentrations of HCV envelope protein E2 in vitro stimulate B-cell expansion via interaction with CD81, a known HCV E2 entry factor [45]. IgG-bound HCV specifically drives the clonal expansion of B-cells secreting IgM-RF; upon chronic HCV infection, immune-complexed HCV stimulates the expansion of V_H-1-69$^+$ B-cells, encoding RF WA [44]. These cells become clonally predominant by continued antigenic exposure (usually over a decade or more), independently of T-cell help [44]. The HCV E2-CD81 interactions could result in a lowered B-cell stimulation threshold, facilitating the secretion of various antibodies, including IgM-RF. Clonal B-cells expansions are demonstrable in the intrahepatic lymphocyte infiltrates, in the bone marrow, and in the peripheral blood mononuclear cells [46, 47]. It is still not understood why such an expansion occurs more readily in chronic HCV, compared to other chronic viral diseases such as hepatitis B virus (HBV) or human immunodeficiency virus (HIV). Increased serum B-cell activating factor (BAFF), a TNF-alpha family member required for B-cell survival has been described in HCV-associated MC [48, 49].

In a limited number of patients (<10%), monoclonal B-cell expansion leading to type II MC may evolve into frank B-cell non-Hodgkin-lymphoma. Transformation from polyclonal B-cell proliferation (type III MC) to oligo/monoclonal B-cell proliferation (type II MC) and to the overt malignant lymphoma is a multistep process probably requiring multiple mutagenic events [50, 51]. The duration of B-cell stimulation caused by infectious or other exogenous agents has been also implicated.

1.4. Pathogenesis of Kidney Injury in HCV-Associated Mixed Cryoglobulinemia. Some evidence support that the kidney injury due to HCV is mediated by cryoglobulins. Cryoglobulins are deposited in the mesangium during their trafficking in the glomerulus. They can also be seen as intense subendothelial IgM deposits by immunofluorescence. Their nephrotoxicity is related to special affinity of the IgM*k*-RF for cellular fibronectin present in the mesangial matrix [52]. It has been possible to induce, in an experimental mouse model, a membranoproliferative glomerulonephritis (MPGN) similar to human cryoglobulinemic glomerulonephritis by intravenous administration of 37°C solubilized type II cryoglobulins from patients with HCV membranoproliferative glomerulonephritis [53]. The monoclonal IgM*k*-RF was isolated from such cryoglobulins, separately injected, and able to deposit in the glomerulus; this suggests a special affinity of IgM*k*-RF for the glomerular structures. It needs to be clarified if the deposition of a monoclonal IgM RF in the glomerulus occurs alone or as mixed IgG-IgM cryoglobulin not bound to HCV or as a complex made of HCV, anti-HCV IgG and IgM*k*-RF. Only the RF isolated from cryoprecipitable type II MC had specific affinity; all the other monoclonal RFs are not able to fix fibronectin.

The typical histopathological lesion is a membrano-proliferative (mesangiocapillary) glomerulonephritis [54]. Cryoglobulins can also be deposited in the glomerular capillaries as eosinophilic thrombi, usually associated with vasculitis and fibrinoid necrosis of the glomeruli. Endothelial injury may be an expression of the direct cytopathic activity of the virus. Cryoglobulins may also induce endothelitis via antiendothelial antibody activity and complement activation leading to overexpression of VCAM-1 and subsequent platelet aggregation [54–56]. Immune complexes containing HCV antigens have been observed in the mesangium of patients with cryoglobulinemia leading to mesangial expansion [57]. The presence of HCV-related proteins in the mesangium has been associated with higher proteinuria, possibly reflecting direct mesangial damage of HCV [54]. An increased expression of tolllike receptors has been found in the mesangial cells target of HCV-related MPGN, but not in those of non-HCV MPGN. Mesangial upregulation of toll-like receptors is linked with strong inflammatory activity [58].

1.5. Clinical Features. Clinically, essential mixed cryoglobulinemia is characterized by the triad of purpura, arthralgias, and weakness. The clinical course of patients with MC is variable: some patients have an indolent course, while others develop vasculitic lesions in various organs. Of particular importance is the development of renal disease, since nephritis represents a hallmark of a severe prognosis. Main extrarenal clinical features of MC include neuropathy, hepatomegaly, sicca syndrome, central nervous system, and gut involvement. Peripheral neuropathy has been mostly described as both a motor and sensory polyneuropathy, mainly distal, and of subacute onset; more rarely, patients may present with the multineuropathy features [59–62]. Less frequently, patients may present with a central nervous system involvement due to cerebral vasculitis [63]. Gastrointestinal manifestations are reported in 7.4% of patients with HCV-MC vasculitis. Abdominal pain, surgical abdomen and/or intestinal bleeding were the main presentation. Patients with gastrointestinal manifestations showed more frequent renal (75% versus 30%; $P = 0.003$) and cardiac involvement (25% versus 2%; $P = 0.006$) and higher cryoglobulin levels (2.2 g/L versus 1.2 g/L; $P = 0.07$) [64]. In many series, the pulmonary involvement was infrequent; however, when pulmonary function was routinely investigated, functional abnormalities related to the immunologic aggression to lung interstitium were seen in 61% of patients [65]. Patients frequently exhibit normal or mild elevation of liver enzymes (60%–70% of cases). Individuals with MC usually show serum positivity for anti-HCV antibodies and HCV RNA in serum. Serum rheumatoid factor (RF), which is positive in 16%–70% of HCV positive patients, is usually increased in the setting of HCV MC; the serum levels of C4 and C1q are usually very low [44].

The clinical syndrome of mixed cryoglobulinemia vasculitis can be associated with both type II and III cryoglobulins. In the rheumatologic surveys, patients with type III MC outnumbered those with type II MC [66]; conversely, surveys based on the description of renal involvement revealed a greater prevalence of type II MC, the monoclonal IgM component being mostly IgM*k* [67]. While in the few cases of type III MC with renal involvement the glomerular lesions were variable and nonspecific, in type II MC, in which IgM*k* was the monoclonal component, a specific well-characterized pattern of glomerular disease has been described, called "cryoglobulinemic glomerulonephritis."

The amount of circulating cryoglobulins is measured as cryocrit, showing various levels in different patients and in the same patients at various times. The relationship between the severity of the extrarenal and renal manifestations and the cryocrit level is still discussed [68]. The frequency of kidney involvement in MC varies from 8% to 58% of patients. In a minority of cases, the renal disease can be the first and unique presenting manifestation which makes the diagnosis of MC possible. More than half of patients have proteinuria and/or hematuria only [67]. A nephritic syndrome is diagnosed in about 20% of cases. Often both nephrotic and nephritis syndromes are simultaneously present. In 10% of patients, an acute oliguric kidney failure is the first indicator of kidney disease. Arterial hypertension is a frequent symptom, affecting more than 50% of patients at the time of diagnosis. This complication is frequently severe and require intense therapy. In many cases, a malignant hypertension is associated with rapidly progressive nephritis, while in others refractory hypertension is independent of the severity of kidney disease [68]. Signs of MC vasculitis usually precede the renal disease for many years; however, in 29% of cases renal and extrarenal involvement are concurrent [67].

The first clinical manifestation of type II mixed cryoglobulinemia usually appear in the fourth of fifth decade of life [69]. Women outnumber men, and MC incidence varies in different geographical areas [69]. The course of MC is usually characterized by periods of extra renal symptoms alternated with periods of quiescence. The exacerbation of extra renal symptoms is often associated with a flare of the renal disease, but it can occur independently. In many patients, renal disease shows an indolent course, and end-stage renal disease requiring dialysis is rare (<10%); patients with cryoglobulinemic nephritis have a poor prognosis mainly because of a high incidence of infectious, end-stage liver, and cardiovascular diseases [68].

Roccatello et al. [70] included 146 patients with cryoglobulinemic nephritis, of whom 87% ($n = 127$) were HCV positive. Type II cryoglobulins (IgG/IgM*k*) occurred in 74.4% of cases. The remainder had type III cryoglobulins. A diffuse MPGN was the most common histological pattern (83%). Cox regression model showed that age, serum creatinine, and proteinuria at onset of kidney disease were associated independently with a risk for developing severe renal failure at followup. Survival at 10 years was about 30% and cardiovascular disease was the cause of death in more than 60% of patients; additional causes of death included infections (10%), hepatic failure (19%), and neoplasia (3%). Kaplan Meier survival curves were worsened by baseline serum creatinine greater than 1.5 mg/dL. Conflicting results had been found in an older study by Tarantino et al. [68] who enrolled 105 patients and showed that the number of deaths caused by infections (21%) and hepatic failure (19%) approached the number of deaths caused by cardiovascular diseases (29%). These opposite findings have been attributed to different use of antibiotics, antiviral agents, or immunosuppressive drugs. In 151 consecutive HCV RNA-positive patients with MC vasculitis prospectively followed up between 1993 and 2009, baseline factors associated with a poor prognosis were severe liver fibrosis (hazard ratio (HR), 5.31), central nervous system (HR, 2.72), kidney (HR, 1.91), and heart involvement (HR, 4.2). Use of antiviral agents was associated with a good prognosis, whereas treatment with immunosuppressant agents had a negative impact. The 1-year, 3-year, 5-year, and 10-year survival rates (from the MC diagnosis) were 96%, 86%, 75%, and 63%, respectively [71].

1.6. Therapy of HCV-Associated Mixed Cryoglobulinemia and HCV-Associated Glomerulonephritis. The discovery of HCV and a better understanding of pathophysiological mechanisms provided the opportunity to control HCV-MC using various approaches: (1) antiviral therapy based on the belief that the underlying infection is driving immune complex formation and resultant vasculitis; (2) B-cell depletion therapy

Table 2: Antiviral treatment of HCV-associated GN: clinical studies.

Authors	SVR	Antiviral therapy, schedule	Reference year
Mazzaro et al. [75]	14% (1/7)	Lymphoblastoid-IFN	2000
Bruchfeld et al. [76]	71% (5/7)	IFN-α-2b + ribavirin (n = 5) Peg-FN-α-2b + ribavirin (n = 2)	2003
Rossi et al. [79]	100% (3/3)	IFN-α-2b + ribavirin	2003
Alric et al. [26]	67% (12/18)	IFN-α + ribavirin (n = 14) Peg-FN-α + ribavirin (n = 4)	2004
Saadoun et al. [80]	59% (13/22)	IFN-α-2b + ribavirin (n = 12) Peg-FN-α-2b + ribavirin (n = 10)	2006
Roccatello et al. [70]	11% (6/55)	IFN (n = 10) IFN + ribavirin (n = 45)	2007
Garini et al. [77]	75% (3/4)	IFN-α + ribavirin (n = 2) Peg-FN-α-2a + ribavirin (n = 2)	2007
Abbas et al. [78]	13% (4/30)	IFN-α + ribavirin	2008
Saadoun et al. [84]	40% (4/10)	Peg-IFN-α-2b + ribavirin	2010
Fabrizi et al.	0.42 (95% CI, 0.24; 0.61)	Pooled analysis	2012

Results have been calculated according to an intention-to-treat (ITT) analysis.
SVR: sustained virological response.

targeting B-cells which produce cryoglobulins, and, (3) non-specific immunosuppressive therapy targeting inflammatory cells present in vasculitic lesions. Potential adverse effects of immunosuppressive therapy with glucocorticoids and cytotoxic drugs on an underlying chronic viral infection are a matter of concern [72–74].

1.6.1. Antiviral Therapy. There are no randomized controlled clinical trials (RCTs) regarding the antiviral treatment of HCV-associated glomerulonephritis. HCV-related GN is usually, but not invariably, associated to mixed cryoglobulinemia and only small-sized observational studies exist [24, 38, 70, 75–80] (Table 2). Initial studies were based on monotherapy with conventional or pegylated interferon (IFN) but the combined regimen, pegylated IFN plus ribavirin, has become the gold standard of HCV treatment. The optimal treatment for chronic HCV genotype 1 is now the triple therapy, peg-IFN plus ribavirin and direct-acting antiviral agents (DAA) such as telaprevir or boceprevir [81, 82], according to novel guidelines [83]. However, no evidence has been made on DAA use in patients with kidney impairment [83].

Overall, available information shows positive results in terms of remission of proteinuria, hematuria and improvement of serum creatinine as a consequence of HCV RNA clearance from serum, and a decrease in circulating cryoglobulin levels. However, HCV eradication has not been obtained in all patients, and the clinical benefit of antiviral therapy is sometimes transient and restricted to patients with low-grade involvement [72–74]. A meta-analysis of controlled clinical trials compared the efficacy and safety of antiviral versus immunosuppressive therapy (corticosteroids alone or with cyclophosphamide) in patients with HCV-related glomerulonephritis [85]. Proteinuria decreased more after antiviral (monotherapy with standard IFN for at least six months) than immunosuppressive therapy, OR 3.12 (95% CI, 0.72; 13.48; $P = 0.06$) (random-effects model). Unfortunately, both treatment regimens failed to significantly improve renal dysfunction. Of note, in all patients with reduction of proteinuria, an HCV RNA clearance from serum was given at the end of antiviral therapy.

Data on the antiviral treatment in the setting of GN-associated with hepatitis C are limited but encouraging results exist; we found by pooled analysis that the frequency of sustained viral response was 0.42, 95% confidence intervals (95% CI), 0.24; 0.61 (random-effects model), with significant heterogeneity ($P < 0.0001$; $I^2 = 85.5\%$). As listed in Table 2, the frequency of sustained viral response was higher after combination therapy (pegylated IFN plus ribavirin) than antiviral therapy based on recombinant IFN (alone or with ribavirin). Kidney involvement is frequently associated with negative clinical response; thus, a 48-week course has been recommended. In 72 consecutive patients with symptomatic HCV-associated mixed cryoglobulinemia [80], peg-IFN-α plus ribavirin ($n = 42$ patients) permitted to achieve a higher rate of complete clinical (67.5% versus 56.3%) and virologic response (62.5% versus 53.1%) as compared with standard IFN-α plus ribavirin ($n = 32$), regardless of HCV genotype and viral load. In multivariate analysis, an early virologic response at month 3 (odds ratio (OR), 3.53) was associated with a complete clinical response of MC vasculitis whereas a glomerular filtration rate (GFR) <70 ml/min (OR 0.18) was negatively linked with a complete clinical response [80].

Antiviral therapy of HCV-associated GN shows some shortcomings that must be weighted. Firstly, the impact of antiviral therapy on long-term outcomes of kidney disease is not well known. Secondly, response to antiviral therapy is usually rather slow as it takes several weeks to obtain viral clearance and clinical remission, whereas rapid renal involvement is not uncommon in these patients. Thirdly, interferon-alpha has been reported to exacerbate proteinuria in some patients with underlying glomerulopathies [86]. Finally, use of ribavirin in patients with glomerular filtration rate less than 50 mL per min per 1.73 m^2 had not been recommended in some guidelines [87] even if preliminary data support ribavirin use in patients with chronic kidney disease and GFR < 50 mL/min/1.73 m^2 in a cautious and well-monitored setting [76].

1.6.2. B-Cell Depletion Therapy. Given the etiologic role of hepatitis C virus infection in the majority of patients with MC, targeting HCV replication by antiviral treatment (interferon plus ribavirin) should be considered the first-line therapy in HCV-related MC and its complications. Recent evidence has given emphasis to the notion that HCV infection represent the "initiation" step followed by the "perpetuation" step where infections, autoantigens, and cell regulation abnormalities support autoimmunity and B-cell lympho-proliferation.

Rituximab (RTX) is a chimeric monoclonal antibody directed to CD20 antigen, a transmembrane protein expressed on pre-B and mature lymphocytes, and is highly effective for *in vivo* B-cell depletion, particularly IgM autoantibody-producing B-cells [72]. Due to its selective activity, rituximab has been used instead of other immunosuppressive approaches such as steroids, cyclophosphamide, plasma exchange, and other cytotoxic drugs. High-dose or prolonged corticosteroid treatment greatly increase morbidity (i.e., myopathy, osteoporosis, major infections) and cyclophosphamide may be hazardous (cytopenia, bladder cancer, and opportunistic infections).

Rituximab was originally approved for the treatment of low-grade B-cell non-Hodgkin's lymphoma (NHL). More recently, it has been used to treat severe hematologic disorders including pure red cell aplasia, haemolytic anaemia, and posttransplant B-lymphoproliferative disorders. Rituximab is usually give intravenously at 375 mg/m^2, once a week for one month. Mixed cryoglobulinemia is featured by chronic stimulation of B lymphocytes by HCV and widespread autoantibody production related to HCV-induced lowering of the cell activation threshold. Thus, MC patients have been considered appropriate candidates for rituximab therapy. Various reports have emphasized its efficacy in the management of symptomatic mixed cryoglobulinemia [88–106]. RTX proved to have great efficacy for the main vasculitic signs (remission of purpura, arthralgias, and improvement of peripheral neuropathy), even if a relapse of mixed cryoglobulinemia has been noted in many patients after completion of therapy. Laboratory features, that is, reduction of cryocrit percentage and RF activity, and increases of C4 levels were consistent with the clinical efficacy.

Two uncontrolled pilot trials have been conducted on RTX use for HCV-associated GN. A total of 11 individuals have been treated. An important decrease in proteinuria was noted by Roccatello et al. (2.18 ± 1.57 versus 0.63 ± 0.4 g/day, $P = 0.04$) [92] and Quartuccio et al. (1.74 ± 1.26 versus 0.5 ± 0.729 g/day, $P = 0.09$) [93]. A concomitant reduction of serum levels of rheumatoid factor was also found in the first (751.1 ± 66 versus 363.8 + 273 IU/L, P = NS) and second study (1, 888.8 ± 1, 80 IU/L versus 1, 414 ± 2.52 IU/L, P = NS). No acute or delayed severe adverse effects were seen. However, clinical relapses of glomerular disease after completion of rituximab therapy were found.

A number of side effects have been reported in patients with HCV-associated mixed cryoglobulinemia treated with rituximab. RTX has no efficacy on HCV viral clearance and an increment of HCV RNA in both unfractionated sera and the cryoprecipitate has been reported by various authors [88]. Reactivation of liver disease related to HBV- or HCV-infections after rituximab therapy has been also shown. We recently reported on a renal transplant recipient with chronic and mild hepatitis C who received standard rituximab therapy for gastric lymphoma [107]. Rituximab was complicated by cholestatic hepatitis C with extremely high HCV RNA levels; liver failure occurred. The patient developed bacterial pneumonia, and respiratory insufficiency was the cause of death. Although other mechanisms could not be excluded, we implicated rituximab in the pathogenesis of cholestatic hepatitis C in our patient. Randomized controlled trials with adequate size and followup are warranted to clarify the risk to benefit ratio for RTX use in HCV-associated mixed cryoglobulinemia patients, particularly those with kidney involvement.

In order to better define the place of rituximab in the therapeutic strategy of HCV-related mixed cryoglobulinemia, some authors have used antiviral therapy with or without rituximab in HCV MC. Two prospective, controlled clinical trials have compared the efficacy and safety of a combination of rituximab followed by peg-IFN-α/ribavirin versus peg-IFN-α/ribavirin for HCV-related mixed cryoglobulinemia. Compared with peg-IFN-α/rituximab ($n = 55$), Saadoun et al. [84] observed that rituximab plus peg-IFN-α/ribavirin ($n = 38$) had a shorter time to clinical remission (5.4 ± 4 versus 8.4 ± 4.7 months, $P = 0.004$) and higher rates of cryoglobulin clearance (68.4% versus 43.6%, $P = 0.001$). They observed a significant reduction of daily proteinuria and hematuria in both the groups; patients treated with rituximab followed by peg-IFN-α/ribavirin also had a significant improvement of kidney function (217.5 ± 47.4 versus 136.9 ± 27 μmol/L, $P = 0.03$), whereas no significant change was noted in the second group (150 ± 30 versus 169.2 ± 44 μmol/L, NS). In the work by Dammacco et al. [108], a complete response was achieved in 54.5% (12/22) of patients who received RTX followed by peg-IFN-α/ribavirin and in 33.3% (5/15) of patients on peg-IFN-α/ribavirin. No significant change in serum creatinine and daily proteinuria in both the groups occurred.

1.6.3. Nonspecific Immunosuppressive Agents. Immunosuppressive agents have been given to MC patients with severe disease manifestations such as membranoproliferative glomerulonephritis, severe neuropathy and other life-threatening complications. A combination of corticosteroids and immunosuppressant such as cyclophosphamide and azathioprine has been used while awaiting the generally slow response to antiviral treatments. In a large retrospective study of 105 patients with cryoglobulinemia vasculitis associated renal disease, 80% were administered corticosteroids and/or cytotoxic agents, while 67% underwent plasma exchange [68]. Despite this aggressive approach, long-lasting remission of the renal disease was achieved in only 14% of cases, and the 10-year survival rate was only 49%.

Corticosteroids, used alone or in addition to IFN-α did not favourably affect the response of HCV-related vasculitis manifestations in two controlled studies [109, 110]. In one randomized trial, methyl-prednisolone alone given for one year was associated with clinical response in 22% of patients, compared with 66% and 71% in patients receiving IFN-α or IFN-α plus methyl-prednisolone, respectively [110]. Low dose corticosteroids may help to control minor intermittent inflammatory signs such as arthralgia but do not succeed in cases of major organ involvement (i.e. neurologic, renal) or in the long-term control of MC vasculitis.

Plasma exchange offers the theoretical advantage of removing the pathogenic cryoglobulins from the circulation in order to avoid the rebound increase in cryoglobulinemia commonly seen after discontinuation of corticosteroids. When used in combination with HCV treatment, three times weekly plasma exchange did not modify the viral response if standard IFN-α was given after each plasma exchange session [111].

1.6.4. Treatment of HCV-Associated Mixed Cryoglobulinemia: Conclusions. Given to the lack of randomized controlled trials, it is difficult to define a standard strategy for the therapy of HCV-related mixed cryoglobulinemia. We recommend an approach tailored on the disease manifestations, and comorbidities. Antiviral therapy with Peg-IFN plus ribavirin is suggested for HCV-MC patients with mild to moderate disease severity and activity (i.e., without rapidly progressive nephritis, motor neuropathy, or other life-threatening complications). In patients presenting with severe, rapidly progressive vasculitic complications (i.e., progressive renal disease, progressive motor neuropathy, extensive skin disease including ulcers and distal necrosis), a combined treatment with high-dose steroids, immunosuppressors and plasma-exchange has been recommended. In the setting of severe/active but not life-threatening complications RTX may now represent the first option. Novel approaches include antiviral regimens with better efficacy and tolerance, and the combination of rituximab plus antiviral agents, provided no new safety concerns are raised using this approach.

Abbreviations

CI: Confidence intervals
DAA: Direct-acting antiviral agents
EMC: Essential mixed cryoglobulinemia
GFR: Glomerular filtration rate
HR: Hazard ratio
HBV: Hepatitis B virus
HCV: Hepatitis C virus
HIV: Human immunodeficiency virus
Ig: Immunoglobulin
MC: Mixed cryoglobulinemia
MPGN: Membranoproliferative glomerulonephritis
NHL: Non-Hodgkin's lymphoma
NS: Not significant
OR: Odds ratio
RF: Rheumatoid factor
RCT: Randomized controlled trial
RTX: Rituximab
SVR: Sustained virological response.

Acknowledgments

This work has been supported in part by the grant "Project Glomerulonephritis," and in the memory of Pippo Neglia.

References

[1] M. Wintrobe and M. Buell, "Hyperproteinemia associated with multiple myeloma: with report of a case in which an extraordinary hyperproteinemia was associated with thrombosis of the retinal veins and symptoms suggesting Raynaud's disease," *Bulletin of the Johns Hopkins Hospital*, vol. 52, no. 2, pp. 156–164, 1933.

[2] A. Lerner and C. Watson, "Studies of cryoglobulins. I. Unusual purpura associated with the presence of a high concentration of cryoglobulin (cold precipitable serum globulins)," *American Journal of Medicine*, vol. 214, no. 4, pp. 410–418, 1947.

[3] M. Meltzer, E. C. Franklin, K. Elias, R. T. McCluskey, and N. Cooper, "Cryoglobulinemia-A clinical and laboratory study. II. Cryoglobulins with rheumatoid factor activity," *The American Journal of Medicine*, vol. 40, no. 6, pp. 837–856, 1966.

[4] J. Brouet, J. Clauvel, F. Danon, M. Klein, and M. Seligmann, "Biologic and clinical significance of cryoglobulins. A report of 86 cases," *American Journal of Medicine*, vol. 57, no. 5, pp. 775–788, 1974.

[5] F. Fabrizi, P. Colucci, C. Ponticelli, and F. Locatelli, "Kidney and liver involvement in cryoglobulinemia," *Seminars in Nephrology*, vol. 22, no. 4, pp. 309–318, 2002.

[6] Q. L. Choo, G. Kuo, A. J. Weiner, L. R. Overby, D. W. Bradley, and M. Houghton, "Isolation of a cDNA clone derived from a blood-borne non-A, non-B viral hepatitis genome," *Science*, vol. 244, no. 4902, pp. 359–362, 1989.

[7] G. Kuo, Q. L. Choo, H. J. Alter et al., "An assay for circulating antibodies to a major etiologic virus of human non-A, non-B hepatitis," *Science*, vol. 244, no. 4902, pp. 362–364, 1989.

[8] M. Pascual, L. Perrin, E. Giostra, and J. A. Schifferli, "Hepatitis C virus in patients with cryoglobulinemia type II," *Journal of Infectious Diseases*, vol. 162, no. 2, pp. 567–569, 1990.

[9] C. Ferri, F. Greco, G. Longombardo et al., "Antibodies to hepatitis C virus in patients with mixed cryoglobulinemia," *Arthritis and Rheumatism*, vol. 34, no. 12, pp. 1606–1610, 1991.

[10] P. Cacoub, T. Poynard, P. Ghillani et al., "MULTIVIRC Group. Multidepartment Virus C: extra-hepatic manifestations of chronic hepatitis C," *Arthritis & Rheumatism*, vol. 42, no. 10, pp. 2204–2212, 1999.

[11] O. Trejo, M. Ramos-Casals, M. García-Carrasco et al., "Cryoglobulinemia: study of etiologic factors and clinical and immunologic features in 443 patients from a single center," *Medicine*, vol. 80, no. 4, pp. 252–262, 2001.

[12] D. Saadoun, J. Sellam, P. Ghillani-Dalbin, R. Crecel, J. C. Piette, and P. Cacoub, "Increased risks of lymphoma and death among

patients with non-hepatitis C virus-related mixed cryoglobulinemia," *Archives of Internal Medicine*, vol. 166, no. 19, pp. 2101–2108, 2006.

[13] J. M. Cruzado, M. Carrera, J. Torras, and J. M. Grinyó, "Hepatitis C virus infection and de Novo glomerular lesions in renal allografts," *American Journal of Transplantation*, vol. 1, no. 2, pp. 171–178, 2001.

[14] J. M. Morales, J. Pascual-Capdevila, J. M. Campistol et al., "Membranous glomerulonephritis associated with hepatitis C virus infection in renal transplant patients," *Transplantation*, vol. 63, no. 11, pp. 1634–1639, 1997.

[15] D. Roth, R. Cirocco, K. Zucker et al., "De novo membranoproliferative glomerulonephritis in hepatitis C virus- infected renal allograft recipients," *Transplantation*, vol. 59, no. 12, pp. 1676–1682, 1995.

[16] H. B. El-Serag, H. Hampel, C. Yeh, and L. Rabeneck, "Extrahepatic manifestations of hepatitis C among United States male veterans," *Hepatology*, vol. 36, no. 6, pp. 1439–1445, 2002.

[17] J. I. Tsui, E. Vittinghoff, M. G. Shlipak, and A. M. O'Hare, "Relationship between hepatitis C and chronic kidney disease: results from the Third National Health and Nutrition Examination Survey," *Journal of the American Society of Nephrology*, vol. 17, no. 4, pp. 1168–1174, 2006.

[18] J. I. Tsui, E. Vittinghoff, M. G. Shlipak et al., "Association of hepatitis C seropositivity with increased risk for developing end-stage renal disease," *Archives of Internal Medicine*, vol. 167, no. 12, pp. 1271–1276, 2007.

[19] L. S. Dalrymple, T. Koepsell, J. Sampson et al., "Hepatitis C virus infection and the prevalence of renal insufficiency," *Clinical Journal of the American Society of Nephrology*, vol. 2, no. 4, pp. 715–721, 2007.

[20] S. M. Moe, A. J. Pampalone, S. Ofner, M. Rosenman, E. Teal, and S. L. Hui, "Association of Hepatitis C virus infection with prevalence and development of kidney disease," *American Journal of Kidney Diseases*, vol. 51, no. 6, pp. 885–892, 2008.

[21] S. K. Asrani, P. Buchanan, B. Pinsky, L. R. Rey, M. Schnitzler, and F. Kanwal, "Lack of association between Hepatitis C infection and chronic kidney disease," *Clinical Gastroenterology and Hepatology*, vol. 8, no. 1, pp. 79–84, 2010.

[22] J. J. Lee, M. Y. Lin, Y. H. Yang, S. N. Lu, H. C. Chen, and S. J. Hwang, "Association of Hepatitis C and B virus infection with CKD in an endemic area in Taiwan: a cross-sectional study," *American Journal of Kidney Diseases*, vol. 56, no. 1, pp. 23–31, 2010.

[23] A. A. Butt, X. Wang, and L. F. Fried, "HCV infection and the incidence of CKD," *American Journal of Kidney Diseases*, vol. 57, no. 3, pp. 396–402, 2011.

[24] C. M. Wyatt, C. Malvestutto, S. G. Coca, P. E. Klotman, and C. R. Parikh, "The impact of hepatitis C virus coinfection on HIV-related kidney disease: a systematic review and meta-analysis," *AIDS*, vol. 22, no. 14, pp. 1799–1807, 2008.

[25] H. Izzedine, D. Sene, P. Cacoub et al., "Kidney diseases in HIV/HCV-co-infected patients," *AIDS*, vol. 23, no. 10, pp. 1219–1226, 2009.

[26] L. Alric, E. Plaisier, S. Thébault et al., "Influence of antiviral therapy in Hepatitis C virus-associated cryoglobulinemic MPGN," *American Journal of Kidney Diseases*, vol. 43, no. 4, pp. 617–623, 2004.

[27] S. Liangpunsakul and N. Chalasani, "Relationship between hepatitis C and microalbuminuria: results from the NHANES III," *Kidney International*, vol. 67, no. 1, pp. 285–290, 2005.

[28] J. F. Huang, W. L. Chuang, C. Y. Dai et al., "Viral hepatitis and proteinuria in an area endemic for hepatitis B and C infections: another chain of link?" *Journal of Internal Medicine*, vol. 260, no. 3, pp. 255–262, 2006.

[29] C. L. Davis, D. R. Gretch, J. D. Perkins et al., "Hepatitis C–associated glomerular disease in liver transplant recipients," *Liver Transplantation and Surgery*, vol. 1, no. 3, pp. 166–175, 1995.

[30] T. Sikaneta, W. W. Williams, R. T. Chung, A. B. Cosimi, and M. Pascual, "Remission of hepatitis C virus-associated cryoglobulinemic glomerulonephritis with interferon alfa-2b and ribavirin combination therapy after liver transplantation," *Transplantation*, vol. 74, no. 12, pp. 1767–1768, 2002.

[31] M. Montalbano, L. Pasulo, A. Sonzogni, G. Remuzzi, M. Colledan, and M. Strazzabosco, "Treatment with pegylated interferon and ribavirin for hepatitis C virus-associated severe cryoglobulinemia in a liver/kidney transplant recipient," *Journal of Clinical Gastroenterology*, vol. 41, no. 2, pp. 216–220, 2007.

[32] P. Cacoub, T. Maisonobe, V. Thibault et al., "Systemic vasculitis in patients with hepatitis C," *Journal of Rheumatology*, vol. 28, no. 1, pp. 109–118, 2001.

[33] S. Beddhu, S. Bastacky, and J. P. Johnson, "The clinical and morphologic spectrum of renal cryoglobulinemia," *Medicine*, vol. 81, no. 5, pp. 398–409, 2002.

[34] S. T. Takyar, D. S. Li, Y. H. Wang, R. Trowbridge, and E. J. Gowans, "Specific detection of minus-strand hepatitis C virus RNA by reverse- transcription polymerase chain reaction on polyA+-purified RNA," *Hepatology*, vol. 32, no. 2, pp. 382–387, 2000.

[35] M. H. V. Sung, S. Shimodaira, A. L. Doughty et al., "Establishment of B-cell lymphoma cell lines persistently infected with hepatitis C virus in vivo and in vitro: the apoptotic effects of virus infection," *Journal of Virology*, vol. 77, no. 3, pp. 2134–2146, 2003.

[36] S. De Vita, V. De Re, D. Sansonno et al., "Lack of HCV infection in malignant cells refutes the hypothesis of a direct transforming action of the virus in the pathogenesis of HCV-associated B-cell NHLs," *Tumori*, vol. 88, no. 5, pp. 400–406, 2002.

[37] S. Marukian, C. T. Jones, L. Andrus et al., "Cell culture-produced hepatitis C virus does not infect peripheral blood mononuclear cells," *Hepatology*, vol. 48, no. 6, pp. 1843–1850, 2008.

[38] R. J. Johnson, D. R. Gretch, W. G. Couser et al., "Hepatitis C virus-associated glomerulonephritis. Effect of α-interferon therapy," *Kidney International*, vol. 46, no. 6, pp. 1700–1704, 1994.

[39] C. Ferri, F. Greco, G. Longombardo et al., "Antibodies to hepatitis C virus in patients with mixed cryoglobulinemia," *Arthritis and Rheumatism*, vol. 34, no. 12, pp. 1606–1610, 1991.

[40] F. Fabrizi, C. Pozzi, M. Farina et al., "Hepatitis C virus infection and acute or chronic glomerulonephritis: an epidemiological and clinical appraisal," *Nephrology Dialysis Transplantation*, vol. 13, no. 8, pp. 1991–1997, 1998.

[41] V. Agnello, R. T. Chung, and L. M. Kaplan, "A role for hepatitis C virus infection in Type II cryoglobulinemia," *The New England Journal of Medicine*, vol. 327, no. 21, pp. 1490–1495, 1992.

[42] P. Cacoub, F. L. Fabiani, L. Musset et al., "Mixed cryoglobulinemia and hepatitis C virus," *American Journal of Medicine*, vol. 96, no. 2, pp. 124–132, 1994.

[43] D. Sansonno, L. Gesualdo, C. Manno, F. P. Schena, and F. Dammacco, "Hepatitis C virus-related proteins in kidney tissue

from hepatitis C virus-infected patients with cryoglobulinemic membranoproliferative glomerulonephritis," *Hepatology*, vol. 25, no. 5, pp. 1237–1244, 1997.

[44] E. D. Charles and L. B. Dustin, "Hepatitis C virus-induced cryoglobulinemia," *Kidney International*, vol. 76, no. 8, pp. 818–824, 2009.

[45] D. Rosa, G. Saletti, E. De Gregorio et al., "Activation of naïve B lymphocytes via CD81, a pathogenetic mechanism for hepatitis C virus-associated B lymphocyte disorders," *Proceedings of the National Academy of Sciences of the United States of America*, vol. 102, no. 51, pp. 18544–18549, 2005.

[46] L. Vallat, Y. Benhamou, M. Gutierrez et al., "Clonal B cell populations in the blood and liver of patients with chronic hepatitis C virus infection," *Arthritis and Rheumatism*, vol. 50, no. 11, pp. 3668–3678, 2004.

[47] E. D. Charles, R. M. Green, S. Marukian et al., "Clonal expansion of immunoglobulin $M^{+}CD27^{+}$ B cells in HCV-associated mixed cryoglobulinemia," *Blood*, vol. 111, no. 3, pp. 1344–1356, 2008.

[48] D. A. Landau, M. Rosenzwajg, D. Saadoun, D. Klatzmann, and P. Cacoub, "The B lymphocyte stimulator receptor-ligand system in hepatitis C virus-induced B cell clonal disorders," *Annals of the Rheumatic Diseases*, vol. 68, no. 3, pp. 337–344, 2009.

[49] M. Fabris, L. Quartuccio, S. Sacco et al., "B-Lymphocyte stimulator (BLys) up-regulation in mixed cryoglobulinaemia syndrome and hepatitis-C virus infection," *Rheumatology*, vol. 46, no. 1, pp. 37–43, 2007.

[50] D. Sene, P. Ghillani-Dalbin, V. Thibault et al., "Longterm course of mixed cryoglobulinemia in patients infected with hepatitis C virus," *Journal of Rheumatology*, vol. 31, no. 11, pp. 2199–2206, 2004.

[51] D. A. Landau, D. Saadoun, L. H. Calabrese, and P. Cacoub, "The pathophysiology of HCV induced B-cell clonal disorders," *Autoimmunity Reviews*, vol. 6, no. 8, pp. 581–587, 2007.

[52] A. Fornasieri, S. Armelloni, P. Bernasconi et al., "High binding of immunoglobulin Mκ rheumatoid factor from type II cryoglobulins to cellular fibronectin: a mechanism for induction of in situ immune complex glomerulonephritis?" *American Journal of Kidney Diseases*, vol. 27, no. 4, pp. 476–483, 1996.

[53] A. Fornasieri, M. Li, S. Armelloni et al., "Glomerulonephritis induced by human IgMK-IgG cryoglobulins in mice," *Laboratory Investigation*, vol. 69, no. 5, pp. 531–540, 1993.

[54] R. S. Barsoum, "Hepatitis C virus: from entry to renal injury—facts and potentials," *Nephrology Dialysis Transplantation*, vol. 22, no. 7, pp. 1840–1848, 2007.

[55] P. Cacoub, P. Ghillani, R. Revelen et al., "Anti-endothelial cell auto-antibodies in hepatitis C virus mixed cryoglobulinemia," *Journal of Hepatology*, vol. 31, no. 4, pp. 598–603, 1999.

[56] G. Kaplanski, T. Maisonobe, V. Marin et al., "Vascular cell adhesion molecule-1 (VCAM-1) plays a central role in the pathogenesis of severe forms of vasculitis due to hepatitis C-associated mixed cryoglobulinemia," *Journal of Hepatology*, vol. 42, no. 3, pp. 334–340, 2005.

[57] D. Sansonno, G. Lauletta, M. Montrone, G. Grandaliano, F. P. Schena, and F. Dammacco, "Hepatitis C virus RNA and core protein in kidney glomerular and tubular structures isolated with laser capture microdissection," *Clinical and Experimental Immunology*, vol. 140, no. 3, pp. 498–506, 2005.

[58] M. Wörnle, H. Schmid, B. Banas et al., "Novel role of toll-like receptor 3 in hepatitis C-associated glomerulonephritis," *American Journal of Pathology*, vol. 168, no. 2, pp. 370–385, 2006.

[59] J. Costa, C. Resende, and M. De Carvalho, "Motor-axonal polyneuropathy associated with hepatitis C virus," *European Journal of Neurology*, vol. 10, no. 2, pp. 183–185, 2003.

[60] F. J. Authier, J. M. Pawlotsky, J. P. Viard, L. Guillevin, J. D. Degos, and R. K. Gherardi, "High incidence of hepatitis C virus infection in patients with cryoglobulinemic neuropathy," *Annals of Neurology*, vol. 34, no. 5, pp. 749–750, 1993.

[61] D. Saadoun, B. Terrier, O. Semoun et al., "Hepatitis C virus associated polyarteritis nodosa," *Arthritis Care and Research*, vol. 63, no. 3, pp. 427–435, 2011.

[62] G. Valli, A. De Vecchi, L. Gaddi, E. Nobile-Orazio, A. Tarantino, and S. Barbieri, "Peripheral nervous system involvement in essential cryoglobulinemia and nephropathy," *Clinical and Experimental Rheumatology*, vol. 7, no. 5, pp. 479–483, 1989.

[63] M. Casato, D. Saadoun, A. Marchetti et al., "Central nervous system involvement in hepatitis C virus cryoglobulinemia vasculitis: a multicenter case-control study using magnetic resonance imaging and neuropsychological tests," *Journal of Rheumatology*, vol. 32, no. 3, pp. 484–488, 2005.

[64] B. Terrier, D. Saadoun, D. Sène, S. Scerra, L. Musset, and P. Cacoub, "Presentation and outcome of gastrointestinal involvement in hepatitis C virus-related systemic vasculitis: a case-control study from a single-centre cohort of 163 patients," *Gut*, vol. 59, no. 12, pp. 1709–1715, 2010.

[65] G. Viegi, E. Fornai, C. Ferri et al., "Lung function in essential mixed cryoglobulinemia: a short-term follow-up," *Clinical Rheumatology*, vol. 8, no. 3, pp. 331–338, 1989.

[66] P. Gorevic, H. Kassab, Y. Levo et al., "Mixed cryoglobulinemia: clinical aspects and long-term follow-up of 40 patients," *American Journal of Medicine*, vol. 69, no. 2, pp. 287–308, 1980.

[67] A. Tarantino, A. De Vecchi, G. Montagnino et al., "Renal disease in essential mixed cryoglobulinaemia. Long-term follow-up of 44 patients," *Quarterly Journal of Medicine*, vol. 50, no. 197, pp. 1–30, 1981.

[68] A. Tarantino, M. Campise, G. Banfi et al., "Long-term predictors of survival in essential mixed cryoglobulinemic glomerulonephritis," *Kidney International*, vol. 47, no. 2, pp. 618–623, 1995.

[69] C. Ferri, "Mixed cryoglobulinemia," *Orphanet Journal of Rare Diseases*, vol. 3, no. 1, article 25, 2008.

[70] D. Roccatello, A. Fornasieri, O. Giachino et al., "Multicenter study on Hepatitis C virus-related cryoglobulinemic glomerulonephritis," *American Journal of Kidney Diseases*, vol. 49, no. 1, pp. 69–82, 2007.

[71] B. Terrier, O. Semoun, D. Saadoun, D. Sène, M. Resche-Rigon, and P. Cacoub, "Prognostic factors in patients with hepatitis C virus infection and systemic vasculitis," *Arthritis and Rheumatism*, vol. 63, no. 6, pp. 1748–1757, 2011.

[72] F. Fabrizi, G. Lunghi, P. Messa, and P. Martin, "Therapy of hepatitis C virus-associated glomerulonephritis: current approaches," *Journal of Nephrology*, vol. 21, no. 6, pp. 813–825, 2008.

[73] N. Perico, D. Cattaneo, B. Bikbov, and G. Remuzzi, "Hepatitis C infection and chronic renal diseases," *Clinical Journal of the American Society of Nephrology*, vol. 4, no. 1, pp. 207–220, 2009.

[74] Kidney Disease, "Improving Global Outcomes. KDIGO clinical practice guidelines for the prevention, diagnosis, evaluation, and treatment of Hepatitis C in chronic kidney disease," *Kidney International*, vol. 73, supplement 109, pp. S1–S99, 2008.

[75] C. Mazzaro, G. Panarello, S. Carniello et al., "Interferon versus steroids in patients with hepatitis C virus-associated cryoglobulinaemic glomerulonephritis," *Digestive and Liver Disease*, vol. 32, no. 8, pp. 708–715, 2000.

[76] A. Bruchfeld, K. Lindahl, L. Ståhle, M. Söderberg, and R. Schvarcz, "Interferon and ribavirin treatment in patients with hepatitis C-associated renal disease and renal insufficiency," *Nephrology Dialysis Transplantation*, vol. 18, no. 8, pp. 1573–1580, 2003.

[77] G. Garini, L. Allegri, F. Iannuzzella, A. Vaglio, and C. Buzio, "HCV-related cryoglobulinemic glomerulonephritis: implications of antiviral and immunosuppressive therapies," *Acta Biomedica de l'Ateneo Parmense*, vol. 78, no. 1, pp. 51–81, 2007.

[78] G. Abbas, S. Hussain, and T. Shafi, "Effect of antiviral therapy on hepatitis C virus related glomerulopathy," *Saudi Journal of Kidney Diseases and Transplantation*, vol. 19, no. 5, pp. 775–780, 2008.

[79] P. Rossi, T. Bertani, P. Baio et al., "Hepatitis C virus-related cryoglobulinemic glomerulonephritis: long-term remission after antiviral therapy," *Kidney International*, vol. 63, no. 6, pp. 2236–2241, 2003.

[80] D. Saadoun, M. Resche-Rigon, V. Thibault, J. C. Piette, and P. Cacoub, "Antiviral therapy for hepatitis C virus-associated mixed cryoglobulinemia vasculitis: a long-term followup study," *Arthritis and Rheumatism*, vol. 54, no. 11, pp. 3696–3706, 2006.

[81] J. G. McHutchison, G. T. Everson, S. C. Gordon et al., "Telaprevir with peginterferon and ribavirin for chronic HCV genotype 1 infection," *The New England Journal of Medicine*, vol. 360, no. 18, pp. 1827–1838, 2009.

[82] C. Hézode, N. Forestier, G. Dusheiko et al., "Telaprevir and peginterferon with or without ribavirin for chronic HCV infection," *The New England Journal of Medicine*, vol. 360, no. 18, pp. 1839–1850, 2009.

[83] G. Ghany, D. Nelson, D. Strader, D. Thomas, and L. Seeff, "An update on treatment of genotype 1 chronic hepatitis C virus infection: 2011 practice guidelines by the American Association for the Study of Liver Diseases," *Hepatology*, vol. 54, no. 4, pp. 1433–1434, 2011.

[84] D. Saadoun, M. R. Rigon, D. Sene et al., "Rituximab plus Peg-interferon-α/ribavirin compared with Peg-interferon-α/ribavirin in hepatitis C-related mixed cryoglobulinemia," *Blood*, vol. 116, no. 3, pp. 326–334, 2010.

[85] F. Fabrizi, A. Bruchfeld, S. Mangano, V. Dixit, P. Messa, and P. Martin, "Interferon therapy for HCV-associated glomerulonephritis: meta-analysis of controlled trials," *International Journal of Artificial Organs*, vol. 30, no. 3, pp. 212–219, 2007.

[86] S. Ohta, H. Yokoyama, T. Wada et al., "Exacerbation of glomerulonephritis in subjects with chronic hepatitis C virus infection after interferon therapy," *American Journal of Kidney Diseases*, vol. 33, no. 6, pp. 1040–1048, 1999.

[87] D. B. Strader, T. Wright, D. L. Thomas, and L. B. Seeff, "Diagnosis, management, and treatment of Hepatitis C," *Hepatology*, vol. 39, no. 4, pp. 1147–1171, 2004.

[88] D. Sansonno, V. De Re, G. Lauletta, F. A. Tucci, M. Boiocchi, and F. Dammacco, "Monoclonal antibody treatment of mixed cryoglobulinemia resistant to interferon α with an anti-CD20," *Blood*, vol. 101, no. 10, pp. 3818–3826, 2003.

[89] F. Zaja, S. De Vita, C. Mazzaro et al., "Efficacy and safety of rituximab in type II mixed cryoglobulinemia," *Blood*, vol. 101, no. 10, pp. 3827–3834, 2003.

[90] E. Ghijsels, E. Lerut, Y. Vanrenterghem, and D. Kuypers, "Anti-CD20 monoclonal antibody (rituximab) treatment for hepatitis C-negative therapy-resistant essential mixed cryoglobulinemia with renal and cardiac failure," *American Journal of Kidney Diseases*, vol. 43, no. 5, pp. e34–e38, 2004.

[91] M. Koukoulaki, S. C. Abeygunasekara, K. G. C. Smith, and D. R. W. Jayne, "Remission of refractory hepatitis C-negative cryoglobulinaemic vasculitis after rituximab and infliximab," *Nephrology Dialysis Transplantation*, vol. 20, no. 1, pp. 213–216, 2005.

[92] D. Roccatello, S. Baldovino, D. Rossi et al., "Long-term effects of anti-CD20 monoclonal antibody treatment of cryoglobulinaemic glomerulonephritis," *Nephrology Dialysis Transplantation*, vol. 19, no. 12, pp. 3054–3061, 2004.

[93] L. Quartuccio, G. Soardo, G. Romano et al., "Rituximab treatment for glomerulonephritis in HCV-associated mixed cryoglobulinaemia: efficacy and safety in the absence of steroids," *Rheumatology*, vol. 45, no. 7, pp. 842–846, 2006.

[94] D. Roccatello, S. Baldovino, D. Rossi et al., "Rituximab as a therapeutic tool in severe mixed cryoglobulinemia," *Clinical Reviews in Allergy and Immunology*, vol. 34, no. 1, pp. 111–117, 2008.

[95] G. Basse, D. Ribes, N. Kamar et al., "Rituximab Therapy for Mixed Cryoglobulinemia in Seven Renal Transplant Patients," *Transplantation Proceedings*, vol. 38, no. 7, pp. 2308–2310, 2006.

[96] A. Braun, T. Neumann, P. Oelzner et al., "Cryoglobulinaemia type III with severe neuropathy and immune complex glomerulonephritis: remission after plasmapheresis and rituximab," *Rheumatology International*, vol. 28, no. 5, pp. 503–506, 2008.

[97] M. Visentini, M. Granata, M. L. Veneziano et al., "Efficacy of low-dose rituximab for mixed cryoglobulinemia," *Clinical Immunology*, vol. 125, no. 1, pp. 30–33, 2007.

[98] S. De Vita, L. Quartuccio, and M. Fabris, "Rituximab in mixed cryoglobulinemia: increased experience and perspectives," *Digestive and Liver Disease*, vol. 39, no. 1, supplement, pp. S122–S128, 2007.

[99] A. Petrarca, L. Rigacci, M. Monti et al., "Improvement in liver cirrhosis after treatment of HCV-related mixed cryoglobulinemia with rituximab," *Digestive and Liver Disease*, vol. 39, no. 1, supplement, pp. S129–S133, 2007.

[100] M. R. Korte, M. J. van Heerde, R. A. de Man, and M. H. G. Betjes, "Rituximab for the treatment of glomerulonephritis in hepatitis C associated cryoglobulinaemia," *Netherlands Journal of Medicine*, vol. 66, no. 1, pp. 27–30, 2008.

[101] D. Saadoun, M. Resche-Rigon, D. Sene, L. Perard, A. Karras, and P. Cacoub, "Rituximab combined with Peg-interferon-ribavirin in refractory hepatitis C virus-associated cryoglobulinaemia vasculitis," *Annals of the Rheumatic Diseases*, vol. 67, no. 10, pp. 1431–1436, 2008.

[102] A. Petrarca, L. Rigacci, P. Caini et al., "Safety and efficacy of rituximab in patients with hepatitis C virus-related mixed cryoglobulinemia and severe liver disease," *Blood*, vol. 116, no. 3, pp. 335–342, 2010.

[103] F. Wink, P. M. Houtman, and T. L. T. A. Jansen, "Rituximab in cryoglobulinaemic vasculitis, evidence for its effectivity: a case report and review of literature," *Clinical Rheumatology*, vol. 30, no. 2, pp. 293–300, 2011.

[104] M. Visentini, S. Ludovisi, A. Petrarca et al., "A phase II, single-arm multicenter study of low-dose rituximab for refractory mixed cryoglobulinemia secondary to hepatitis C virus infection," *Autoimmunity Reviews*, vol. 10, no. 11, pp. 714–719, 2011.

[105] C. Ferri, P. Cacoub, C. Mazzaro et al., "Treatment with rituximab in patients with mixed cryoglobulinemia syndrome: results of multicenter cohort study and review of the literature," *Autoimmune Reviews*, vol. 11, no. 1, pp. 48–55, 2011.

[106] S. De Vita, L. Quartuccio, M. Isola et al., "A randomized controlled trial of rituximan for the treatment of severe cryoglobulinemic vasculitis," *Arthritis & Rheumatism*, vol. 64, no. 3, pp. 843–853, 2012.

[107] F. Fabrizi, P. Martin, A. Elli et al., "Hepatitis C virus infection and rituximab therapy after renal transplantation," *International Journal of Artificial Organs*, vol. 30, no. 5, pp. 445–449, 2007.

[108] F. Dammacco, F. A. Tucci, G. Lauletta et al., "Pegylated interferon-α, ribavirin, and rituximab combined therapy of hepatitis C virus-related mixed cryoglobulinemia: a long-term study," *Blood*, vol. 116, no. 3, pp. 343–353, 2010.

[109] R. Misiani, P. Bellavita, D. Fenili et al., "Interferon alfa-2a therapy in cryoglobulinemia associated with hepatitis C virus," *The New England Journal of Medicine*, vol. 330, no. 11, pp. 751–756, 1994.

[110] F. Dammacco, D. Sansonno, J. H. Han et al., "Natural interferon-α versus its combination with 6-methyl-prednisolone in the therapy of type II mixed cryoglobulinemia: a long-term, randomized, controlled study," *Blood*, vol. 84, no. 10, pp. 3336–3343, 1994.

[111] P. Hausfater, P. Cacoub, U. Assogba, P. Lebon, and J. C. Piette, "Plasma exchange and interferon-alpha pharmacokinetics in patients with hepatitis C virus-associated systemic vasculitis," *Nephron*, vol. 91, no. 4, pp. 627–630, 2002.

6

Adjudication of the Alleged Role of Vitamin D in the Antimicrobial Pathway

Gerald M. Higa,[1] Jason Hicks,[2] and Christopher Isabella[2]

[1] *Schools of Pharmacy and Medicine and the Mary Babb Randolph Cancer Center, West Virginia University, Morgantown, WV 26506, USA*
[2] *School of Pharmacy, West Virginia University, Morgantown, WV 26506, USA*

Correspondence should be addressed to Gerald M. Higa; ghiga@hsc.wvu.edu

Academic Editors: P. Bouvet, J. A. Castro, and Y. Chagnon

Dynamic interactions between microorganism and host have evolved in such a way that while microbial pathogens are the cause of many human infections, a symbiotic relationship is also known to exist. Another important anomaly is that exposure to pathogenic organisms does not necessarily result in development of clinical disease. The latter conclusion infers that susceptibility to infectious disease can be modified by host-related factors. Arguably the two most prominent factors are genetic variability and immunologic status of the exposed individual. Because of the Human Genome and the HapMap projects, developments in genotyping technology have brought the possibility of identifying associations between specific genetic alterations and common diseases closer to reality. In addition, a growing body of evidence suggests vitamin D has an important contributory role in the antimicrobial pathway.

1. Introduction

Epidemiologic, biologic, and even genotypic data convincingly demonstrate the essential role of microorganisms in the genesis of many human infections; even so, exposure alone does not necessarily result in development of clinical disease. Inherent in this technically accurate paradox is that while the former supports the well-established link between microbial pathogens and infectious diseases, the latter infers that disease susceptibility can be modified by extramicrobial factors [1–3]. Arguably, the most important "other" factor is adaptive and innate immunity of the exposed individual. Furthermore, accumulating data indicate that alterations of immune responsiveness are partly dependent on genetic factors [4]. For example, in addition to the one gene-one infection paradigm such as the Duffy-null genotype, Fy^{a-b-} (the most common genotype among those of black African heritage), and resistance to malaria [5], there is also evidence which supports the association between one gene with multiple types of infections or multiple genes with a single type of infection [6]. Hence, susceptibility to infection can be characterized by a construct that involves not only gene expression patterns of the host but also that of the microorganism, both of which continue to adapt in response to external stimuli. A plausible extension of this concept relates to the involvement of vitamin D in immunomodulation and the role the vitamin appears to have in a number of infectious diseases.

These preparatory comments notwithstanding, it seems counter-intuitive to suggest that results of laboratory and clinical research can actually increase the uncertainty of what is already a controversy in medicine. Yet, this conclusion is apparently true for vitamin D. Now, perhaps even more than nearly a century ago when the first investigational studies were conducted to elucidate the etiology of rickets [7], research has revealed that the beneficial effects of the vitamin D endocrine system may extend beyond the musculoskeletal system. Indeed, a profound holistic effect on well-being has been linked to a number of nonclassic actions of the vitamin (Figure 1) [8, 9]. This paper focuses on our increased, though by no means complete, understanding of the vitamin-D-dependent antimicrobial pathway and attempts to adjudicate published evidence regarding the vitamin's alleged role in altering host susceptibility to infections.

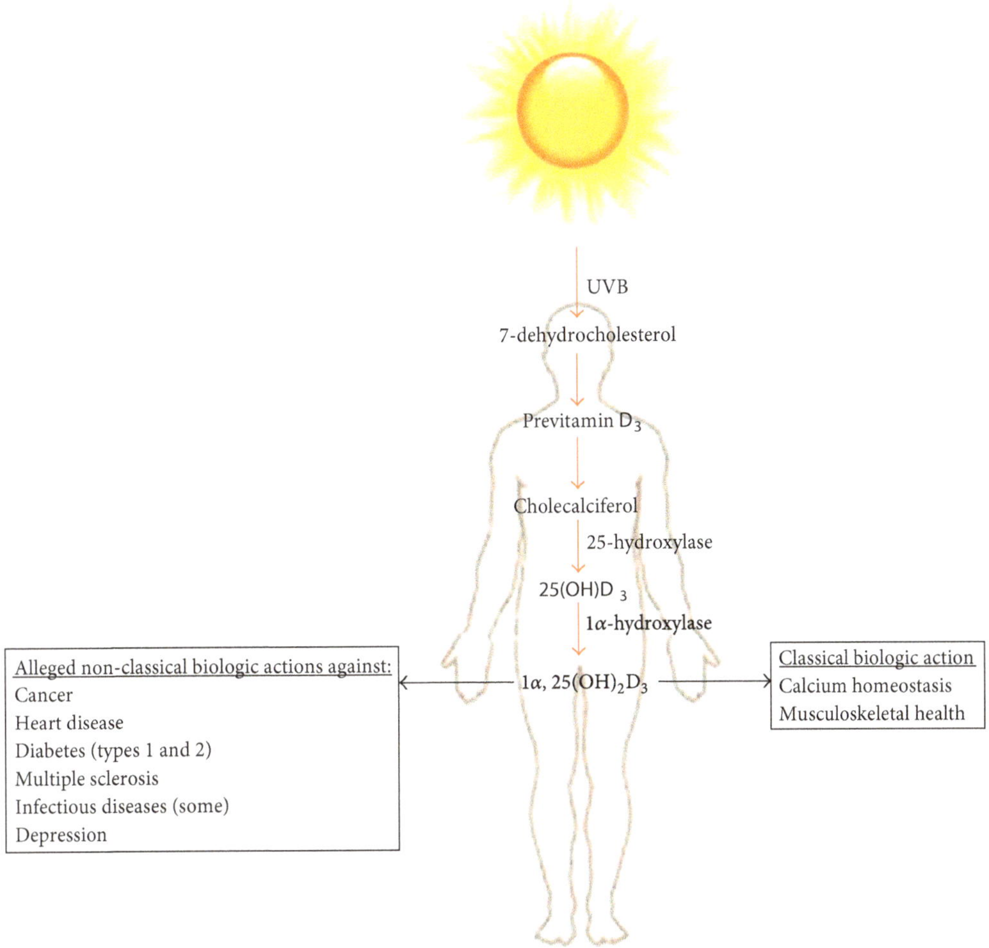

FIGURE 1: Synthesis and biologic actions of vitamin D_3. A number of nontraditional roles are linked to adverse consequences of vitamin D deficiency.

2. Vitamin D Status and Health

Although the Endocrine Society strongly recommends using serum 25(OH)D levels to classify vitamin D status in humans [10] there is still some inconsistency regarding the cut-off point that distinguishes sufficient from insufficient levels of the vitamin. Even the recommended sufficient range of 25–80 ng/mL, which was extracted from previous data that did not account for sun exposure, race, age, and geographic latitude, may not necessarily apply to the noncalcemic effects for which the vitamin purportedly has a biological role. Nonetheless, there is evidence, when collectively analyzed, which suggests an association between vitamin D and risk of dying from any cause. One such meta-analysis involved over 57,000 subjects, the majority of who were postmenopausal women, examined the potential benefits of vitamin D supplementation [11]. Among those in the vitamin-supplemented intervention groups, serum 25(OH)D levels were up to five-fold higher compared to the control group. Over an adjusted mean followup of nearly six years 4,777 deaths occurred. Despite daily doses of supplemental vitamin D, which ranged between 300 international units (IUs) and 2,000 (IU), the intervention groups had a 7% reduction in relative risk of dying from any cause compared to the control groups. Although the association between low vitamin D levels and mortality was not statistically significant, the relatively small risk reduction may nevertheless be clinically relevant as deaths due to cardiovascular- and diabetes-related complications (diseases that may be impacted by low vitamin D) claim the lives of approximately 435,000 American women annually [12].

Because serum levels appear to be correlated with physiological and pathological musculoskeletal outcomes [13], it is tempting to speculate that the vitamin's effect in the antimicrobial pathway would also depend merely on maintaining sufficient levels of 25(OH)D. While this belief may have some validity, it also grossly oversimplifies an immensely intricate pharmacological process. And in order to enhance reader appreciation of this complex phenomenon, an overview of the basic biology and molecular pharmacology of vitamin D is presented.

3. Basic Biology of Vitamin D

Plant-derived ergosterol and dermal-derived 7-dehydrocholesterol are the precursors of ergocalciferol (D_2) and cholecalciferol (D_3), respectively, the two major forms of vitamin D. However, most of the body's vitamin requirement is acquired through ultraviolet B sunlight-cleavage of 7-dehydrocholesterol resulting in D_3, the predominant, though biologically inert, isoform of the vitamin. Conversion to the metabolically active hormone, $1\alpha,25(OH)_2D_3$, requires two hydroxylation steps, first in the liver and then the kidney. Although some uncertainty still exists regarding the specific enzymes involved in the bioactivation process, cytochrome (CY) P2R1 has been shown to possess very potent hepatic 25-hydroxylase activity [14] while CYP27B1 appears to be the primary renal 1α-hydroxylase [15, 16].

The site-specific hydroxylation reactions differ in one major way. While hepatic production of 25(OH)D is partially, and inversely, influenced by serum vitamin D levels, renal activation to the bioactive hormone is a stringently regulated process. This disparity may also explain a pharmacologic inconsistency related to the metabolite that mediates vitamin D toxicity. Instead of the bioactive hormone, it has been reported that the 25-hydroxy metabolite appears to mediate the toxic manifestations [17]. This finding is somewhat surprising because 25(OH)D exhibits two features that would suggest, otherwise, (1) a very high affinity for vitamin-D-binding protein (VDBP) and (2) a low affinity for the vitamin D receptor (VDR). Using $CYP27B1^{-/-}$ (knockout) mice, which do not have the capacity to produce the biologically active hormone, Deluca and colleagues observed similar degrees of vitamin D intoxication in both null and wild-type mice given large doses of D_3. Severe toxic hypercalcemia occurred with serum levels of 25(OH)D ranging between 800 to 1000 ng/mL. Even more interesting was the finding that while 25(OH)D is biologically inactive at normal serum concentrations, gene assays revealed that, at levels of 400 ng/mL, the metabolite became transcriptionally active. This finding is consistent with other *in vitro* data showing that at high concentrations, the bioactivity of $25(OH)D_3$ mimics $1\alpha,25(OH)_2D_3$ [18].

4. Molecular Pharmacology of Vitamin D

Conversion of D_3 to $1\alpha,25(OH)_2D_3$ is a relatively simple process compared to translation of the hormone's effects which involves a number of intricate steps and additional factors. Since a high percentage of circulating steroid hormones are bound to soluble proteins, it is well appreciated that extracellular factors can influence the vitamin's pharmacokinetic and pharmacodynamic properties. One soluble factor is VDBP, which exhibits hierarchical binding with the greatest affinity for $25(OH)D_3$, the major circulating form of the vitamin; the binding affinity for D_3 and $1\alpha,25(OH)_2D_3$ is at least ten-fold lower [19]. Studies using $VDBP^{-/-}$ mice revealed that deficiency of the binding protein resulted in lower $25(OH)D_3$ and $1\alpha,25(OH)_2D_3$ levels due to increased clearance of the unbound metabolites compared to wild-type mice [20]. After eight weeks of consuming a vitamin-D-deficient diet, $VDBP^{-/-}$ mice developed secondary hyperparathyroidism and manifested evidence of osteoporosis; neither of these signs were observed in $VDBP^{+/+}$ mice. And because VDBP purportedly facilitates delivery of activated vitamin to target tissue [21], the bound complexes could also serve as a circulating reservoir, which could contribute to the dynamic regulation of vitamin-D-related effects.

Attached to plasma membranes of vitamin-D-target tissue, a second group of proteins facilitates entry of VDBP-bound molecules [22]. However, the binding protein is not absolutely essential for internalization of the sterol. Furthermore, internal trafficking of $25(OH)D_3$ does not appear to be a random process as members of the heat shock protein 70 family act as intracellular chaperones that determine whether the metabolites are destined for enzymatic degradation or biochemical interaction with the VDR [23]. One important concept related to the latter interaction is an apparent misnomer associated with the designation "bioactive metabolite" because $1\alpha,25(OH)_2D_3$ is devoid of biological activity in the absence of the VDR [24]. In essence, the VDR is the requisite component that enables hormonal stimulus to be molecularly transcribed into hormonal effect. The significance of this principle should not be underestimated as the receptor belongs to a superfamily of nuclear factors that target genes at the transcriptional level [24]. Although a highly conserved zinc finger region essential for high-affinity binding to vitamin D response elements (VDREs) in target genes and a bridge region connecting the ligand-binding and DNA-binding domains are common to all members of the family, the VDR incorporates two unique differences [25]. First, the absence of the ligand-independent activation factor (AF)-1 motif in the N-terminus transcriptional-activating domain; second, the presence of an extraloop (not found in any other nuclear receptor) between the second and third helices in the C-terminus ligand-binding domains [26]. The functional relevance of these differences is still unclear. Even though our understanding of the receptor multiplex is incomplete, multidimensional constructs have made it possible to better appreciate and even visualize the delicate precision of the hormone-receptor interaction [27].

The primal event of hormone binding activates a sequence of events which includes induction of conformational changes in the receptor, activation of intrinsic AF-2, dissociation from heat shock proteins, phosphorylation, dimerization, and ultimately transcription [28]. Of note, the highly conserved amino acid sequence of AF-2 is especially significant as single point mutations within this short core motif have been shown to disrupt receptor transcriptional activity [29]. In addition, and unlike the homodimers formed by sex steroid hormone receptors, ligand-bound VDRs preferentially form heterodimers, particularly with one of three retinoid X receptors (RXR) [30].

The molecular basis by which the hormone-VDR complex interacts with nuclear transcriptional elements is extraordinarily more complicated than the foregoing events as recruitment of additional comodulators has been shown to be necessary in order to "fine tune" hormonal activity. It is important to emphasize that activation or repression of transcription depends on the balance of the recruited coregulatory components. Both types of transcriptional activity are best illustrated using 1α,25$(OH)_2$D actions on bone although similar mechanisms may apply to the alleged non-classical effects of the vitamin. For instance, while genes that regulate calcium homeostasis (i.e., *CaT1*, calcium transport protein 1; *calbindin-D* $_{9K}$) have been identified, the manner in which this takes place appears to depend on a number of precise interactions involving numerous coactivator complexes. Activation of targeted genes requires the presence of two chromatin remodeling complexes known as SWI/SNF-A (switching defective/sucrose non-fermenting) and SWI/SNF-B as well as coactivators of the p160 family including SRC-1, SRC-2 and SRC-3 (steroid receptor coactivator-1, 2, 3), and DRIP (vitamin D_3 receptor-interacting protein) [31, 32]. All of the SRCs contain two activation domains, AD1 and AD2, which serve as binding sites for p300 and CARM1 (coactivator-associated arginine methyltransferase 1) [33]. The interaction between the SRC/DRIP complexes and the AF-2 domain of the VDR promotes recruitment of two epigenetic proteins to the receptor. Together with the SRC complexes, histone acetylases and methyltransferases disrupt the stability of DNA, which allow transcriptional output of the target genes.

Negative feedback is also a unique characteristic of the endocrine system. Molecular evidence suggests that part of the mechanism for self-attenuation of receptor-mediated signaling depends on the presence of corepressors. Two of the most well-known repressors of VDR-mediated transcriptional activity are NCor (nuclear corepressor) and SMRT (silencing mediator of retinoid and thyroid receptor) [34]. Notably, interactions between the VDR-NCoR and VDR-Alien complexes do not appear to involve the receptor's AF-2 domain, a finding dissimilar to the VDR-SRC coactivators mentioned previously. The implications of the different interfaces relate to the possibility that transcriptional repression may not result simply from competitive occupation of specific binding sites on DNA response elements but rather the presence of functionally different pathways for repressing transcriptional activity [35].

Another mechanism by which VDR-mediated transcriptional activity can be suppressed is somewhat of an anomaly. An endogenous protein known as VDRE-binding protein (BP) has been shown to have paradoxical effects on the regulation of DNA transcription. In the *absence* of 1α,25$(OH)_2$D-bound VDR, VDRE-BP interacts with the same target gene promoter response elements and induces nuclear transcription [36]. However, overexpression of this binding protein can inhibit the formation of the receptor dimer-transactivating complex, thus suppressing transcriptional activity [37]. In essence, an intrinsic cellular program initiated by hormones follows a blueprint for the repetitive remodeling of chromatin, regulates the process of gene transcription, and determines specific endocrine effects on target tissue. The complexity of this conclusion can be further appreciated by the notion that vitamin D is certain to be only one functional component, albeit a very small one, of a dynamic, interactive, and adaptive process within the antimicrobial pathway.

5. Vitamin D and Infectious Diseases

Seldom has a compound labeled as a nutritional substance commanded as much attention as vitamin D. Aside from its role in the promotion of bone health, a measure that best supports this conclusion is the number of publications related to the extraskeletal effects of the vitamin. One area of keen interest is the pharmacologic effects and biologic relevance of the vitamin-D-dependent antimicrobial pathway.

Even before reports related to the presence of the VDR in human leukocytes were published [38], a link was loosely established between 1α,25$(OH)_2$D and osteoclasts, which appeared at sites of active bone resorption [39]. Because cells of the monocyte/macrophage lineage are precursors of osteoclasts [40], it was hypothesized, and subsequently demonstrated that, like glucocorticoids [41], 1α,25$(OH)_2$D could induce terminal differentiation of myeloid leukemic blasts [42, 43]. Although the underlying mechanism of their differentiating effects on both mouse and human leukemia cell lines was not known, it had been postulated that both hormones interacted with specific cytoplasmic receptors in the leukemic cells [44].

Soon thereafter, numerous publications indicated a prominent inhibitory effect of 1α,25$(OH)_2$D on specific subsets of CD4+ T-helper cells. Not only did the hormone have the ability to suppress IL-2-mediated T-cell proliferation and function [45], the hormone could also inhibit γ-interferon gene transcription [46]. Notably, the suppressive effects on cell-mediated components of the immune response were somewhat disparate as inhibition of T-helper lymphocytes was much greater than the repressive effects on T-suppressor cell activity [47]. Laboratory studies subsequently demonstrated cellular components of the nonspecific immune system could also be influenced by vitamin D [48]. In two early reports, investigators showed that innate immunity was mediated, in part, by an apparent association between activation of Toll-like receptors (TLRs) and expression of antimicrobial peptides, though the biological mechanism remained elusive [49, 50].

5.1. Mycobacterium sp. Further investigation of monocytes stimulated with a truncated synthetic lipo-peptide derived from *Mycobacterium tuberculosis* (TLR2/1L) identified the *VDR* gene as one of two candidate genes that may be involved in the antimicrobial response of these cells. Pursuit of this finding with elegant *in vitro* studies indicated that the vitamin D pathway was the key intermediary between TLRs and innate host defense peptides [51]. In their study, Liu and colleagues demonstrated that monocytes activated by TLRs upregulated intracellular expression of both CYP27B1 and VDR. However, anticipated amplification of a number of genes downstream of the VDR, including the *cathelicidin antimicrobial peptide* (*CAMP*) gene, was not observed. Notably, the absence of *CAMP* mRNA was not due to expression of a dysfunctional VDR but rather insufficient intracellular amounts of bioactive vitamin D. Even though the latter conclusion appears inconsistent with the increased expression of 1α-hydroxylase (CYP27B1), its validity is supported by addition of 1α,25$(OH)_2D_3$, which resulted in a dose-dependent increase in expression of activated cathelicidin as well as a direct antimicrobial effect against *M. tuberculosis*.

More recently, additional effects linking VDR-signaling with innate immunity have been observed including induction of lysosomal function and β-defensin 4 (DEFB4) [52, 53]. Collectively, these effects take on even greater significance when coupled with the finding that the antimicrobial response was dependent on the presence of sufficient vitamin D levels. This was aptly demonstrated in a laboratory study involving monocytes cultured in medium containing either fetal calf serum (FCS) or human serum [51]. Notably, addition of TLR2/1L resulted in cathelicidin being upregulated only in monocytes maintained in media containing human serum. Because *cathelicidin* is a target gene of a functional vitamin D pathway, one plausible explanation relates to the five-fold greater amount of 25$(OH)D_3$ in normal human serum compared to FCS. Validation of this belief was achieved with the demonstration that expression of cathelicidin occurred only when 25$(OH)D_3$ and TLR2/1L were added simultaneously to FCS. These findings also suggested that the TLR and vitamin D pathways do not merely intersect but rather converge to fortify host defense mechanisms against microbial pathogens.

The significance of vitamin D sufficiency in laboratory models of antimicrobial response to *M. tuberculosis* has clinical correlates as well. The authors of a very recent paper sought to determine the extent to which susceptibility to active tuberculosis was associated with vitamin D deficiency among HIV-positive and HIV-negative black South Africans [54]. Exceeding the importance related to the finding that 63% of the participants were vitamin D deficient (defined as <20 ng/mL) was the apparent relationship between vitamin deficiency and increased susceptibility to active tuberculosis (TB) in both cohorts of subjects; HIV-infected (odds ratio [OR] = 5.6, 95% CI, 2.7–11.6; $P < 0.001$) and HIV-uninfected (OR = 5.2, 95% CI, 2.8–9.7; $P < 0.001$). Of interest also, reporting of new TB cases varied inversely following the three-month period with the highest and lowest mean serum 25$(OH)D_3$ concentrations.

Additional *in vivo* evidence of a link between vitamin D and the innate immune response has been obtained from subjects infected with *M. leprae*, another intracellular pathogen [55]. The two forms in which leprosy present clinically enabled investigation of biological mechanisms that could account for their differences in disease severity. Molecular analysis of sample lesions from subjects with either the progressive lepromatous or the self-limited tuberculoid forms of leprosy indicated expression of a number of microribonucleic acids (miRNAs), one of which was miRNA21 (mir21). Expressed primarily in infected monocytes of those with the more severe form of the disease, mir21 was capable of downregulating TLR2/1-induced expression of *CYP27B1*. Increased expression of mir21 in monocytes cultured from lepromatous lesions was also associated with silencing of the genes responsible for encoding CAMP and DEFB4. The strong link between mir21 and the two vitamin-D-dependent antimicrobial peptides was confirmed using *mir* $21^{-/-}$-infected monocytes with restoration of CAMP and DEFB4 expression, and TLR2/1 activity against the bacterium. These immunologic findings may partially explain the more aggressive course of the lepromatous subtype.

Even though these same investigators recently suggested that vitamin D_3 supplementation may be immunologically advantageous to humans [55], addition of the vitamin to the treatment of leprosy has actually been advocated for approximately 100 years [56]. Nonetheless, the rationale for this recommendation may be strengthened as new information related to vitamin-D-dependent immune mechanisms is elucidated.

5.2. Hepatitis C Virus. A high prevalence of vitamin D deficiency among patients with severe hepatic impairment should not necessarily be surprising as the liver is the site of the initial hydroxylation reaction. This conclusion is supported by numerous investigators who reported such an association regardless of the underlying cause of liver disease [57, 58]. Even though a similar association among subjects infected with the hepatitis C virus (HCV) was not unexpected, investigators found an interesting nuance in patients with chronic HCV infection [59]. While impaired liver function is likely the primary cause of vitamin D deficiency, Lange and colleagues suggest extrahepatic factors may also be involved. Although circumstantial, the evidence is nonetheless notable. For example, a higher incidence of vitamin D deficiency was observed in patients with chronic hepatitis C, even those without fibrotic changes in the liver, compared to controls; second, published data indicate that hydroxylation of cholecalciferol can be inhibited or impaired by viral induction of inflammatory cytokines; third, the finding that circulating 25(OH)D levels increased after eradication of the virus [60].

In addition, the link between vitamin D and HCV is strengthened by correlative evidence showing a significantly higher sustained virologic response (SVR, defined as undetectable serum HCV RNA 24 weeks posttherapy) rates to anti-viral therapy among patients who did not have severe vitamin D deficiency [59, 61]. That the improved SVR may be partially due to a direct antiviral effect of vitamin D is supported by a recent publication [62]. Using a hepatoma cell line, findings related to the effect of vitamin D in HCV-infected cells are worthy of comment. First, addition of HCV to various concentrations of vitamin D-treated cells resulted in dose-dependent inhibition of HCV production. That this inhibitory effect involved the vitamin D pathway was supported by increased expression of a number of downstream targets including the *CYP27B1* gene, 1α,25$(OH)_2D$, VDR mRNA, and 24-hydroxylase. The last finding, upregulation of *CYP24A1*, the gene encoding 24-hydroxylase, represents one potential confounding element of this study. Even though production of the bioactive metabolite is stringently controlled by hormone-induced upregulation of the gene responsible for its own catabolism and downregulation of

CYP27B1, the only significant finding in vitamin-D-treated cells infected with HCV, was reduced expression of the catalytic enzyme. Hence, part of the inhibitory effect of vitamin D on HCV production can be explained by higher hormone concentrations (or more prolonged duration of activity) in the virus-infected cells. Another notable finding of this study was the effect of vitamin D on the innate interferon (INF) signaling pathway. In contrast to the minimal effect of both D_3 and $1\alpha,25(OH)_2D_3$ in noninfected cells, a significant increase in *INF-β* gene expression was observed in virus-infected cells. Functionality of INF-β was correlated with induction of the INF-signaling gene *MxA*. These data provide reasonably compelling evidence that vitamin D may have a direct antiviral effect which may be partly mediated by inducing endogenous INFs.

The above data are partially counterbalanced by inconsistencies related to 25(OH)D levels and virologic response rates. Although two separate groups reported direct correlations between vitamin D levels and viral responses only in patients infected with HCV genotype 2-3 [59, 63], a third study reported the same correlation in HCV genotype 1 patients [64].

5.3. Human Immunodeficiency Virus (HIV)-1. Juxtaposed to the preceding findings are data which also demonstrate that components of the adaptive immune system can be suppressed by vitamin D [52, 65–67]. As such, the disease caused by HIV-1 could also be affected. The apparent inconsistent effect on the two arms of the immune systems can be reconciled by critically examining both laboratory and epidemiological data. It is well known that resting, unstimulated T helper cells can undergo further differentiation to Th_0, Th_1, or Th_2 cells. Each helper cell subset is distinguished by their characteristic pattern of lymphokines produced [68]. For example, when CD4+ cells were cocultured with $1\alpha,25(OH)_2D$, the Th_1 subset was shown to be the most sensitive to the hormone's inhibitory effect, thus suppressing IL-2 production [69]. Interestingly, by blocking antigen-presenting cell secretion of IL-12, the hormone was also able to further antagonize Th_1 cell activation [70]. Nevertheless, these effects can be beneficial. For example, vitamin D may have therapeutic application when suppression of adaptive elements such as Th_1 and IL-12, which have central roles in the pathogenesis of diseases such as solid organ rejection and multiple sclerosis, is desirable. In addition, the vitamin also has a critical role in *killing* intracellular pathogens by an antimicrobial process known as autophagy or programmed cell death-2 [67]. Although not restricted to *M. tuberculosis*, destruction of HIV-1 may also be induced by this process [71].

Even though there are no convincing data to support a *causal* relationship between vitamin D and the pathogenesis of HIV, correlative evidence of an association between vitamin deficiency and clinical progression/all-cause mortality among HIV-infected people does exist. One of the most recently published studies included 2,000 randomly selected subjects from a large international cohort of HIV-infected individuals who met specific study criteria [72]. Of the total number of subjects, 25(OH)D levels were available from 1985 persons; these subjects were segregated into three groups based on acceptable threshold values of vitamin D. For descriptive purposes and statistical analyses, the individual groups were labeled "lowest," "middle," and "higher," which corresponded to 25(OH)D levels of ≤12 ng/mL, 12.1–20 ng/mL, and >20 ng/mL, respectively. Each group had similar percentages of persons based on a number of demographic characteristics. Kaplan-Meier curves of HIV infection progressing to AIDS and AIDS-related death were significantly lower among those in the middle and higher tertiles compared to subjects in the lowest vitamin D tertile. However, non-AIDS-related deaths were significantly reduced only in the higher tertile group. Another relatively large study was conducted to determine whether any correlation existed between baseline vitamin D status and three disease-related endpoints in HIV-infected pregnant women [73]. Vitamin D levels were known for 885 of the 1,078 women enrolled. In contrast to the previous study, vitamin D status was categorized as "insufficient" and "sufficient" with cut-off 25(OH)D thresholds of <32 ng/mL and ≥32 ng/mL, respectively. After a median follow-up period of nearly six years, the data indicated that pregnant women classified as having insufficient vitamin D levels had a significantly higher rate of disease progressing to stage III or higher as well as the development of severe anemia; $P = 0.01$ for both endpoints. While a relationship between vitamin D status and all-cause mortality was not observed, a significantly lower risk of dying was correlated with the highest 25(OH)D quintile approximating >55 ng/mL compared to women at the other extreme with levels <20 ng/mL.

Inherent in the above studies are a number of issues that need to be addressed. First, the relationship between low vitamin D levels and poorer clinical outcomes should be construed as correlative rather than causal. This conclusion is partially supported by methodological parameters of both studies in which 25(OH)D levels were measured in patients already infected with HIV. Hence, it is unknown to what extent the disease may have influenced vitamin D levels. Reverse-causation bias may also occur if advanced stage or progressive disease reduces sun exposure or adversely affects dietary intake, both of which could negatively impact vitamin D status. Nonetheless, and regardless of vitamin D classification, most of the subjects in both studies had early stage disease and similar CD4 T-cell counts when baseline vitamin D levels were measured. Although both of these factors weaken the notion of reverse causation, the evidence still does not establish a cause-effect relationship. Second, since the majority of subjects involved in one study were relatively young and the other restricted to mid-gestational pregnant women, both study populations may not have been truly representative of the whole cohort of HIV-infected patients. These nuances aside, it is of interest that concomitant anti-retroviral therapy (ART) did not appear to impact the results as the majority of patients in one study [72] were prescribed ART while the other not [73]. Other than drug-induced alteration of vitamin D metabolism, the effectiveness of ART subordinates a disease-related cause of vitamin D deficiency. Third, compelling data have been published that directly correlates skeletal health with circulating 25(OH)D levels

[74]. In their study, Priemel and colleagues analyzed bone integrity by histomorphometric examination of 675 human bone marrow biopsy specimens. In this cohort of German adults, increased osteoid volume, surface, and thickness, which are pathologic markers of mineralization defects were not present when 25(OH)D levels exceed 30 ng/mL. The clinical relevance of this finding parallels the HIV study which used a cutoff point of ≥32 ng/mL to distinguish sufficient from insufficient vitamin D levels. However, this was not corroborated by the EuroSIDA study which showed that slower progression to AIDS or death correlated with 25(OH)D levels >12 ng/mL. Even though both assay systems used to quantify 25(OH)D levels measured only the D_3 metabolite, it is unlikely that unmeasured 25(OH)D_2 contributed to the notable differences which correlated vitamin D status with the observed clinical outcomes. What the findings do suggest is the vitamin D status that correlates with optimal bone health may not be the same for enhanced immune function.

Data published within the past 15 years appear to provide provocative, though circumstantial, evidence to support the allegation that vitamin D status may influence host susceptibility to infectious diseases. The veracity of this conclusion is limited by the critical role of the VDR, a receptor that interfaces with diseases substantially different from skeletal development and bone mineralization. And because of its functional importance, herculean efforts have been made to identify *VDR* gene polymorphisms (*VDRGP*) that could have predictive or prognostic value.

6. VDRGP and Infections

Even though published epidemiologic data suggest that susceptibility to TB involves a complex interaction between genetic variability and environmental and cultural factors [75, 76], nutritional components, especially with regards to vitamin D, have also been reported to be associated with the risk of the disease. In a small study involving 126 *untreated* patients with TB and 116 healthy contacts who were sensitized, but did not have any clinical or radiographic evidence of the disease, vitamin D deficiency was observed in 67% and 26% of patients with active TB and healthy contacts, respectively, $P = 0.008$ [77]. These data notwithstanding, the association between vitamin D deficiency and the pathogenesis of TB is somewhat inconsistent with the observation that not all TB-infected individuals are vitamin D deficient. This finding suggests that defects in other components of the vitamin D-signaling pathway may increase the risk for, and/or progression of, the disease. One putative mechanism may involve the *VDR* gene (Figure 2). In order to address the issue whether an interaction between *VDRGP* and serum vitamin D concentrations influenced the susceptibility to the disease was also investigated. Two of the most well-studied *VDR* polymorphisms indicated that neither *Taq1* nor *Fok1* restriction enzymes alone was associated with serum vitamin D levels; however, the finding that 6.6% and 12%, (OR = 0.53; 95% CI, 0.31–0.88; $P = 0.01$), of the TB case and control patients, respectively, carried the VDR-*tt* genotype indicated that homozygosity of the *t* allele was associated with clinical resistance to the disease [78]. These findings are partially corroborated by a more recent publication involving native South Americans [79]. Among two Paraguayan populations examined, individuals harboring the VDR-TT genotype were significantly less able to mount a delayed-type hypersensitivity response to antigen challenge.

Besides *Fok1* in the 5′ regulatory region of the *VDR* gene, single nucleotide polymorphisms (SNPs) of Cdx2 may extend to HIV and *M. tuberculosis* infections as well. The most well-characterized SNP of this transcription factor is *Cdx2-A* and *Cdx2-G* depending on whether adenine or guanine is at position −3791 base pairs relative to the transcription start site of *VDR* gene. In a study to determine the association between Cdx2 genotype and susceptibility to HIV and TB infection, Alagarasu et al. reported the frequency of the *Cdx2-G/A* genotype was significantly increased in HIV-positive individuals compared to healthy controls (OR = 1.89, 95% CI 1.14–3.15; $P = 0.012$) [80]. Interestingly, extended genotype frequency analysis indicated that the loose association between the *GA* haplotype and protection against HIV infection could be strengthened by the presence of two copies of that specific haplotype.

Perhaps more notable was the observation that three restriction fragment length polymorphisms (RFLP), *Bsm*I, *Apa*I, and *Taq*I, detected in the 3′ untranslated region (UTR) of the *VDR* gene, appear to have better correlation with susceptibility to or protection against HIV infection. Genomic DNA was amplified by polymerase chain reaction for allelic discrimination of the three restriction sites. Individual RFLPs are defined by capital letters (i.e., *B, A, T*) in the absence of the restriction site; lower case letters of the same are used when the restriction sites were present. As such, the *BAt* haplotype was associated with increased susceptibility, while the *bAT* haplotype conferred protection. These findings are consistent with earlier published data showing that subjects harboring the *BAt* haplotype had decreased production of interleukin-10 (IL-10), a lymphokine with known inhibitory effects against HIV [81]. On the other hand, increased expression of 1L-10 and other antiviral chemokines coupled with downregulation of HIV coreceptor in individuals with the *bAT* haplotype are associated with defective VDR signaling and protection against HIV. Perhaps of equal importance was the association between the increased frequency of the *BAt* haplotype and the increased susceptibility to pulmonary TB in HIV-infected patients [80].

VDR gene polymorphisms continue to be relevant in order to explain the apparent disparity between vitamin action and risk of disease. One frequently occurring DNA sequence variation involves the *Bsm*1 restriction enzyme. The prevalence of the *Bsm*1 polymorphism was determined in a cohort of 185 HIV-1-seropositive individuals; the results were then correlated with disease susceptibility and progression [82]. Compared to the *VDR-Bb* and *VDR-bb* genotypes, *BB* homozygotes have identical alleles with absent restriction sites, which negatively impact the ability to synthesize the full-length VDR protein. Notably, the *VDR-BB* genotype was correlated with more rapid progression to both CD4 counts

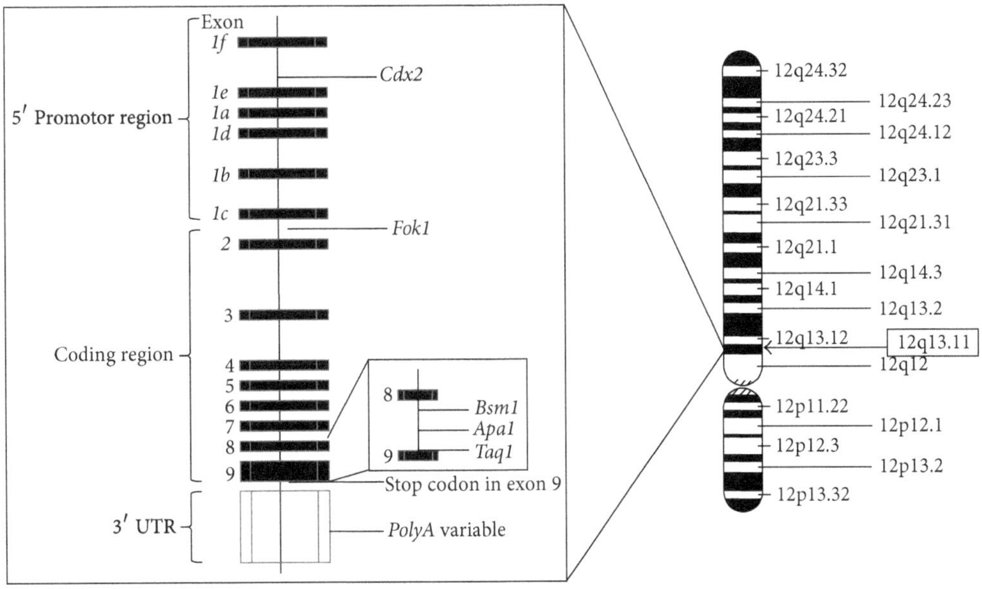

Figure 2: Locations of the *VDR* gene on chromosome 12 (right); and some of the currently known VDR polymorphisms (left). The gene has nine exons, eight of which (numbers 2–9) encode proteins and number one designated (*1a–1f*) contains six untranslated subunits.

<200 cells/uL and acquired immunodeficiency syndrome (AIDS). Although the influence of the *Bsm*1 polymorphism on VDR protein function and signaling is largely unknown, the authors speculated that persons who harbored the *VDR-BB* genotype were less responsive to the immunosuppressive action of vitamin D, which could enhance Th_1 cell activation and survival and enable a more efficient process by which the virus infected these cells.

One other interesting finding involving *Apa*1 has been reported in subjects infected with T-cell lymphotropic virus type-1 (HTLV-1) who are at risk for developing a complication known as HTLV-1-associated myelopathy (HAM). However, the observation that only a very small percentage of patients actually do suggests host factors may play an important role. In a relatively recent paper Japanese investigators genotyped the three RFLPs mentioned previously plus the *Fok*1 RFLP in patients with and without HAM [83]. Genomic analysis of 247 individuals indicated no difference in *Fok*1, *Bsm*I, and *Taq*I genotypic or allelic frequencies among the 118 subjects with HAM and 129 seropositive controls. However, a significant difference in ApaI genotypes (i.e., *AA*, 3.9%; *Aa*, 43%; *aa*, 53.1%) was found. Upon further investigation of an additional 89 subjects with HAM (and 95 seropositive controls) a significant association was observed between females with the *AA* genotype and lower risk of developing HAM ($P = 0.029$). Although linkage disquilibrium between *Fok*1 and *Apa*1 was not apparent, cross-genotyping between the two RFLPs appeared to further clarify the protective effect, which was restricted to those who were genotypically *AA* and *Ff* for the VDR polymorphism. This finding is notable in that the frequencies of the lowest genotype was associated with the highest genotype suggesting that development of HAM would be somewhat higher were it not for the heterozygous *Fok*1 genotype.

Leprosy susceptibility has been reported to be associated with distinct loci of chromosomes 6, 10, 17, 20 and 21. The caveat is that a specific locus may not be a risk factor for all forms of leprosy and may not confer increased risk across individuals differing in ethnicity. For example, the identification of PARK2 and PACRG at 6q25 and q26, respectively, as major leprosy risk genes in two populations, but not a third, highlights the heterogeneity of risk alleles for infectious diseases across different ethnic groups. In addition, a specific locus identified at 10p13 was confirmed as a risk factor for paucibacillary leprosy, but not overall leprosy susceptibility [84]. However, a followup study involving families from Southeast Asia and Brazil identified two SNPs in the mannose receptor 1 gene (*MRC1*) located in the 10p13 region that were associated with multibacillary leprosy and leprosy overall but not with paucibacillary disease [85]. The lack of an association with paucibacillary disease in that study suggests that the causative gene at the 10p13 locus has not yet been identified.

The *Taq*1 RFLP of the *VDR* gene has also been linked to one of two subtypes of infections caused by *M. leprae* [86]. Compared to control, homozygosity of the *t* allele was found to be significantly increased in subjects with tuberculoid leprosy (OR = 3.22, CI = 1.47 – –7.13; $P = 0.001$). In contrast, the lepromatous form of the disease occurred more frequently in subjects with the *TT* genotype (OR = 1.67, CI = 1.02–2.75; $P = 0.03$) compared to controls. An extension of these disparate findings encompasses a possible, though not exclusive, association between *Taq*1 genotype and the immunomodulatory role of vitamin D. Far more complex than the implied simplicity of this conclusion is the signature adaptive immune response to the bacterial pathogen, cell-mediated in patients with tuberculoid leprosy and humoral in those with lepromatous disease. Not precisely known is how the genotypes influence the selective TH_1 and TH_2-type responses.

What appears to be absolutely clear (at least with regard to common *VDRGPs*) is that the amount of discordance which already exists in the only absolutely agreed upon biological role of vitamin D will likely complicate confirming the vitamin's role in other metabolic pathways as well. This conclusion is supported by studies showing interethnic differences in bone mineral density (BMD). Results of an analysis of *VDRGP* in Mexican-American Caucasian women indicated not only a change in the amino acid sequence of the VDR protein but also a correlation with BMD [87]. Using the Fok1 enzyme to cleave a 265 bp region in exon 2 resulted in three *Fok1* genotypes, *FF*, *Ff*, and *ff*. Women with the *ff* genotype had significantly lower BMD at the lumbar spine compared to women with the *FF* genotype ($P = 0.01$); and after two years of followup, BMD in the femoral neck decreased significantly in those with the *ff* genotype compared to the *FF* genotype (−4.7% versus −0.5%, $P = 0.005$). The results of this study were among the earliest to suggest that a functional *VDRGP* was apparently responsible for the observed difference. In contrast, another study involving pre- and postmenopausal Japanese women investigated whether genotyping *Fok1*, Apa1, and Taq1 alleles could also predict BMD [88]. In order to minimize potential confounding factors, the authors targeted a sample size large enough to have sufficient statistical power and a sample representative of the study population, utilized instruments assessing BMD and DNA that were valid and reliable, and controlled for factors such as anthropometric indices, race, and lifestyle. Notwithstanding these precautionary measures, their findings were inconsistent with the previous study with regards to *Fok1* polymorphism, which did not have an independent effect on BMD.

Even more compelling evidence indicates that hypermethylated CpG (cytosine-guanine dinucleotide) regions in the *VDR* gene promotor region can, by silencing gene expression, disrupt normal vitamin D signaling. This epigenetic phenomenon may help explain the apparent resistance of tumor cells. Co-cultured with the bioactive hormone, differences in VDR transcripts and intensity of methylated CpGs were observed in breast cancer and normal breast epithelial cells [89]. An important correlative finding was that demethylation induced by inhibition of DNA methyltransferase increased expression of full-length VDR mRNA and a number of *VDRE*-genes, including 1α-hydroxylase, p21 (cyclin-dependent kinase inhibitor 1), and C/EBP (CCAAT-enhancer-binding proteins). The relative importance of the latter two relates to their function as tumor suppressors genes. Hence, epigenetic alterations may be another biological mechanism which contributes to vitamin D resistance in spite of adequate 25(OH)D levels.

7. Conclusion

A hallmark characteristic of human infections is that development of clinical disease does not necessarily follow exposure to microbial pathogens. This feature implies that intersubject susceptibility to infectious diseases depends on multiple factors including the microorganism, environment, heredity, and host immune status. Because of the immunoregulatory role of the bioactive hormone, vitamin D may have a significant influence on the antimicrobial pathway. While published studies provide strong correlative evidence that links vitamin D status to infections, functional genomic aberrations of the vitamin D pathway are not always as clear or consistent. The reality is that DNA is a relatively simple construct; yet tethered to this scaffold is an extraordinarily dynamic genome, still malleable by the forces of mutation. This belief is especially important as gene expression patterns of microorganisms and hosts are certain to be altered continuously as an adaptive response to external stimuli. As such and as change is certain, the microbial and human genomes will continue to evolve in unpredictable ways, necessitating, and even demanding, periodic reexamination of preexisting dogma.

References

[1] F.-R. Zhang, W. Huang, S.-M. Chen et al., "Genomewide association study of leprosy," *The New England Journal of Medicine*, vol. 361, no. 27, pp. 2609–2618, 2009.

[2] S. Davila, V. J. Wright, C. C. Khor et al., "Genome-wide association study identifies variants in the CFH region associated with host susceptibility to meningococcal disease," *Nature Genetics*, vol. 42, no. 9, pp. 772–776, 2010.

[3] J. L. Troyer, G. W. Nelson, J. A. Lautenberger et al., "Genome-wide association study implicates $PARD_3B$-based AIDS restriction," *Journal of Infectious Diseases*, vol. 203, no. 10, pp. 1491–1502, 2011.

[4] E. A. Van Der Eijk, E. Van De Vosse, J. P. Vandenbroucke, and J. T. Van Dissel, "Heredity versus environment in tuberculosis in twins: the 1950s United Kingdom Prophit Survey—Simonds and Comstock revisited," *American Journal of Respiratory and Critical Care Medicine*, vol. 176, no. 12, pp. 1281–1288, 2007.

[5] K. M. VanBuskirk, E. Sevova, and J. H. Adams, "Conserved residues in the Plasmodium vivax Duffy-binding protein ligand domain are critical for erythrocyte receptor recognition," *Proceedings of the National Academy of Sciences of the United States of America*, vol. 101, no. 44, pp. 15754–15759, 2004.

[6] J. L. Casanova and L. Abel, "Human genetics of infectious diseases: a unified theory," *The EMBO Journal*, vol. 26, no. 4, pp. 915–922, 2007.

[7] E. Mellanby, "An experimental investigation on rickets," *The Lancet*, vol. 193, no. 4985, pp. 407–412, 1919.

[8] A. G. Pittas, J. Lau, F. B. Hu, and B. Dawson-Hughes, "Review: the role of vitamin D and calcium in type 2 diabetes. A systematic review and meta-analysis," *The Journal of Clinical Endocrinology and Metabolism*, vol. 92, no. 6, pp. 2017–2029, 2007.

[9] F. P. Boscoe and M. J. Schymura, "Solar ultraviolet-B exposure and cancer incidence and mortality in the United States, 1993—2002," *BMC Cancer*, vol. 6, article 264, 2006.

[10] M. F. Holick, N. C. Binkley, H. A. Bischoff-Ferrari et al., "Evaluation, treatment, and prevention of vitamin D deficiency: an endocrine society clinical practice guideline," *The Journal of Clinical Endocrinology and Metabolism*, vol. 96, no. 7, pp. 1911–1930, 2011.

[11] P. Autier and S. Gandini, "Vitamin D supplementation and total mortality: a meta-analysis of randomized controlled trials," *Archives of Internal Medicine*, vol. 167, no. 16, pp. 1730–1737, 2007.

[12] Center for Disease Control and Prevention, National Vital Statistics System: LCWK10: Deaths, Percent of Total Deaths and Rank Order for 113 Selected Causes of Death, by Race and Sex: United States, 2001-06, http://www.cdc.gov/nchs/nvss/mortality/lcwk10.htm.

[13] R. P. Heaney, "Functional indices of vitamin D status and ramifications of vitamin D deficiency," *The American Journal of Clinical Nutrition*, vol. 80, no. 6, supplement, pp. 1706S–1709S, 2004.

[14] R. M. Shepard and H. F. Deluca, "Plasma concentrations of vitamin D_3 and its metabolites in the rat as influenced by vitamin D_3 or 25-hydroxyvitamin D_3 intakes," *Archives of Biochemistry and Biophysics*, vol. 202, no. 1, pp. 43–53, 1980.

[15] K. I. Takeyama, S. Kitanaka, T. Sato, M. Kobori, J. Yanagisawa, and S. Kato, "25-Hydroxyvitamin D_3 1α-hydroxylase and vitamin D synthesis," *Science*, vol. 277, no. 5333, pp. 1827–1830, 1997.

[16] D. W. Nebert and F. J. Gonzalez, "P450 genes: structure, evolution, and regulation," *Annual Review of Biochemistry*, vol. 56, pp. 945–993, 1987.

[17] H. F. Deluca, J. M. Prahl, and L. A. Plum, "1,25-Dihydroxyvitamin D is not responsible for toxicity caused by vitamin D or 25-hydroxyvitamin D," *Archives of Biochemistry and Biophysics*, vol. 505, no. 2, pp. 226–230, 2011.

[18] T. C. Chen, K. Persons, M. R. Uskokovic, R. L. Horst, and M. F. Holick, "An evaluation of 1,25-dihydroxyvitamin D_3 analogues on the proliferation and differentiation of cultured human keratinocytes, calcium metabolism and the differentiation of human HL-60 cells," *Journal of Nutritional Biochemistry*, vol. 4, no. 1, pp. 49–57, 1993.

[19] N. E. Cooke and J. G. Haddad, "Vitamin D binding protein (Gc-globulin)," *Endocrine Reviews*, vol. 10, no. 3, pp. 294–307, 1989.

[20] F. F. Safadi, P. Thornton, H. Magiera et al., "Osteopathy and resistance to vitamin D toxicity in mice null for vitamin D binding protein," *The Journal of Clinical Investigation*, vol. 103, no. 2, pp. 239–251, 1999.

[21] J. F. McLeod and N. E. Cooke, "The vitamin D-binding protein, α-fetoprotein, albumin multigene family: detection of transcripts in multiple tissues," *The Journal of Biological Chemistry*, vol. 264, no. 36, pp. 21760–21769, 1989.

[22] H. Birn, J. C. Fyfe, C. Jacobsen et al., "Cubilin is an albumin binding protein important for renal tubular albumin reabsorption," *The Journal of Clinical Investigation*, vol. 105, no. 10, pp. 1353–1361, 2000.

[23] J. S. Adams, H. Chen, R. F. Chun et al., "Novel regulators of vitamin D action and metabolism: lessons learned at the Los Angeles Zoo," *Journal of Cellular Biochemistry*, vol. 88, no. 2, pp. 308–314, 2003.

[24] D. J. Mangelsdorf, C. Thummel, M. Beato et al., "The nuclear receptor super-family: the second decade," *Cell*, vol. 83, no. 6, pp. 835–839, 1995.

[25] L. P. Freedman, B. F. Luisi, Z. R. Korszun, R. Basavappa, P. B. Sigler, and K. R. Yamamoto, "The function and structure of the metal coordination sites within the glucocorticoid receptor DNA binding domain," *Nature*, vol. 334, no. 6182, pp. 543–546, 1988.

[26] A. W. Norman, D. Adams, E. D. Collins, W. H. Okamura, and R. J. Fletterick, "Three-dimensional model of the ligand binding domain of the nuclear receptor for 1α,25-dihydroxy-vitamin D_3," *Journal of Cellular Biochemistry*, vol. 74, no. 3, pp. 323–333, 1999.

[27] N. Rochel, J. M. Wurtz, A. Mitschler, B. Klaholz, and D. Moras, "The crystal structure of the nuclear receptor for vitamin D bound to its natural ligand," *Molecular Cell*, vol. 5, no. 1, pp. 173–179, 2000.

[28] O. Wrange, P. Eriksson, and T. Perlmann, "The purified activated glucocorticoid receptor is a homodimer," *The Journal of Biological Chemistry*, vol. 264, no. 9, pp. 5253–5259, 1989.

[29] B. Durand, M. Saunders, C. Gaudon, B. Roy, R. Losson, and P. Chambon, "Activation function 2 (AF-2) of retinoic acid receptor and 9-cis retinoic acid receptor: presence of a conserved autonomous constitutive activating domain and influence of the nature of the response element on AF-2 activity," *The EMBO Journal*, vol. 13, no. 22, pp. 5370–5382, 1994.

[30] A. Staal, A. J. Van Wijnen, J. C. Birkenhäger et al., "Distinct conformations of vitamin D receptor/retinoid X receptor-alpha heterodimers are specified by dinucleotide differences in the vitamin D-responsive elements of the osteocalcin and osteopontin genes," *Molecular Endocrinology*, vol. 10, no. 11, pp. 1444–1456, 1996.

[31] M. Stern, R. Jensen, and I. Herskowitz, "Five SWI genes are required for expression of the HO gene in yeast," *Journal of Molecular Biology*, vol. 178, no. 4, pp. 853–868, 1984.

[32] C. Rachez, M. Gamble, C. P. B. Chang, G. B. Atkins, M. A. Lazar, and L. P. Freedman, "The DRIP complex and SRC-1/p160 coactivators share similar nuclear receptor binding determinants but constitute functionally distinct complexes," *Molecular and Cellular Biology*, vol. 20, no. 8, pp. 2718–2726, 2000.

[33] D. Chen, S. M. Huang, and M. R. Stallcup, "Synergistic, p160 coactivator-dependent enhancement of estrogen receptor function by CARM1 and p300," *The Journal of Biological Chemistry*, vol. 275, no. 52, pp. 40810–40816, 2000.

[34] R. Sánchez-Martínez, A. Zambrano, A. I. Castillo, and A. Aranda, "Vitamin D-dependent recruitment of corepressors to vitamin D/retinoid X receptor heterodimers," *Molecular and Cellular Biology*, vol. 28, no. 11, pp. 3817–3829, 2008.

[35] P. Polly, M. Herdick, U. Moehren, A. Baniahmad, T. Heinzel, and C. Carlberg, "VDR-Alien: a novel, DNA-selective vitamin D_3 receptorcorepressor partnership," *The FASEB Journal*, vol. 14, no. 10, pp. 1455–1463, 2000.

[36] J. E. Arbelle, H. Chen, M. A. Gacad, E. A. Allegretto, J. W. Pike, and J. S. Adams, "Inhibition of vitamin D receptor-retinoid X receptor-vitamin D response element complex formation by nuclear extracts of vitamin D-resistant new world primate cells," *Endocrinology*, vol. 137, no. 2, pp. 786–789, 1996.

[37] H. Chen, B. Hu, E. A. Allegretto, and J. S. Adams, "The vitamin D response element-binding protein: a novel dominant-negative regulator of vitamin D-directed transactivation," *The Journal of Biological Chemistry*, vol. 275, no. 45, pp. 35557–35564, 2000.

[38] D. M. Provvedini, C. D. Tsoukas, L. J. Deftos, and S. C. Manolagas, "1,25-Dihydroxyvitamin D_3 receptors in human leukocytes," *Science*, vol. 221, no. 4616, pp. 1181–1183, 1983.

[39] H. Rasmussen and P. Bordier, *The Physiological and Cellular Basis of Metabolic Bone Disease*, Williams & Wilkins, Baltimore, Md, USA, 1974.

[40] D. A. Fischman and E. D. Hay, "Origin of osteoclasts from mononuclear leucocytes in regenerating newt limbs," *The Anatomical record*, vol. 143, pp. 329–337, 1962.

[41] J. Lotem and L. Sachs, "Induction of specific changes in the surface membrane of myeloid leukemic cells by steroid hormones," *International Journal of Cancer*, vol. 15, no. 5, pp. 731–740, 1975.

[42] E. Abe, C. Miyaura, and H. Sakagami, "Differentiation of mouse myeloid leukemia cells induced by 1α,25-dihydroxyvitamin D_3," *Proceedings of the National Academy of Sciences of the United States of America*, vol. 78, no. 8, pp. 4990–4994, 1981.

[43] C. Miyaura, E. Abe, and T. Kuribayashi, "1α,25-dihydroxyvitamin D_3 induces differentiation of human myeloid leukemia cells," *Biochemical and Biophysical Research Communications*, vol. 102, no. 3, pp. 937–943, 1981.

[44] Y. Honma, T. Kasukabe, J. Okabe, and M. Hozumi, "Glucocorticoid binding and mechanism of resistance in some clones of mouse myeloid leukemic cells resistant to induction of differentiation by dexamethasone," *Journal of Cellular Physiology*, vol. 93, no. 2, pp. 227–235, 1977.

[45] W. F. C. Rigby, T. Stacy, and M. W. Fanger, "Inhibition of T lymphocyte mitogenesis by 1,25-dihydroxyvitamin D_3 (calcitriol)," *The Journal of Clinical Investigation*, vol. 74, no. 4, pp. 1451–1455, 1984.

[46] H. Reichel, H. P. Koeffler, A. Tobler, and A. W. Norman, "1α,25-Dihydroxyvitamin D_3 inhibits γ-interferon synthesis by normal human peripheral blood lymphocytes," *Proceedings of the National Academy of Sciences of the United States of America*, vol. 84, no. 10, pp. 3385–3389, 1987.

[47] J. M. Lemire, J. S. Adams, and V. Kermani-Arab, "1,25-dihydroxyvitamin D_3 suppresses human T helper/inducer lymphocyte activity in vitro," *The Journal of Immunology*, vol. 134, no. 5, pp. 3032–3035, 1985.

[48] J. S. Adams, S. Ren, P. T. Liu et al., "Vitamin D-directed rheostatic regulation of monocyte antibacterial responses," *The Journal of Immunology*, vol. 182, no. 7, pp. 4289–4295, 2009.

[49] S. Tauszig, E. Jouanguy, J. A. Hoffmann, and J. L. Imler, "Toll-related receptors and the control of antimicrobial peptide expression in *Drosophila*," *Proceedings of the National Academy of Sciences of the United States of America*, vol. 97, no. 19, pp. 10520–10525, 2000.

[50] S. Thoma-Uszynski, S. Stenger, O. Takeuchi et al., "Induction of direct antimicrobial activity through mammalian toll-like receptors," *Science*, vol. 291, no. 5508, pp. 1544–1547, 2001.

[51] P. T. Liu, S. Stenger, H. Li et al., "Toll-like receptor triggering of a vitamin D-mediated human antimicrobial response," *Science*, vol. 311, no. 5768, pp. 1770–1773, 2006.

[52] J. M. Yuk, D. M. Shin, H. M. Lee et al., "Vitamin D_3 induces autophagy in human monocytes/macrophages via cathelicidin," *Cell Host and Microbe*, vol. 6, no. 3, pp. 231–243, 2009.

[53] M. Fabri, S. Stenger, D. M. Shin et al., "Vitamin D is required for IFN-gamma-mediated antimicrobial activity of human macrophages," *Science Translational Medicine*, vol. 3, no. 104, pp. 1–10, 2011.

[54] A. R. Martineau, S. Nhamoyebonde, T. Oni et al., "Reciprocal seasonal variation in vitamin D status and tuberculosis notifications in Cape Town, South Africa," *Proceedings of the National Academy of Sciences of the United States of America*, vol. 108, no. 47, pp. 19013–19017, 2011.

[55] P. T. Liu, M. Wheelwright, R. Teles et al., "MicroRNA-21 targets the vitamin D-dependent antimicrobial pathway in leprosy," *Nature Medicine*, vol. 18, no. 2, pp. 267–273, 2012.

[56] L. Rogers, "Chaulmoogra oil in leprosy and tuberculosis," *The Lancet*, vol. 1, pp. 1178–1180, 1921.

[57] M. PcDuarte, M. L. F. Farias, H. S. M. Coelho et al., "Calcium-parathyroid hormone-vitamin D axis and metabolic bone disease in chronic viral liver disease," *Journal of Gastroenterology and Hepatology*, vol. 16, no. 9, pp. 1022–1027, 2001.

[58] J. George, H. K. Ganesh, S. Acharya et al., "Bone mineral density and disorders of mineral metabolism in chronic liver disease," *World Journal of Gastroenterology*, vol. 15, no. 28, pp. 3516–3522, 2009.

[59] C. M. Lange, J. Bojunga, E. Ramos-Lopez et al., "Vitamin D deficiency and a CYP27B1-1260 promoter polymorphism are associated with chronic hepatitis C and poor response to interferon-alfa based therapy," *Journal of Hepatology*, vol. 54, no. 5, pp. 887–893, 2011.

[60] P. Bellecave, M. Sarasin-Filipowicz, O. D. Sarasin-Filipowicz et al., "Cleavage of mitochondrial antiviral signaling protein in the liver of patients with chronic hepatitis c correlates with a reduced activation of the endogenous interferon system," *Hepatology*, vol. 51, no. 4, pp. 1127–1136, 2010.

[61] D. Bitetto, C. Fabris, E. Fornasiere et al., "Vitamin D supplementation improves response to antiviral treatment for recurrent hepatitis C," *Transplant International*, vol. 24, no. 1, pp. 43–50, 2011.

[62] M. Gal-Tanamy, L. Bachmetov, A. Ravid et al., "Vitamin D: an innate antiviral agent suppressing hepatitis C virus in human hepatocytes," *Hepatology*, vol. 54, no. 5, pp. 1570–1579, 2011.

[63] A. Nimer and A. Mouch, "Vitamin D improves viral response in hepatitis C genotype 2-3 naïve patients," *World Journal of Gastroenterology*, vol. 18, no. 8, pp. 800–805, 2012.

[64] S. Petta, C. Camma, C. Scazzone et al., "Low vitamin d serum level is related to severe fibrosis and low responsiveness to interferon-based therapy in genotype 1 chronic hepatitis C," *Hepatology*, vol. 51, no. 4, pp. 1158–1167, 2010.

[65] B. D. Mahon, A. Wittke, V. Weaver, and M. T. Cantorna, "The targets of vitamin D depend on the differentiation and activation status of CD4 positive T cells," *Journal of Cellular Biochemistry*, vol. 89, no. 5, pp. 922–932, 2003.

[66] S. Chen, G. P. Sims, X. C. Xiao, Y. G. Yue, S. Chen, and P. E. Lipsky, "Modulatory effects of 1,25-dihydroxyvitamin D_3 on human B cell differentiation," *The Journal of Immunology*, vol. 179, no. 3, pp. 1634–1647, 2007.

[67] D. M. Shin, J. M. Yuk, H. M. Lee et al., "Mycobacterial lipoprotein activates autophagy via TLR2/1/CD14 and a functional vitamin D receptor signalling," *Cellular Microbiology*, vol. 12, no. 11, pp. 1648–1665, 2010.

[68] T. R. Mosmann and R. L. Coffman, "TH1 and TH2 cells: different patterns of lymphokine secretion lead to different functional properties," *Annual Review of Immunology*, vol. 7, pp. 145–173, 1989.

[69] W. F. C. Rigby, S. Denome, and M. W. Fanger, "Regulation of lymphokine production and human T lymphocyte activation by 1,25-dihydroxyvitamin D_3. Specific inhibition at the level of messenger RNA," *The Journal of Clinical Investigation*, vol. 79, no. 6, pp. 1659–1664, 1987.

[70] J. M. Lemire, "Immunomodulatory actions of 1,25-dihydroxyvitamin D_3," *Journal of Steroid Biochemistry and Molecular Biology*, vol. 53, no. 1–6, pp. 599–602, 1995.

[71] O. V. Vieira, R. E. Harrison, C. C. Scott et al., "Acquisition of Hrs, an essential component of phagosomal maturation, is impaired by mycobacteria," *Molecular and Cellular Biology*, vol. 24, no. 10, pp. 4593–4604, 2004.

[72] J. P. Viard, J. C. Souberbielle, O. Kirk et al., "Vitamin D and clinical disease progression in HIV infection: results from the EuroSIDA study," *AIDS*, vol. 25, no. 10, pp. 1305–1315, 2011.

[73] S. Mehta, E. Giovannucci, F. M. Mugusi et al., "Vitamin D status of HIV-infected women and its association with hiv disease progression, anemia, and mortality," *PLoS ONE*, vol. 5, no. 1, Article ID e8770, 2010.

[74] M. Priemel, C. Von Domarus, T. O. Klatte et al., "Bone mineralization defects and vitamin D deficiency: histomorphometric analysis of iliac crest bone biopsies and circulating 25-hydroxyvitamin D in 675 patients," *Journal of Bone and Mineral Research*, vol. 25, no. 2, pp. 305–312, 2010.

[75] C. M. T. Greenwood, T. M. Fujiwara, L. J. Boothroyd et al., "Linkage of tuberculosis to chromosome 2q35 loci, including NRAMP1, in a large Aboriginal Canadian family," *American Journal of Human Genetics*, vol. 67, no. 2, pp. 405–416, 2000.

[76] R. Bellamy, N. Beyers, K. P. W. J. McAdam et al., "Genetic susceptibility to tuberculosis in Africans: a genome-wide scan," *Proceedings of the National Academy of Sciences of the United States of America*, vol. 97, no. 14, pp. 8005–8009, 2000.

[77] R. J. Wilkinson, M. Llewelyn, Z. Toossi et al., "Influence of vitamin D deficiency and vitamin D receptor polymorphisms on tuberculosis among Gujarati Asians in west London: a case-control study," *The Lancet*, vol. 355, no. 9204, pp. 618–621, 2000.

[78] R. Bellamy, C. Ruwende, T. Corrah et al., "Tuberculosis and chronic hepatitis B virus infection in Africans and variation in the vitamin D receptor gene," *Journal of Infectious Diseases*, vol. 179, no. 3, pp. 721–724, 1999.

[79] A. K. Wilbur, L. Salter Kubatko, A. M. Hurtado, K. R. Hill, and A. C. Stone, "Vitamin D receptor gene polymorphisms and susceptibility *M. tuberculosis* in Native Paraguayans," *Tuberculosis*, vol. 87, no. 4, pp. 329–337, 2007.

[80] K. Alagarasu, P. Selvaraj, S. Swaminathan, G. Narendran, and P. R. Narayanan, "5′ regulatory and 3′ untranslated region polymorphisms of vitamin D receptor gene in south Indian HIV and HIV-TB patients," *Journal of Clinical Immunology*, vol. 29, no. 2, pp. 196–204, 2009.

[81] P. Selvaraj, M. Vidyarani, K. Alagarasu, S. Prabhu Anand, and P. R. Narayanan, "Regulatory role of promoter and 3′ UTR variants of vitamin D receptor gene on cytokine response in pulmonary tuberculosis," *Journal of Clinical Immunology*, vol. 28, no. 4, pp. 306–313, 2008.

[82] Y. Barber, C. Rubio, E. Fernández, M. Rubio, and J. Fibla, "Host genetic background at CCR5 chemokine receptor and vitamin D receptor loci and human immunodeficiency virus (HIV) type 1 disease progression among HIV-seropositive injection drug users," *Journal of Infectious Diseases*, vol. 184, no. 10, pp. 1279–1288, 2001.

[83] M. Saito, N. Eiraku, K. Usuku et al., "ApaI polymorphism of vitamin D receptor gene is associated with susceptibility to HTLV-1-associated myelopathy/tropical spastic paraparesis in HTLV-1 infected individuals," *Journal of the Neurological Sciences*, vol. 232, no. 1-2, pp. 29–35, 2005.

[84] M. T. Mira, A. Alcaïs, H. Van Thuc et al., "Susceptibility to leprosy is associated with *PARK2* and *PACRG*," *Nature*, vol. 427, no. 6975, pp. 636–640, 2004.

[85] A. Alter, L. De Léséleuc, N. Van Thuc et al., "Genetic and functional analysis of common MRC1 exon 7 polymorphisms in leprosy susceptibility," *Human Genetics*, vol. 127, no. 3, pp. 337–348, 2010.

[86] S. Roy, A. Frodsham, B. Saha, S. K. Hazra, C. G. N. Mascie-Taylor, and A. V. S. Hill, "Association of vitamin D receptor genotype with leprosy type," *Journal of Infectious Diseases*, vol. 179, no. 1, pp. 187–191, 1999.

[87] C. Gross, T. R. Eccleshall, P. J. Malloy, M. L. Villa, R. Marcus, and D. Feldman, "The presence of a polymorphism at the translation initiation site of the vitamin D receptor gene is associated with low bone mineral density in postmenopausal Mexican-American women," *Journal of Bone and Mineral Research*, vol. 11, no. 12, pp. 1850–1855, 1996.

[88] A. Morita, M. Iki, Y. Dohi et al., "Prediction of bone mineral density from vitamin D receptor polymorphisms is uncertain in representative samples of Japanese women. The Japanese population-based osteoporosis (JPOS) study," *International Journal of Epidemiology*, vol. 33, no. 5, pp. 979–988, 2004.

[89] R. Marik, M. Fackler, E. Gabrielson et al., "DNA methylation-related vitamin D receptor insensitivity in breast cancer," *Cancer Biology and Therapy*, vol. 10, no. 1, pp. 44–53, 2010.

7

Using Risk Models to Improve Patient Selection for High-Risk Vascular Surgery

Philip P. Goodney[1, 2]

[1] Section of Vascular Surgery, Dartmouth-Hitchcock Medical Center, 1 Medical Center Drive, Lebanon, NH 03766, USA
[2] Dartmouth-Hitchcock Medical Center, The Dartmouth Institute for Health Policy and Clinical Practice, Hanover, NH 03765, USA

Correspondence should be addressed to Philip P. Goodney; philip.goodney@gmail.com

Academic Editors: A. Kalangos and M. Morasch

Vascular surgeons frequently perform procedures aimed at limiting death, stroke, or amputation on patients who present with diseases such as aortic aneurysms, carotid atherosclerosis, and peripheral arterial occlusive disease. However, now more than ever surgeons must balance the potential benefits associated with these interventions with the risks of physiologic insult for these elderly patients, who often have significant comorbidity burdens and the potential for costly complications. In this paper, we highlight how regional and national datasets can help surgeons identify which patients are most likely to benefit from vascular operations and which patients are most likely to suffer complications in the postoperative period. By using these guidelines to improve patient selection, our risk models can help patients, physicians, and policymakers improve the clinical effectiveness of surgical and endovascular treatments for vascular disease.

1. Introduction

Vascular surgeons frequently perform procedures aimed at limiting death, stroke, or amputation on patients who present with diseases such as aortic aneurysms, carotid atherosclerosis, and peripheral arterial occlusive disease [1]. These operations, whether they involve repair of an aneurysmal segment of aorta [2], bypass of an occluded artery in the leg [3], or removal of atherosclerotic plaque in a carotid artery [4], all serve a palliative purpose. The operations themselves, of course, do not cure atherosclerosis. Rather, they serve to mitigate its effects and limit its manifestations during the remainder of the patient's life. In other words, they must prevent death from ruptured aneurysms, limit limb loss from lower extremity vascular disease, and provide prophylaxis from stroke from carotid atherosclerosis.

However, given the current cost constraints in health care, surgeons must, now more than ever, balance the potential benefits associated with these surgical interventions with alternative strategies [5, 6]. They must consider, against the background of medical alternatives, the physiologic insult that surgery entails in these elderly patients, who often carry with them significant comorbidity burdens [7–10]. One of the most important elements in effectively utilizing expensive, morbid procedures, such as thoracic aneurysm repair, lower extremity bypass, and carotid endarterectomy, is to perform these procedures on patients who will benefit from the procedure and not suffer complications from it.

While "good patient selection" may sound like a simple objective, achieving good patient selection remains a constantly evolving and sometimes elusive goal. New, less invasive endovascular alternatives can change the risk profile of an operation, such as thoracic endovascular grafting for thoracic aortic aneurysms [11]. New medications, such as high-dose statins and antiplatelet agents, can enhance the durability and effectiveness of lower extremity bypass procedures [12]. And both of these changes—less invasive alternatives and new medical adjuncts—have influenced which patients undergo, and garner benefit from carotid revascularization [13, 14].

To best select patients for these high-risk operations, surgeons need data that incorporates these complex covariates in their decision-making algorithms. In this paper, we highlight how regional and national datasets can help surgeons identify which patients are most likely to benefit from these operations and which patients are most likely to suffer complications in the postoperative period. By using these guidelines to improve patient selection, our risk models can help patients, physicians, and policymakers improve the clinical effectiveness of surgical and endovascular treatments for vascular disease [15–18].

Herein, we will use three illustrative examples—(1) survival following thoracic aneurysm repair [19], (2) amputation following lower extremity bypass [20], and (3) stroke following carotid revascularization [21]—to demonstrate how we can use past experience to inform which patients should be selected for vascular surgery in the future.

2. Predicting Survival following Thoracic Aneurysm Repair

2.1. An Overview: What Is at Stake in Thoracic Aneurysm Repair? Given the significant potential for morbidity and mortality involved with descending thoracic aortic aneurysm (TAA) repair, surgeons have sought to balance the chance of dying from aneurysm rupture with the risk of surgical intervention [22–25]. Thoracic endovascular repair (TEVAR) has further complicated this relationship [26, 27], as this less-invasive intervention has expanded the pool of patients who are physiologically able to undergo surgery. Subsequently, single-center, regional, and national studies have described a significant increase of utilization of TEVAR, with a significant short-term benefit in perioperative mortality.

Several reports have described similar mid-term survival following open repair and TEVAR. However, these studies have been limited to single institution series from centers of excellence, or results from industry-sponsored trials and registries [23, 28], and only one clinical trial has reported five-year outcomes [26, 27]. Little population-based data describing TEVAR and open TAA repair is available that allows examination of survival differences for distinct TAA, especially across rupture status at presentation, or by repair type [28]. In this summary of our prior work, we describe our efforts in comparing perioperative and long-term mortality in the contemporary, real-world practice of open TAA repair and TEVAR.

2.2. Establishing a Cohort of Patients Who Underwent Repair of TAA. First, using Medicare claims, we created a cohort of patients who underwent a broad range of thoracic aortic procedures, as defined by the ICD-9 codes [29]. Next, we selected from this cohort those patients who underwent TEVAR and open repair of TAA. As outlined in Figure 1, we eliminated all claims that were not contained in the Medicare Denominator File as well as patients not at least aged 66. We required patients to have at least one year of Medicare eligibility prior to surgery and used this time period to establish comorbidities and construct patient-specific Charlson scores [30, 31]. In addition to the procedural codes for TAA, we required that each patient has a diagnosis code for TAA. We excluded any patient with diagnosis codes for ascending thoracic aortic aneurysm, or with procedural codes for cardiopulmonary bypass occurring with circulatory arrest, and patients with thoracoabdominal aneurysms, thoracic aortic dissections, and "other" aortic pathology from our analysis, as these entities are clinically distinct from TAA. Finally, we examined the effect of changes in practice pattern over time. First, in prior work [32], we demonstrated that between 1998 and 2003, a significant increase in the use of TEVAR occurred. Before 2003, fewer than 10% of all intact TAA were repaired using TEVAR. After 2003, more than 10% of all intact TAAs were repaired with TEVAR, and this rate grew to 27% by 2007. We studied the effect of time across this pattern using time-dependent analyses. We followed this cohort over time to establish our two main outcome measures: perioperative and long-term survival, using one- and five-year survival rates. First, to define perioperative mortality, we sought to capture all deaths occurring in the period following surgery. We defined perioperative mortality as death occurring within the index hospitalization (regardless of postoperative day), as well as any death within thirty days (irrespective of inpatient or outpatient status). Second, survival at one and five years was established using the Medicare Denominator file to establish the date of death. We censored those patients who survived until the end of our analysis (at December 31, 2007).

Finally, we used a survivor function wherein age, gender, race, era of procedure, and Charlson score [30] were adjusted using a Cox proportional hazards model to estimate survival. This allowed comparison of survival estimates, adjusted to reflect survival within the strata of minimal patient-level risk within each group [33]. For ruptured patients, we stratified our Cox models by repair type and calculated hazard ratios for the remaining covariates. Additionally, we used propensity matching methods to create similar cohorts for survival analysis [34]. First, we generated a propensity score for the likelihood of undergoing TEVAR, based on a multivariable logistic model that described the association between preoperative patient characteristics and the choice to perform TEVAR. Within a sample of patients between age 65 and 75 who underwent surgery during the latter 4 years of our study period, we matched patients by age and comorbidity. This allowed us to generate two cohorts that were matched in terms of age, gender, race, era of procedure, comorbidities that constitute the Charlson score, as well as the Charlson score itself.

2.3. Comparison of Outcomes by Procedure Type. In this analysis, we studied 12,573 Medicare patients who underwent open procedures and 2,732 patients who underwent TEVAR (Figure 1). By presentation status, 13,998 patients presented for surgery with intact TAA (11,565 open repair, 2,433 TEVAR), while 1,307 patients underwent surgery for ruptured TAA (1,008 open repair, 299 TEVAR). Several demographic differences existed between open repair and TEVAR patients with intact TAA. First, patients undergoing TEVAR were significantly older than patients undergoing open repair (75.9 years versus 73.8 years, $P < 0.0001$). Second, the proportion of male patients was slightly higher among patients undergoing TEVAR than open repair (58.7 versus 55.4%, $P < 0.0001$).

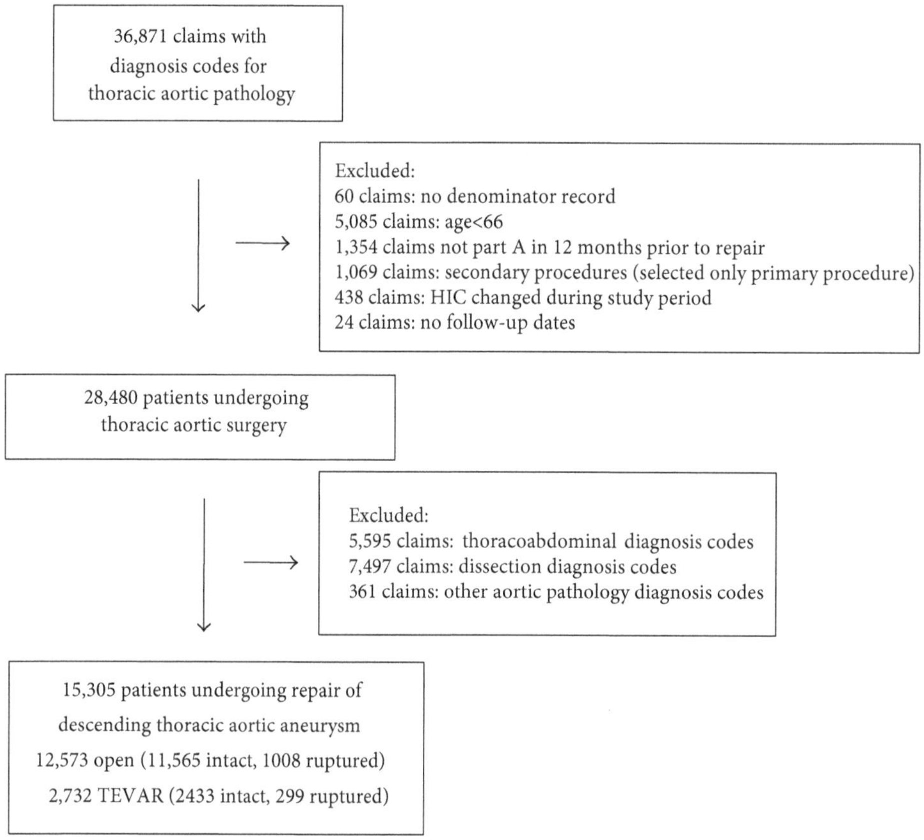

Figure 1: Establishing the cohort of patients undergoing TAA repair.

In terms of outcomes the lowest perioperative mortality rate occurred in patients undergoing repair of intact TAA using TEVAR (6.1% (95% CI 5.1–7.0%)). While the perioperative mortality rate for open repair was slightly higher (7.1% (95% CI 6.7–7.6%)), the clinical magnitude of this difference was small and borderline in terms of statistical significance ($P = 0.07$). Among patients presenting with ruptured thoracic aneurysms, perioperative mortality was 28.4% (95% CI 23.2–33.5%) for TEVAR and 45.6% (95% CI 42.5–48.7%) for open repair ($P = 0.0001$). Crude long-term survival varied by presentation (intact versus ruptured) as well as repair type (open repair versus TEVAR) is shown in Figure 2(a). Even though patients with intact TAA selected for TEVAR had lower perioperative mortality, patients selected for open repair reclaimed the survival advantage within the first year after surgery (1-year survival by life table analysis: 87% open repair (95% CI 86–88%), 82% TEVAR (95% CI 80–83%), log rank $P = 0.001$). This survival advantage continued to accumulate over time, as seen in our five-year survival data (5-year survival by life table analysis: 72% (95% CI 71–73%)) open repair, 62% TEVAR (95% CI 60–65%, log rank $P = 0.001$). This survival advantage was also seen in patients who underwent repair of ruptured TAA (Figure 2(b)). After five years, by life table analysis, fewer than 30% of patients were alive after repair of their ruptured TAA, irrespective of the type of repair (26% (95% CI 23–30%) open repair, 23% (95%CI 16–32%) TEVAR, log rank $P = 0.37$). Our results were similar, even in analyses adjusted for age, sex, race, era of procedure, and other comorbidities.

In other adjusted analyses, we used propensity matching to create matched cohorts. These cohorts of patients were similar in terms of patient characteristics available for measurement in administrative claims and who underwent either open repair or TEVAR. In these groups, perioperative mortality was statistically similar in patients undergoing TEVAR compared to open repair (4.5% (95% CI 2.8–6.2%) open repair versus 4.2% (95% CI 2.5–5.8) TEVAR, $P = 0.78$). Any difference in perioperative mortality incurred by TEVAR disappeared within the first year postoperatively. Late survival was significantly worse in patients undergoing TEVAR (Figure 2(c)). By life table analysis at five years' postoperatively, late survival was significantly worse in patients undergoing TEVAR (73% (95% CI 68–76%)) than open repair (81% (95% CI 77–85%)) within the propensity-matched cohort (log rank $P = 0.007$). And lastly, our outcomes remained similar, even if we stratified by before or after FDA approval of TEVAR procedures.

2.4. Implications of Our Findings, by Procedure Type. The competing mortalities of observation and open surgical repair for TAA have been investigated for several decades. However, the effect of TEVAR on survival remains less well studied. Our study examined survival following open repair and TEVAR in national, real-world practice and found that,

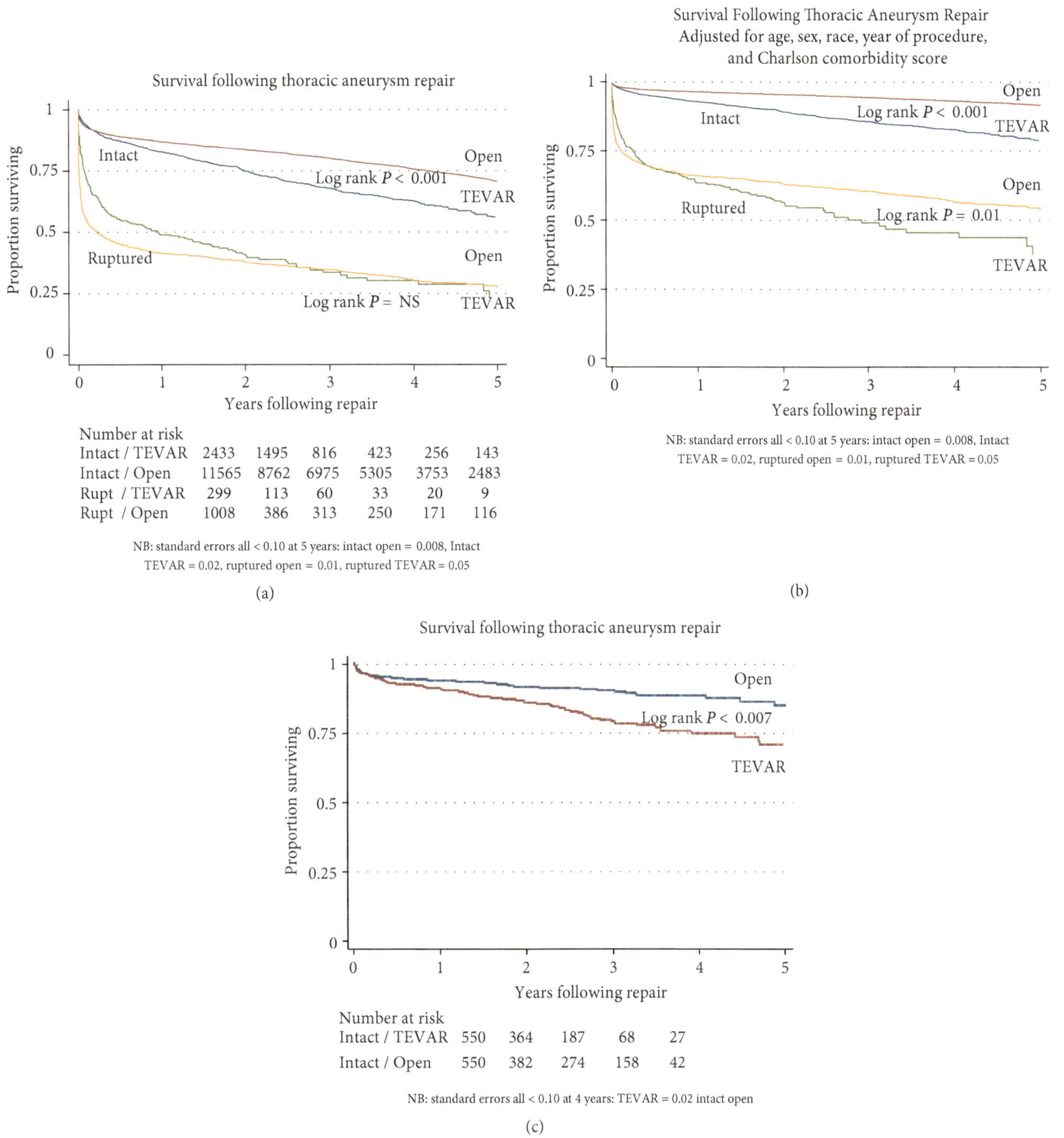

FIGURE 2: (a) Unadjusted five-year survival in thoracic aneurysms, by procedure type and diagnosis. (b) Adjusted five-year survival in thoracic aneurysms, by procedure type and diagnosis. Results represent male, nonblack patients under age of 75 with Charlson score < 2, performed after 2003. (c) Propensity-matched five-year survival in thoracic aneurysms, by procedure type. These patients represent a randomly selected, propensity-matched sample of low-risk patients who are at equal likelihood of undergoing either open repair or TEVAR.

while perioperative mortality is lower in TEVAR, patients selected for TEVAR have worse long-term survival than patients selected for open repair. These results suggest that higher risk patients are being offered TEVAR and that some do not benefit based on long-term survival. This study demonstrates that the treatment of TAA follows a similar course to infrarenal AAA, with one important exception. As with infrarenal AAA, we found a survival advantage in short-term mortality for patients who undergo TEVAR as compared to open repair. Further, as with infrarenal AAA, any survival advantage gained in the perioperative period following endovascular repair was lost within two years after surgery. But unlike infrarenal AAA, adjusted survival at five years was significantly worse for patients selected for TEVAR as compared to open repair. Therefore, the widespread application of TEVAR has resulted in a cohort of patients who may have previously not undergone surgery, but now undergo TEVAR. Patients selected for TEVAR achieve worse survival than patients undergoing open repair, and many of these deaths occur within the first two years after TEVAR. These deaths could be due to the selection of "sicker" patients for TEVAR, although our finding of poorer survival following TEVAR persists, even in propensity-matched analyses that account for differences in patient risk measurable using administrative claims. Alternatively, these differences in survival could be explained by device-related complications occurring within the first five years following surgery.

Survival following aortic aneurysm surgery has been a topic of extensive study, but primarily in patients with infrarenal abdominal aortic aneurysm (AAA) [35, 36]. Several randomized trials [37–39] have demonstrated lower perioperative mortality with endovascular techniques. It is well known that patients who experience late death following infrarenal AAA repair most commonly die from cardiopulmonary comorbidities unrelated to their aneurysm, and relatively few experience aneurysm-related death, in either open or endovascular repair [40]. As with patients with infrarenal AAA, we suspect that the loss of survival advantage is secondary to patient-level comorbidities. For example, in the EVAR-2 trial [41], survival was similar among patients treated with endovascular repair and patients who did not undergo repair. The data available from our study supports this presumption, as TEVAR patients tend to be older and have higher comorbidity scores than the patients selected for open repair. However, it is important to acknowledge that our findings are based solely on administrative claims, and our analysis is therefore limited in terms of clinical detail.

This study provides an important focus on the data used to demonstrate the efficacy of endovascular repair of TAA [42, 43]. First, when compared to data from TEVAR clinical trials (Table 1), it is evident that perioperative mortality is higher in "real-world" practice than in the centers of excellence where the clinical trials were performed. Second, in real-world practice, patients selected for open repair had better survival that the surgical controls used in clinical trials (72% five-year survival in Medicare, 67% five-year survival in the single trial that reported this measure). Collectively, these two differences resulted in the disparity in conclusions between our study, wherein TEVAR patients fared significantly worse at five years and the clinical trial, wherein outcomes were similar at five years. Given the findings in our study and others, there is little evidence to suggest that long-term survival is better in patients selected for TEVAR as compared to open surgical repair, and it may in fact be worse [44].

In conclusion, the consistent short-term survival advantage offered by TEVAR disappears within the first two years after surgery. These results suggest that higher risk patients are being offered TEVAR and that some do not benefit based on long-term survival. Patient selection in TEVAR requires better risk stratification to better select patients for this new procedure.

3. Lower Extremity Bypass: How Do We Select Patients Who Will Avoid Amputation?

3.1. Introduction. Now, we turn our attention to a different type of vascular disease. Lower extremity peripheral arterial disease (PAD) affects over 8 million Americans, with significant associated morbidity and mortality [45–49]. Significant morbidity and mortality are encountered when elderly, medically complex patients undergo prolonged, invasive arterial reconstruction [47, 49]. One of the key elements in minimizing morbidity and mortality is optimal patient selection, especially in the current era wherein endovascular alternatives may exist [50]. To this end, we examined the risk factors associated with amputation or graft occlusion one year after surgery.

3.2. Studying a Cohort of Lower Extremity Bypass Patients Using a Regional Dataset. In this analysis, we utilized data collected prospectively by the Vascular Study Group of Northern New England (VSGNNE), a regional cooperative quality improvement initiative developed in 2002 to study regional outcomes in vascular surgery. Further details on this registry have been published previously [51] and described in detail at vsgnne.org. Our unit of analysis was the bypass graft. Our main outcome measure was a combined measure of either permanent graft occlusion (loss of secondary patency) or major amputation (above or below knee) following surgery. Between January 1, 2003, and December 31, 2006, we identified 2,036 patients in our database that underwent 2,301 bypass procedures. Graft patency and major amputation rates were determined at several stages: first preoperatively, then at discharge following surgery, and again at 1 year postoperatively. Major amputation was defined as above-knee amputation or below-knee amputation. This outcome was assessed both at discharge and again at one-year followup.

We used life table analysis given that not all follow-up data was obtained at exactly one year. Patients who died within one year of surgery were censored after their date of death. Risk factors found by univariate analysis to be associated with a P value of <0.1 were then used in a multivariate Cox proportional hazards model. This model was then used to calculate hazard ratios (HRs) and 95% confidence intervals (CIs) for ability to ambulate one year after surgery. To examine the validity of our risk prediction model, we constructed our risk model from the data obtained between 2003 and 2006. We then applied the risk model to the data acquired from the VSG sites in 2007. Lastly, using our model, we predicted a one-year amputation/occlusion rate for each patient, based on that patient's individual risk factor profile. We also compared results across centers, based on the characteristics of the patients treated at each center. The predictive ability of each model was then evaluated by generating an observed-to-expected outcome ratio across the range of risk identified.

3.3. Outcomes and Their Association with Amputation. In our study, 2,036 patients underwent lower extremity bypass in

TABLE 1: Outcomes at 30 days, 1 year, and 5 years, by repair type and study.

Repair type	Outcome measure	Medicare 1998–2007	TAG [43]	VALOR [42]	TX2 [11]
Open repair	In hospital/30-day mortality	7.1%	6.4%	8.0%	6.0%
	1-year survival	87%	78%	79%	88%
	5-year survival	72%	67%	—	—
TEVAR	In hospital/30-day mortality	6.1%	1.2%	2.0%	1.9%
	1-year survival	82%	82%	84%	84–94%
	5-year survival	62%	68%	—	—

Northern New England at one of the 11 centers participating in our registry. Patients were most commonly male (67%), aged 70–80 (30%), and nearly all were Caucasian. Nearly all patients had a history of either prior or current smoking (82%). About half of patients had a history of diabetes, 40% had coronary disease, and nearly a third had a history of COPD. Indication for surgery was claudication in 25% of patients, while the remaining patients had critical ischemia. In claudicants, one-year primary patency was 79% and secondary patency 87%. However, one-year primary and secondary patency was significantly lower (73 and 81%, respectfully) in patients with critical limb ischemia. As expected, limb salvage rates in our cohort were lower in patients with critical limb ischemia compared to claudication (86% versus 98%, $P < 0.0001$). Of 143 major amputations (8% of all bypasses) that occurred in our cohort, 17% were performed in patients who had a patent bypass graft. Similarly, 277 graft occlusions were noted in our cohort, of which 42% resulted in amputation. Our combined amputation or permanent graft occlusion rate was 3% at discharge and 16% at 1 year, by life table analysis.

In univariate analyses, several physiologic parameters such as advanced age, diabetes, and hypertension were associated with amputation or graft occlusion at 1 year. Additionally, functional parameters such as baseline ambulatory status prior to surgery, living status prior to surgery, and presence of tissue loss were also highly closely correlated with loss of graft patency or amputation at 1 year. The factors associated with amputation or graft occlusion at one year are shown in Table 2. These were of age less than 50, nonambulatory status preoperatively, dialysis dependence, diabetes, critical limb ischemia, conduit requiring venovenostomy, tarsal target, and nursing home residence preoperatively. The likelihood of amputation or graft occlusion at one year varied from less than 0.5% in patients with no risk factors to nearly 30% in patients with three or more risk factors (Figure 3).

Lastly, to examine the validity of our risk prediction model, we constructed our risk model from the data obtained between 2003 and 2006 and applied the risk model to the data acquired from the VSG sites in 2007 (Figure 4). We found that our model performed well in discriminating risk. For example, patients with no risk factors had no episodes of graft occlusion or amputation, while those patients with three or more risk factors had a 30% incidence of amputation or graft occlusion. Differences between groups were statistically significant (<0.002). This risk prediction models allow benchmarking and facilitate comparison of risk-adjusted outcomes across centers as part of quality improvement efforts. To this end, we used our risk prediction model to calculate expected amputation/occlusion rates across centers and compared observed results with the expected results using O/E ratios. Predicted risks of amputation or graft occlusion varied from 3% at our lowest risk centers to 19% at the highest risk center.

TABLE 2: Multivariate predictors of amputation or graft occlusion 1 year following lower extremity bypass.

Variable	Hazard ratio	95% CI	*P* value
Age			
<40	**1.4**	**0.4–4.7**	**0.645**
40–49	1.9	1.2–3.1	0.007
50–59	**1.2**	**0.8–1.7**	**0.424**
60–69	**1.2**	**0.8–1.7**	**0.334**
70+	**1**	**0.7–1.5**	**0.757**
Nonambulatory preoperatively	1.6	1–2.5	0.044
Dialysis	1.6	1.1–2.2	0.008
Diabetes	1.6	1.1–2.5	0.029
Critical limb ischemia	1.7	1.3–2.3	0.0001
Two vein segments	2	1.4–2.8	0.0001
Tarsal target for bypass	2.5	1.2–5.3	0.021
Nursing home residence	2.8	1.3–6	0.011

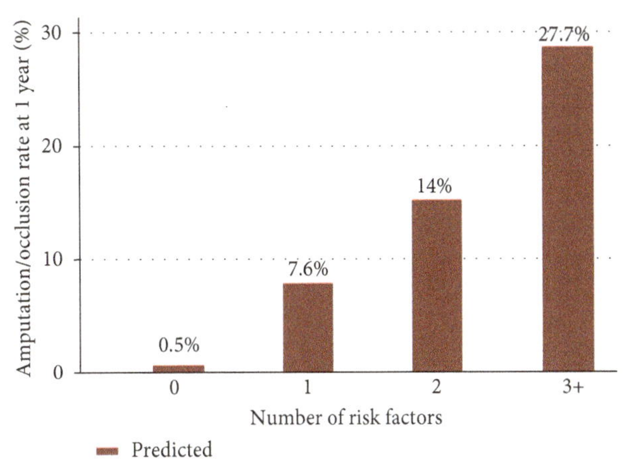

FIGURE 3: Predicted risk of amputation or graft occlusion, by the number of risk factors.

3.4. *Implications of Our Findings for Patient Selection in Lower Extremity Bypass.*

This review of factors associated

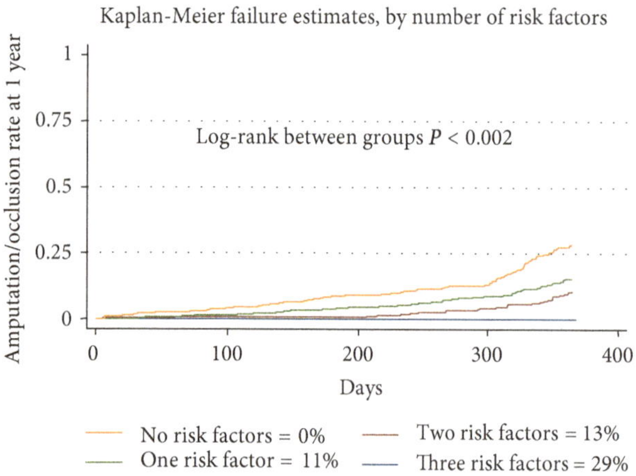

FIGURE 4: Validation of the risk prediction model using data from the VSGNE from 2007.

with amputation or graft occlusion found that eight risk factors allow surgeons to predict which patients are at risk for graft occlusion or major amputation within one year following surgery. Additionally, this model allowed us to establish benchmarks for performance and compare risk-adjusted long-term outcomes within our region.

Prior investigators have recently studied clinical risk factors identified with a variety of different outcomes following lower extremity bypass [52–55]. In several single-center studies, ranging in size from 128 to 468 patients, investigators identified a variety of angiographic grading systems, as well as variables such as gender, conduit type, diabetes, and tissue loss, that were all predicted poor results in terms of graft patency. Further, Schanzer et al. analyzed a highly selected population of patients undergoing lower extremity bypass to determine predictors of amputation-free survival. They found that age, end-stage renal disease, critical limb ischemia, anemia, and advanced coronary artery disease were associated with decreased amputation-free survival one year after surgery. While these models are slightly different than the findings in our study, we believe both models will be helpful to both surgeons and patients in their preoperative discussions weighing the risks and benefits of surgery.

Our study, because it focuses on a predominantly white population, offers limited insight into racial effects on amputation risk. Peripheral vascular disease is more common in African Americans than any other racial group, and African American race has been widely identified as a risk factor for heart disease, stroke, and lower extremity vascular disease [56]. African Americans have poorer outcomes with lower extremity revascularization and overall are much more likely to undergo amputation [57–59]. In national studies, the Dartmouth Atlas Project has documented that African Americans underwent amputations at a rate nearly five times that of whites −4.17 per 1,000 African American Medicare patients, compared to 0.88 per 1,000 white Medicare patients [56]. Efforts to identify and address these disparities in care are ongoing and will be important to those surgeons caring for patients with vascular disease.

Patients and surgeons can use this risk model not only to guide their expectations for success with bypass surgery but to also weigh the risks and benefits when considering surgery or endovascular intervention. Patients with only 1 or 2 risk factors have excellent outcomes in terms of graft patency and limb salvage, and in these patients bypass surgery represents a durable and effective treatment for both claudication and critical limb ischemia. However, in patients with 3 or more risk factors, nearly 1 in 3 will not have a patent graft or an intact limb within a year of their surgery. As to whether open bypass surgery or endovascular interventions should be used first, while many believe an "endovascular first" strategy should be employed [50, 60, 61], practice patterns vary significantly, and best practices have yet to be established with high quality evidence. We believe future comparative effectiveness research and clinical trials are necessary to address this question directly.

But in addition to helping surgeons predict amputation risk, one of the main goals of the VSGNE is to study and improve the care of vascular surgery patients. By comparing risk adjusted outcomes, surgeons can set benchmarks and compare results across centers. By studying those centers that do things well, surgeons can identify processes of care that contribute towards the best outcomes. Then, by widely implementing these processes of care, we hope to improve our results across the region. This model has been used effectively in cardiac surgery [62, 63], myocardial infarction care [64, 65], and in the treatment of pulmonary disease [66] and cancer [67]. In addition to our ongoing efforts in quality improvement in lower extremity bypass surgery, we are applying similar strategies in improving results after carotid endarterectomy in our region [21].

In conclusion, this study identified several risk factors that allow surgeons to predict which patients are at risk for amputation or graft occlusion following lower extremity bypass. Moreover, this model permits benchmarking and comparison of results across hospitals, key activities within our quality improvement initiative, which aims to use these data to broadly improve vascular care for patients at risk for amputation.

4. Carotid Atherosclerosis: Who Will Benefit from Carotid Revascularization?

4.1. Introduction: Who Is at Risk for Stroke during and after CEA? Finally, we turn our attention to one last, and hotly debated, vascular territory—the carotid artery. While many believe that carotid endarterectomy, or surgical removal of plaque from the carotid arteries, can prevent stroke, debate has persisted for more than three decades as to which patients are best served by undergoing this procedure. Many investigators have studied risk factors associated with stroke or death following carotid endarterectomy (CEA), with the intent of improving preoperative assessment and patient selection [68–73]. Across these studies, the most consistent risk factor found to predict stroke or death following CEA has been preoperative neurologic symptoms (Table 3). Other variables associated with increased operative risk have

TABLE 3: Previous studies analyzing risk of stroke/death following CEA.

Author	Year	*n*, study type	Risk factors
Musser et al.	1994	562 patients, single center, retrospective series	AF, emergent operation, PVCs, intraop hypotension, ESRD
Goldstein et al.	1998	1,160 patients, multicenter, retrospective administrative database	Female, age over 75, CHF
Rothwell et al.	1999	2,060 patients, multicenter, prospective trial	Symptomatic status, DM, recent MI Plaque characteristics
Frawley et al.	2000	1,000 patients, single center retrospective series	Female gender
Kresowik et al.	2001	10,561 patients, retrospective chart review of medicare beneficiaries	Aspirin/ticlopidine use, heparin use, patch angioplasty
Tu et al.	2003	6,038 patients, regional retrospective database	Symptomatic status, AF, contralateral occlusion, CHF, DM
Nicolaides et al.	2005	1,115 patients, prospective clinical trial	Symptomatic status, degree of stenosis, creatinine

AF: atrial fibrillation; MI: myocardial infarction; PVC: premature ventricular contractions; ESRD: end stage renal disease; CHF: congestive heart failure; DM: diabetes mellitus.

included emergent operation [74], renal failure [75], and diabetes [72]. Interestingly, preoperative antiplatelet medications were found to be protective in only one of these models [76], despite evidence that such therapy reduces stroke risk associated with CEA [77, 78]. And, as with our efforts in lower extremity revascularization, another role for risk prediction models is to allow comparison of risk-adjusted outcomes among different centers. An important element in surgical quality improvement is to establish benchmarks for performance [79–82]. Most outcome benchmarks require risk adjustment, to account for potential differences in patient populations that could influence outcomes [83], and multivariate risk prediction models are developed to account for differences in patient characteristics when comparing outcomes [84, 85].

4.2. Selecting a Cohort of Carotid Endarterectomy Patients Using a Regional Dataset. As with the project described earlier, we included only patients in the Vascular Study Group of New England but in this analysis included those who underwent primary CEA (excluding redo operations or those combined with coronary bypass grafting). We selected 30-day postoperative stroke or death as our main outcome measure. The determination of major or minor stroke was made according to these definitions by the nurse clinician or trained research assistant responsible for entering the data into the database at each participating institution. Operative volume categories were defined using cutpoints guided by prior studies [86–88], modified to create terciles of approximately equal size from our dataset. In order to predict 30-day postoperative stroke or death, we initially performed univariate comparisons between our main outcome measures and many patient level variables. We selected appropriate patient preoperative variables for comparison based on previous publications [87, 89–92]. We generated a multivariate model, using backwards stepwise multivariate logistic regression, which was used to generate odds ratios and 95% confidence intervals for 30-day postoperative stroke or death. We used the resulting model to calculate an expected stroke/death rate for each patient, based on that particular patient's characteristics.

4.3. Outcomes and Their Association with Stroke or Death. Overall, we studied 2,714 patients undergoing 3,092 primary CEAs. Most patients were males, with a history of smoking and hypertension, and nearly half were symptomatic. We observed, across 3,092 CEAs, 38 minor strokes, 14 major strokes, and 8 deaths, 5 of which were stroke related, within 30 days of the index procedure (30-day stroke or death rate = 1.8%); 5 of the 52 strokes (10%) and 2 of the 8 deaths (25%) were reported after discharge but before 30 days.

We found that, on univariate analysis, emergent operation, contralateral internal carotid artery (ICA) occlusion, ipsilateral cortical symptoms (both TIA and stroke), congestive heart failure, performance of a completion study, and ICA stenosis <60% all were associated with increased risk of 30-day stroke or death. By multivariate analysis, emergent procedure, contralateral ICA occlusion, pre-operative ipsilateral cortical stroke, congestive heart failure, and age over 70 were associated with a significantly higher risk of stroke or death, while preoperative ASA or clopidogrel use was protective (Table 4). We examined the impact and additive effects of the number of risk factors present (Figure 5). In patients with 0-1 of these risk factors, the risk of stroke or death was less than 1%. However, when patients had 3 or more risk factors, the risk of stroke or death increased to nearly 5%. When expected stroke or death rates were compared to the observed stroke or death rates, excellent correlation was observed ($r = 0.96$). The model was found to have reasonable discriminative ability (area under ROC curve 0.71). Finally, in benchmarking analyses across the 8 hospitals in our region, the expected stroke/death rate ranged from 1.5% to 2.0%, while observed results varied from 0% to over 4%. Two hospitals had O/E ratios greater than 1, indicating a higher observed 30-day stroke and death rate than expected.

TABLE 4: Multivariate analysis of factors associated with thirty-day stroke/death after CEA.

Variable	Odds ratio	95% CI	*P* value
Age over 70 years	1.3	0.8–2.3	0.315
Contralateral ICA occlusion	2.8	1.3–6.2	0.009
Antiplatelet agent use	0.4	0.2–0.9	0.02
Congestive heart failure	1.6	1.1–2.4	0.03
Emergent procedure (within 6 hours of admission)	7.0	1.8–26.9	0.004
Preoperative ipsilateral cortical symptoms (stroke)	2.4	1.1–5.1	0.02

Area under ROC: 0.71; TIA: transient ischemia attack.

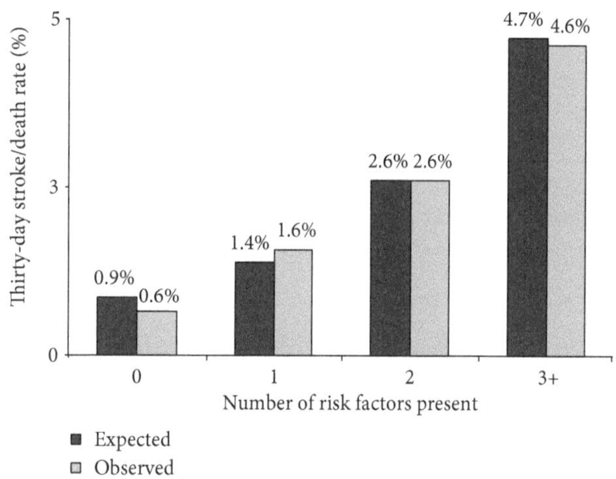

FIGURE 5: Comparison of observed and expected 30-day stroke/death rate. Risk factors include emergent procedure, preoperative ipsilateral stroke, age over 70, lack of antiplatelet agent, contralateral ICA occlusion, and congestive heart failure.

4.4. Implications of Our Findings for Patient Selection in Carotid Endarterectomy. In our study of contemporary carotid surgical revascularization, we identified emergent procedure, contralateral ICA occlusion, preoperative cortical stroke, congestive heart failure, increased age, and (lack of) antiplatelet agent use as predictive of postoperative 30-day stroke or death following CEA. Our model describes several risk factors reported in previous studies, with similar effect sizes. Two prior models reported odds ratios of 30-day stroke or death of 1.8 for contralateral ICA occlusion, which is similar in magnitude to our odds ratio of 2.8 [18, 87]. These same studies [70, 72] also reported that ipsilateral cerebral symptoms increased the risk of stroke and death nearly twofold, similar to our finding of an odds ratio of 2.4 for preoperative ipsilateral stroke. Patients with pre-operative stroke before CEA have been shown to be at higher risk for postoperative stroke, independent of whether or not they have TIAs at the time of CEA [93]. And finally, emergent CEA, usually indicated for free-floating thrombus or crescendo symptoms, has been well described as having worse surgical outcomes compared to routine or urgent carotid endarterectomy [94], in keeping with our findings.

Our study found a protective effect with antiplatelet therapy. The benefit of ASA to reduce postoperative stroke or death was shown in the North American Symptomatic Carotid Endarterectomy Trial [91], as well as a small randomized trial showed that stroke rates were reduced with lower dose perioperative ASA (81 mg/day) versus placebo [95]. Moreover, the ASA and Carotid Endarterectomy (ACE) trial [96] further emphasized the benefit of low-dose ASA. Finally, Kresowik et al. noted a significant reduction in stroke or death with the use of preoperative antiplatelet therapy in review of over 10,000 Medicare beneficiaries undergoing CEA between 1995 and 1996 [76]. Other antiplatelet agents have not been as extensively studied in terms of their benefit for stroke reduction after CEA, but recent studies of clopidogrel provide evidence that perioperative embolization is reduced [97, 98]. Given this evidence, one might assume that nearly all patients undergoing carotid revascularization are on antiplatelet medication. However, a recent study from The Netherlands indicated that only 66% of patients undergoing CEA were on preoperative antiplatelet agents, showing the opportunity for improvement using this simple process [77]. Even within our region, prior to starting our quality improvement efforts, only 73% of patients undergoing CEA were on antiplatelet agents. However, this percentage has increased to over 93% after dedicated efforts to improve this process measure across our participating centers [51]. We feel that our regional efforts in quality improvement have helped in this process, a technique that has been successfully used to improve processes of care by cardiac surgeons in our region [99].

We found it interesting that our study found no influence of surgeon or hospital volume on outcome; this is likely a type II error, given prior publications in this area [86–88]. Most studies that found a surgeon volume effect for CEA outcome required hundreds of surgeons and tens of thousands of patients to find a relatively small effect [86, 87], while we studied a relatively small number of surgeons performing approximately 3,000 CEAs. And finally, we found our stroke rates to be relatively low in our analysis, and we found little measurable benefit in statin therapy [100–102]. These findings may reflect a type II error, and future work will investigate these endpoints as our sample size increases.

In conclusion, we identified factors associated with 30-day stroke or death following CEA using our regional prospective database. Surgeons can easily preoperatively "risk-stratify" patients by considering these easily available variables (emergent nature of procedure, contralateral ICA occlusion, preoperative ipsilateral cortical stroke, congestive heart failure, and age). From a quality improvement perspective, risk adjustment models like this allow valuable benchmarking among different centers and help regional collaboratives improve practice.

5. Summary

As we have demonstrated in these three examples, improving patient selection for high-risk vascular surgery involves a complex interaction between patient-level variables, procedure-related covariates, and insight the patient's underlying short- and long-term risk of adverse outcomes, all within the context of their life expectancy. As technology improves, analytic techniques evolve and our understanding of detailed regional and national datasets expands, we hope to eventually arrive at a time and place in vascular surgery where surgeons will know, *before* an intervention is performed, if their choice to perform surgery is the right one. And while a "crystal ball" that is able to predict surgical outcomes may seem like a far-fetched idea, it may not be as far off as you think.

Acknowledgment

This paper incorporates, with permission, excerpts, tables, andfigures from three previously published manuscripts.

References

[1] A. T. Hirsch, Z. J. Haskal, N. R. Hertzer et al., "ACC/AHA 2005 Practice Guidelines for the management of patients with peripheral arterial disease (lower extremity, renal, mesenteric, and abdominal aortic): a collaborative report from the American Association for Vascular Surgery/Society for Vascular Surgery, Society for Cardiovascular Angiography and Interventions, Society for Vascular Medicine and Biology, Society of Interventional Radiology, and the acc/aha task force on practice guidelines (writing committee to develop guidelines for the management of patients with peripheral arterial disease): endorsed by the american association of cardiovascular and pulmonary rehabilitation; national heart, lung, and blood institute; society for vascular nursing; transatlantic inter-society consensus; and vascular disease foundation," *Circulation*, vol. 113, no. 11, pp. e463–e654, 2006.

[2] S. D. Killeen, E. J. Andrews, H. P. Redmond, and G. J. Fulton, "Provider volume and outcomes for abdominal aortic aneurysm repair, carotid endarterectomy, and lower extremity revascularization procedures," *Journal of Vascular Surgery*, vol. 45, no. 3, pp. 615–626, 2007.

[3] J. H. Ix and M. H. Criqui, "Epidemiology and diagnosis of peripheral arterial disease in patients with chronic kidney disease," *Advances in Chronic Kidney Disease*, vol. 15, no. 4, pp. 378–383, 2008.

[4] R. A. Hanel, A. R. Xavier, J. F. Kirmani, A. M. Yahia, and A. I. Qureshi, "Management of carotid artery stenosis: comparing endarterectomy and stenting," *Current Cardiology Reports*, vol. 5, no. 2, pp. 153–159, 2003.

[5] C. Mihalopoulos, D. A. Cadilhac, M. L. Moodie et al., "Development and application of Model of Resource Utilization, Costs, and Outcomes for Stroke (MORUCOS): an Australian economic model for stroke," *International Journal of Technology Assessment in Health Care*, vol. 21, no. 4, pp. 499–505, 2005.

[6] E. H. Morreim, "Managed care, ethics, and academic health centers: maximizing potential, minimizing drawbacks," *Academic Medicine*, vol. 72, no. 5, pp. 332–340, 1997.

[7] A. Berni, A. Giuliani, F. Tartaglia et al., "Effect of vascular risk factors on increase in carotid and femoral intima-media thickness. Identification of a risk scale," *Atherosclerosis*, vol. 216, no. 1, pp. 109–114, 2011.

[8] M. S. Conte, "Understanding objective performance goals for critical limb ischemia trials," *Seminars in Vascular Surgery*, vol. 23, no. 3, pp. 129–137, 2010.

[9] J. B. Dimick, S. L. Chen, P. A. Taheri, W. G. Henderson, S. F. Khuri, and D. A. Campbell Jr., "Hospital costs associated with surgical complications: a report from the private-sector National Surgical Quality Improvement Program," *Journal of the American College of Surgeons*, vol. 199, no. 4, pp. 531–537, 2004.

[10] J. B. Dimick, W. B. Weeks, R. J. Karia, S. Das, and D. A. Campbell Jr., "Who pays for poor surgical quality? Building a business case for quality improvement," *Journal of the American College of Surgeons*, vol. 202, no. 6, pp. 933–937, 2006.

[11] J. S. Matsumura, R. P. Cambria, M. D. Dake, R. D. Moore, L. G. Svensson, and S. Snyder, "International controlled clinical trial of thoracic endovascular aneurysm repair with the Zenith TX2 endovascular graft: 1-year results," *Journal of Vascular Surgery*, vol. 47, no. 2, pp. 247–257, 2008.

[12] A. Schanzer, N. Hevelone, C. D. Owens, J. A. Beckman, M. Belkin, and M. S. Conte, "Statins are independently associated with reduced mortality in patients undergoing infrainguinal bypass graft surgery for critical limb ischemia," *Journal of Vascular Surgery*, vol. 47, no. 4, pp. 774–781, 2008.

[13] P. P. Goodney and R. J. Powell, "Carotid artery stenting: What have we learned from the clinical trials and registries and where do we go from here?" *Annals of Vascular Surgery*, vol. 22, no. 1, pp. 148–158, 2008.

[14] P. P. Goodney, M. L. Schermerhorn, and R. J. Powell, "Current status of carotid artery stenting," *Journal of Vascular Surgery*, vol. 43, no. 2, pp. 406–411, 2006.

[15] S. R. G. Finlayson, J. D. Birkmeyer, M. F. Fillinger, and J. L. Cronenwett, "Should endovascular surgery lower the threshold for repair of abdominal aortic aneurysms?" *Journal of Vascular Surgery*, vol. 29, no. 6, pp. 973–985, 1999.

[16] M. R. Harrigan, J. U. Howington, R. A. Hanel, L. R. Guterman, and L. N. Hopkins, "Patient selection for revascularization in cervical carotid artery disease: angioplasty and stenting versus endarterectomy," *The American Heart Hospital Journal*, vol. 2, no. 1, pp. 8–15, 2004.

[17] Z. Luo, J. C. Gardiner, and C. J. Bradley, "Applying propensity score methods in medical research: pitfalls and prospects," *Medical Care Research and Review*, vol. 67, no. 5, pp. 528–554, 2010.

[18] P. M. Rothwell and C. P. Warlow, "Prediction of benefit from carotid endarterectomy in individual patients: a risk-modelling study," *The Lancet*, vol. 353, no. 9170, pp. 2105–2110, 1999.

[19] P. P. Goodney, L. Travis, F. L. Lucas et al., "Survival after open versus endovascular thoracic aortic aneurysm repair in an observational study of the medicare population," *Circulation*, vol. 124, no. 24, pp. 2661–2669, 2011.

[20] P. P. Goodney, B. W. Nolan, A. Schanzer et al., "Factors associated with amputation or graft occlusion one year after lower extremity bypass in northern New England," *Annals of Vascular Surgery*, vol. 24, no. 1, pp. 57–68, 2010.

[21] P. P. Goodney, D. S. Likosky, and J. L. Cronenwett, "Factors associated with stroke or death after carotid endarterectomy in Northern New England," *Journal of Vascular Surgery*, vol. 48, no. 5, pp. 1139–1145, 2008.

[22] J. S. Coselli, "Thoracoabdominal aortic aneurysms: experience with 372 patients," *Journal of Cardiac Surgery*, vol. 9, no. 6, pp. 638–647, 1994.

[23] M. F. Conrad, R. S. Crawford, J. K. Davison, and R. P. Cambria, "Thoracoabdominal aneurysm repair: a 20-year perspective," *Annals of Thoracic Surgery*, vol. 83, no. 2, pp. S856–S861, 2007.

[24] E. S. Crawford, K. R. Hess, E. S. Cohen, J. S. Coselli, and H. J. Safi, "Ruptured aneurysm of the descending thoracic and thoracoabdominal aorta: analysis according to size and treatment," *Annals of Surgery*, vol. 213, no. 5, pp. 417–426, 1991.

[25] E. S. Crawford, L. G. Svensson, J. S. Coseli, H. J. Safi, and H. R. Hess, "Surgical treatment of aneurysm and/or dissection of the ascending aorta, transverse aortic arch, and ascending aorta and transverse aortic arch. Factors influencing survival in 717 patients," *Journal of Thoracic and Cardiovascular Surgery*, vol. 98, no. 5, pp. 659–674, 1989.

[26] J. A. Cowan Jr., J. B. Dimick, P. K. Henke, T. S. Huber, J. C. Stanley, and G. R. Upchurch Jr., "Surgical treatment of intact thoracoabdominal aortic aneurysms in the United States: hospital and surgeon volume-related outcomes," *Journal of Vascular Surgery*, vol. 37, no. 6, pp. 1169–1174, 2003.

[27] J. A. Cowan Jr., J. B. Dimick, R. M. Wainess, P. K. Henke, J. C. Stanley, and G. R. Upchurch Jr., "Ruptured thoracoabdominal aortic aneurysm treatment in the United States: 1988 to 1998," *Journal of Vascular Surgery*, vol. 38, no. 2, pp. 319–322, 2003.

[28] M. F. Conrad, E. A. Ergul, V. I. Patel, V. Paruchuri, C. J. Kwolek, and R. P. Cambria, "Management of diseases of the descending thoracic aorta in the endovascular era: a medicare population study," *Annals of Surgery*, vol. 252, no. 4, pp. 603–609, 2010.

[29] Current procedural technology manual, 2010.

[30] L. I. Iezzoni, *Risk Adjustment for Measuring Health Care Outcomes*, Health Administration Press, Ann Arbor, Mich, USA, 1994.

[31] S. M. Kieszak, W. D. Flanders, A. S. Kosinski, C. C. Shipp, and H. Karp, "A comparison of the Charlson Comorbidity Index derived from medical record data and administrative billing data," *Journal of Clinical Epidemiology*, vol. 52, no. 2, pp. 137–142, 1999.

[32] S. T. Scali, R. J. Feezor, C. K. Chang, and D. H. Stone, "Safety of elective management of synchronous aortic disease with simultaneous thoracic and aortic stent graft placement," *Journal of Vascular Surgery*, vol. 56, no. 4, pp. 957.e1–964.e1, 2012.

[33] S. J. Pocock, T. C. Clayton, and D. G. Altman, "Survival plots of time-to-event outcomes in clinical trials: good practice and pitfalls," *The Lancet*, vol. 359, no. 9318, pp. 1686–1689, 2002.

[34] P. R. Rosenbaum and D. B. Rubin, "The central role of the propensity score in observational studies for causal effects," *Biometrika*, vol. 70, no. 1, pp. 41–55, 1983.

[35] M. L. Schermerhorn, S. R. G. Finlayson, M. F. Fillinger et al., "Life expectancy after endovascular versus open abdominal aortic aneurysm repair: results of a decision analysis model on the basis of data from EUROSTAR," *Journal of Vascular Surgery*, vol. 36, no. 6, pp. 1112–1120, 2002.

[36] M. L. Schermerhorn, A. J. O'Malley, A. Jhaveri, P. Cotterill, F. Pomposelli, and B. E. Landon, "Endovascular versus open repair of abdominal aortic aneurysms in the medicare population," *New England Journal of Medicine*, vol. 358, no. 5, pp. 464–474, 2008.

[37] R. M. Greenhalgh, L. C. Brown, G. P. Kwong, J. T. Powell, and S. G. Thompson, "Comparison of endovascular aneurysm repair with open repair in patients with abdominal aortic aneurysm (evar trial 1), 30-day operative mortality results: randomised controlled trial," *The Lancet*, vol. 364, no. 9437, pp. 843–848, 2004.

[38] R. M. Greenhalgh, D. J. Allison, P. R. F. Bell et al., "Endovascular repair of aortic aneurysm in patients physically ineligible for open repair," *New England Journal of Medicine*, vol. 362, no. 20, pp. 1872–1880, 2010.

[39] J. D. Blankensteijn, S. E. C. A. de Jong, M. Prinssen et al., "Two-year outcomes after conventional or endovascular repair of abdominal aortic aneurysms," *New England Journal of Medicine*, vol. 352, no. 23, pp. 2398–2405, 2005.

[40] P. P. Goodney, D. Tavris, F. L. Lucas, T. Gross, E. S. Fisher, and S. R. G. Finlayson, "Causes of late mortality after endovascular and open surgical repair of infrarenal abdominal aortic aneurysms," *Journal of Vascular Surgery*, vol. 51, no. 6, pp. 1340–1347, 2010.

[41] "Endovascular aneurysm repair and outcome in patients unfit for open repair of abdominal aortic aneurysm (EVAR trial 2): randomised controlled trial," *The Lancet*, vol. 365, no. 9478, pp. 2187–2192, 2005.

[42] R. M. Fairman, F. Criado, M. Farber et al., "Pivotal results of the medtronic vascular talent thoracic stent graft system: the VALOR trial," *Journal of Vascular Surgery*, vol. 48, no. 3, pp. 546–554, 2008.

[43] M. S. Makaroun, E. D. Dillavou, G. H. Wheatley, and R. P. Cambria, "Five-year results of endovascular treatment with the Gore TAG device compared with open repair of thoracic aortic aneurysms," *Journal of Vascular Surgery*, vol. 47, no. 5, pp. 912–918, 2008.

[44] J. S. Cho, S. E. A. Haider, and M. S. Makaroun, "Endovascular therapy of thoracic aneurysms: gore TAG trial results," *Seminars in Vascular Surgery*, vol. 19, no. 1, pp. 18–24, 2006.

[45] M. M. McDermott, "The magnitude of the problem of peripheral arterial disease: epidemiology and clinical significance," *Cleveland Clinic Journal of Medicine*, vol. 73, supplement 4, pp. S2–S7, 2006.

[46] A. B. Newman, L. Shemanski, T. A. Manolio et al., "Ankle-arm index as a predictor of cardiovascular disease and mortality in the Cardiovascular Health Study," *Arteriosclerosis, Thrombosis, and Vascular Biology*, vol. 19, no. 3, pp. 538–545, 1999.

[47] R. Nowygrod, N. Egorova, G. Greco et al., "Trends, complications, and mortality in peripheral vascular surgery," *Journal of Vascular Surgery*, vol. 43, no. 2, pp. 205–216, 2006.

[48] B. Sigvant, K. Wiberg-Hedman, D. Bergqvist et al., "A population-based study of peripheral arterial disease prevalence with special focus on critical limb ischemia and sex differences," *Journal of Vascular Surgery*, vol. 45, no. 6, pp. 1185–1191, 2007.

[49] L. Norgren, W. R. Hiatt, J. A. Dormandy et al., "Inter-society consensus for the management of peripheral arterial disease (TASC II)," *Journal of Vascular Surgery*, vol. 45, no. 1, pp. S5–S67, 2007.

[50] D. J. Adam, J. D. Beard, T. Cleveland et al., "Bypass versus angioplasty in severe ischaemia of the leg (BASIL): multicentre, randomised controlled trial," *The Lancet*, vol. 366, no. 9501, pp. 1925–1934, 2005.

[51] J. L. Cronenwett, D. S. Likosky, M. T. Russell, J. Eldrup-Jorgensen, A. C. Stanley, and B. W. Nolan, "A regional registry for quality assurance and improvement: the Vascular Study Group of Northern New England (VSGNNE)," *Journal of Vascular Surgery*, vol. 46, no. 6, pp. 1093–1102, 2007.

[52] F. Biancari, A. Albäck, L. Ihlberg, I. Kantonen, M. Luther, and M. Lepäntalo, "Angiographic runoff score as a predictor of outcome following femorocrural bypass surgery," *European Journal of Vascular and Endovascular Surgery*, vol. 17, no. 6, pp. 480–485, 1999.

[53] P. J. Rossi, C. L. Skelly, S. L. Meyerson et al., "Redo infrainguinal bypass: factors predicting patency and limb salvage," *Annals of Vascular Surgery*, vol. 17, no. 5, pp. 492–502, 2003.

[54] A. Schanzer, J. Mega, J. Meadows, R. H. Samson, D. F. Bandyk, and M. S. Conte, "Risk stratification in critical limb ischemia: derivation and validation of a model to predict amputation-free survival using multicenter surgical outcomes data," *Journal of Vascular Surgery*, vol. 48, no. 6, pp. 1464–1471, 2008.

[55] B. Toursarkissian, M. D'Ayala, D. Stefanidis et al., "Angiographic scoring of vascular occlusive disease in the diabetic foot: relevance to bypass graft patency and limb salvage," *Journal of Vascular Surgery*, vol. 35, no. 3, pp. 494–500, 2002.

[56] *Dartmouth Atlas Cardiovascular and Thoracic Health Care*, Manning Selvage & Lee, 1998.

[57] M. S. Conte, D. F. Bandyk, A. W. Clowes, G. L. Moneta, H. Namini, and L. Seely, "Risk factors, medical therapies and perioperative events in limb salvage surgery: observations from the PREVENT III multicenter trial," *Journal of Vascular Surgery*, vol. 42, no. 3, pp. 456–464, 2005.

[58] M. S. Conte, D. F. Bandyk, A. W. Clowes et al., "Results of PREVENT III: a multicenter, randomized trial of edifoligide for the prevention of vein graft failure in lower extremity bypass surgery," *Journal of Vascular Surgery*, vol. 43, no. 4, pp. 742–751, 2006.

[59] F. L. Lucas, T. A. Stukel, A. M. Morris, A. E. Siewers, and J. D. Birkmeyer, "Race and surgical mortality in the United States," *Annals of Surgery*, vol. 243, no. 2, pp. 281–286, 2006.

[60] A. T. Hirsch, "Treatment of peripheral arterial disease—extending "intervention" to 'therapeutic choice,'" *New England Journal of Medicine*, vol. 354, no. 18, pp. 1944–1947, 2006.

[61] B. W. Nolan, S. Finlayson, A. Tosteson, R. J. Powell, and J. L. Cronenwett, "The treatment of disabling intermittent claudication in patients with superficial femoral artery occlusive disease-Decision analysis," *Journal of Vascular Surgery*, vol. 45, no. 6, pp. 1179–1184, 2007.

[62] W. C. Nugent, "Clinical applications of risk-assessment protocols in the management of individual patients," *Annals of Thoracic Surgery*, vol. 64, pp. S68–S72, 1997.

[63] G. T. O'Connor, J. D. Birkmeyer, L. J. Dacey et al., "Results of a regional study of modes of death associated with coronary artery bypass grafting," *Annals of Thoracic Surgery*, vol. 66, no. 4, pp. 1323–1328, 1998.

[64] W. L. Holman, M. Sansom, C. I. Kiefe et al., "Alabama coronary artery bypass grafting project: results from phase II of a statewide quality improvement Initiative," *Annals of Surgery*, vol. 239, no. 1, pp. 99–109, 2004.

[65] I. A. Scott, "Optimising care of acute myocardial infarction: results of a regional quality improvement project," *Journal of Quality in Clinical Practice*, vol. 20, no. 1, pp. 12–19, 2000.

[66] G. T. O'Connor, H. B. Quinton, R. Kahn et al., "Case-mix adjustment for evaluation of mortality in cystic fibrosis," *Pediatric Pulmonology*, vol. 33, no. 2, pp. 99–105, 2002.

[67] M. A. O'Grady, E. Gitelson, R. F. Swaby et al., "Development and implementation of a medical oncology quality improvement tool for a regional community oncology network: the Fox Chase Cancer Center partners initiative," *Journal of the National Comprehensive Cancer Network*, vol. 5, no. 9, pp. 875–882, 2007.

[68] H. J. M. Barnett, R. W. Gunton, M. Eliasziw et al., "Causes and severity of ischemic stroke in patients with internal carotid artery stenosis," *Journal of the American Medical Association*, vol. 283, no. 11, pp. 1429–1436, 2000.

[69] P. B. Gorelick, R. L. Sacco, D. B. Smith et al., "Prevention of a first stroke: a review of guidelines and a multidisciplinary consensus statement from the National Stroke Association," *Journal of the American Medical Association*, vol. 281, no. 12, pp. 1112–1120, 1999.

[70] P. M. Rothwell, "Risk modeling to identify patients with symptomatic carotid stenosis most at risk of stroke," *Neurological Research*, vol. 27, supplement 1, pp. S18–S28, 2005.

[71] P. M. Rothwell, J. Slattery, and C. P. Warlow, "A systematic review of the risks of stroke and death due to endarterectomy for symptomatic carotid stenosis," *Stroke*, vol. 27, no. 2, pp. 260–265, 1996.

[72] J. V. Tu, H. Wang, B. Bowyer, L. Green, J. Fang, and D. Kucey, "Risk factors for death or stroke after carotid endarterectomy: observations from the ontario carotid endarterectomy registry," *Stroke*, vol. 34, no. 11, pp. 2568–2573, 2003.

[73] P. A. Wolf, W. B. Kannel, P. Sorlie, and P. McNamara, "Asymptomatic carotid bruit and risk of stroke. The Framingham study," *Journal of the American Medical Association*, vol. 245, no. 14, pp. 1442–1445, 1981.

[74] D. J. Musser, G. G. Nicholas, and J. F. Reed, "Death and adverse cardiac events after carotid endarterectomy," *Journal of Vascular Surgery*, vol. 19, no. 4, pp. 615–622, 1994.

[75] S. K. Kakkos, A. N. Nicolaides, M. Griffin et al., "Factors associated with mortality in patients with asymptomatic carotid stenosis: results from the ACSRS study," *International Angiology*, vol. 24, no. 3, pp. 221–230, 2005.

[76] T. F. Kresowik, D. Bratzler, H. R. Karp et al., "Multistate utilization, processes, and outcomes of carotid endarterectomy," *Journal of Vascular Surgery*, vol. 33, no. 2, pp. 227–235, 2001.

[77] A. Assadian, U. Eidher, C. Senekowitsch et al., "Antiplatelet therapy prior to carotid endarterectomy—still room for improvement," *Vasa*, vol. 35, no. 2, pp. 96–100, 2006.

[78] D. L. Bhatt, S. R. Kapadia, C. T. Bajzer et al., "Dual antiplatelet therapy with clopidogrel and aspirin after carotid artery stenting," *Journal of Invasive Cardiology*, vol. 13, no. 12, pp. 767–771, 2001.

[79] E. A. Halm, C. Lee, and M. R. Chassin, "Is volume related to outcome in health care? A systematic review and methodologic critique of the literature," *Annals of Internal Medicine*, vol. 137, no. 6, pp. 511–520, 2002.

[80] M. Pine, H. S. Jordan, A. Elixhauser et al., "Enhancement of claims data to improve risk adjustment of hospital mortality," *Journal of the American Medical Association*, vol. 297, no. 1, pp. 71–76, 2007.

[81] D. Teres and T. L. Higgins, "What if your hospital informatics department could provide a severity adjuster?" *Critical Care Medicine*, vol. 28, no. 10, pp. 3570–3571, 2000.

[82] M. B. El-Tamer, B. M. Ward, T. Schifftner, L. Neumayer, S. Khuri, and W. Henderson, "Morbidity and mortality following breast cancer surgery in women: national benchmarks for standards of care," *Annals of Surgery*, vol. 245, no. 5, pp. 665–671, 2007.

[83] E. P. Brass and W. R. Hiatt, "Review of mortality and cardiovascular event rates in patients enrolled in clinical trials for claudication therapies," *Vascular Medicine*, vol. 11, no. 3, pp. 141–145, 2006.

[84] R. K. H. Wyse and K. M. Taylor, "Using the STS and multinational cardiac surgical databases to establish risk-adjusted benchmarks for clinical outcomes," *Heart Surgery Forum*, vol. 5, no. 3, pp. 258–264, 2002.

[85] E. D. Peterson, E. R. DeLong, L. H. Muhlbaier et al., "Challenges in comparing risk-adjusted bypass surgery mortality results: results from the Cooperative Cardiovascular Project," *Journal of the American College of Cardiology*, vol. 36, no. 7, pp. 2174–2184, 2000.

[86] J. D. Birkmeyer, T. A. Stukel, A. E. Siewers, P. P. Goodney, D. E. Wennberg, and F. L. Lucas, "Surgeon volume and operative mortality in the United States," *New England Journal of Medicine*, vol. 349, no. 22, pp. 2117–2127, 2003.

[87] J. A. Cowan Jr., J. B. Dimick, B. G. Thompson, J. C. Stanley, and G. R. Upchurch, "Surgeon volume as an indicator of outcomes after carotid endarterectomy: an effect independent of specialty practice and hospital volume," *Journal of the American College of Surgeons*, vol. 195, no. 6, pp. 814–821, 2002.

[88] P. J. E. Holt, J. D. Poloniecki, I. M. Loftus, and M. M. Thompson, "Meta-analysis and systematic review of the relationship between hospital volume and outcome following carotid endarterectomy," *European Journal of Vascular and Endovascular Surgery*, vol. 33, no. 6, pp. 645–651, 2007.

[89] J. F. Toole, "Endarterectomy for asymptomatic carotid artery stenosis," *Journal of the American Medical Association*, vol. 273, no. 18, pp. 1421–1428, 1995.

[90] E. Ballotta, L. Renon, G. da Giau, B. Barbon, O. Terranova, and C. Baracchini, "Octogenarians with contralateral carotid artery occlusion: a cohort at higher risk for carotid endarterectomy?" *Journal of Vascular Surgery*, vol. 39, no. 5, pp. 1003–1008, 2004.

[91] K. D. Calligaro, "Impact of clinical pathways on hospital costs and early outcome after major vascular surgery," *Journal of Vascular Surgery*, vol. 22, no. 6, pp. 649–660, 1995.

[92] C. Warlow, B. Farrell, A. Fraser, P. Sandercock, and J. Slattery, "Randomised trial of endarterectomy for recently symptomatic carotid stenosis: final results of the MRC European Carotid Surgery Trial (ECST)," *The Lancet*, vol. 351, no. 9113, pp. 1379–1387, 1998.

[93] M. Eliasziw, J. Y. Streifler, J. D. Spence, A. J. Fox, V. C. Hachinski, and H. J. M. Barnett, "Prognosis for patients following a transient ischemic attack with and without a cerebral infarction on brain CT," *Neurology*, vol. 45, no. 3 I, pp. 428–431, 1995.

[94] A. F. Bhatti, L. R. Leon, N. Labropoulos et al., "Free-floating thrombus of the carotid artery: literature review and case reports," *Journal of Vascular Surgery*, vol. 45, no. 1, pp. 199–205, 2007.

[95] B. Lindblad, N. H. Persson, R. Takolander, and D. Bergqvist, "Does low-dose acetylsalicylic acid prevent stroke after carotid surgery? A double-blind, placebo-controlled randomized trial," *Stroke*, vol. 24, no. 8, pp. 1125–1128, 1993.

[96] D. W. Taylor, H. J. M. Barnett, R. B. Haynes et al., "Low-dose and high-dose acetylsalicylic acid for patients undergoing carotid endarterectomy: a randomised controlled trial," *The Lancet*, vol. 353, no. 9171, pp. 2179–2184, 1999.

[97] D. A. Payne, C. I. Jones, P. D. Hayes, A. R. Naylor, and A. H. Goodall, "Therapeutic benefit of low-dose clopidogrel in patients undergoing carotid surgery is linked to variability in the platelet adenosine diphosphate response and patients' weight," *Stroke*, vol. 38, no. 9, pp. 2464–2469, 2007.

[98] D. A. Payne, C. I. Jones, P. D. Hayes et al., "Beneficial effects of clopidogrel combined with aspirin in reducing cerebral emboli in patients undergoing carotid endarterectomy," *Circulation*, vol. 109, no. 12, pp. 1476–1481, 2004.

[99] D. J. Malenka and G. T. O'Connor, "The northern new England cardiovascular disease study group: a regional collaborative effort for continuous quality improvement in cardiovascular disease," *The Joint Commission Journal on Quality Improvement*, vol. 24, no. 10, pp. 594–600, 1998.

[100] B. A. Perler, "The effect of statin medications on perioperative and long-term outcomes following carotid endarterectomy or stenting," *Seminars in Vascular Surgery*, vol. 20, no. 4, pp. 252–258, 2007.

[101] M. J. McGirt, B. A. Perler, B. S. Brooke et al., "3-Hydroxy-3-methylglutaryl coenzyme A reductase inhibitors reduce the risk of perioperative stroke and mortality after carotid endarterectomy," *Journal of Vascular Surgery*, vol. 42, no. 5, pp. 829–836, 2005.

[102] J. Kennedy, H. Quan, A. M. Buchan, W. A. Ghali, and T. E. Feasby, "Statins are associated with better outcomes after carotid endarterectomy in symptomatic patients," *Stroke*, vol. 36, no. 10, pp. 2072–2076, 2005.

8

Homeostatic Imbalance in Epithelial Ducts and Its Role in Carcinogenesis

Katarzyna A. Rejniak[1,2]

[1] *Depatment of Integrated Mathematical Oncology, H. Lee Moffitt Cancer Center and Research Institute, 12902 Magnolia Drive, Room SRB-4 24000G, Tampa, FL 33612, USA*
[2] *Department of Oncologic Sciences, College of Medicine, University of South Florida, Tampa, FL 33612, USA*

Correspondence should be addressed to Katarzyna A. Rejniak; kasia.rejniak@moffitt.org

Academic Editors: P. Bates and M. Mottolese

An epithelial duct is a well-defined multicellular structure composed of tightly packed cells separating and protecting body compartments that are used for enzyme secretion and its transport across the internal. The structural and functional integrity (homeostasis) of such ducts is vital in carrying many life functions (breathing, lactation, production of hormones). However, the processes involved in maintaining the homeostatic balance are not yet fully understood. On the other hand, the loss of epithelial tissue architecture, such as filled lumens or ductal disorganization, are among the first symptoms of the emerging epithelial tumors (carcinomas). Using the previously developed biomechanical model of epithelial ducts: *IBCell*, we investigated how different signals and mechanical stimuli imposed on individual epithelial cells can impact the homeostatic (im)balance and integrity of the whole epithelial tissue. We provide a link between erroneous responses of individual epithelial cells to specific signals and the emerging ductal morphologies characteristic for preinvasive cancers observed in pathology specimens, or characteristic for multicellular structures arising from mutated cells cultured *in vitro*. We summarize our finding in terms of altered properties of epithelial cell polarization, and discuss the relative importance of various polarization signals on the formation of tumor-like multicellular structures.

1. Introduction

Epithelia are one of the most abundant tissues in the human body and cover all cavities and surfaces of many organs, including the bronchi and alveoli of the lungs, breast ducts and lobules, gastrointestinal crypts, reproductive urinary tracts, and the endocrine glands. In their mature form, the simple epithelia (in contrast to stratified, multilayered tissues) are organized into monolayer sheets of tightly packed polarized cells that enclose lumens (either empty or filled with milk, semen, or air) to prevent leakage of molecules from one side of the epithelia to the other. The overall structure and properties of these well-organized multicellular systems emerge from physical interactions and chemical signals shared locally between individual neighboring cells. However, the processes involved in keeping the epithelial tissue integrity over the span of human lifetime are not yet fully understood.

On one hand, certain control mechanisms are required that ensure tissue stabilization (e.g., via cell differentiation). On the other hand, some degree of adaptability to a range of conditions (e.g., stress or damage) is needed. All critical decisions regulating epithelial tissue integrity, such as initiation of cell growth, selection of the axis of cell division, or the induction of cell death, may be influenced by actions of neighboring cells and interactions between the cells and their dynamically evolving microenvironment. This includes diverse set of forces, such as compressive, tensile, or hydrostatic pressures, each of which plays a part in shaping the tissue [1–3]. The way in which cells respond to forces is dictated by their physical properties. In fact, cells are both elastic and viscous, meaning that they deform in a time-dependent manner upon applied forces and can return towards their initial form following removal of the stresses. Cells can also exert forces on their neighbors. Epithelial cells develop specialized cell-cell connections, such as adherens junctions, that mechanically attach cells to one another. Similarly, cell surface receptors, such as integrins, transmit forces from the external environment. Additionally, cells develop gap junctions that mediate the passage of chemical and electrical signals between neighboring cells and provide a mechanism for coordinating the activities of individual cells in the tissue. Thus, mechanical signals sensed by the cell result in activation of intracellular biochemical signaling pathways (the process called mechanotransduction), that in turn regulate cell behavior [4, 5].

This complex interplay allows for the emergence of more robust multicellular systems that can tolerate both external and internal perturbations [6]. Normal epithelial cells can adapt to certain perturbations in biochemical, genetic, and physical cues sensed from their immediate microenvironment. However, there are limitations to this plasticity, and when cell responses are compromised, they may induce a malignant behavior, such as filling the hollow ductal lumen with mutated cells and breaking through the basement membrane, that results in loss of tissue homeostasis. For example, early preinvasive forms of epithelial cancers, such as breast ductal carcinoma *in situ* (DCIS) or prostatic intraepithelial neoplasia (PIN), are both characterized by filled ductal lumens and ductal epithelium disorganization. Thus, the disruption of normal epithelial tissue architecture is one of the initial symptoms of progression to epithelial tumors [7]. It has been shown that changes in extracellular matrix structure, its stiffness, and mechanics can promote or suppress formation of malignant multicellular spheroids in 3D cell cultures [8, 9]. The physical forces and differences in cellular mechanics provide essential cues driving cell differentiation, growth, or death. In these cases, biomechanics underlies the abilities of the cell as well as the tissue to carry out normal function in health or to malfunction in disease. From this perspective, the emergence of preinvasive cancers can be viewed as tissue homeostatic imbalance in which the natural symbiosis between cellular and microenvironmental components is perturbed.

We previously developed a biomechanical computational model of deformable cells, *IBCell* (the Immersed Boundary model of a Cell, see appendix), that was used to test various cell-cell and cell-microenvironment interactions in the self-organizing polarized cysts. Here, we extend this mathematical framework to include alterations in mechanical stimuli responsible for cell epithelial polarization to investigate how this pressure imbalance impacts the overall tissue integrity.

2. Results

Tissue homeostatic balance emerges from the integration of multiple subcellular, intercellular, extracellular, chemical, and physical signals and constraints. Understanding how this normal form and function of the tissues is maintained is vital for recognizing which elements play the key roles during transition from normal epithelia to preinvasive tumors. We previously developed a biomechanical model, *IBCell*, of the formation of normal epithelial acini (the 3D *in vitro* cultures resembling hollow epithelial cysts) and discussed both the necessary and sufficient conditions for their self-organization [10, 11]. In this approach, each epithelial cell is modeled as a deformable body with the fluid-like cytoplasm and an elastic membrane, equipped with a set of discrete receptors/sensors distributed along the cell boundary. Five types of receptors are considered here: growth, death, apical, lateral, and basal (see Figure 1), and, based on the configuration of its receptors, the cell undergoes one of several possible life processes: growth, division, apoptotic death, or epithelial polarization. For instance, the cell requires that a certain number of growth or death receptors to be active in order to initiate the process of growth or death, respectively. The *IBCell* receptors are meant to resemble the biological role of cell membrane receptors; however, some simplifications need to be introduced in the computational model. The biological receptors are highly dynamic and can be relocated or created in response to extracellular signals. The *IBCell* receptors are immobile, but their role can be modified (activated) based on local cues. The default state of all *IBCell* receptors is *growth*, but their status will be changed to *lateral*, if two cells are close to one another and develop the cell-cell adhesion link. The receptor's role will change to *basal*, if the level of the extracellular matrix (ECM) proteins in its vicinity is high enough to provide cell-ECM adhesion. The receptor will be activated as *apical* when the epithelial cell becomes polarized and develops the apical membrane domain. Finally, the receptor's status will be changed to *death* when the cell loses its adhesive connection with polarized cells. A particular cell life process will be initiated depending on whether the number of active receptors reaches a predefined threshold.

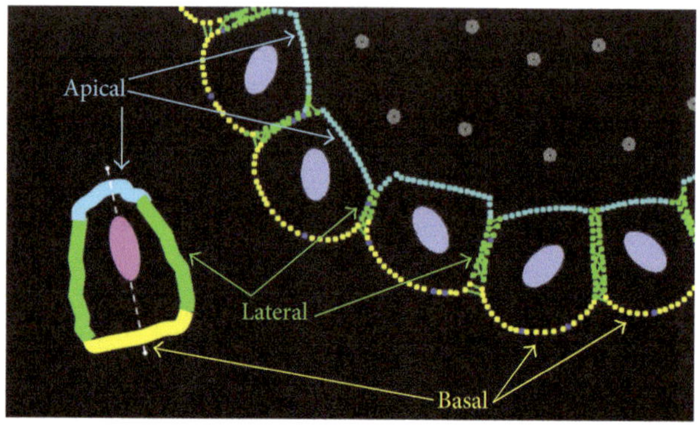

Figure 1: Schematics of the *IBCell* polarized epithelium. An epithelially polarized cell contains three membrane domains: lateral (green) in contact with other cells in the epithelium, basal (yellow) in contact with the extracellular matrix (ECM), and lateral (cyan) in contact with the lumen. These membrane domains in *IBCell* are composed of corresponding boundary points (receptors). *IBCell* contains also growth (blue) and death (grey) receptors. Colors of cell nuclei: viable cells (purple) and dying cells (red). Inset: a graphical representation of a polarized cell and its three different membrane domains.

These thresholds define cell intrinsic sensitivity to extrinsic signals.

The fundamental feature of tissue epithelial architecture a well-defined apical-basolateral polarity of all individual cells (defined as asymmetrical distribution of cell components, especially membrane proteins). The membrane of epithelial cells is composed of noncoalescent apical and basolateral domains—with the apical side facing the lumen, the lateral sides adhering to other cells, and the basal side attached to the underlying basement membrane. In *IBCell*, epithelial polarity is acquired by developing three distinct membrane compartments (Figure 1): basal, defined by cell membrane receptors contacting the external media (red); lateral, defined by cell receptors being in contact with other cells (green); apical, composed of markers facing the hollow lumen (cyan). Depending on the tissue of origin, the hollow lumen may be a result of cell death (MCF10A breast cells [12, 13]) or vacuolar exocytosis (MDCK kidney cells [14]). Cell apoptotic death is modeled in *IBCell* by placing point sinks and sources along the membrane of the whole cell to release fluid from the cell interior to the extracellular space. In contrast, cell growth is modeled by locating point sources and sinks of fluid in such a way to increase the amount of fluid inside the cell (see the appendix for more details). Critical decisions regulating epithelial tissue integrity, such as cell growth, division, or death, can be triggered by signals from the neighboring cells and from the microenvironment. We will illustrate here how changes in cellular responses to such cues sensed by the host cells via their different membrane receptors may result in the disruption of epithelial tissue morphology. Specifically, we will use *IBCell* to examine how epithelial morphologies are changing as a result of disrupted or altered cellular responses to different constrains arising from cell epithelial polarization, such as ECM, apical, lateral, and death signals controlling cell mitosis, adhesion, or death.

2.1. Development of Normal Epithelial Cysts. Polarized cells forming the epithelial tissue are of cubical or columnar shape with three well-defined membrane domains each with specific proteins and lipids. However, the relative proportions of surface areas of these membrane sides are not known, and it is not known how changes in distribution of membrane-specific proteins can influence the epithelial development and maintenance. In order to identify the ranges of apical, lateral, and basal receptors in normally formed epithelial cells, we simulated the development of several self-organized epithelial cysts. One realization of our model is shown in Figure 2. The presented developmental stages are consistent with 3D *in vitro* cultures derived from nontumorigenic epithelial cell lines, for example, breast cells MCF10A that form hollow mammospheres [15, 16], prostate cells RWPE-1 that produce one-layered acini [17], or ovarian OVCAR-5 cells growing in a cyst-like form [18]. The acinar structure is formed from a single cell that upon consecutive divisions gives rise to an aggregate of randomly oriented cells consisting of two cell populations: outer cells having contact with the external medium and inner cells surrounded entirely by other cells. Subsequently, cells in the outer layer develop an apical-basal polarity and form a monolayer of epithelial cells. This is followed by apoptotic death of inner cells, resulting in the formation of the hollow lumen and in stabilization of the epithelial structure (Figure 2(a)). All final epithelial cells have been analyzed in order to quantify the percentage of various cell membrane receptors that guarantee proper cell polarization in the model (Figure 2(b)).

On average, in our simulations of polarized epithelial ducts, each polarized cell contains about 30% of ECM receptors forming the basal membrane domain that is in contact with the external medium (such as matrigel *in vitro* or the extracellular matrix *in vivo*). Lateral domains composed of cell-cell adhesive receptors (such as cadherins or tight junctions) contain about half of all receptors and are divided between lateral sides being in contact with two adjacent cells. Most of the final epithelial cells in *IBCell* are of cuboidal shape; thus, their apical sides are composed of quite large numbers of apical markers (~25%). The active growth receptors in the final stable configurations are very rare (about 2% per cell, and many cells have no active growth receptors at all) in contrast to earlier stages when active growth receptors (blue) are dominant over other kinds of receptors. These values have been used in subsequent simulations for testing how changes in a particular signaling mechanism (from ECM, other cells, and lumen) lead to morphological alternations in epithelial structures.

2.2. Alterations in ECM Signals. During the development of epithelial tissues, the outer (basal) cells secrete various proteins, such as collagens and laminins, that accumulate in the form of a stiff supportive basement membrane (BM) surrounding the whole structure [15]. Epithelial cells are capable of attaching to the basement membrane through the special cell-ECM transmembrane receptors, such as integrins. In *IBCell*, the formation of BM is modeled by accumulating ECM proteins and changing the role of cell receptors from *growth* to *basal* (ECM) receptors (Figure 2 and the appendix). However, when the ECM receptors in the host cell are downregulated, their role is changed back to the default state: *growth*. Thus, the ratio of growth receptors increases, and the cell is able to reenter the proliferation process. Since all other signals (lateral and apical) are assumed to be unchanged, the growing cells divide in a typical epithelial fashion, that is, orthogonal to the lumen. It has been reported in [19] that normal epithelial cells acquire two different orientations of cell division: either orthogonal or parallel to the lumen. The orthogonal division along the basal-apical axis results in two luminally positioned daughter cells and leads to duct expansion. In our simulation, the elevated cell proliferation accompanied with basal-apical orientation of cell division axis results in the emergence of a new tubular duct sprout shown in Figure 3(a). This is consistent with experiments showing initiation and outgrowth of cell cohorts forming new tubule-like structures in the three-dimensional cultures of Madin-Darby canine kidney (MDCK) epithelial cells [20].

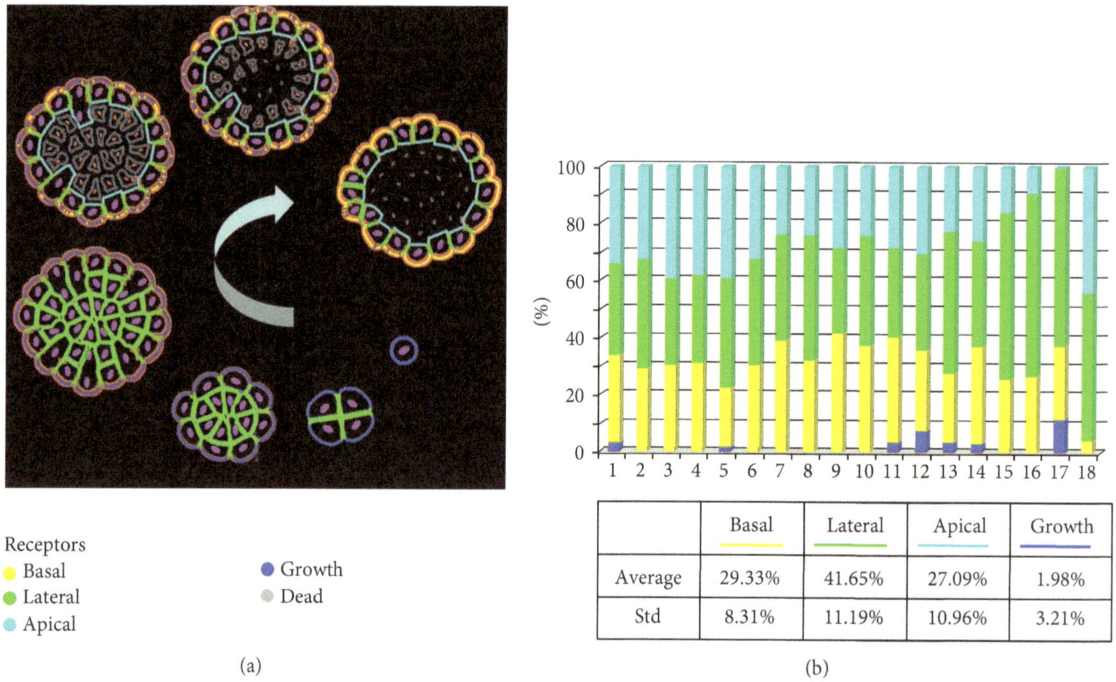

	Basal	Lateral	Apical	Growth
Average	29.33%	41.65%	27.09%	1.98%
Std	8.31%	11.19%	10.96%	3.21%

FIGURE 2: Emergence of polarized cells during normal epithelium development. (a) Sequence of consecutive stages in the development of normal epithelium from a single cell to a one layer of polarized cells enclosing the hollow lumen. (b). Distributions of membrane receptors in each polarized cell forming the final one-layered epithelial structure. Cell membrane receptors are color-coded identically in (a) and (b). The red bands surrounding the multicellular structures in (a) represent accumulation of ECM proteins.

Immersed Boundary Equations.

$$\rho\left(\frac{\partial \mathbf{u}(\mathbf{x},t)}{\partial t} + (\mathbf{u}(\mathbf{x},t)\cdot\nabla)\,\mathbf{u}(\mathbf{x},t)\right) = -\nabla p(\mathbf{x},t) + \mu\Delta\mathbf{u}(\mathbf{x},t) + \frac{\mu}{3\rho}\nabla s(\mathbf{x},t) + \mathbf{f}(\mathbf{x},t), \tag{1}$$

$$\rho\nabla\cdot\mathbf{u}(\mathbf{x},t) = s(\mathbf{x},t), \tag{2}$$

$$\mathbf{f}(\mathbf{x},t) = \int_\Gamma \mathbf{F}(l,t)\,\delta(\mathbf{x}-\mathbf{X}(l,t))\,dl \tag{3}$$

$$\mathbf{F}(l,t) = \mathscr{F}_*\frac{\|\mathbf{X}(l_*,t)-\mathbf{X}(l,t)\| - \mathscr{L}_*}{\|\mathbf{X}(l_*,t)-\mathbf{X}(l,t)\|}(\mathbf{X}(l_*,t)-\mathbf{X}(l,t)), \tag{4}$$

$$s(\mathbf{x},t) = \sum_{k\in\Xi^+} S^+(\mathbf{Y}_k,t)\,\delta(\mathbf{x},\mathbf{Y}_k) + \sum_{k\in\Xi^-} S^-(\mathbf{Z}_m,t)\,\delta(\mathbf{x},\mathbf{Z}_m), \tag{5}$$

$$\frac{\partial\mathbf{X}(l,t)}{\partial t} = \mathbf{u}(\mathbf{X}(l,t),t) = \int_\Omega \mathbf{u}(\mathbf{x},t)\,\delta(\mathbf{x}-\mathbf{X}(l,t))\,dx, \tag{6}$$

$$\frac{\partial\gamma(\mathbf{X}(l,t))}{\partial t} = \kappa_1\mathbf{X}(l,t) - \kappa_2\gamma(\mathbf{X}(l,t)). \tag{7}$$

2.3. Alterations in ECM and Apical Signals. We have previously hypothesized [21] that disruption in both cell-ECM adhesion signals and apical signals results in the loss of tissue homeostatic balance and initiation of cell hyperplastic growth, leading to both luminal filling and invasion of the surrounding tissue (Figure 3(b)). If such changes are only present locally in one epithelial cell, the remaining cells can still form a functional duct. However, if more cells are affected, the overall cluster morphology resembles more an unorganized multicellular spheroid. Similar results have been shown experimentally when the ECM stiffness was modified that resulted in alterations of ECM signaling and in the loss of cell epithelial polarity leading to growth of aberrant multicellular structures [22]. In contrast, when certain oncogenes were overexpressed in individual cells growing within the organotypic mammary acini, the mutated cells were able to initiate luminal outgrowth without disrupting the ductal structure [23].

2.4. Alterations in Apical Signals. We used *IBCell* to simulate a case when a randomly chosen single cell loses its apical markers. This resulted in an elevated ratio of growth receptors leading to reinitiation of cell proliferation process. Since all other signals (lateral and basal) were unchanged, the host cell was able to maintain its basal and lateral membrane domains. As a result, all growing cells were dividing in a typical epithelial fashion (orthogonal to the lumen), and the duct integrity was preserved. However, the elevated cellular proliferation with preserved orientation of cell division led together to bending of the duct towards the side with abnormal apical signals producing a concaved cleft (Figure 3(c)).

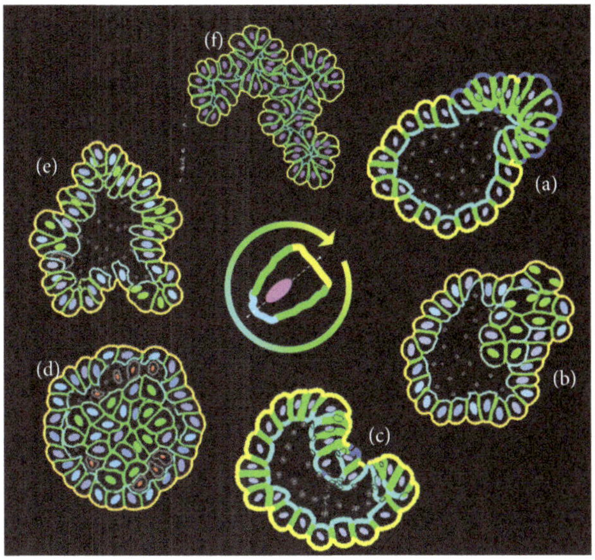

FIGURE 3: Irregular multicellular morphologies arising after disruption of certain epithelialpolarization signals. Upon dysregulation of one of more of basal, lateral, or apical signals, an individual cell may lose its ability to properly polarize that in turn may result in the emergence of irregular acinar morphologies. The altered signals are identified by a color on the inner circle: yellow-basal (ECM) signals; cyan-apical signals; green-lateral signals. The center picture shows schematics of a polarized cell with typical distribution of cell membrane receptors.

Prolonged growth would lead to the closure of the luminal space and to the collapse of the whole duct. Whether similar processes can occur in epithelial ducts in the living organisms has not been documented. However, the process of cleft formation has been observed, for example, during salivary glands morphogenesis, although not in the hollow ducts but in the glands fully filled with cells [24].

2.5. Alterations in Apical and Death Signals. Normal development of epithelial cysts requires clearance of the luminal space from all inner cells. Different processes could be responsible for this selective cell removal, however, it has been shown experimentally that cell apoptotic death is the necessary contributor to the formation and maintenance of the empty luminal space [25]. This form of cell death is induced on purpose and often called *programmed cell death*. However, it is not known how the process of lumen clearance is triggered. We previously used *IBCell* to test the hypothesis that apoptotic death arises in cells directly attached to the polarized cells and is initiated upon the formation of the apical membrane domain and disassembly of the adhesive links between polarized and inner cells [11]. Here, we simulate an opposite scenario. When cell response to apical signal is altered in such a way that cell apoptotic death in adjacent cells is not initiated, these cells can sense free space in their vicinity and reinitiate the growth process. As a result, the inner lumen space can be repopulated (Figure 3(d)). This kind of escape from tissue homeostatic balance leads to the formation of mutants resembling ductal carcinoma *in situ*, a noninvasive form of ductal tumors characterized by intact overall ductal structure with filled luminal space [7].

2.6. Alterations in Lateral but Not Basal and Apical Signals. We previously showed in [11] that in order to form round regular ductal structures, the orientation of mitotic spindle poles and the axis of cell division need to be coordinated in *IBCell*. The expansion of the epithelial layer of cells requires symmetrical cell division (along the apical-basal axis) resulting in two luminally positioned daughter cells. In contrast, asymmetrical cell division (parallel to the basement membrane and/or lumen) gives rise to one basally and one luminally positioned daughter cell and culminates in either cell differentiation or its apoptosis. As a result, the dying cell contributes to lumen expansion. The rule of choosing one of the directions was based on cell shape, with the asymmetrical direction chosen when the cell was elongated along the basal-apical axis. Cell elongation might be due, for example, to the pressure of tightly packed neighboring cells or may arise from cell-cell adhesion forces. Here, we simulated the case when epithelial cells in the duct gained the proliferative phenotype due to disruption in cell-cell lateral signaling followed by acquiring additional growth receptors. However, we assumed that the basal and apical signals are not altered, so the growing cells will divide symmetrically. This leads to increased lateral tension and results in duct bending (Figure 3(e)), because an excess of epithelial cells is not accompanied by the expansion of the lumen inside the duct.

2.7. Alterations in Lateral and Apical Signals. Our final simulation (Figure 3(f)) tests a scenario when all cell divisions in the developing structure are symmetrical, that is, orthogonal to the basal membrane domain. In this case, all cells have minuscule apical sides and almost no luminal space. Since the lateral signals are altered, the cells have excess of growth receptors and proliferate continuously leading to the formation of highly irregular multicellular structure with no detectable lumen. The importance of the orientation of cell division axis was investigated experimentally in 3D cultures of MDCK cells [26], where it was shown that if the angle between apico-basal axis and the spindle axis (which is perpendicular to the axis of cell division) is less than 45°, the formation of inner lumen is suppressed.

3. Discussion

Maintaining the structural homeostatic balance in tissues is essential for their proper function. Certain changes in tissue architecture do take place even in an adult healthy organism, but there are constrains in terms of the amount of disruption the cells and tissues can withstand, and how long they are exposed to the disruption clues. For example, it has been determined, based on morphological identification of both mitotic and apoptotic events [27], that cell turnover in lobules of the normal human breast undergoes significant cyclical changes during the menstrual cycle, with the peak for apoptosis occurring 3 days after the peak for mitosis. An even more spectacular example of a controlled tissue structure remodeling is the process of involution—a programmed destruction and removal of the breast epithelial ducts that were generated during pregnancy to enable milk production. This postlactation regression involves a massive death of epithelial cells and remodeling of epithelial ducts to their prepregnant state and function [28]. However, uncontrolled homeostatic imbalance may lead to nonreversible changes in tissue microarchitecture and subsequently to its malignancy.

Cancer is a genetic disease, but the mutated cell manifests its tumorous characteristics by changing its physical behavior. For instance, the invasive cell must overcome adhesive forces exerted by the neighboring cells, apply repulsive forces to break through the basement membrane surrounding the epithelial duct, and utilize pulling and pushing forces to actively move through the extracellular matrix. Thus, in addition to indispensible functions of genetics programs, all cells and tissues are also shaped by mechanical forces and stresses. Tumor progression is characterized by an incremental stiffening of the tissue. In fact, breast self-exam, the preliminary cancer screening method, looks for unusual differences in tissue density and stiffness, such as lumps or nodules.

On the other hand, homeostatic mechanisms are built using the cells' existing molecular and signaling machinery as well as the architecture of the tissue and other physical constraints. Despite their general robustness against the most common perturbations, some genetic mutations and certain changes in tissue architecture could disrupt homeostasis. Moreover, there is increasing experimental evidence showing that the restoration of tissue organization is able to repress the malignant phenotype of genetically aberrant cells. For example, when mouse embryonal carcinoma cells (which form malignant tumors upon subcutaneous injection) were fused with normal blastocysts, they were able to give rise to phenotypically normal cancer-free mouse [29]. Also, malignant T4-2 cells forming disorganized continuously proliferating colonies can be reverted to near-normal phenotype when grown in the presence of integrin-blocking antibodies. These reverted T4-2 cells formed regular growth-arrested acinar structures with restored apico-basal polarity, reorganized actin cytoskeleton, and were able to remain quiescent for up to 1 month in culture [30].

We have shown using the biomechanical model of epithelial ducts, *IBCell*, that alterations in cell intrinsic responses to extrinsic signals lead to the loss of tissue integrity if such microenvironmental perturbations are exerted in a persistent and/or prolonged way. When cell epithelial character is disturbed by changes in the expression of certain cell membrane receptors or markers, the uncontrolled growth is triggered leading to aberrations in the epithelial duct structure (altered lateral and/or apical signaling), or to the emergence of microinvasions (misread ECM signaling). These examples show that microscopic changes in cell mechanics, extracellular matrix structure, and cell-matrix interactions can dysregulate molecular mechanisms of mechanotransduction. Thus, the physical basis for epithelial cancer initiation might be attributed to either altered force balance on cellular or tissue level or the perturbed cellular responses to various mechanical stimuli.

Appendix

Mathematical Model

The *IBCell* was introduced in [31] to model early tumor development and subsequently applied to investigate the sufficient and necessary conditions for the formation and stability of hollow epithelial acini, three-dimensional multicellular culture systems that recapitulate the structure and function of epithelial mammary cysts [10, 11]. In this model, the eukaryotic cell is represented as a two-dimensional fully deformable body, and its structure includes an elastic plasma membrane modeled as a network of linear springs that define cell shape and encloses the viscous incompressible fluid representing the cytoplasm and providing cell mass. These individual cells can interact with other cells and with the environment via a set of discrete membrane receptors located on the cell boundary. In particular, each boundary point can be engaged in adhesion either with one of the neighboring cells or with the extracellular matrix, and cell membrane receptors can be used to sense the presence of other cells or extracellular matrix in the local cell vicinity. The host cell can initiate certain cell-life processes, such as proliferation, division, apoptotic death, or epithelial polarization, based on its membrane receptors signature (a distribution of growth, death, apical, cell-cell, and cell-ECM adhesion receptors). More precisely, cell growth is modeled by placing point sources and sinks around the cell boundary to model transport of fluid through the cell membrane, and, once the cell area is doubled, the contractile ring is formed by introducing springs between opposite points on the cell boundary that upon contraction split the cell into two daughters. Cell epithelial polarity is acquired by developing three distinct cell membrane domains: basal, defined by cell membrane receptors contacting the external media; lateral, defined by cell receptors being in contact with other cells; apical, facing the hollow lumen. Cell apoptotic death is modeled by placing point sinks and sources along the membrane of the whole cell to release fluid from the cell interior to the extracellular space. The *IBCell* model is based on the immersed boundary framework and governed by (1)–(7).

In this system, (1) is the Navier-Stokes equation of a viscous incompressible fluid defined on the Cartesian grid $x = (\mathbf{x_1}, \mathbf{x_2})$, where p is the fluid pressure, μ is the fluid viscosity, ρ is the fluid density, s is the local fluid expansion, and f is the external force density. Equation (2) is the law of mass balance. Interactions between the fluid and the material points $X(l,t)$, on cell boundaries Γ and at point sources $\mathbf{Y_k}$ and sinks $\mathbf{Z_m}$ placed in the cell local microenvironment, are defined in (4), (5), (6). Here, the force density $\mathbf{F}(l,t)$ defined on cell boundaries, and the sources $S^{+}(\mathbf{Y_k},t)$ and sinks $S^{-}(\mathbf{Z_m},t)$ defined in the cell microenvironment, are applied to the fluid using the two-dimensional Dirac delta function δ, while all material boundary points $X(l,t)$ are carried along with the fluid. The boundary forces $\mathbf{F}(l,t)$ arise from elastic properties of cell boundaries, from cell-to-cell adhesion, and from contractile forces splitting a cell during its division. The sources $S^{+}(\mathbf{Y_k},t)$ and sinks $S^{-}(\mathbf{Z_m},t)$ are chosen such that they balance around each cell separately.

The kinetics of ECM proteins $\gamma(x,t)$ is defined along the cell boundaries and include: constant secretion (at a rate k_1) along the cells' basal domains and its decay (at a rate k_2) around all cells' boundaries. More details on the mathematical formulation of *IBCell* and the implementation of cell-life processes can be found in [31]. The model is implemented in Fortran with all graphical routines executed using Matlab. A typical simulation of developing acinar structures, like these presented here, lasts up to 6 hours on the one-processor desktop computer. The corresponding *in vitro* experiments take about 24–30 days. The *IBCell* simulations can be found at http://www.rejniak.net/ under research option, and the code may be obtained from the author upon request.

Acknowledgment

This work was partially supported by the NIH-NCI Integrative Cancer Biology Program (ICBP), (U54CA113007).

References

[1] C. C. Dufort, M. J. Paszek, and V. M. Weaver, "Balancing forces: architectural control of mechanotransduction," *Nature Reviews Molecular Cell Biology*, vol. 12, no. 5, pp. 308–319, 2011.

[2] J. I. Lopez, I. Kang, W. You, D. M. McDonald, and V. M. Weaver, "In situ force mapping of mammary gland transformation," *Integrative Biology*, vol. 3, pp. 910–921, 2011.

[3] H. Huang, R. D. Kamm, and R. T. Lee, "Cell mechanics and mechanotransduction: pathways, probes, and physiology," *American Journal of Physiology*, vol. 287, no. 1, pp. C1–C11, 2004.

[4] K. S. Kolahi and M. R. K. Mofrad, "Mechanotransduction: a major regulator of homeostasis and development," *Wiley Interdisciplinary Reviews: Systems Biology and Medicine*, vol. 2, no. 6, pp. 625–639, 2010.

[5] D. E. Jaalouk and J. Lammerding, "Mechanotransduction gone awry," *Nature Reviews Molecular Cell Biology*, vol. 10, no. 1, pp. 63–73, 2009.

[6] H. Kitano, "Cancer robustness: tumour tactics," *Nature*, vol. 426, no. 6963, p. 125, 2003.

[7] J. Debnath and J. S. Brugge, "Modelling glandular epithelial cancers in three-dimensional cultures," *Nature Reviews Cancer*, vol. 5, no. 9, pp. 675–688, 2005.

[8] M. J. Bissell, D. C. Radisky, A. Rizki, V. M. Weaver, and O. W. Petersen, "The organizing principle: microenvironmental influences in the normal and malignant breast," *Differentiation*, vol. 70, no. 9-10, pp. 537–546, 2002.

[9] P. Lu, V. N. Weaver, and Z. Werb, "The extracellular matrix: a dynamic niche in cancer progression," *The Journal of Cell Biology*, vol. 196, pp. 395–406, 2012.

[10] K. A. Rejniak and A. Anderson, "A computational study of the development of epithelial acini. I. Sufficient conditions for the formation of a hollow structure," *Bulletin of Mathematical Biology*, vol. 70, no. 3, pp. 677–712, 2008.

[11] K. A. Rejniak and A. Anderson, "A computational study of the development of epithelial acini. II. Necessary conditions for structure and lumen stability," *Bulletin of Mathematical Biology*, vol. 70, no. 5, pp. 1450–1479, 2008.

[12] M. J. Reginato and S. K. Muthuswamy, "Illuminating the center: mechanisms regulating lumen formation and maintenance in mammary morphogenesis," *Journal of Mammary Gland Biology and Neoplasia*, vol. 11, no. 3-4, pp. 205–211, 2006.

[13] A. A. Mailleux, M. Overholtzer, and J. S. Brugge, "Lumen formation during mammary epithelial morphogenesis: insights from in vitro and in vivo models," *Cell Cycle*, vol. 7, no. 1, pp. 57–62, 2008.

[14] D. M. Bryant and K. E. Mostov, "From cells to organs: building polarized tissue," *Nature Reviews Molecular Cell Biology*, vol. 9, no. 11, pp. 887–901, 2008.

[15] J. Debnath, S. K. Muthuswamy, and J. S. Brugge, "Morphogenesis and oncogenesis of MCF-10A mammary epithelial acini grown in three-dimensional basement membrane cultures," *Methods*, vol. 30, no. 3, pp. 256–268, 2003.

[16] C. M. Nelson and M. J. Bissell, "Modeling dynamic reciprocity: engineering three-dimensional culture models of breast architecture, function, and neoplastic transformation," *Seminars in Cancer Biology*, vol. 15, no. 5, pp. 342–352, 2005.

[17] D. R. Tyson, J. Inokuchi, T. Tsunoda, A. Lau, and D. K. Ornstein, "Culture requirements of prostatic epithelial cell lines for acinar morphogenesis and lumen formation in vitro: role of extracellular calcium," *Prostate*, vol. 67, no. 15, pp. 1601–1613, 2007.

[18] F. Xu, J. Celli, I. Rizvi, S. Moon, T. Hasan, and U. Demirci, "A three-dimensional in vitro ovarian cancer coculture model using a high-throughput cell patterning platform," *Biotechnology Journal*, vol. 6, no. 2, pp. 204–212, 2011.

[19] D. J. Ferguson, "An ultrastructural study of mitosis and cytokinesis in normal "resting" human breast," *Cell and Tissue Research*, vol. 252, no. 3, pp. 581–587, 1988.

[20] L. E. O'Brien, M. M. P. Zegers, and K. E. Mostov, "Building epithelial architecture: Insights from three-dimensional culture models," *Nature Reviews Molecular Cell Biology*, vol. 3, no. 7, pp. 531–537, 2002.

[21] V. Quaranta, K. A. Rejniak, P. Gerlee, and A. Anderson, "Invasion emerges from cancer cell adaptation to competitive microenvironments: quantitative predictions from multiscale mathematical models," *Seminars in Cancer Biology*, vol. 18, no. 5, pp. 338–348, 2008.

[22] D. T. Butcher, T. Alliston, and V. M. Weaver, "A tense situation: forcing tumour progression," *Nature Reviews Cancer*, vol. 9, no. 2, pp. 108–122, 2009.

[23] C. T. Leung and J. S. Brugge, "Outgrowth of single oncogene-expressing cells from suppressive epithelial environments," *Nature*, vol. 482, pp. 410–414, 2012.

[24] J. Harunaga, J. C. Hsu, and K. M. Yamada, "Dynamics of salivary gland morphogenesis," *Journal of Dental Research*, vol. 90, pp. 1070–1077, 2011.

[25] J. Debnath, K. R. Mills, N. L. Collins, M. J. Reginato, S. K. Muthuswamy, and J. S. Brugge, "The role of apoptosis in creating and maintaining luminal space within normal and oncogene-expressing mammary acini," *Cell*, vol. 111, no. 1, pp. 29–40, 2002.

[26] A. E. Rodriguez-Fraticelli, S. Vergarajauregui, D. J. Eastburn et al., "The Cdc42 GEF intersectin 2 controls mitotic spindle orientation to form the lumen during epithelial morphogenesis," *Journal of Cell Biology*, vol. 189, no. 4, pp. 725–738, 2010.

[27] D. J. P. Ferguson and T. J. Anderson, "Morphological evaluation of cell turnover in relation to the menstrual cycle in the "resting" human breast," *British Journal of Cancer*, vol. 44, no. 2, pp. 177–181, 1981.

[28] C. J. Watson, "Involution: apoptosis and tissue remodelling that convert the mammary gland from milk factory to a quiescent organ," *Breast Cancer Research*, vol. 8, no. 2, pp. 203–207, 2006.

[29] B. Mintz and K. Illmensee, "Normal genetically mosaic mice produced from malignant teratocarcinoma cells," *Proceedings of the National Academy of Sciences of the United States of America*, vol. 72, no. 9, pp. 3585–3589, 1975.

[30] V. M. Weaver, S. Lelièvre, J. N. Lakins et al., "$\beta 4$ integrin-dependent formation of polarized three-dimensional architecture confers resistance to apoptosis in normal and malignant mammary epithelium," *Cancer Cell*, vol. 2, no. 3, pp. 205–216, 2002.

[31] K. A. Rejniak, "An immersed boundary framework for modelling the growth of individual cells: an application to the early tumour development," *Journal of Theoretical Biology*, vol. 247, no. 1, pp. 186–204, 2007.

9

Within-Niche Constant Selection of *Drosophila* Inversions?

José M. Álvarez-Castro and Gonzalo Alvarez

Department of Genetics, University of Santiago de Compostela, Avenida Carvalho Calero s/n, 27002 Lugo, Galiza, Spain

Correspondence should be addressed to José M. Álvarez-Castro; jose.alvarez.castro@usc.es

Academic Editors: C. Jodice, T. Shikano, and A. Taylor-Robinson

Extensive and fruitful work is being devoted for more than 70 years to elucidate the fine points of the maintenance of inversion polymorphisms of the genus *Drosophila*. Recent studies have resumed selection in heterogeneous environments (or niches) as a major underlying mechanism for these balanced polymorphisms. In those studies, constant selection within niches is assumed throughout although this assumption is since long known not to hold. In the present communication it is sustained that the results in those studies are robust in the face of this fact. To that end, this communication deals with a particular long-lasting question within this topic—whether the minimal model of constant viability selection (MCV, assuming frequency-, sex-, and stage-independent adaptive values) suffices to reproduce the trajectories of frequencies of Drosophila chromosomal arrangements observed in experimental populations along generations under homogeneous environments. Fitness estimates are here obtained from published trajectories of frequencies using a maximum likelihood approach, and relevant literature is revised in the light of these new analyses, pointing to an affirmative answer to that question.

1. Introduction

Dobzhansky's fundamental finding that natural selection acts on polymorphic chromosomal inversions of *Drosophila* flies [1–3] was path-breaking in evolutionary biology and bestowed plenty of delightful work upon geneticists for years to come [4]. In particular, it triggered a long-term line of work to elucidate the particular, strong mechanism(s) of selection underlying the inversion polymorphisms that were maintained both under natural and (often) under experimental conditions [5, 6]. The first hypothesis to test was the heterozygote types (heterokaryotypes) having higher adaptive values than the homozygote types (homokaryotypes) assuming the model of constant viability (MCV), which was referred to as heterosis [7, 8]. The plausibility of this hypothesis did not only come from its simplicity, but also because no discrepancies were initially found between the predicted trajectories assuming heterosis and the observed data [5, 6, 8]. Subsequently, more thorough assessments were designed in order to definitely reveal the role of heterosis in the maintenance of the *Drosophila* inversion polymorphisms.

The least-squares and goodness-of-fit-based methods to estimate constant adaptive values from experimental runs [6, 9, 10] were replaced by more convenient maximum likelihood (ML) approaches [11, 12]. However, when applying these methods to real data, the results were not conclusive. For some experiments, the trajectories predicted using the estimated adaptive values would fit the data well, whereas statistically significant departures between the observed and the predicted trajectories would be found for others [12–14]. Further ML methods were then designed to account for more realistic selection regimes involving stage- and sex-dependent adaptive values [15, 16]. However, the data requirements increase with the number of parameters, and the information content the observed trajectories of frequencies can bear is limited. Consequently, Prout [17, 18] proposed that this puzzle would have to be broken up into more accessible pieces, which turned researchers in this field to estimate separate fitness components in competition experiments (reviewed in [19–21]). This line of research revealed the maintenance of *Drosophila* inversion polymorphisms not to be ruled simply by heterosis. In fact, selection has been shown to take capricious enough appearances that can simultaneously be frequency-, sex-, and stage-dependent, as rare male advantage [22, 23].

The integrative approach proposed by Prout [15, 17, 18, 24] consists in modelling the trajectories of frequency of *Drosophila* inversions along generations using the fitness-component estimates obtained in competition experiments. This strategy has recently shown a more than reasonably good fit of predicted-to-observed trajectories, using from the last ones only their starting points [25, 26]. However, this positive result is not sufficient for completely understanding the balanced inversion polymorphisms of *Drosophila's* natural populations, with individuals migrating among niches with different selection pressures [27–30]. In fact, *Drosophila* inversions being affected by selection in heterogeneous environments have been originally pointed out by Dobzhansky [2] as the cause of the altitudinal clines of their frequencies. Kirkpatrick and Barton [31] have more recently inspected the ecological and genetic mechanisms underlying the evolution of these clines and emphasized the potential of inversions for the adaptation of populations to local environments (i.e., niches). More to the point, Schaeffer [32] has recently estimated adaptive values of inversions for the six niches identified for *Drosophila pseudoobscura* in the southwestern USA, using a model of selection-migration balance.

In order to address the complexity of niche-dependent selection in those recent studies, the MCV has been used to describe selection within niches (or localities). However, *Drosophila* inversions are since long known to be affected by more complex modes of selection—as pointed out above. Consequently, the question of whether the reliability of those results is spoiled by the assumption of within-niche constant selection is here addressed. Dobzhansky's unresolved concern on whether the MCV fits the changes in frequency of *Drosophila* inversions [6] is thus revisited. More precisely, is the MCV (in spite of not being causative) appropriate to accurately reproduce the changes in frequency of *Drosophila* chromosomal arrangements along generations under constant environments? Previous studies on this subject are here reviewed in the light of new analyses of published data.

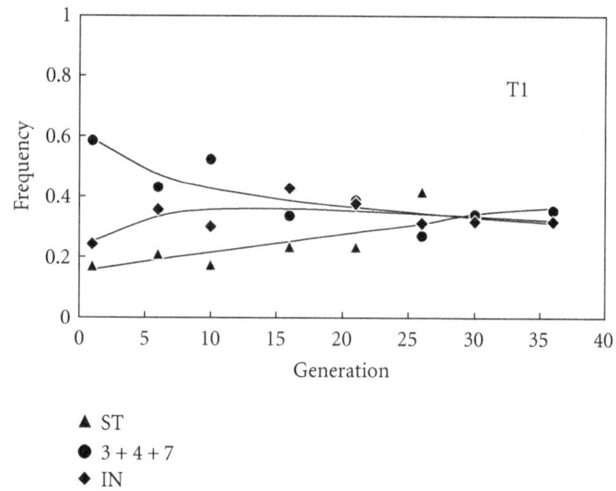

FIGURE 1: Observed frequencies (symbols) of arrangements of the O chromosome along generations of experimental population T1 of *Drosophila subobscura* [33] and predicted trajectories (lines) using ML estimates of frequency-, sex-, and stage-independent adaptive values and initial frequencies from the observed frequencies.

2. Methods

Estimates of stage-, sex-, and frequency-independent adaptive values and initial frequencies of three-allele karyotypic classes are here obtained from experimental populations of *Drosophila subobscura* [33] using an implementation of DuMouchel and Anderson's [12] unconditional ML method. The de Frutos' [33] datasets are of the same kind as the ones generated for using this ML method [12–14, 34, 35]—to this regard, it is in particular important to note that the experimental population sizes are large relative to the sample sizes so that the sample procedure does not strongly affect the population frequencies of subsequent generations [36]. The required implementation consists in estimating the initial frequencies, due to the experimental populations having been started from wild individuals with unknown frequencies [33]. This implementation was reported to have already been applied to other datasets [13, 14], although not yet described.

For a k-allele genetic system, the MCV expresses the gene frequencies of zygotes of generation $(t+1)$, $p_i(t+1)$, $i = 1, \ldots, k$, in terms of the frequencies at the previous generation and the adaptive values $p_i(t)$, ω_{ij}, $i, j = 1, \ldots, k$, respectively, using the following recurrence equations:

$$p_i(t+1) = \frac{F_i(t)}{D(t)}, \quad i = 1, \ldots, k, \tag{1}$$

where $F_i(t) = p_i(t)\sum_{j=1}^{k} p_j(t)\omega_{ij}$, $i = 1, \ldots, k$, and $D(t) = \sum_{l,m=1}^{k} p_l(t)p_m(t)\omega_{lm}$. The vector of independent parameters to estimate is $\mathbf{E} = (p_1(0), \ldots, p_{k-1}(0), \omega_{11}, \ldots, \omega_{kk-1})^{\mathrm{T}}$, where the superindex T stands for transpose. The remaining frequency, $p_k(0)$, is defined by all frequencies having to sum up to one, and the remaining adaptive value, ω_{kk}, is defined by $\sum_{ij\in V}\omega_{ij} = k(k+1)/2$ where V is the set of the $k(k+1)/2$ adaptive values.

The data are the observed gene frequencies in zygotes of subsequent, not necessarily consecutive, generations $x_i(t)$, $i = 1, \ldots, k$, $t \in X$, and the number of genes sampled for each generation, $n(t)$, $t \in X$, where X is the set of all observed generations. Thus, the likelihood function is $\prod_{t\in X}\prod_{i=1}^{k} p_i(t)^{x_i(t)}$. Hence, its logarithm is

$$L = c + \sum_{t\in X}\sum_{i=1}^{k} x_i(t)\log p_i(t), \tag{2}$$

where c is a constant.

The ML estimate of the vector $\mathbf{E}$ can be computed iteratively from an attempting initial value $\mathbf{E}^{(u)}$, using Newton's iteration algorithm $\mathbf{E}^{(u+1)} = \mathbf{E}^{(u)} + \mathbf{I}^{-1}\cdot\mathbf{S}$ [37, 38], where the likelihood vector is $\mathbf{S} = (\partial L/\partial \varepsilon)_{\varepsilon \in \mathbf{E}} = (\sum_{t\in X}\sum_{i=1}^{k}(x_i(t)/p_i(t))(\partial p_i(t)/\partial\varepsilon))_{\varepsilon\in\mathbf{E}}$, using (2), and the information matrix is $\mathbf{I} = (\sum_{t\in X} n(t)\sum_{i=1}^{k}[((\partial p_i(t)/\partial\delta)(\partial p_i(t)/\partial\varepsilon))/p_i(t)])_{\delta,\varepsilon\in\mathbf{E}}$. In these expressions, the derivatives of the gene frequencies along generations with respect to the parameters to estimate can be computed recursively, from (1), as

$$\frac{\partial p_i(t+1)}{\partial\varepsilon} = \frac{\partial F_i(t)}{\partial\varepsilon}\frac{1}{D(t)} - \frac{F_i(t)}{[D(t)]^2}\frac{\partial D(t)}{\partial\varepsilon}, \quad \varepsilon\in\mathbf{E}, \quad i = 1,\ldots,k, \tag{3}$$

where

$$\frac{\partial D(t)}{\partial\varepsilon} = \sum_{i=1}^{k}\frac{\partial F_i(t)}{\partial\varepsilon}, \quad \varepsilon\in\mathbf{E},$$

$$\frac{\partial F_i(t)}{\partial p_r(0)} = \sum_{j=1}^{k}\left[\omega_{ij}\left(p_i(t)\frac{\partial p_j(t)}{\partial p_r(0)} + p_j(t)\frac{\partial p_i(t)}{\partial p_r(0)}\right)\right], \quad r = 1,\ldots,k-1,$$

$$\frac{\partial F_i(t)}{\partial\omega_{lm}} = \sum_{j=1}^{k}\left[p_i(t)\,p_j(t)\frac{\partial\omega_{ij}}{\partial\omega_{lm}} + \omega_{ij}\left(p_i(t)\frac{\partial p_j(t)}{\partial\omega_{lm}} + p_j(t)\frac{\partial p_i(t)}{\partial\omega_{lm}}\right)\right], \quad lm\in V\setminus\{kk\}. \tag{4}$$

The recursive process is initiated using that the frequencies at time $t = 0$ are independent of the adaptive values and that $\partial p_i(0)/\partial p_r(0)$ equals $1, -1$, and 0, when $i = r$, $i = k$, and otherwise, respectively.

3. Results

The ML method described above succeeded to converge to a vector of positive estimates for only three out of the ten populations of *Drosophila subobscura* sampled along several generations by de Frutos [33]—the ones labelled as H2, T1, and P2 (Figures 1 and 2). These estimates are shown in Table 1 together with the results of a statistical test assessing the goodness of fit between the observed trajectories of frequencies and the ones predicted using the estimates. For populations H2 and T1, only a few of the multiple scrutinizing starting values have led to local convergence of the ML method, which reflects that the information content of the data is not optimal and the estimates are therefore not robust. In particular, H2 has a lower number of generations sampled than the other two populations and T1 has lower efforts of per generation samples than P2 (cf. sample sizes in [33]) and was funded at frequencies closer to the equilibrium (cf. Figures 1 and 2). In any event, the fact that populations associated to weak estimates (with only local convergence of the ML method) display statistically significant departures between the observed trajectories and the ones predicted by the estimates, using a goodness-of-fit test (Table 1), does not prove that the model cannot fit more informative data.

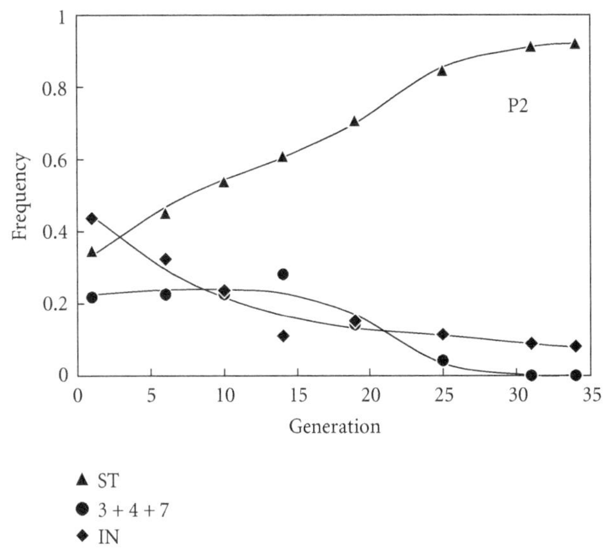

FIGURE 2: Observed frequencies and predicted trajectories of population P2 (same specifications as in legend of Figure 1).

The key to address this problem is thus the performance the predictions show at populations for which global convergence to meaningful adaptive values evidences the good quality of the data. In point of fact, such data is scarce in the literature. Fortunately, however, this actually is the case for population P2 (Figure 2), where global convergence of the ML method described above has led to robust estimates of selective values (Table 1). In fact, the predicted trajectories for population P2 (Figure 2) seem to provide the best possible approximation to the data—the only mismatch attracting visual attention happens at generation 14, at which the least sampling effort for this population has been made [33]. This visual appreciation is in accordance with the results of the statistical tests. It is noteworthy that sample size is higher for P2 than for T1 [33] and that the larger the sample sizes, the higher the power to detect discrepancies between the predicted and the observed trajectories by the goodness-of-fit test [39]. In spite of that, no significant discrepancies occur for population P2 (Table 1). Therefore, these results clearly point to the estimation procedure to generate predicted trajectories that fit the data extremely well—whenever applied to datasets that are informative enough to provide robust estimates.

These results enable us to provide a coherent interpretation of the results reported in the literature for the inversion polymorphism of *Drosophila pseudoobscura* [12–14, 34, 35]. Indeed, reinterpreting those works has been a major motivation for us to use the same methodology. DuMouchel and Anderson [12] found no discrepancies between predicted (under the MCV) and observed trajectories in diallelic populations, but statistically significant discrepancies in multiallelic populations (in which similar sampling efforts were

TABLE 1: ML estimates of frequency-, sex-, and stage-independent adaptive values, ω_{ij}, and initial frequencies, $p_i(1)$, from observed frequencies of arrangements of the *O* chromosome along generations of experimental populations of *Drosophila subobscura* [33], goodness of fit, χ^2, and degrees of freedom, df, to test the adequacy of the selection model to the data and equilibrium frequencies, $\widehat{p}_i$, predicted by the estimates.

Population	Arrangement[(a)]	$p_i(1) \pm \sigma_{pi(1)}$	$\omega_{1j} \pm \sigma_{\omega 1j}$	$\omega_{2j} \pm \sigma_{\omega 2j}$	$\omega_{3j} \pm \sigma_{\omega 3j}$	χ^2	df	$\widehat{p}_i$
	O_{ST}	0.040 ± 0.011	0.936 ± 0.456	1.450 ± 1.672	1.083 ± 0.206	17.373***	3	0.424
H2	O_{3+4+7}	0.735 ± 0.026		0.367 ± 3.462	1.707 ± 4.584			0.338
	O_{IN}	0.225 ± 0.024			0.456 ± 3.108			0.238
	O_{ST}	0.158 ± 0.022	1.030 ± 0.115	1.045 ± 0.083	1.107 ± 0.259	26.105***	7	0.596
T1	O_{3+4+7}	0.590 ± 0.032		0.812 ± 0.078	1.240 ± 0.225			0.171
	O_{IN}	0.252 ± 0.029			0.766 ± 0.308			0.233
	O_{ST}	0.333 ± 0.024	1.069 ± 0.041	0.613 ± 0.103	1.045 ± 0.043	8.072	7	1
P2	O_{3+4+7}	0.225 ± 0.019		1.963 ± 0.286	0.551 ± 0.219			0
	O_{IN}	0.443 ± 0.029			0.759 ± 0.125			0

(a)The less frequent arrangements are pulled together into the category O_{IN}, which is dominated by arrangements O_{3+4} or O_7 [33].
$^{***}P < 0.001$.

made in spite of the increasing number of parameters to estimate). Accordingly, statistically significant discrepancies between predicted and observed data were found by Watanabe et al. [13] in a highly parameterized genetic system (four-allele populations in which also the initial frequencies had to be estimated), whereas Anderson et al. [14] obtained good fit using lesser parameterized models (triallelic populations) and taking special care in sampling a considerable number of generations ahead of the equilibrium.

Overall, a comprehensive view of the estimation of selection (with the MCV) of *Drosophila* inversions from changes in frequency along generations can be summarized in two points. On the one hand, the statistical discrepancies found at populations between observed trajectories and the ones predicted with non robust estimates reflect that the amount of information content of many datasets is not in accordance with the number of parameters to estimate. On the other hand, the systematic fit of trajectories predicted by a reasonably small amount of estimates obtained from reasonably high-quality data (ensuing global convergence of the estimation procedure to meaningful values) proves that the constant (stage-, sex-, and frequency-independent) model of selection suffices to describe the observed trajectories of inversion frequencies within niches.

4. Discussion

Several recent studies have dealt with intraniche constant selection of *Drosophila* inversions as a black-box model to investigate how selection works across niches [31, 32]. This practice is in accordance with Prout's [17, 18] proposal of addressing, in turn, separate aspects of this problem. Schaeffer [32], in particular, provides evidence for selection in heterogeneous environments to be a crucial mechanism in the maintenance of inversion polymorphisms in *Drosophila* populations of the southwestern USA. He shows that models assuming constant adaptive values that do not display heterosis within niches can fit data on balanced polymorphisms in natural populations of *Drosophila pseudoobscura*. The adaptive values obtained under the different environments are then used to reproduce the equilibrium frequencies through recursions using the MCV with selection-migration balance, assuming different migration rates and migration schemes.

The motivation for the present communication is that the results just mentioned can be questioned by arguing that, within environments, adaptive values of *Drosophila* inversions are known not to be constant at all but stage-, sex-, and frequency-dependent, as explained in the Introduction section. Interestingly, the reasoning behind these results does not exactly rely on the MCV entailing the true mechanism of selection within the different niches. To be precise, Schaeffer's [32] results rely instead on the MCV being able to accurately reproduce the changes in inversion frequencies along generations of flies within each niche. Therefore, the apparent contradiction coming from using the MCV as a simplifying assumption vanishes under the outcome of this communication—the MCV, although non causative, suffices to reproduce the changes in frequency of *Drosophila* inversions that are due to selection within niches. Thus, a critical step has here been worked out that is needed to sustain previous results that have been published concerning the maintenance of *Drosophila* inversion polymorphisms.

It is not astonishing that the question of whether the MCV would fit *Drosophila* inversions frequencies lasted long. Indeed, when this subject was first addressed, the MCV was still regarded as a potential causative mechanism—instead of as a black-box model—for *Drosophila* inversion polymorphisms and heterosis comprised an appealing explanation to *Drosophila* balanced polymorphisms, as explained in the Introduction section. This fact must have initially encouraged researchers to address the estimation of adaptive values in all kinds of populations (including rather complex ones) and to progressively abandon this line of work as the evidences of complex modes of selection of inversions became stronger. As a consequence—and despite several indications advised for the design of experiments to estimate constant-selection parameters from trajectories of frequency (see, e.g., [12])—the *Drosophila* literature does not in the end provide many datasets that can lead to robust estimates. Rather, the experimental datasets often involve three or more alleles and entail the initial frequencies as parameters to estimate.

In the present communication it was actually necessary to reduce the complexity of the original data towards a triallelic system by pooling the less frequent arrangements into the category O_{IN}. This is one of the factors putatively precluding most of the populations of de Frutos [33] to lead to global convergence of the ML method. On the other hand, the fitness estimate obtained for population P2 predicting the fixation of one arrangement, O_{ST} (Table 1), is an occasional fact (several inversions are often maintained in experimental populations, see, e.g., [21]) that actually facilitates the convergence of the estimation procedure—since it facilitates that a higher number of generations involving changes in frequency occur before the equilibrium is attained (cf. Figures 1 and 2). Incidentally, the estimates obtained by the ML method are consistent with the output of all populations since they correctly predict whether the multiallelic polymorphism would be maintained or not (see the equilibrium frequencies predicted from the estimates of adaptive values in Table 1), which reinforces our main conclusion—the MCV can be used to obtain adaptive values that approximate well the trajectories of frequencies of *Drosophila* inversions within niches, as long as there is enough data available for the ML method to provide robust estimates.

In any case, it must be recalled that the good fit of the MCV to the inversion frequencies cannot be argued to endorse heterosis as the causative factor of the maintenance of the *Drosophila* inversion polymorphisms. As pointed out above, numerous studies found complex modes of selection to occur in the maintenance of *Drosophila* inversion polymorphisms reviewed in [19–21]. Furthermore, the stage-, sex-, and frequency-dependent fitness estimates obtained in competition experiments of *Drosophila pseudoobscura* have been successfully used to replicate the trajectories of frequencies of experimental populations along generations [25], which supports those multifaceted fitness estimates—instead of the minimal MCV with heterosis—as the selection mechanisms underlying the maintenance of inversion polymorphisms in experimental populations. Similarly, it cannot be argued that selection in heterogeneous environments is the only force maintaining the polymorphisms, since other balancing forces (different from heterosis) are known to act within niches.

Dobzhansky's fundamental finding that *Drosophila* inversions are affected by strong selective forces in natural populations via seasonality [1] and altitudinal clines [2] gave rise to extensive, fruitful research in evolutionary biology during Dobzhansky's life and shortly after his passing reviewed in [21]. This topic keeps on improving nowadays our insight in new scientific challenges, as shown, for instance, through the assessment of global climate change by shifts of latitudinal clines of *Drosophila* inversion polymorphisms [40] and through the understanding of speciation mechanisms that may underlie the origin of humans [41]. On the whole (although dealing here only with what is related to the maintenance of *Drosophila* inversion polymorphisms), Dobzhanky's bequest keeps on bestowing plenty of motivating challenges upon geneticists for times to come.

Abbreviations

MCV: Model of constant viability
ML: Maximum likelihood.

Acknowledgments

J. M. Álvarez-Castro acknowledges Arnaud Le Rouzic for having triggered the completion of this communication. This work has been supported by the autonomous government Xunta de Galicia through a fellowship from the Secretaría Xeral de Desenvolvemento and an "Isidro Parga Pondal" contract.

References

[1] T. Dobzhansky, "Genetics of natural populations IX. Temporal changes in the composition of populations of *Drosophila pseudoobscura*," *Genetics*, vol. 28, no. 2, pp. 162–186, 1943.

[2] T. Dobzhansky, "Genetics of natural populations XVI. Altitudinal and seasonal changes produced by natural selection in certain populations of *Drosophila pseudoobscura*," *Genetics*, vol. 33, pp. 158–176, 1948.

[3] T. Dobzhansky, "Evolutionary oscillations in *D. pseudoobscura*," in *Ecological Genetics and Evolution*, R. Greed, Ed., pp. 109–133, Blackwell, Oxford, UK, 1971.

[4] B. Charlesworth, "The good fairy godmother of evolutionary genetics," *Current Biology*, vol. 6, no. 3, p. 220, 1996.

[5] T. Dobzhansky, "Genetics of natural populations. XIX. Origin of heterosis through natural selection in populations of *Drosophila pseudoobscura*," *Genetics*, vol. 35, no. 3, pp. 288–302, 1950.

[6] S. Wright and T. Dobzhansky, "Genetics of natural populations. XII. Experimental reproduction of some of the changes caused by natural selection in certain populations of *Drosophila pseudoobscura*," *Genetics*, vol. 31, no. 2, pp. 125–156, 1946.

[7] T. Dobzhansky, *Genetics and the Origin of Species*, Columbia University Press, New York, NY, USA, 1937.

[8] T. Dobzhansky and O. Pavlovsky, "Indeterminate outcome of certain experiments of *Drosophila* populations," *Evolution*, vol. 7, pp. 198–210, 1953.

[9] T. Dobzhansky and H. Levene, "Development of heterosis through natural selection in experimental populations of *Drosophila pseudoobscura*," *American Naturalist*, vol. 85, no. 823, pp. 247–264, 1951.

[10] H. Levene, O. Pavlovsky, and T. Dobzhansky, "Interaction of the adaptive values in polymorphic experimental populations of *Drosophila-pseudoobscura*," *Evolution*, vol. 8, no. 4, pp. 335–349, 1954.

[11] L. L. Cavalli, "The analysis of selection courves," *Biometrics*, vol. 6, pp. 208–220, 1950.

[12] W. H. DuMouchel and W. W. Anderson, "The analysis of selection in experimental populations," *Genetics*, vol. 58, no. 3, pp. 435–449, 1968.

[13] T. Watanabe, W. W. Anderson, T. Dobzhansky, and O. Pavlovsky, "Selection in experimental populations of *Drosophila pseudoobscura* with different initial frequencies of chromosomal variants," *Genetical Research*, vol. 15, no. 1, pp. 123–129, 1970.

[14] W. W. Anderson, T. Dobzhansky, and O. Pavlovsky, "A natural population of *Drosophila* transferred to a laboratory environment," *Heredity*, vol. 28, no. 1, pp. 101–107, 1972.

[15] T. Prout, "The estimation of fitnesses from population data," *Genetics*, vol. 63, no. 4, pp. 949–967, 1969.

[16] J. Wilson, "Experimental design in fitness estimation," *Genetics*, vol. 66, no. 3, pp. 555–567, 1970.

[17] T. Prout, "The relation between fitness components and population prediction in *Drosophila* I, The estimation of fitness components," *Genetics*, vol. 68, pp. 127–149, 1971.

[18] T. Prout, "The relation between fitness components and population prediction in *Drosophila* II. Population prediction," *Genetics*, vol. 68, pp. 151–167, 1971.

[19] D. Sperlich and P. Pfriem, "Chromosomal polymorphism in natural and experimental populations," in *The Genetics and Biology of Drosophila*, M. Ashburner, H. L. Carson, and J. N. Thompson Jr., Eds., vol. 3e, pp. 257–309, Academy Press, London, UK, 1986.

[20] C. B. Krimbas and J. R. Powell, *Drosophila Inversion Polymorphism*, CRC Press, Boca Raton, Fla, USA, 1992.

[21] J. R. Powell, *Progress and Prospects in Evolutionary Biology. The Drosophila Model*, Oxford University Press, Oxford, UK, 1997.

[22] L. Ehrman, B. Spassky, O. Pavlovsky, and T. Dobzhansky, "Sexual selection, geotaxis, and chromosomal polymorphism in experimental populations of *Drosophila subobscura*," *Evolution*, vol. 19, pp. 337–346, 1965.

[23] C. Petit and L. Ehrman, "Sexual selection in *Drosophila*," *Evolutionary Biology*, vol. 3, pp. 177–223, 1969.

[24] T. Prout, "The estimation of fitness from genotypic frequencies," *Evolution*, vol. 19, pp. 546–551, 1965.

[25] J. M. Álvarez-Castro and Ö. Carlborg, "The yank of Dobzhansky's bequest," *Evolutionary Biology*, vol. 35, no. 3, pp. 176–181, 2008.

[26] J. M. Alvarez-Castro and G. Alvarez, "Models of general frequency-dependent selection and mating-interaction effects and the analysis of selection patterns in *Drosophila* inversion polymorphisms," *Genetics*, vol. 170, no. 3, pp. 1167–1179, 2005.

[27] M. A. Riley, M. E. Hallas, and R. C. Lewontin, "Distinguishing the forces controlling genetic variation at the Xdh locus in *Drosophila pseudoobscura*," *Genetics*, vol. 123, no. 2, pp. 359–369, 1989.

[28] S. W. Schaeffer and E. L. Miller, "Estimates of gene flow in *Drosophila pseudoobscura* determined from nucleotide sequence analysis of the alcohol dehydrogenase region," *Genetics*, vol. 132, no. 2, pp. 471–480, 1992.

[29] M. Kovacevic and S. W. Schaeffer, "Molecular population genetics of X-linked genes in *Drosophila pseudoobscura*," *Genetics*, vol. 156, no. 1, pp. 155–172, 2000.

[30] S. W. Schaeffer, M. P. Goetting, M. Kovacevic et al., "Evolutionary genomics of inversions in *Drosophila pseudoobscura*: evidence for epistasis," *Proceedings of the National Academy of Sciences of the United States of America*, vol. 100, no. 14, pp. 8319–8324, 2003.

[31] M. Kirkpatrick and N. Barton, "Chromosome inversions, local adaptation and speciation," *Genetics*, vol. 173, no. 1, pp. 419–434, 2006.

[32] S. W. Schaeffer, "Selection in heterogeneous environments maintains the gene arrangement polymorphism of *Drosophila pseudoobscura*," *Evolution*, vol. 62, no. 12, pp. 3082–3099, 2008.

[33] R. de Frutos, "Changes of chromosomal polymorphism in experimental cage populations of *Drosophila subobscura*," *Genetica*, vol. 49, no. 2-3, pp. 139–151, 1978.

[34] W. W. Anderson, C. Oshima, T. Watanabe, T. Dobzhansky, and O. Pavlovsky, "Genetics of natural populations. XXXIX. A test of the possible influence of two insecticides on the chromosomal polymorphism in *Drosophila pseudoobscura*," *Genetics*, vol. 58, no. 3, pp. 423–434, 1968.

[35] O. Pavlovsky and T. Dobzhansky, "Genetics of natural populations. XXXVII. The coadapted system of chromosomal variants in a population of *Drosophila pseudoobscura*," *Genetics*, vol. 53, no. 5, pp. 843–854, 1966.

[36] A. R. Templeton, "Analysis of selection in populations observed over a sequence of consecutive generations - I. Some one locus models with a single, constant fitness component per genotype," *Theoretical and Applied Genetics*, vol. 45, no. 5, pp. 179–191, 1974.

[37] R. Elandt-Johnson, *Probability Models and Statistical Methods in Genetics*, John Willey & Sons, London, UK, 1971.

[38] B. S. Weir, *Genetic Data Analysis*, Sinnauer Associates, Sunderland, Mass, USA, 1990.

[39] R. R. Sokal, F. J. Rohlf, and Biometry, *The Principles and Practice of Statistics in Biological Research*, W. H. Freeman and Company, New York, NY, USA, 3rd edition, 1995.

[40] P. A. Umina, A. R. Weeks, M. R. Kearney, S. W. McKechnie, and A. A. Hoffmann, "Evolution: a rapid shift in a classic clinal pattern in *Drosophila* reflecting climate change," *Science*, vol. 308, no. 5722, pp. 691–693, 2005.

[41] F. J. Ayala and M. Coluzzi, "Chromosome speciation: humans, *Drosophila*, and mosquitoes," *Proceedings of the National Academy of Sciences of the United States of America*, vol. 102, supplement 1, pp. 6535–6542, 2005.

10

Free-Radical Polymer Science Structural Cancer Model: A Review

Richard C. Petersen

Department of Biomaterials and Biomedical Engineering, The University of Alabama at Birmingham, SDB 539, 1919 7th Avenue South, Birmingham, AL 35294, USA

Correspondence should be addressed to Richard C. Petersen; richbme@uab.edu

Academic Editors: S. Fukushige, K. Jung, and S.-Y. Shieh

Polymer free-radical lipid alkene chain-growth biological models particularly for hypoxic cellular mitochondrial metabolic waste can be used to better understand abnormal cancer cell morphology and invasive metastasis. Without oxygen as the final electron acceptor for mitochondrial energy synthesis, protons cannot combine to form water and instead mitochondria produce free radicals and acid during hypoxia. Nonuniform bond-length shrinkage of membranes related to erratic free-radical covalent crosslinking can explain cancer-cell pleomorphism with epithelial-mesenchymal transition for irregular membrane borders that "ruffle" and warp over stiff underlying actin fibers. Further, mitochondrial hypoxic conditions produce acid that can cause molecular degradation. Subsequent low pH-activated enzymes then provide paths for invasive cell movement through tissue and eventually blood-born metastasis. Although free-radical crosslinking creates irregularly shaped membranes with structural actin-polymerized fiber extensions as filopodia and lamellipodia, due to rapid cell division the overall cell modulus (approximately stiffness) is lower than normal cells. When combined with low pH-activated enzymes and lower modulus cells, smaller cancer stem cells subsequently have a large advantage to follow molecular destructive pathways and leave the central tumor. In addition, forward structural spike-like lamellipodia protrusions can leverage to force lower-modulus cancer cells through narrow openings. By squeezing and deforming even smaller to allow for easier movement through difficult passageways, cancer cells can travel into adjacent tissues or possibly metastasize through the blood to new tissue.

1. Introduction

Cancer Fundamentals. Cancer is a pathological condition related to malignant uncontrolled rapid cell growth proliferation, invasive cell movement into adjacent tissues, and occasional metastatic spread through blood and lymph to more distant locations [1–4]. Conversely, benign tumors represent uncontrolled cell growth that does not invade other tissues [1–4]. Cancers are the result of progressive accumulations in genetic mutations through cell interactions with carcinogens such as tobacco, sunlight, radiation, infectious microbes, or certain chemicals/material [1–4]. Some genetic changes can be added by being passed along from one generation to another to increase cancer risk [1–4]. Although normal cells have limits to replication or the number of cell divisions to control growth by apoptosis cell death when necessary with a cascade of caspase enzymes, cancer cells can develop almost limitless uncontrolled growth after at least four genetic mutations [1–4], Figure 1.

Cancer cells can thus become less prone to death so that unneeded cells develop to form extra tissue known as tumors [1–4]. However, benign tumors that localize and do not invade adjacent tissue are not cancer [1–4]. Benign tumors are further often encapsulated by connective tissue [1, 4]. Conversely, malignant tumors invade adjacent tissues and can enter the blood stream to attack other organs by metastasis [1, 2, 4]. In order to become motile and invade into other tissues, major genetic cell traits change involving mutation through a process termed the epithelial-mesenchymal transition (EMT) [4]. Several important cellular alterations occur during EMT to include loss of integrin attachment between cytoskeleton actin fibers with adjacent cells and subsequent motility with invasiveness [4]. Further, EMT is characterized by large variations in cell shape that comprise loss of spheroid rounding

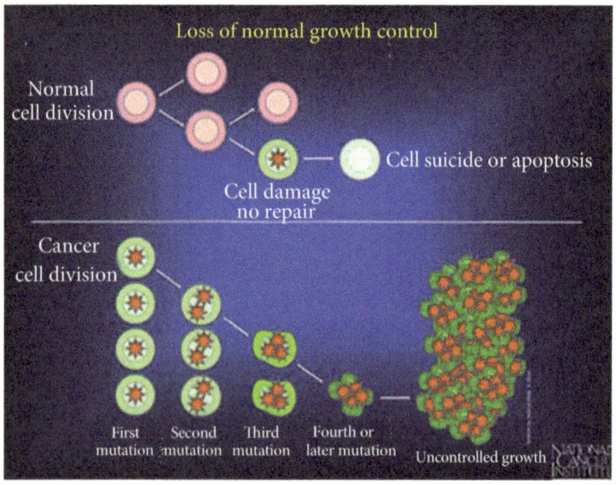

FIGURE 1: Normal cells control growth by programmed death known as apoptosis. Cancer cells conversely build genetic mutations that can result in uncontrolled growth after at least the fourth mutation. (With permission from the National Institutes of Health/Department of Health and Human Services).

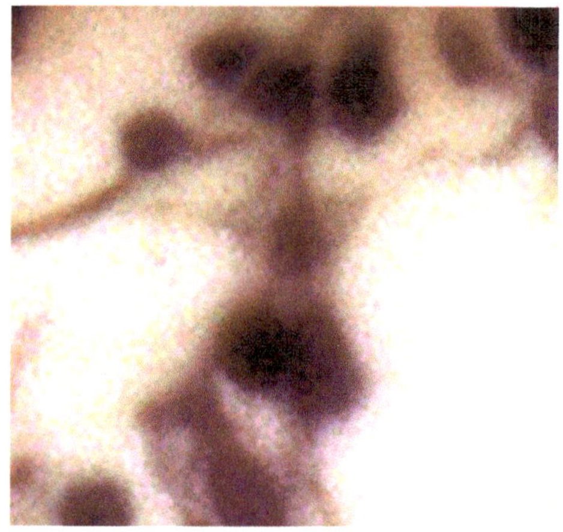

FIGURE 2: Mesenchymal stem cell with more lightly stained nucleus in bone marrow central to differentiating preosteoblastic stem cells above and below the stellate cell acquired during histomorphometry analysis.

with formation of spindle-shaped or fibroblast-like cells and irregular membrane borders especially at the invasive tumor edge [4]. EMT may also consist of possible long growth processes [4]. During EMT, cells dedifferentiate from the normal tissue phenotype toward the more primitive mesenchymal stem cell [4]. To better understand EMT by comparison between carcinoma cells derived from the epithelium with smooth normal cell membranes tightly bound together, a classical stellate mesenchymal stem cell with membrane extensions is isolated free in bone marrow extracellular space and surrounded by advancing differentiated preosteoblastic stem cells, Figure 2.

A more complete list of cancer causing risk factors includes the following.

(1) Age increases cancer risk probably by additive effects of genetic mutation and exposures [1, 3, 4].

(2) Tobacco is the most widely known cause of death and directly related to an extremely high level of cancer mortality. About 20–30 percent of all cancer deaths are related to tobacco. Cancers that increase in risk with smoking are found in the lung (highest percent of cancer-related deaths), mouth, throat, larynx, esophagus, stomach, pancreas, bladder, kidney, cervix, and in the blood with myeloid leukemia [1–5].

(3) Ultraviolet (UV) light from the sun or other sources for tanning can initiate aging and eventually cancer [1, 3, 4, 6].

(4) Ionizing radiation from radioactive sources such as nuclear explosions increases cancer for leukemia, the thyroid, breast, lung and stomach, and radon gas formed in the earth to increase lung cancer. Other sources of radiation include X-rays and cosmic rays from space [1, 3, 4, 7].

(5) Chemicals and materials from a multitude of various sources can increase cancer risk from arsenic, asbestos, styrene, benzene, benzidine, cadmium, nickel, or vinyl chloride. Carcinogenesis by chemicals was shown to occur by an initiation step with a primary application and then an irritation step that promotes cancer [1, 3, 4, 8].

(6) Infectious microbes like viruses and bacterium can even exist as a subclinical reservoir for long periods [1, 3, 4, 9].

(7) Hormones such as estrogen increase the severity for breast cancer while estrogen reduced and androgen increased prostate cancer severity [1, 3, 4, 10].

(8) Familial DNA genetic alterations where added and passed on from one generation to another [1, 4].

(9) Alcohol with more than 2 drinks per day for a long time increases the risk for cancer of the liver, mouth, throat, larynx, esophagus, and breast [1, 3, 4].

(10) Diet with high levels of fat can increase cancer risk for the colon, uterus, and prostate. Antioxidant nutrients have alternatively shown decreased risks for cancer [1, 3, 4, 11].

(11) Sedentary life style with lack of physical activity is related to overweight factors leading to cancer of the colon, esophagus, breast, kidney, and uterus [1, 3, 4].

(12) Hypoxia and ischemia from low molecular oxygen concentrations resulting in mitochondrial free radicals and acid are more general biological conditions that exist for cancer cellular activity [2, 4, 12–16]. Subsequent tumors exhibit anaerobic metabolism that produces energy without oxygen in hypoxic microenvironments [4, 12–16]. Conversely, normal tissues use oxygen for aerobic mitochondrial energy synthesis [1, 12–18].

2. Hypoxic Free Radicals and Polymerization

Mitochondria create electrons from different fuel sources of the body that flow through a series of protein enzymes and other mobile electron carriers [17, 18]. These electrons through the mitochondrial electron transport chain combine with molecular oxygen and protons to form water [17, 18]. However, imperfect formation of water by mitochondria during hypoxic low O_2 states produces free-radical reactive oxygen species (ROS) as superoxide ($O_2^{\bullet-}$), hydrogen peroxide (H_2O_2), and hydroxyl radicals ($^{\bullet}OH$) [15, 18–21]. Other reactive free-radical species can also be formed as well [19]. By definition, a free radical is a molecule that contains an unpaired electron which is highly unstable and seeks out another electron for a stable covalent bond pair [15, 22–24]. Subsequent hypoxic free-radical species are then involved in damage to lipids, proteins, and DNA [15, 18, 19, 24]. As a result, hypoxic low-oxygen concentrations of tumors emphasize the strong influence that free radicals play during the development of cancer such that reactive oxygen species are considered oncogenic [1, 12–16, 20].

In terms of similarities with a basic chemistry understanding for molecular pathobiology, polymer science unsaturated alkene chain-growth free-radical covalent bond formation with increased liquid/resin viscosity by molecular crosslinking toward solid structure produces irregular shrinkage patterns [22]. Further, from polymer science free radicals polymerize unsaturated resins to produce increased material modulus (or stiffness) with higher density measured as reduced bulk volume percent from shorter interatomic bond distances [22, 25–27]. In fact, the most characteristic subsequent manifestations of overall polymerization crosslinking is material shrinkage with some internal stresses and warpage [22, 25–27]. A highly common free-radical cure method in past has been a resin system with styrene monomer and dibenzoyl peroxide, depicted in Figure 3, to illustrate free-radical reactive secondary sequence by crosslinking across a carbon-carbon (C=C) vinyl double bond [22].

During similar structure-related hypoxic free-radical pathobiology, cell pleomorphism occurs as part of cancer cell EMT by irregular invaginated lipid membranes containing extensive folds associated with possible new lipid polymerization chemistry [22, 28] in the presence of membrane ruffles [4]. EMT pleomorphism further includes extreme differences in cell shapes/sizes [4] related to increased overall tumor mass density from a stiffer (or higher modulus) denser stroma of fibrotissue [4, 29, 30]. In advanced carcinomas EMT-dedifferentiated desmoplastic stroma produces a harder denser overall tumor mass related to a more aggressive grade of cancer that in time becomes an acellular collagenous extracellular matrix [4]. Relative to free-radical covalent bond formation to produce material structure, increasing density surface oxidation crosslinking of rubber reduces oxygen diffusion into the deeper subsurface layers [31].

Pertinent to cancer pathophysiology, capillary distance has been measured in tissue showing a respective decrease in both oxygen concentration and pH [4, 14, 32], where increasing hypoxic mitochondrial electron-transport free radicals would be expected to produce some biologic structure from covalent bonding. As increased biologic structure limits O_2 diffusion more, a new fall in pH with lower O_2 would be expected by interfering even further with capillary diffusion of molecules. Because oxygen is fundamentally critical to prevent cell death, tumors found over 0.2 mm away from blood vessels fail to grow [4, 14, 32] which is the approximate distance for O_2 diffusion through living tissue before a zero concentration develops [4, 14, 32]. The low pH eventually becomes an overall result of lactic acid production by anaerobic mitochondria glycolysis energy synthesis [4, 14]. On the other hand, throughout efficient aerobic cellular respiration in the mitochondria, oxygen is fundamental during energy synthesis to form water from the electron respiratory transport chain and proton gradient [21, 33–35]. Part of mitochondrial respiratory aerobic energy synthesis includes one of the most well-studied enzymes ever with cytochrome c that was identified in earliest National Cancer Institute research, Figure 4. The enzyme cytochrome c is part of the electron transport chain and localizes in the intermembrane space but can leak into the cytosol to participate in cell death by apoptosis with the caspase enzymes [1–4].

During hypoxia, cells switch to anaerobic glycolysis to produce lactic acid [14], but with alternate aerobic respiration energy synthesis reactive oxygen species with other free radicals and also protons start to form [21, 33–35]. However, cancer cells can adapt to hypoxia by high glucose uptake with anaerobic glycolysis and lactic acid production to minimize free radical formation from the mitochondria [4, 14, 16, 36]. Subsequent hypoxic cancer conditions then not only produce large amounts of free radicals [4, 15] but also contribute to acid formation for a much lower pH microenvironment [4, 14, 16, 36]. Through a mechanism known as the Warburg effect [14, 16, 36], cancer cells continue to produce energy by aerobic glycolysis even with O_2 present [14, 16, 36] possibly as mentioned before as an adaptive mechanism to help limit hypoxic free-radical formation by the mitochondria [36]. Free radicals may represent a potentially more serious threat than lower pH since free-radical molecular structure through the rapid chemistry of covalent crosslinking limits oxygen diffusion progressively as a primary source for cancer pathology through continual increasing levels of free radicals and acids from oxidatively stressed mitochondria.

In addition to chronic infections with widespread inflammatory cells, chronic inflammation has been recognized as a major common cause of cancer promotion that further involves free radicals [3, 4, 19, 37, 38]. Sources of chronic inflammation can include microbial/viral infections or toxic/allergic substances and also obesity [3, 4, 19, 37, 38]. Dysplasia occurs in chronic inflammation and also in benign growths before premalignant cell proliferation [4, 37, 38]. Cells that invade through the basement membrane are then considered malignant [4, 37, 38]. Pleomorphism occurs as a sign of dysplasia with cells displaying large variations in cell sizes and shape morphologies with unusually large deeply stained nuclei [4, 37, 38]. Mitotic cellular division is also high such that the increased possibility of malignant transformation through EMT can occur by benign cells

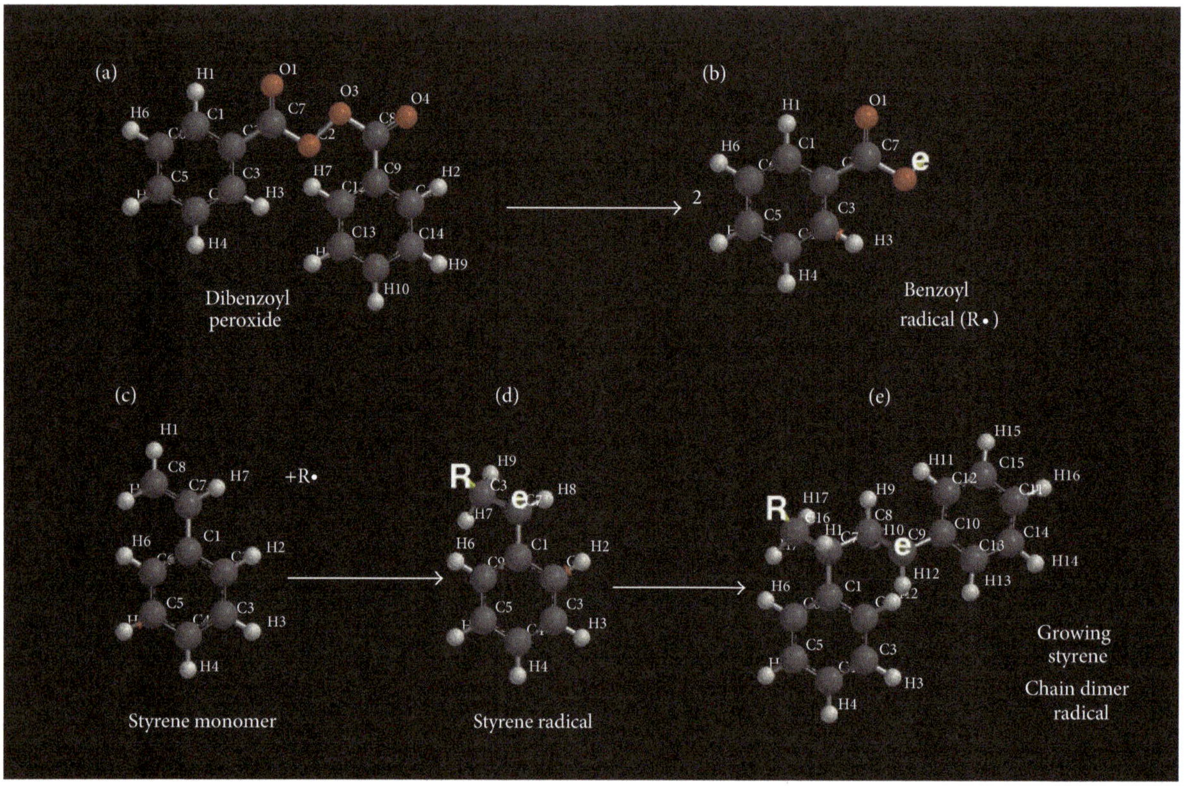

FIGURE 3: (a) Dibenzoyl peroxide commonly known as benzoyl peroxide or BPO dissociates into two molecules to provide (b) benzoyl free radicals (R$^\bullet$). (c) In liquid form, styrene monomer with vinyl-group C7 and C8 (C=C) double pi (π) bond upper left of molecule is attacked by R$^\bullet$ to add a benzoyl group on one of the carbon atoms. (d) Subsequent styrene radical formation depicted by "e" on the opposite vinyl carbon atom can now enter into a reaction with a new styrene molecule C=C vinyl group. (e) A second styrene molecule can add the benzoyl-styrene radical on the C=C vinyl group for the growing chain to form a free radical again as "e" on the opposite vinyl carbon atom. Free-radical additions through the liquid styrene monomer C=C vinyl groups continue the polymerization process by the reactive secondary sequence method a multitude of times to eventually form a solid.

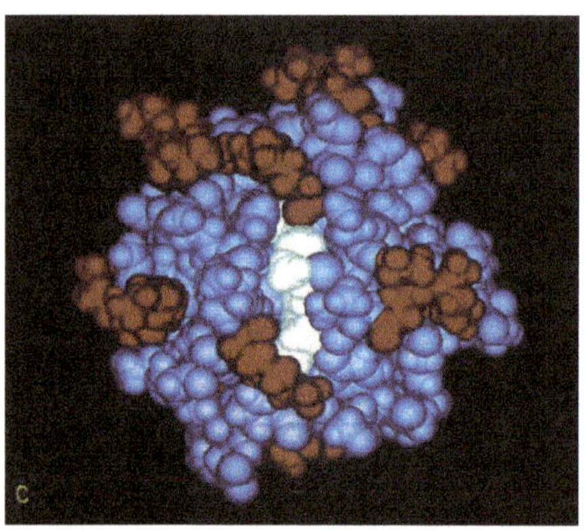

FIGURE 4: Image depicting cytochrome c which is a small soluble globular protein used in the mitochondrial electron transfer chain that carries electrons as radicals with other mobile transporter carriers ultimately to combine with oxygen and protons to form water [4, 17, 18]. (With permission from the National Institutes of Health/Department of Health and Human Services).

unrestrained from normal process in the dysplastic states [4, 37, 38]. In addition, inflammatory cells mediate cancer progression through free radicals that can mutate DNA, produce epigenetic alternations with DNA methylation, increase cell proliferation, oxidize lipids, crosslink proteins, and promote angiogenesis [4, 19].

3. Other Important Fundamentals in the Study of Cancer

(1) Angiogenesis or blood vessel development was shown to be an important part of tumor expansion that could be used as a pharmaceutical chemotherapeutic anti-cancer target. Later research showed the pathology that tumors produce factors to encourage angiogenesis with new abnormal blood vessels to support cancer growth. Tumors cannot increase to more than 1-2 mm in diameter without growing blood vessels to bring in oxygen and nutrients [2, 4].

(2) Apoptosis is a normal cell physiologic death that helps to prevent unwanted cell growth. However, tumors on the other hand contain cancer cells with mutations that prevent normal apoptosis. Cells lacking apoptosis death regulatory pathways are then more resistant to death in addition to chemotherapeutic cancer cytotoxic agents [4, 39].

(3) Tumors secrete protease enzymes that degrade collagen protein to provide exits for entering the blood stream and metastasizing to more distant tissue sites [2, 4, 14, 40].

(4) DNA methylation can turn a gene off [3, 4, 41–44]. Hydrogen abstraction has been commonly identified as part of a free-radical lipid peroxidation breakdown process that produces characteristic biomarkers. Since breaking a carbon-carbon bond requires much less energy than breaking a hydrogen-carbon bond [22, 23], highly reactive methyl and other small acyl-free radicals could be considered as sources for DNA methylation during periods of lipid peroxidation or during hypoxia with the generation of free-radical electrons and acid [22].

(5) Tumor suppressor genes inhibit cell proliferation and are targets of carcinogenesis when such genes are inactivated. For example, proteins from several viruses bind to a tumor suppressor gene to stop manifestation of downstream functional activities to subsequently promote cancer. The most common tumor suppressor gene is the p53 gene that initiates apoptosis through the p53 protein [4, 45–47].

(6) Protooncogenes code for cell growth or proliferation and can mutate to become oncogenes to cause cancer, Figure 5. Common proto-oncogenes can code for growth factor proteins, cytoplasmic enzymes, membrane receptors with tyrosine kinase enzymes, or transcription factors in the nucleus for cell division [4, 48–50].

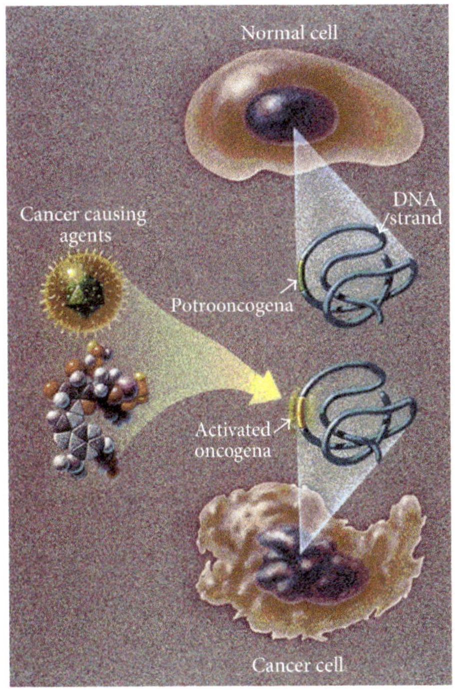

FIGURE 5: National Cancer Institute illustration shows the stages of how a normal round cell is converted to a cancer cell with shape irregularities for both the nuclear and plasma cell membranes when an oncogene becomes activated. (With permission from the National Institutes of Health/Department of Health and Human Services).

4. Irregular Membrane Ruffling by Free-Radical Crosslinking

In order to better simplify cancer fundamentals into a molecular biology polymer approach for an easier mechanistic understanding theory of cellular and tissue changes during carcinogenesis, figures in imaging from the National Cancer Institute are helpful. A typical National Cancer Institute consensus illustration, Figure 5, depicts the basic morphology that a cancer cell has irregular borders with membrane wrinkling as ruffling when compared to the identical normal rounded cell. In addition, Figure 5 shows how an oncogene is activated by a cancer causing agent so that instead of normal cell division, oncogenic cellular DNA damage causes cancer. Cancer cell nuclei are also misshapen into strange unusual irregular shapes compared to the normal rounded oval nuclei with smooth borders. For a plausible explanation regarding the membrane irregular borders with ruffling in cancer cells, free radicals need some understanding. As a constant source, free radicals produced during hypoxia are found at high levels in cancer cells [1, 12–16]. Further, excessive free radicals as reactive oxygen species attack unsaturated fatty acids found as lipids in cell membranes with carbon-carbon (C=C) double bonds [22, 24].

One of the most characteristic features for free-radical covalent bonding in a liquid to increase viscoelastic solid structure with increased modulus and density properties becomes most apparent in materials that polymerize by electron-pair chain-growth polymerization as the linear/volumetric cure shrinkage [22, 25–27, 51, 52]. In fact, free radicals are engineered for specific materials science application to crosslink molecules with consequent cure shrinkage and possibly warpage as one the most distinguishing material problems of extensive polymer electron-pair bonding [22, 51, 52]. Because shrinkage is not necessarily perfect with inhomogeneous material, nonuniform electron pairing in curing in addition to increasing the modulus can create residual internal stresses to produce warpage of materials that weakens parts [51, 52]. Warpage is particularly accentuated during free-radical polymer curing with thin film coatings of variable thickness without good support [52]. As covalent single sigma (σ) bonds form by replacing C=C pi (π) bonds during reactive secondary sequence chain growth [22, 25–27], polymer chains draw together from more distant van der Waals intermolecular attraction forces and chain-entanglement equilibrium distances to closer covalent distances with increasing chain entanglement that reduce bulk volume by linear/volumetric cure shrinkage [22, 25–27]. Free-radical double-bond conversion to single bonds is thermodynamically favorable and forms an exothermic polymerization even without extra energy added at room temperature [51]. Consequently, solutions of unsaturated lipids that undergo thermoset free-radical chain growth will

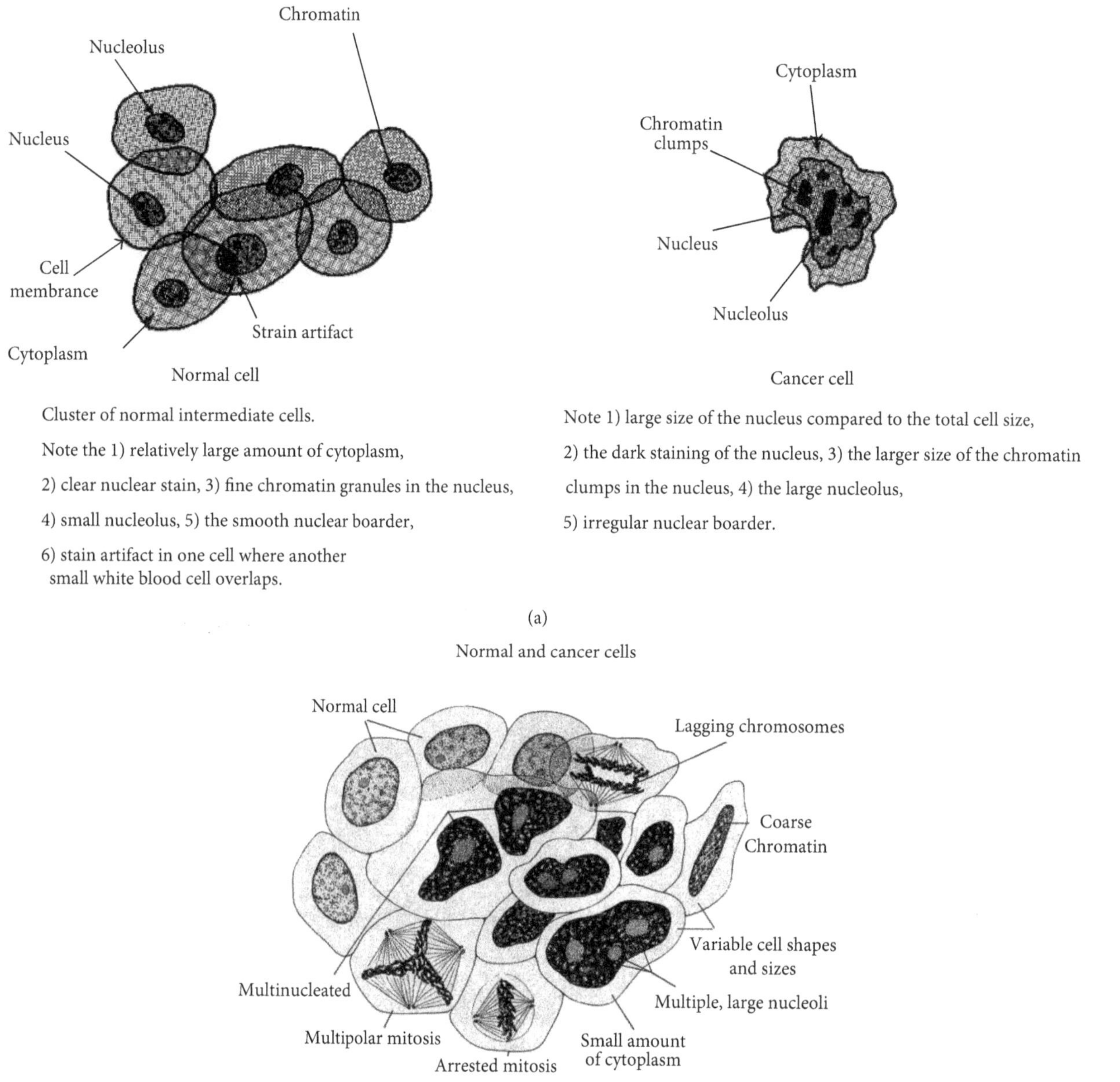

FIGURE 6: (a) Graphics and description comparing normal round cells and cancer cells with both irregular nuclear and plasma cell membranes (With permission from the National Institutes of Health/Department of Health and Human Services). (b) The round normal and cancerous characteristics with warped irregular borders are identified. (With permission from the National Institutes of Health/Department of Health and Human Services).

also produce linear/volumetric cure shrinkage without added energy [22, 25–27, 51, 52].

Cytoskeleton actin fibers provide tensile strength and support to the cell [4] so that the composite plasma cell membrane with lipid oils and phosphate groups offers conditions that maintain separate mediums to accentuate free-radical polymerization warping particularly as an outer veil thin film. Hydrocarbon lipid molecules drawn together at a rounder border would require some invagination to wrinkle inward especially when combined with coupling to underlying rigid fibers resulting in the possible explanation for common ruffling irregular membrane appearances of cancer cells depicted in consensus National Cancer Institute Figures 5, 6(a), 6(b), and 7(a)–7(d). Lipid oil with an unsaturated linoleic/oleic fatty acid combination for free-radical crosslinking has previously demonstrated a wrinkling and warpage during a solidification polymerization process [22]. As well as irregular plasma cell membrane borders on the outer periphery of a cancer cell, the nuclear membranes are misshapen and nuclear to cytoplasm ratios increase [36, 37]. In addition to normal cell round morphology changing by EMT to irregular membrane border patterns with invaginations in cancer, other common findings are presented as basic consensus for changes in cancer cells through the National

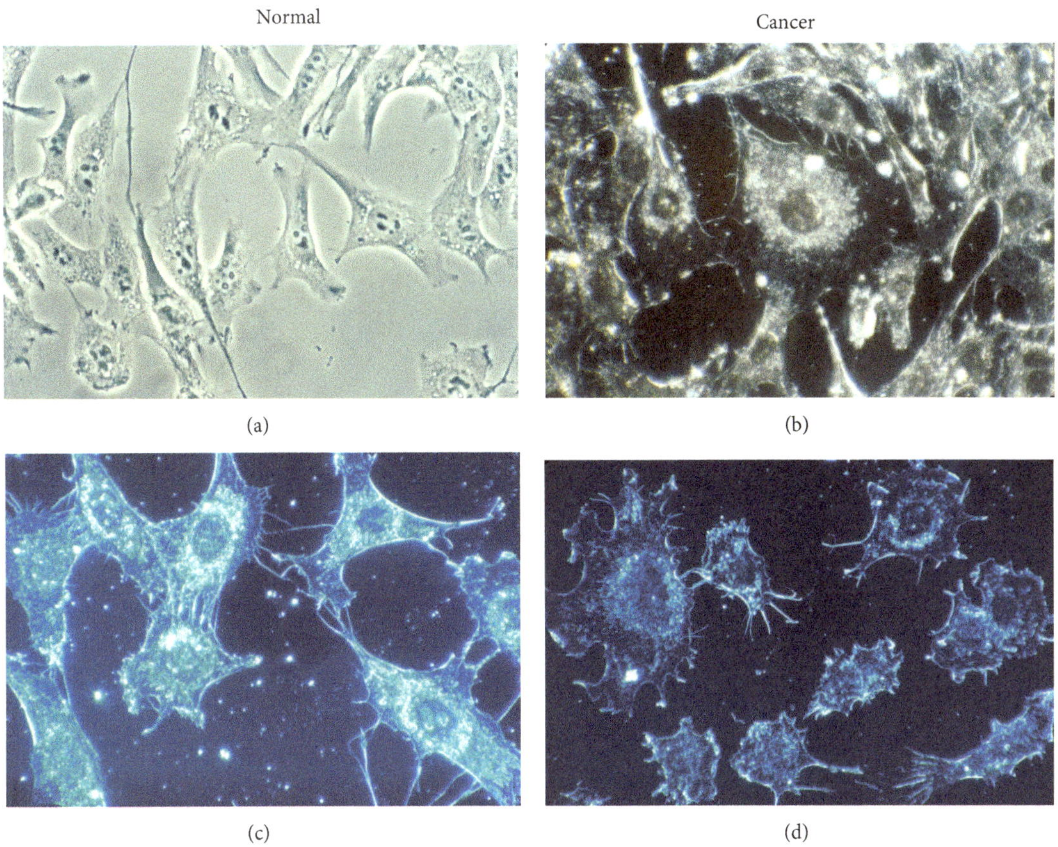

FIGURE 7: Normal cells on the left and cancer cells with more spike-like membrane extensions on the right in culture from human connective tissue. At a magnification of 500x, the cells were illuminated by darkfield amplified contrast technique. (a) Normal cells compared to (b) cancer cells. (c) Normal Cells compared to (d) cancer cells (with permission from the National Institutes of Health/Department of Health and Human Services).

Cancer Institute with two separate illustrations, Figures 6(a) and 6(b), as.

(1) darker staining nucleus,

(2) coarse chromatin and clumping,

(3) more irregular nuclear border,

(4) less cytoplasm and larger nuclei,

(5) multinucleated,

(6) variable pleomorphism in cell sizes and shapes.

Cell cultures that show normal cells with smoother membrane outlines compared to cancer cells with more irregular membranes help to document the plasma cell membrane spike-type extensions that form deeper invaginated irregular borders as part of the EMT with transformation to cancer, Figures 7(a)–7(d).

Another more common intracellular organelle membrane feature possibly related to covalent C=C double-bond crosslink shrinkage and thin-film warpage [52] includes the most distinctive inner membrane features of the mitochondria with the high convolutions called cristae [17, 18, 33–35], Figures 8(a) and 8(b). The convoluted mitochondrial cristae that make up the inner membrane serve to create an impermeable confining larger surface area for important biologic electron interactions during aerobic respiratory energy synthesis [17, 18, 33–35]. Subsequent electron flow during energy synthesis [17, 18, 33–35] should further be an extreme source for free-radical lipid crosslinking through C=C double bonds to provide the structural convolutions noted in the mitochondria. The mitochondrial interior inside the inner membrane is a gel of approximately 50% protein [18]. Most of the mitochondrial protein studies thus far are not fibers but rather soluble or globular enzymes [17, 18, 33–35] that would not provide cytoskeleton-type support like structural fibers in a composite [51]. During crosslink shrinkage by high concentrations of free radicals from the electron transport chain, the lipid hydrocarbons would accentuate warpage into convolutions of the thin-film inner membrane without the more stable influence from reinforcing stacked planar fibers provided by the plasma cell membrane or nuclear membrane.

Proteins contain ionizable groups on the terminal carboxylic acid end, the terminal amino end, and many side chain groups to function as buffers [18]. Proteins also generally exist with a negative charge at physiologic pH 7.2 [18]. Since proteins maintain a negative charge intracellularly and are further the major blood buffer as part of the plasma [17], the ideal medium is available to sequester radicals from the mitochondrial electron transport chain and buffer protons

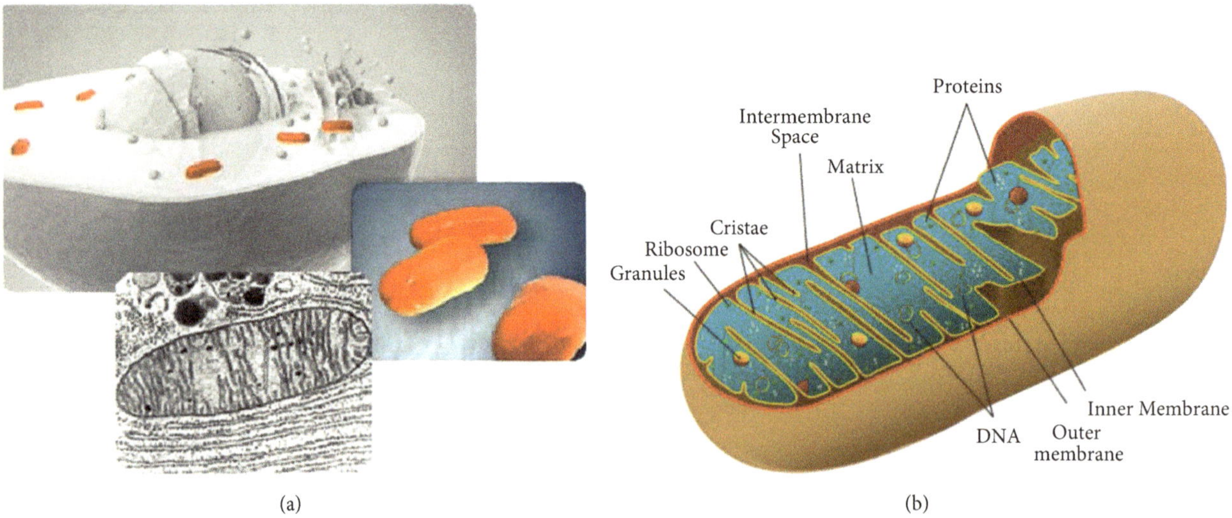

FIGURE 8: Mitochondrial inner membrane cristae (a) 3D illustration upper left shows spheroidal mitochondria in red located peripherally circumferential around the nucleus and SEM below showing convoluted cristae. (b) Mitochondrion illustration with tortuous cristae ((a) with permission from the National Institutes of Health/Department of Health and Human Services).

from the proton gradient in the form of the multiple protein enzymes that help synthesize energy aerobically by oxygen with water as the final product. In fact, amino acid side chains on hemoglobin protein [53] and even in short peptides [54, 55] are known to sequester radicals with tyrosine, histidine, and cysteine residues [54, 55]. Further, radicals can be delocalized from a side chain into the peptide bond [54, 55]. Although the spin density for radical delocalization from a side chain into the peptide bond atoms is small for pentapeptides, projections could be large depending on peptide bond conformational changes or electrostatics [55]. In addition, proteins could increase radical delocalization through the much higher numbers of peptide bonds than a small peptide molecule so that radicals from the electron mitochondrial transport chain could be stabilized for even longer periods than normal radical intermediates studied thus far. So, instead of radicals disseminating into different pathologies constantly, much longer induction periods would be made available by proteins acting as antioxidants, but nevertheless could still become oversaturated eventually to act as an electron pool or source for free-radical damaging properties. Still, free-radical crosslinking of the mitochondrial inner membrane would help explain the extreme convolutions that structure into an impermeable medium.

5. Cell Movement and Lamellipodia

A state-of-the-art scanning electron microscope (SEM) shows the intricate details for irregular plasma cell membrane borders that form ruffling and an extensive network of structural spike-like ridges that project long distances, Figure 9(a). A more complete conception of an SEM 3D-enhanced National Cancer Institute image shows how a cancer cell and its long processes called lamellipodia move on a cellular tissue surface, Figure 9(b). Carcinogenesis requires cell movement with EMT and cell shape changes for metastasis and invasion [2, 4, 56]. Subsequent cell movement involves reactive oxygen species that includes H_2O_2 as common denominators for the formation of the hydroxyl-free ($^{\bullet}OH$) radical which in turn creates protrusions at the cell edges [57, 58]. Cell movement is directed through extracellular chemical gradients by chemotaxis [2, 4, 59]. Free radicals that form as a constant source from reactive oxygen species including H_2O_2 have been shown to act as key chemotactic factors to regulate chemoattractants that bind to cell membranes with actin polymerization for cell migration toward H_2O_2 and other reactive oxygen species [60–62]. Further, the traveling cell is polarized by microtubules radiating from the centrosome near the nucleus to the outer cell edges [63, 64] to grow actin protrusions with adhesions between the extracellular matrix that contract in the forward direction [4, 57, 63, 64]. The cell protrusions are long lamellipodia extensions and short focal adhesive filopodia constructed from actin fibers that polymerize at the advancing forward edge [4, 57, 64]. Conversely, depolymerization of actin occurs away from the advancing cell edge [4, 57, 64]. Cytoskeleton microtubule and actin fibers are polarized positively near the cell membrane to elongate [57, 64] and negatively by microtubules toward the organizing centrosome center near the nucleus [56, 65]. A strong long-range static electric field develops on the mitochondria and also on the microtubules that lie in close contact [66] resulting in a possible delocalization mechanism for the electron transport chain during periods of mitochondrial oxidative stress. Polymerization of actin fibers at the plus end forms protrusions that contain focal adhesions with the extracellular matrix so contractions provide forward movement [4, 57, 63, 64]. In addition, depolymerization occurs at the negative ends of the actin fibers on the rear edge of cell movement for release of focal adhesions and in addition making actin monomers available to be recycled for polymerization at the forward positive actin protrusive end [4, 57, 64].

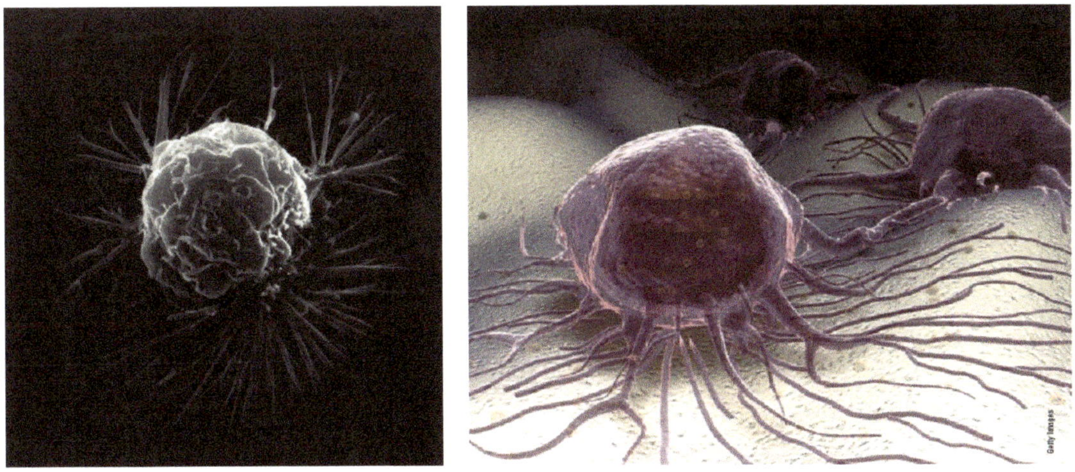

(a) (b)

FIGURE 9: (a) SEM of a breast cancer cell that clearly shows both the soft petals of membrane ruffling and much longer lamellipodia spiking extensions. (b) A scanning electron microscopic 3D-enhanced NIH image of cancer cells and lamellipodia spike processes on a cellular tissue surface (with permission from the National Institutes of Health/Department of Health and Human Services).

Free-radical crosslinking and agglomeration with weaker secondary bonding previously described account for atoms, molecules, and larger molecular chains being drawn together [22, 25–27, 51, 52] to provide a possible mechanism for forward movement in the contraction process. Lipid peroxidation products with low molecular weights and a C=C double bond have demonstrated high crosslinking with both unsaturated fatty acids [22] and protein [67]. Further, a polyunsaturated fatty acid with 6 C=C double bonds has been shown to activate cells as a chemoattractant to migrate during reorganization of actin fiber in lamellipodia using a strong free-radical oxidant as peroxinitrate [68], with strong free-radical crosslinking indication for contraction through covalent bond shrinkage [22]. In addition to lipid free-radical crosslinking across C=C double bonds as a reactive secondary sequence, amino acid side chains of protein are modified at about 50 percent of the residue by the hydroxyl-free radical formed from H_2O_2 [69]. Further, proteins are found to agglomerate or crosslink most notably through the amino acid tyrosine [70, 71] with metal-catalyzed reactions [70].

While most cancer cells studied through the National Institute of Health figures presented demonstrate extensive spike protrusions that could greatly interfere with movement and prevent leakage through a small tissue pore, the more aggressive cancer cells have a smaller membrane area that allows the lower modulus cells to more easily squeeze through and penetrate small openings in the endothelium [72]. Nevertheless, membrane protrusions are most frequent on the leading edge of cancer cells during metastasis movement [73]. Formation of the leading edge with cytoskeleton actin fibers that shape lamellipodia [4, 73] is only about 200 nanometers thick [4, 74, 75]. In addition, the actin fibers orient along the axis of the membrane protrusions so that the modulus is highest to resist deformations in the lamellipodia plane and much lower in the perpendicular plane [73]. As a result, the leading lamellipodia edge can push with leverage through the smallest openings and still deform on the sides to start squeezing through extremely narrow spaces for escape into new tissue [73]. Fiber polarizations from the negative centrosome end near the nucleus to the positively charged plasma cell membrane side [63–65] are thought to be responsible for the forward polymerization of the actin fibers during cell movement [57, 63, 64]. As such, electrons conducted from microtubules into actin fibers by highly charged mitochondria [66] overstressed under hypoxic conditions should accumulate at accentuated levels through the electron transport chain deprived of oxygen that could help account for a portion of the free radical polymerization mechanisms with actin fibers. In fact, actin has been shown to restructure under free radical conditions with H_2O_2 to increase cell motility [76]. Regarding H_2O_2 ability to polymerize actin by free-radical chain lengthening mechanisms, H_2O_2 has proven to be an exceptional initiator for free-radical polymerization in polyester resin formulations [77]. By related free-radical reactive oxygen species biological chemistry, actin polymerization has also been observed in macrophages exposed to oxidized low-density lipids [78]. Further, high levels of H_2O_2 and other reactive oxygen species are found in various cancer cells [79].

6. Nucleus Changes with Free-Radical DNA Methylation

Cancer initiation and progression have been linked to increasing free-radicals following oxidative stress and reactive oxygen species that are continuously produced by mitochondria during cell metabolism [4, 15, 79–81]. Cancer cells are characterized by increased reactive oxygen species and accumulation while the mitochondria are considered the major source for reactive oxygen species [81]. Subsequent hypoxic mitochondrial free-radical species are then involved in damage to lipids, proteins, and DNA [4, 15, 18, 19, 24, 81]. As a result, hypoxic low oxygen concentrations of tumors emphasize the strong influence that free radicals play during the development of cancer such that reactive oxygen species are considered oncogenic [1, 12–16, 20, 81]. A major role for free radicals produced by hypoxia or ischemia through mitochondrial metabolism includes crosslinking with either simple electron pairing or as extensive reactive secondary sequence C=C double-bond chain growth. A major effect of free-radical crosslinking molecules is a characteristic volumetric shrinkage and warpage [22, 25–27, 51, 52]. By similar free-radical crosslink chemistry, biologic crosslinking could explain the coarse or clumping chromatin depicted in Figures 6(a)-6(b), coupling of DNA to DNA or DNA to protein [15], abnormal cell shrinkage with warpage and irregular membrane borders [4, 37, 38, 59, 66], membrane ruffling [4], protein agglomeration with insoluble accumulation [15, 70, 71], and actin polymerization [76]. Also, as the nuclear membrane structures, a greater amount of the cell is constrained within the nucleus [37, 38, 59].

In addition to genetic DNA alterations or changes in the DNA sequence [4, 14], epigenetics that alter the gene slightly further influence cancer growth and metastasis [4, 80]. Hypoxia is already accepted as a general condition that promotes tumors [14, 82, 83], supports cancer recurrence [83], intensifies malignancy [14, 82, 83], increases metastases [14, 83, 84], and inhibits chemo/radio therapies [14, 83]. The main epigenetic change is by DNA methylation that can be linked to hypoxic-free radical environments with acyl-radical breakdown products [4, 22, 41–44, 85]. Molecular breakdown is further a well-known biomarker when free radicals accumulate with unsaturated lipid fatty acids [86–89] especially when combined with lower pH acid [22] that occurs during hypoxia in mitochondrial metabolism [22]. Further, thermodynamics for bond dissociations studied for lipid peroxidation favors acyl radical formation over hydrogen bond dissociation as a key source for DNA methylation [22]. Hypermethylation of DNA subsequently causes gene silencing of particular importance for tumor suppressor genes [4, 80]. Oxidation of DNA is another risk factor for mutation that modifies bases to favor cancer [4]. Subsequent long-term stages of hypoxic-related free radicals particularly seen with chronic inflammation then account for advanced chromosomal damage with DNA base substitutions particularly through purine replacement by a pyrimidine termed a $G \rightarrow T$ transversion, DNA crosslinks, and chromosomal breaks [4].

7. Metastasis

Although a cancer tumor can invade adjacent tissue directly, most cancer deaths occur by metastasis to distant tissue through the blood [2, 4, 14]. Metastasis takes place through an extremely biocomplex sequence of events in several stages, Figures 10(a) and 10(b). Biocomplexity is a hallmark of cancer that involves both a low pH acidic environment [4, 14] and free radicals [4, 15, 79–81] produced from hypoxic conditions [4, 14, 82–84, 90]. Metastasis further involves cell motility with EMT cell shape changes [4] and also destructive tissue breakdown by pH-activated protein enzymes [4, 14, 91]. Further, focal contacts develop between the extracellular matrix and filopodia that extend as short spikes off the advancing lamellipodia lengthening arms [4]. Microtubules polarized by electric fields influenced through close association with mitochondria [66] have capability to conduct electrons or transport free radical species rapidly to the plasma cell membrane. Free radicals available as a result of low oxygen concentrations leaking from the electron transport chain can then help to provide adhesive bonds by electron pairing and secondary bonding forces during cell migration through focal contacts with the filopodia. In fact, unsaturated lipids that have C=C double bonds with reactive secondary sequence capability [22] are known to influence cell adhesion by focal contacts with the extracellular matrix [92].

The first advanced invasive stage involves attachment of cancer cells from the primary tumor to the basement membrane of local blood vessel endothelial cells [4]. Endothelial cells compose a single layer that wraps around to form a tube inside the blood vessels which are further depicted in Figure 10(b). The next stage involves local breakdown of the endothelial cell barrier by cancer cell protease enzymes filled with both free radicals and acids [4, 93, 94]. As a related biocomplex event, the oxidation of the amino acid cysteine by reactive oxygen species H_2O_2 includes disulfide crosslinks that are involved with metastasis and reduced enzyme activity [95].

Cancer cells with greater metastasis potential have a lower modulus and lower viscosity than normal cells with the ability to deform more in addition to the pleomorphic smaller sizes with less cell membrane area [50, 91, 96]. Cell stiffness increases with organized actin fibers of the cytoskeleton and during cancer transformation actin fibers are disrupted into irregular networks that results in a lower modulus or less stiff, more deformable cell [96]. Conversely, overall increased tumor tissue density is a risk factor for cancer [30, 97, 98]. Increasing stroma density is further characterized by increased collagen deposition [98] that provides better traction forces with focal adhesions to promote cell migration for metastasis [30, 99]. Also, cells tend to migrate toward stiffer substrates [99]. Through a similar reference to cell structure, cancer cell pseudopods with high modulus actin fibers [4] provide stiff leverage movement through narrow gaps to invade other tissue, Figure 11. But, in opposition again with another molecular biology reverse structural-related mechanism, tissue degradation from cancer hypoxic-associated lower pH with protease enzymes removes intercellular adhesion to more easily release cells from the primary tumor and to carve out space for invading cancer cells [4]. Consequently, the smaller cancer cells with lower moduli can subsequently be freed from the primary tumor to move through small openings [100] produced by the common protease breakdown and enter the blood stream. On the other hand, as larger cancer cells invade, metastasis then most commonly progresses when cells get trapped in capillaries to spread into new tissue [4].

8. Protease Enzymes

Cancers revert by EMT to more primitive less differentiated cells with increased acid production [4, 14]. Subsequent

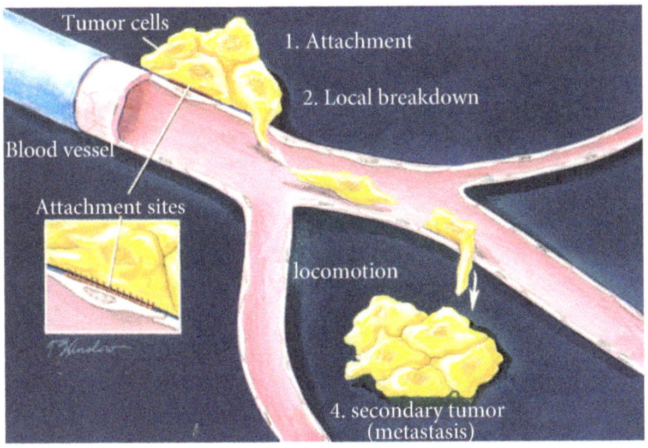

(a)

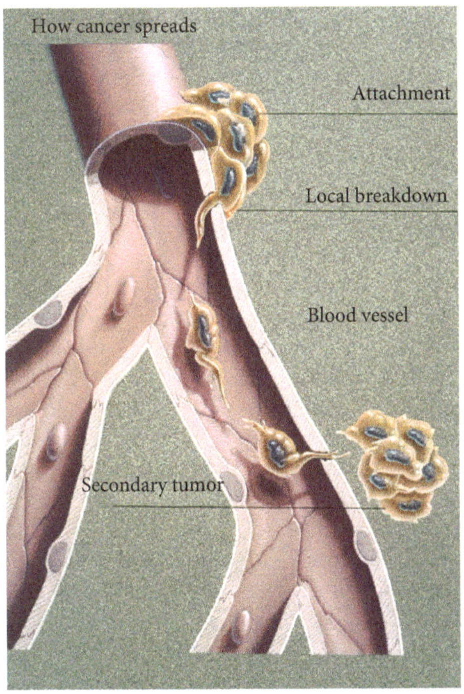

(b)

FIGURE 10: (a) Schematic drawing for the stages of metastasis (1) attachment (2) local breakdown with lamellipodia penetration into a blood vessel (3) locomotion with lamellipodia to exit from blood vessel (4) secondary tumor. (b) Once metastatic cells are attached to the vessel wall basement membrane (a physical barrier that separates tissue components), cancer can break through with stiff lamellipodia on the leading edge and the help of protease enzymes. Cancer cells then move through the blood stream enabling them to spread to other parts of the body. A secondary tumor may subsequently form at another site in the body. (With permission from the National Institutes of Health/Department of Health and Human Services).

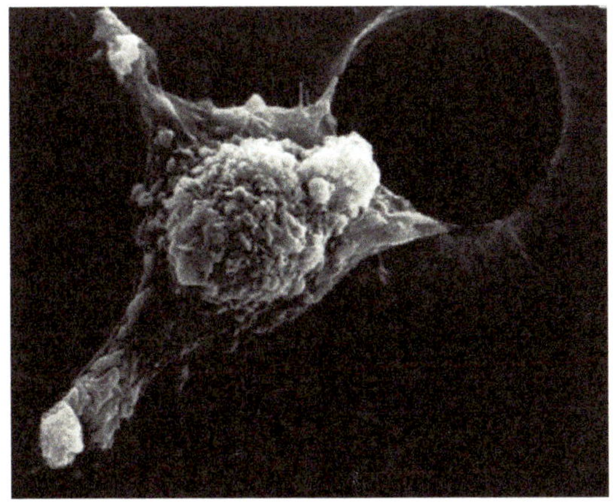

FIGURE 11: SEM of a cancer cell movement through a man-made hole involves "arms" or pseudopodia, termed lamellipodia, enabling them to migrate to other parts of the body. Locomotion cell motility is integral to the entire process of invasive metastasis. (With permission from the National Institutes of Health/Department of Health and Human Services).

protease enzymes activated by acid due to related hypoxic conditions are responsible for degrading structural fibers of the extracellular matrix [4, 14, 91]. As the extracellular matrix is broken down under hypoxic conditions at a much lower pH than normal, cancer cells can initiate paths through the extracellular matrix for cancer cell migration to spread and eventually detach into areas occupied by dying cells [4, 14]. Cancer cells can eventually even use the surrounding dead cells for a nutrition source during rapid cell proliferation by intracellular means with oncogene expression of enzymes linked to membrane receptors [4]. Further, in an unusual biocomplexity, cancer cells are able to induce stromal cells such as fibroblasts to produce H_2O_2 reactive oxygen species and lactate acid through metabolic anaerobic glycolysis to increase invasiveness [4, 14, 72]. In addition, although the pH of the interstitial fluid in the extracellular matrix surrounding a cancer tumor is lower than physiologic pH, the cancer cytosol is either neutral to slightly basic so that cancer cells develop a stronger advantage over the surrounding normal cells in the stroma [14]. Since chronic inflammation is a major cause of cancer [19, 85], inflammatory cells attracted to dead cells surrounding the cancer network would then be expected to increase free radicals further above the high levels observed in hypoxic cancer tissues [79].

Cancer cell adaptation to high free-radical concentrations and the extreme lower pH in the surrounding extracellular matrix at a much superior level to normal cells [4, 14] must require buffering. Since proteins delocalize radicals [101] and generally exist with a negative charge at physiologic pH 7.2 [18] to maintain a negative charge of protein intracellularly [17] and further are the main buffers in the blood [17], increased oncogene protein expression at the plasma cell membrane level [4] might explain superior cancer cell buffering. Of particular interest in buffering low pH extracellular matrix microenvironments are protein kinase enzymes in the cytosol associated with hydrophobic protein membrane receptors [4]. In fact, the majority of cancers are associated even through intracellular protein kinase to membrane receptor ligand binding with the extracellular matrix by phosphorylations on intracellular tyrosine amino acid residues [4, 102, 103]. Phosphate then is the important recognized intracellular buffer [17]. Thus, the cancer cell can be protected from harsh low pH microenvironment conditions with excellent membrane receptor buffering systems that respond rapidly through protein radical delocalization in addition to counteracting high acid concentrations from the extracellular side of the plasma cell membrane.

Membrane receptor signaling into the cell from the extracellular matrix is subsequently associated with EMT cancer progression that changes cell shape, promotes proliferation, and increases cell motility for invasive properties [4, 102, 103]. Subsequent rapid molecular signals could be transferred by proteins at the outer cell membrane into the cell in the form of instantaneous radicals and low molecular weight acids by relative fast mechanisms. Tyrosine kinase membrane receptors then not only act as ligands for binding growth factors and extracellular matrix [4, 102, 103], but further provide intracellular kinases [4, 102, 103] for enzyme activity. Tyrosine kinase enzymes linked to membrane receptors would be able to efficiently continue the breakdown of molecules already being degraded across the membrane in the extracellular matrix at low pH as nutrition sources for cancer with increasing well-organized catalytic nutritional mechanisms. In addition, oxidative mechanisms by reactive oxygen species exist at low pH in the extracellular matrix to dissociate C=C bonds on lipids that might normally be difficult to disrupt [22].

During the extravasation process where cancer cells escape the blood vessels [4], protease enzymes released into the blood stream or incorporated in metastatic cancer cells as a continuation of the original EMT process [4, 102, 103] might be expected to assist the breakdown of endothelial cells at distant locations. The low modulus cancer cell can then deform to squeeze and push through small openings with high-modulus protrusions into distant tissue sites. Although invasive cancer cell movement requires proteases for degradation of the extracellular matrices forming tube-like tracks for lamellipodia extensions, subsequent actin-protein-like buffering by the lamellipodia with cell rounding allows more extensive amoeba-type movement in matrix gaps [104]. When cancer cells enter the lymphatic system, the metastasis occurs in the lymph nodes or continues on to the blood stream [4]. Cancer cells can further become trapped in capillaries and enter organs to form the secondary tumor [4]. Because cancer cells are pleomorphic and contain much larger and much smaller cells than normal, some larger cancer cells become trapped in capillaries [4], while smaller cells can easily enter even more distant sites through openings created possibly by tumor proteases.

9. Cancer Chemotherapeutic Research

A high percent of cancers metastasize or occur within inoperable tissue that result in the majority of deaths [4, 14] and are untreatable by surgical incision so that radiation treatment or chemotherapy is necessary [4, 14]. Chemotherapy is often considered because cancers proliferate faster than normal cells so that drugs interfering with fast growing tissue cells should eradicate cancer cells [14]. However, treatment may aggravate the tumor microenvironment and make cancer cells worse [14]. Further, because chemotherapeutic agents must kill cancer cells that survive beyond apoptotic events, toxicity is extremely high to normal cells [14]. To place cancer chemotherapeutic treatment in better perspective concerning killing cancer cells, images showing cancer cell death can help, Figures 12(a)–12(f).

An immune response by many sacrificial macrophages is required to kill a single cancer cell *in vitro*. Once the cancer cell is detected, macrophages will attach to the larger cancer cell to absorb the hypoxic mitochondrial metabolic wastes of acid and free radicals and reinject such toxins back into the cancer cell. The macrophages then die with the cancer cell. However, as malignant tumor proliferation becomes successful, cancer cells can use macrophages, or tumor associated macrophages (TAMs), to help destroy normal cells with proteases and further assist tumors by bringing in endothelial cells, capillaries, and needed oxygen as part of the cancer growth and invasive process [4].

10. Regenerative Medicine Pharmaceutical Prodrugs

From the free-radical polymer-based cancer model developed, a new class of safe and effective regenerative medicine prodrugs could evolve that reduce the original problems associated with hypoxic conditions [4, 14, 85–88, 90] by mitochondrial free radicals [4, 12, 15, 79–81] and acid [4, 12, 14, 72]. Further, cancers are noted to have a measurable acidic extracellular matrix microenvironment [4, 14, 72]. Although reactive oxygen species are thought to promote cancer [4, 15, 35, 79–81], clinical trials using vitamins to reduce the free radicals associated with cancer suggest that nutrient antioxidant supplements are not effective in reducing risks during treatment [105, 106]. Problems already identified with nutrient supplements include high reactive secondary C=C crosslinks with vitamin A and β-carotene and nonantioxidant activity by vitamin E that may possibly provide alternative benefits as a viscosity reducer of lipids [22]. Due to poor efforts in reducing the pathology of cancer by vitamin therapy, antioxidants are not recommended during cancer treatment so as not to offset chemotherapeutic free-radical-related killing toxicity [105].

Free-radical inhibitors engineered to prevent premature crosslinks in polymer resins and highly active monomers [22, 107] could be initiated as adjunctive treatments with medical treatments for cancer. In fact, the hydroquinone/benzoquinone system has already been used in the prodrug treatment of hypoxic tumors [108]. Free radicals produced under tumor hypoxic conditions that create structures at the molecular, fiber, cell, and pathological tissue levels would not only increase the vicious cycle of hypoxic pathology by interfering with oxygen deliver but also interfere with pharmaceutical drug transport during treatment. In addition, free radicals are involved in the polymerization process for actin fiber development that creates protrusive lamellipodia structures for advanced EMT cancer cell movement, tissue invasion, and vascular metastasis [57]. Further, the hypoxic

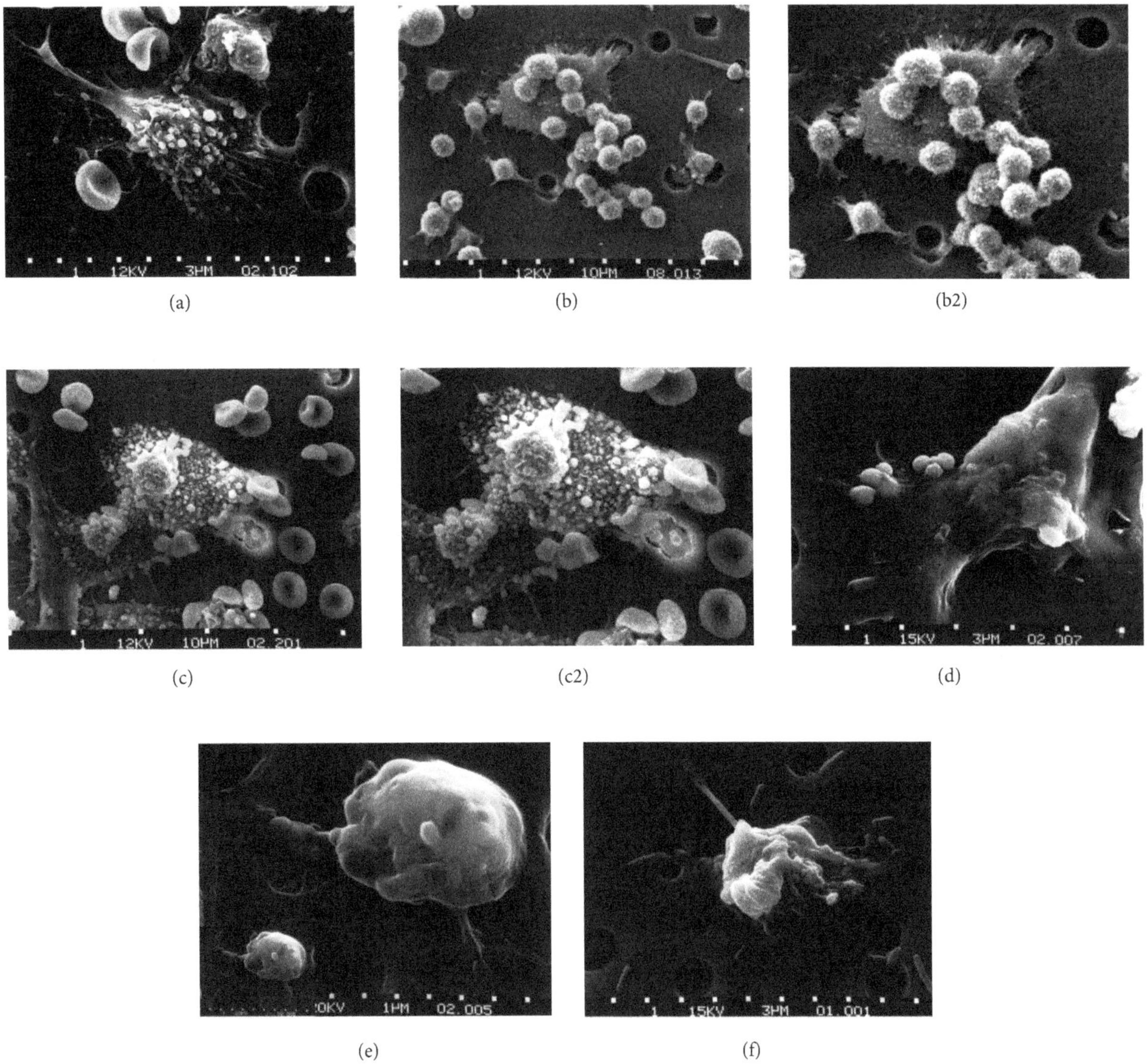

FIGURE 12: Six-step sequence showing the death of a cancer cell. (a) One cancer cell is migrating through a hole of a matrix-coated membrane from the top to the bottom, simulating natural migration of an invading cancer cell between, and sometimes through, the vascular endothelium. Notice the spikes or pseudopodia that are characteristic of an invading cancer cell. A film coat containing red blood cells, lymphocytes, and macrophages is added to the bottom of the membrane. (b) A group of macrophages identify the cancer cell as foreign matter and start to stick to the cancer cell, which still has its spikes. (b2) enlarged for relative cancer cell size comparisons for approximate equal magnifications between Figures (a), (b2), (c2), (d), (e) inset lower left, and (f). (c) Macrophages begin to fuse with, and inject toxins into, the cancer cell. The cancer cell starts rounding up and loses its spikes. (c2) enlarged for cancer cell size comparisons. (d) As the macrophage cells become smooth, the cancer cell appears lumpy in the last stage before it dies. (e) Lumps covering the cancer cell surface are actually the macrophages fused within the cancer cell with inset at lower left for cancer cell size comparisons showing a great reduction in size. (f) The cancer cell then loses its morphology, shrinks up more, and dies. (With permission from the National Institutes of Health/Department of Health and Human Services).

tumor environment produces high levels of free radicals that have been implicated in angiogenesis [109].

Hypoxia is linked with a low pH and an acidic extracellular matrix microenvironment to genetic cell instability [4, 14, 110]. Mutation rates increase at lower pH with chromosomal breaks, chromosome gaps, chromosome exchanges (translocations), DNA over replication and gene amplification, gene expression changes, and lower cell survival [14, 110]. Cancers further resist chemotherapy and radiotherapy with lower pH acidic tissues in the tumor and the extracellular matrix [14, 110]. In addition, the cancer cell is neutral or slightly basic, whereas the extracellular matrix is acidic that prevents the use of weak base drugs [14, 110]. The cancer cell membrane excludes weak base drugs from entering the cell, allows nonpolar neutral drugs to enter, and increases permeability to weakly acidic drugs [14, 110]. To counteract acids for weak base drug delivery, the pH gradient at the cancer cell membrane can be eliminated in some mouse animal models with sodium bicarbonate ad libitum and through peritoneal injections [14, 110]. Other agents known to induce metabolic alkalosis in humans have further been recommended for adjunct chemotherapy to overcome hypoxic acidity in the tumor microenvironment [110].

11. Summary

Hypoxia initiates mitochondrial free radicals formed through the electron transport chain in addition to acid from the proton gradient. Multiple types of initiating events that interfere with oxygen to the mitochondria exist as cancer causing agents/environments. Free radicals are delocalized from the mitochondria for electron-pair bonding of proteins and initiate reactive secondary sequence chain growth of lipids with C=C double bonds to form structure at the molecular and cellular levels. Subsequent covalent crosslinking by electron-pair bonds can block oxygen to the mitochondria in an ever increasing vicious cycle of chronic free-radical production that can expand to the tissue level. Irregular cancer cell membrane borders are the result of free-radical lipid crosslink shrinkage and warpage that wrinkle and pucker the membranes inward when electron pairs bond. As membrane lipid chains come much closer together by electron-pair covalent-bond crosslinking and fit better onto the underlying cytoskeleton, structural actin fibers might also crosslink and wrinkle by shrinking inward. Hypoxic conditions that produce mitochondrial waste as acid and free radicals activate latent globular proteins into efficient molecular degrading enzymes. Enzymatic degradation is further modified by free radicals delocalized into globular proteins to buffer lower pH conditions formed by mitochondrial acids. Even when cancer cells switch to anaerobic glycolysis, high levels of lactate acid form to be easily measured in the extracellular matrix. Degradation by enzymes includes manifestations of multiple mutations in addition to epigenetic changes most notable involving carbon-carbon lipid bond dissociations to methylate DNA and silence tumor suppressor genes. Although DNA mutations, low pH enzyme activity, and free radical crosslinking drive most cells toward senescence and apoptosis, some cells survive through increasing levels of more incompatible environments to eventually produce immortal cancer cells through a genetic EMT. With EMT increasing toward more primitive cancer cell types, mitochondrial hypoxia and increased production from the electron transport chain and proton gradient are subsequent driving forces for cancer cell growth rather than cell death. Also, even when anaerobic glycolysis switches over, free radicals still form at high levels along with lactate acid to lower the surrounding pH for the extracellular matrix. Cancer proliferating cells have lower modulus than normal cells; whereby more cell growth occurs within the nucleus. Cells with lower modulus deform easier to invade local tissue and metastasize. Tissue invasion is increased by protease enzymes activated by hypoxic mitochondrial acid and free radicals. Metastasis finally occurs with more protease enzymes and high modulus membrane lamellipodia extensions that provide leverage and allow low modulus cells to deform through narrow openings in the blood vessel basement membrane. Lamellipodia growth increases with free radicals formed under hypoxic conditions through H_2O_2-elevated polymerization of actin fibers. Further, small membrane filipodia extensions especially off the lamellipodia protrusions provide focal adhesion points to pull cancer cells forward by contracting with the extracellular matrix as minor stronger primary covalent and much weaker secondary bonds form in a manner somewhat similar to cure-shrinkage contraction that occurs during covalent bond polymerization. Angiogenesis responsiveness to hypoxic tumor environment allows cells to survive. Cancer risks associated with obesity and caloric intake especially with dietary fats can now be better defined through risk factors involved in atherosclerosis of blood vessels that cause hypoxia and ischemia to tissue. Resultant decreased oxygen during cell metabolism produce mitochondrial free radicals and acid that are then directly involved in cancer. Other risk factors for cancer should also be defined in terms of possible ischemia and hypoxia at the mitochondrial level. The microenvironment surrounding the cancer tumor can eventually become hostile with free radicals and acid to an extent that macrophage killing is subverted to TAM tumors that might be better controlled toward health with free-radical inhibitors/antioxidants and various buffers. Finally, by acknowledging the original sources of pathology that include hypoxic mitochondrial free radicals and acid, corrective and preventive measures to remove or offset the initiating factors could be more easily done.

Abbreviations

C=C:	Carbon-carbon double bond
sigma (σ):	Single bond
pi (π):	Double bond
EMT:	Epithelial-mesenchymal transition
TAM:	Tumor-associated macrophage.

Acknowledgments

Thanks are given to the National Institutes of Health/Department of Health and Human Services for the many state-of-the-art figures presented here. The funding is done through the National Institutes of Health Grant no. T32DE14300. Director Patricia F. Lott, Center for Metabolic Bone Disease-Histomorphometry, and Molecular Analysis Core Laboratory, The University of Alabama at Birmingham, National Institutes of Health Grant no. P30-AR46031 and Wavefunction Spartan Software, Newport Beach, CA, USA are also acknowledged.

References

[1] National Cancer Institute/National Institutes of Health/Department of Health and Human Services, *What You Need To Know About Cancer*, NIH, 2006.

[2] T. S. Deisboeck and G. S. Stamatakos, *Multiscale Cancer Modeling*, Chapman & Hall/ CRC Press, Boca Raton, Fla, USA, 2011.

[3] B. Kwabi-Addo and T. L. Lindstrom, *Cancer Causes and Controversies*, Praeger, Barbara, Calif, USA, 2011.

[4] R. A. Weinberg, *The Biology of Cancer*, Garland Science, New York, NY, USA, 2007.

[5] R. Doll and A. B. Hill, "Lung cancer and other causes of death in relation to smoking: a second report on the mortality of British doctors," *British Medical Journal*, vol. 233, pp. 1071–1076, 1956.

[6] G. M. Findlay, "Ultra-violet light and skin cancer," *The Lancet*, vol. 212, no. 5491, pp. 1070–1073, 1928.

[7] H. J. Muller, "The production of mutations by X-rays," *Proceedings of the National Academy of Sciences of the United States of America*, vol. 14, no. 9, pp. 714–726, 1928.

[8] I. Berenblum, "The mechanism of carcinogenesis. A study of the significance of cocarcinogenic action and related phenomena," *Cancer Research*, vol. 1, article 807, 1941.

[9] J. G. Kidd and P. Rous, "The carcinogenic effect of a papilloma virus on the tarred skin of radibts: II Major factors determining the phenomenon: the manifold effects of tarring," *The Journal of Experimental Medicine*, vol. 68, pp. 529–562, 1938.

[10] C. Huggins and C. V. Hodges, "Studies on prostatic cancer: I. The effect of castration, of estrogen and of androgen injection on serum phosphatases in metastatic carcinoma of the prostate," *Cancer Research*, vol. 1, article 293, 1941.

[11] A. Tanenbaum and H. Silverstone, "The influence of the degree of caloric restriction on the formation of skin tumors and hepatomas in mice," *Cancer Research*, vol. 9, no. 12, pp. 724–727, 1949.

[12] O. Warburg, K. Posener, and E. Negelein, "The metabolism of the cancer cell," *Biochemische Zeitschrift*, vol. 152, pp. 319–344, 1924.

[13] S. Weinhouse, O. Warburg, D. Burk, and A. L. Schade, "On respiratory impairment in cancer cells," *Science*, vol. 124, no. 3215, pp. 269–270, 1956.

[14] R. J. Gillies, *The Tumour Microenvironment: Causes and Consequences of Hypoxia and Acidity*, Novartis Foundation Symposium 240, John Wiley & Sons, New York, NY, USA, 2001.

[15] J. C. Stavridis, *Oxidation: the Cornerstone of Carcinogenesis*, Springer, New York, NY, USA, 2008.

[16] V. C. Fogg, N. J. Lanning, and J. P. MacKeigan, "Mitochondria in cancer: at the crossroads of life and death," *Chinese Journal of Cancer*, vol. 30, no. 8, pp. 526–539, 2011.

[17] L. Sherwood, *Human Physiology*, Thompson Brooks/Cole, Belmont, Calif, USA, 5th edition, 2004.

[18] R. Harvey and D. Ferrier, *Biochemistry*, Wolters Kluwer/Lippincott Williams & Wilkins, Philadelphia, Pa, USA, 5th edition, 2011.

[19] A. J. Schetter, N. H. H. Heegaard, and C. C. Harris, "Inflammation and cancer: interweaving microRNA, free radical, cytokine and p53 pathways," *Carcinogenesis*, vol. 31, no. 1, pp. 37–49, 2009.

[20] J. Wang and J. Yi, "Cancer cell killing via ROS: to increase or decrease, that is a question," *Cancer Biology and Therapy*, vol. 7, no. 12, pp. 1875–1884, 2008.

[21] M. P. Murphy, "How mitochondria produce reactive oxygen species," *Biochemical Journal*, vol. 417, no. 1, pp. 1–13, 2009.

[22] R. C. Petersen, "Reactive secondary sequence oxidative pathology polymer model and antioxidant tests," *International Journal of Pure and Applied Chemistry*, vol. 2, no. 4, pp. 247–285, 2012.

[23] J. McMurry, *Organic Chemistry*, Thomson/Brooks/Cole, Belmont, Calif, USA, 6th edition, 2004.

[24] J. M. Lü, P. H. Lin, Q. Yao, and C. Chen, "Chemical and molecular mechanisms of antioxidants: experimental approaches and model systems," *Journal of Cellular and Molecular Medicine*, vol. 14, no. 4, pp. 840–860, 2010.

[25] X. A. J. Peacock and A. Calhoun, *Polymer Chemistry Properties and Applications*, Hanser, Munich, Germany, 2006.

[26] I. Mironi-Harpaz, M. Narkis, and A. Siegmann, "Peroxide crosslinking of a styrene-free unsaturated polyester," *Journal of Applied Polymer Science*, vol. 105, no. 2, pp. 885–892, 2007.

[27] Y. Wang, L. Woodworth, and B. Han, "Simultaneous measurement of effective chemical shrinkage and modulus evolutions during polymerization," *Experimental Mechanics*, vol. 51, no. 7, pp. 1155–1169, 2011.

[28] D. Recupero, L. Annaratone, F. Maletta, and G. Bussolati, "Nuclear shape in papillary thyroid carcinoma: a role for lamin b receptor?" *Romanian Journal of Morphology and Embryology*, vol. 51, no. 4, pp. 615–620, 2010.

[29] V. A. McCormack and I. Dos Santos Silva, "Breast density and parenchymal patterns as markers of breast cancer risk: a meta-analysis," *Cancer Epidemiology Biomarkers and Prevention*, vol. 15, no. 6, pp. 1159–1169, 2006.

[30] C. M. Kraning-Rush, J. P. Califano, and C. A. Reinhart-King, "Cellular traction stresses increase with increasing metastatic potential," *PLoS ONE*, vol. 7, no. 2, Article ID e32572, 2012.

[31] G. Y. Li and J. L. Koenig, "FTIR imaging of oxidation of polyisoprene 2. The role of N-phenyl-N′-dimethyl-butyl-p-phenylenediamine antioxidant," *Polymer Degradation and Stability*, vol. 81, no. 3, pp. 377–385, 2003.

[32] G. Helmlinger, F. Yuan, M. Dellian, and R. K. Jain, "Interstitial pH and pO_2 gradients in solid tumors *in vivo*: high-resolution measurements reveal a lack of correlation," *Nature Medicine*, vol. 3, no. 2, pp. 177–182, 1997.

[33] J. Michael and S. Sircar, *Fundamentals of Medical Physiology*, Thieme, New York, NY, USA, 2011.

[34] B. Alberts, A. Johnson, J. Lewis, M. Raff, K. Roberts, and P. Walters, *Molecular Biology of the Cell*, Garland Science, New York, NY, USA, 4th edition, 2002.

[35] L. Stryer, *Biochemistry*, W. H. Freeman and Company, New York, NY, USA, 4th edition, 1995.

[36] J. B. Wenger, S. Y. Chun, D. T. Dang, H. Luesch, and L. H. Dang, "Combination therapy targeting cancer metabolism," *Medical Hypotheses*, vol. 76, no. 2, pp. 169–172, 2011.

[37] N. J. Vardaxis, *A Textbook of Pathology*, Elsevier, New York, NY, USA, 2010.

[38] S. L. Robbins and M. Angell, *Basic Pathology*, WB Saunders, Philadelphia, Pa, USA, 1971.

[39] J. F. Kerr, A. H. Wyllie, and A. R. Currie, "Apoptosis: a basic biological phenomenon with wide-ranging implications in tissue kinetics," *British Journal of Cancer*, vol. 26, no. 4, pp. 239–257, 1972.

[40] L. A. Liotta, K. Tryggvason, and S. Garbisa, "Metastatic potential correlates with enzymatic degradation of basement membrane collagen," *Nature*, vol. 284, no. 5751, pp. 67–68, 1980.

[41] P. A. Jones and S. M. Taylor, "Cellular differentiation, cytidine analogs and DNA methylation," *Cell*, vol. 20, no. 1, pp. 85–93, 1980.

[42] A. Loveless, "Possible relevance of O-6 alkylation of deoxyguanosine to the mutagenicity and carcinogenicity of nitrosamines and nitrosamides," *Nature*, vol. 223, no. 5202, pp. 206–207, 1969.

[43] P. F. Swann and P. N. Magee, "Nitrosamine-induced carcinogenesis. The alklylation of nucleic acids of the rat by N-methyl-N-nitrosourea, dimethylnitrosamine, dimethyl sulphate and methyl methanesulphonate," *Biochemical Journal*, vol. 110, no. 1, pp. 39–47, 1968.

[44] M. Bignami, M. O'Driscoll, G. Aquilina, and P. Karran, "Unmasking a killer: DNA O^6-methylguanine and the cytotoxicity of methylating agents," *Mutation Research*, vol. 462, no. 2-3, pp. 71–82, 2000.

[45] P. Whyte, K. J. Buchkovich, J. M. Horowitz et al., "Association between an oncogene and an anti-oncogene: the adenovirus E1A proteins bind to the retinoblastoma gene product," *Nature*, vol. 334, no. 6178, pp. 124–129, 1988.

[46] J. M. Nigro, S. J. Baker, A. C. Preisinger et al., "Mutations in the p53 gene occur in diverse human tumour types," *Nature*, vol. 342, no. 6250, pp. 705–708, 1989.

[47] S. J. Baker, E. R. Fearon, J. M. Nigro et al., "Chromosome 17 deletions and p53 gene mutations in colorectal carcinomas," *Science*, vol. 244, no. 4901, pp. 217–221, 1989.

[48] C. J. Tabin, S. M. Bradley, and C. I. Bargmann, "Mechanism of activation of a human oncogene," *Nature*, vol. 300, no. 5888, pp. 143–149, 1982.

[49] E. P. Reddy, R. K. Reynolds, E. Santos, and M. Barbacid, "A point mutation is responsible for the acquisition of transforming properties by the T24 human bladder carcinoma oncogene," *Nature*, vol. 300, no. 5888, pp. 149–152, 1982.

[50] E. Taparowsky, Y. Suard, and O. Fasano, "Activation of the T24 bladder carcinoma transforming gene is linked to a single amino acid change," *Nature*, vol. 300, no. 5894, pp. 762–765, 1982.

[51] S. T. Peters, *Handbook of Composites*, Chapman and Hall, New York, NY, USA, 2nd edition, 1998.

[52] K. M. B. Jansen, J. Vreugd de, and L. J. Ernst, "Analytical estimate for curing-induced stress and warpage in coating layers," *Journal of Applied Polymer Science*, vol. 126, pp. 1623–1630, 2012.

[53] L. J. Deterding, D. C. Ramirez, J. R. Dubin, R. P. Mason, and K. B. Tomer, "Identification of free radicals on hemoglobin from its self-peroxidation using mass spectrometry and immuno-spin trapping: observation of a histidinyl radical," *The Journal of Biological Chemistry*, vol. 279, no. 12, pp. 11600–11607, 2004.

[54] I. Ayala, K. Range, D. York, and B. A. Barry, "Spectroscopic properties of tyrosyl radicals in dipeptides," *Journal of the American Chemical Society*, vol. 124, no. 19, pp. 5496–5505, 2002.

[55] I. R. Vassiliev, A. R. Offenbacher, and B. A. Barry, "Redox-active tyrosine residues in pentapeptides," *Journal of Physical Chemistry B*, vol. 109, no. 48, pp. 23077–23085, 2005.

[56] T. Vinogradova, P. M. Miller, and I. Kaverina, "Microtubule network asymmetry in motile cells: role of Golgi-derived array," *Cell Cycle*, vol. 8, no. 14, pp. 2168–2174, 2009.

[57] U. Lindberg, R. Karlsson, I. Lassing, C. E. Schutt, and A. S. Höglund, "The microfilament system and malignancy," *Seminars in Cancer Biology*, vol. 18, no. 1, pp. 2–11, 2008.

[58] A. San Martín and K. K. Griendling, "Redox control of vascular smooth muscle migration," *Antioxidants and Redox Signaling*, vol. 12, no. 5, pp. 625–640, 2010.

[59] L.-E. Copstead and J. Banasik, *Pathophysiology*, Elsevier Saunders, St. Louis, Mo, USA, 6th edition, 2005.

[60] Z. Li, M. Hannigan, Z. Mo et al., "Directional Sensing Requires $G\beta\gamma$-Mediated PAK1 and PIXα-Dependent Activation of Cdc42," *Cell*, vol. 114, no. 2, pp. 215–227, 2003.

[61] H. Hattori, K. K. Subramanian, J. Sakai, Y. Jia, Y. Li, T. F. Porter et al., "Small-molecule screen identifies reacive oxygen species as key regulators of neutorphil chemotaxis," *PNAS*, vol. 107, no. 8, pp. 3546–3551, 2010.

[62] F. Parisi and M. Vidal, "Epithelial delamination and migration: lessons from Drosophila," *Cell Adhesion & Migration*, vol. 5, no. 4, pp. 366–372, 2011.

[63] A. I. M. Barth, H. Y. Caro-Gonzalez, and W. J. Nelson, "Role of adenomatous polyposis coli (APC) and microtubules in directional cell migration and neuronal polarization," *Seminars in Cell and Developmental Biology*, vol. 19, no. 3, pp. 245–251, 2008.

[64] E. W. Dent, S. L. Gupton, and F. B. Gertler, "The growth cone cytoskeleton in axon outgrowth and guidance," *Cold Spring Harbor Perspectives in Biologyl*, vol. 3, no. 3, article 42, 2010.

[65] B. D. Ratner, A. S. Hoffman, F. J. Schoen, and J. E. Lemons, *Biomaterials Science*, Elsevier, San Diego, Calif, USA, 2004.

[66] J. Pokorný, A. Jandová, M. Nedbalová et al., "Mitochondrial metabolism-neglected link of cancer transformation and treatment," *Prague Medical Report*, vol. 113, no. 2, pp. 81–94, 2012.

[67] X. Zhu, M. M. Gallogly, J. J. Mieyal, V. E. Anderson, and L. M. Sayre, "Covalent cross-linking of glutathione and carnosine to proteins by 4-oxo-2-nonenal," *Chemical Research in Toxicology*, vol. 22, no. 6, pp. 1050–1059, 2009.

[68] S. Saraswathy, G. Wu, and N. A. Rao, "Retinal microglial activation and chemotaxis by docosahexaenoic acid hydroperoxide," *Investigative Ophthalmology and Visual Science*, vol. 47, no. 8, pp. 3656–3663, 2006.

[69] H. Zhang, B. C. Gau, L. M. Jones, I. Vidavsky, and M. L. Gross, "Fast photochemical oxidation of proteins for comparing structures of protein-ligand complexes: the calmodulin-peptide model system," *Analytical Chemistry*, vol. 83, no. 1, pp. 311–318, 2011.

[70] R. Torosantucci, O. Mozziconacci, V. Sharov, C. Schöneich, and W. Jiskoot, "Chemical modifications in aggregates of recombinant human insulin induced by metal-catalyzed oxidation: covalent cross-linking via michael addition to tyrosine oxidation products," *Pharmaceutical Research*, vol. 29, no. 8, pp. 2276–2293, 2012.

[71] R. A. Dunlop, R. T. Dean, and K. J. Rodgers, "The impact of specific oxidized amino acids on protein turnover in J774 cells," *Biochemical Journal*, vol. 410, no. 1, pp. 131–140, 2008.

[72] E. M. Darling, S. Zauscher, J. A. Block, and F. Guilak, "A thin-layer model for viscoelastic, stress-relaxation testing of cells using atomic force microscopy: do cell properties reflect metastatic potential?" *Biophysical Journal*, vol. 92, no. 5, pp. 1784–1791, 2007.

[73] F. Fleischer, R. Ananthakrishnan, S. Eckel et al., "Actin network architecture and elasticity in lamellipodia of melanoma cells," *New Journal of Physics*, vol. 9, article 420, 2007.

[74] V. C. Abraham, V. Krishnamurthi, D. Lansing Taylor, and F. Lanni, "The actin-based nanomachine at the leading edge of migrating cells," *Biophysical Journal*, vol. 77, no. 3, pp. 1721–1732, 1999.

[75] E. Atilgan, D. Wirtz, and S. X. Sun, "Morphology of the lamellipodium and organization of actin filaments at the leading edge of crawling cells," *Biophysical Journal*, vol. 89, no. 5, pp. 3589–3602, 2005.

[76] Y. Qian, J. Luo, S. S. Leonard et al., "Hydrogen peroxide formation and actin filament reorganization by Cdc42 are essential for ethanol-induced *in vitro* angiogenesis," *The Journal of Biological Chemistry*, vol. 278, no. 18, pp. 16189–16197, 2003.

[77] B. Gawdzik, J. Księżopolski, and T. Matynia, "Synthesis of new free-radical initiators for polymerization," *Journal of Applied Polymer Science*, vol. 87, no. 14, pp. 2238–2243, 2003.

[78] Y. I. Miller, D. S. Worrall, C. D. Funk, J. R. Feramisco, and J. L. Witztum, "Actin polymerization in macrophages in response to oxidized LDL and apoptotic cells: role of 12/15-lipoxygenase and phosphoinositide 3-kinase," *Molecular Biology of the Cell*, vol. 14, no. 10, pp. 4196–4206, 2003.

[79] M. Ushio-Fukai and Y. Nakamura, "Reactive oxygen species and angiogenesis: NADPH oxidase as target for cancer therapy," *Cancer Letters*, vol. 266, no. 1, pp. 37–52, 2008.

[80] M. J. Hitchler and F. E. Domann, "Metabolic defects provide a spark for the epigenetic switch in cancer," *Free Radical Biology and Medicine*, vol. 47, no. 2, pp. 115–127, 2009.

[81] C. L. Grek and K. D. Twe, "Redox metabolism and malignancy," *Current Opinion in Pharmacology*, vol. 10, no. 4, pp. 362–368, 2010.

[82] M. Höckel and P. Vaupel, "Tumor hypoxia: definitions and current clinical, biologic, and molecular aspects," *Journal of the National Cancer Institute*, vol. 93, no. 4, pp. 266–276, 2001.

[83] P. Vaupel, "The role of hypoxia-induced factors in tumor progression," *Oncologist*, vol. 9, no. 5, pp. 10–17, 2004.

[84] D. M. Brizel, S. P. Scully, J. M. Harrelson et al., "Tumor oxygenation predicts for the likelihood of distant metastases in human soft tissue sarcoma," *Cancer Research*, vol. 56, no. 5, pp. 941–943, 1996.

[85] S. P. Hussain and C. C. Harris, "Inflammation and cancer: an ancient link with novel potentials," *International Journal of Cancer*, vol. 121, no. 11, pp. 2373–2380, 2007.

[86] G. W. Burton, K. H. Cheeseman, T. Doba, K. U. Ingold, and T. F. Slater, "Vitamin E as an antioxidant *in vitro* and *in vivo*," *Ciba Foundation symposium*, vol. 101, pp. 4–18, 1983.

[87] G. W. Burton, K. H. Cheeseman, T. Doba, K. U. Ingold, and T. F. Slater, "Vitamin E as an antioxidant *in vitro* and *in vivo*," in *Ciba Foundation Symposium 101, Biology of Vitamin E*, Pitman, London, UK, 1983.

[88] N. A. Porter, S. E. Caldwell, and K. A. Mills, "Mechanisms of free radical oxidation of unsaturated lipids," *Lipids*, vol. 30, no. 4, pp. 277–290, 1995.

[89] C. Schneider, "An update on products and mechanisms of lipid peroxidation," *Molecular Nutrition and Food Research*, vol. 53, no. 3, pp. 315–321, 2009.

[90] X. Lu and Y. Kang, "Hypoxia and hypoxia-inducible factors: master regulators of metastasis," *Clinical Cancer Research*, vol. 16, no. 24, pp. 5928–5935, 2010.

[91] V. Swaminathan, K. Mythreye, E. Tim O'Brien, A. Berchuck, G. C. Blobe, and R. Superfine, "Mechanical Stiffness grades metastatic potential in patient tumor cells and in cancer cell lines," *Cancer Research*, vol. 71, no. 15, pp. 5075–5080, 2011.

[92] G. L. Johanning, "Modulation of breast cancer cell adhesion by unsaturated fatty acids," *Nutrition*, vol. 12, no. 11-12, pp. 810–816, 1996.

[93] Y. Yang, H. Hong, Y. Zhang, and W. Cai, "Molecular imaging of proteases in cancer," *Cancer Growth Metast*, vol. 17, no. 2, pp. 13–27, 2009.

[94] J. Kim, W. Yu, K. Kovalski, and L. Ossowski, "Requirement for specific proteases in cancer cell intravasation as revealed by a novel semiquantitative PCR-based assay," *Cell*, vol. 94, no. 3, pp. 353–362, 1998.

[95] E. Lee, J. Jeong, S. E. Kim, E. J. Song, S. W. Kang, and K. J. Lee, "Multiple functions of Nm23-H1 are regulated by oxido-reduction system," *PLoS ONE*, vol. 4, no. 11, Article ID e7949, 2009.

[96] W. Xu, R. Mezencev, B. Kim, L. Wang, J. McDonald, and T. Sulchek, "Cell stiffness is a biomarker of the metastatic potential of ovarian cancer cells," *PLoS ONE*, vol. 7, no. 10, Article ID e46609, 2012.

[97] S. Ghosh, T. Kang, H. Wang, Y. Hu, and R. Li, "Mechanical phenotype is important for stromal aromatase expression," *Steroids*, vol. 76, no. 8, pp. 797–801, 2011.

[98] K. Hoyt, B. Castaneda, M. Zhang et al., "Tissue elasticity properties as biomarkers for prostate cancer," *Cancer Biomarkers*, vol. 4, no. 4-5, pp. 213–225, 2008.

[99] L. Trichet, J. Le Digabel, R. J. Hawkins et al., "Evidence of a large-scale mechanosensing mechanism for cellular adaptation to substrate stiffness," *Proceedings of the National Academy of Sciences of the United States of America*, vol. 109, no. 18, pp. 6933–6938, 2012.

[100] E. M. Darling, S. Zauscher, J. A. Block, and F. Guilak, "A thin-layer model for viscoelastic, stress-relaxation testing of cells using atomic force microscopy: do cell properties reflect metastatic potential?" *Biophysical Journal*, vol. 92, no. 5, pp. 1784-1791, 2007.

[101] R. A. Marcus and N. Sutin, "Electron transfers in chemistry and biology," *Biochimica et Biophysica Acta*, vol. 811, no. 3, pp. 265–322, 1985.

[102] Y. H. Soung, J. L. Clifford, and J. Chung, "Crosstalk between integrin and receptor tyrosine kinase signaling in breast carcinoma progression," *BMB Reports*, vol. 43, no. 5, pp. 311–318, 2010.

[103] R. R. Valiathan, M. Marco, B. Leitinger, C. G. Kleer, and R. Fridman, "Discoidin domain receptor tyrosine kinases: new players in cancer progression," *Cancer and Metastasis Reviews*, vol. 31, no. 1-2, pp. 295–321, 2012.

[104] K. Wolf, I. Mazo, H. Leung et al., "Compensation mechanism in tumor cell migration: mesenchymal-amoeboid transition after blocking of pericellular proteolysis," *Journal of Cell Biology*, vol. 160, no. 2, pp. 267–277, 2003.

[105] American Cancer Society, "Nutrition and physical activity guidelines for cancer survivors," *CA—Cancer Journal for Clinicians*, vol. 62, no. 4, pp. 275–276, 2012.

[106] M. Goodman, R. M. Bostick, O. Kucuk, and D. P. Jones, "Clinical trials of antioxidants as cancer prevention agents: past, present, and future," *Free Radical Biology and Medicine*, vol. 51, no. 5, pp. 1068–1084, 2011.

[107] F. Rodriquez, *Principles of Polymer SystemsEdition*, Taylor & Francis, Washington, DC, USA, 4th edition, 1996.

[108] M. Jaffar, N. Abou-Zeid, L. Bai et al., "Quinone bioreductive prodrugs as delivery agents," *Current Drug Delivery*, vol. 1, no. 4, pp. 345–350, 2004.

[109] S. J. Ralph, S. Rodríguez-Enríquez, J. Neuzil, E. Saavedra, and R. Moreno-Sánchez, "The causes of cancer revisited: "Mitochondrial malignancy" and ROS-induced oncogenic transformation—why mitochondria are targets for cancer therapy," *Molecular Aspects of Medicine*, vol. 31, no. 2, pp. 145–170, 2010.

[110] N. Raghunand and R. J. Gillies In:, "pH and chemotherapy," in *The Tumour Microenvironment: Causes and Consequence of Hypoxia and Acidity*, Novartis Foundation Symposium 240, pp. 199–211, Wiley, Chichester, UK, 2001.

11

Genetic Aspects of Congenital and Idiopathic Scoliosis

Philip F. Giampietro

Waisman Center, University of Wisconsin-Madison, 1500 Highland Avenue, Madison, WI 53705, USA

Correspondence should be addressed to Philip F. Giampietro; pfgiampietro@pediatrics.wisc.edu

Academic Editors: F. Acosta, T. M. George, and S. Rasmussen

Congenital and idiopathic scoliosis represent disabling conditions of the spine. While congenital scoliosis (CS) is caused by morphogenic abnormalities in vertebral development, the cause(s) for idiopathic scoliosis is (are) likely to be varied, representing alterations in skeletal growth, neuromuscular imbalances, disturbances involving communication between the brain and spine, and others. Both conditions are characterized by phenotypic and genetic heterogeneities, which contribute to the difficulties in understanding their genetic basis that investigators face. Despite the differences between these two conditions there is observational and experimental evidence supporting common genetic mechanisms. This paper focuses on the clinical features of both CS and IS and highlights genetic and environmental factors which contribute to their occurrence. It is anticipated that emerging genetic technologies and improvements in phenotypic stratification of both conditions will facilitate improved understanding of the genetic basis for these conditions and enable targeted prevention and treatment strategies.

1. Introduction

Advances in developmental biology have enabled improvements in the understanding of spine development and have provided contributions that enhance our understanding of genetic and environmental factors that are associated with congenital and idiopathic scoliosis. This paper will focus on salient features of both forms of scoliosis and highlight research focusing on genetic and environmental mechanisms for their occurrence.

2. Definitions and Epidemiology of Scoliosis

Idiopathic scoliosis (IS) is defined by the Scoliosis Research Society (http://www.srs.org/) as a lateral curvature of the spine of 10° or greater for which no cause can be determined. There is evidence that genetic and environmental factors are likely to play a role in the occurrence of both as described herin, although the mechanism responsible for this is uncertain at the present time. This rotational deformity is measured in the forward bending position by an inclinometer, and the scoliometer as an angle of trunk rotation (ATR).

The incidence of idiopathic scoliosis (IS) in the general population ranges from 2% to 3%, varying with the definition of the magnitude of the curve. Population studies indicate that 11.1% of 1st degree relatives are affected, compared to 2.4% of 2nd degree, and 1.1% of 3rd degree relatives [1]. By age 16, 0.6% of affected people will have required active treatment with a full-time thoracolumbar-sacral orthosis (TLSO) or surgical correction with instrumentation [2, 3]. Older IS subclassification is based on the age of presentation categorized as: (1) infantile (birth to age 3 years), (2) juvenile (age 3 to 11 years), and (3) adolescent (11 years and older).

These subclassifications are sometimes useful clinically, but have no established genetic basis. Age-specific genetic markers have not been identified for IS, and the current concept of scoliosis is that the disorder develops continuously between the juvenile years and adolescence. Hence, in this paper, the term IS is used in most situations without attempt to distinguish juvenile and adolescent subtypes. The incidence of IS for treatable curves defined as 25° or greater is greater in females than in males with a ratio of 2 : 1, respectively. Gender differences may underlie scoliotic curve progression.

Congenital scoliosis (CS) is a form of spinal curvature which is due to the presence of an underlying congenital vertebral malformation (CVM).

The estimated frequency of CVM in the general population is in the range of 0.13–0.5/1,000 [4]. Vertebral malformations most commonly include hemivertebrae (half of a vertebrae), additional vertebrae, vertebral bar (an abnormality of vertebral separation during development), butterfly, and wedge-shaped vertebrae illustrated in Figures 1 and 2. Vertebral malformations may represent an isolated finding, occur in association with other renal, cardiac, or spinal cord malformations, or occur as part of an underlying syndrome or chromosomal abnormality. Autopsy of fetuses with anencephaly and myelomeningocele demonstrates the presence of cervical and thoracic CVM, suggesting a related etiology for both neural tube defects and CVM [5].

Frequently encountered syndromes associated with CVM include the following:

(i) Alagille syndrome (peripheral pulmonic stenosis, cholestasis, facial dysmorphism);

(ii) Jarcho-Levin syndrome (short trunk dwarfism, multiple vertebral and rib defects with posterior rib fusion);

(iii) Klippel-Feil syndrome (short neck, low posterior hairline, and fusion of cervical vertebrae), hemifacial microsomia (associated with craniofacial anomalies including microtia);

(iv) Goldenhar syndrome (hemifacial microsomia and epibulbar dermoids); and

(v) VACTERL syndrome (vertebral malformations, anal atresia, cardiac malformations, tracheo-esophageal fistula, renal, and radial anomalies, and limb defects).

3. Vertebral Development and Genes Involved

Vertebral bodies are derived from somites through a recurrent process of budding off from the presomitic mesoderm mediated by cyclical expression of FGF, Wnt, and Notch signaling pathway genes [8]. A "clock and wavefront" model for somitogenesis was originally proposed by Cooke and Zeeman in 1976 [9]. In this model the "clock" represents an oscillator which connects presomitic mesodermal cells, and the "wave" represents a region of "rapid cellular change" in which transition to somite development occurs, presumably mediated by some type of gradient.

A similar mechanism of oscillation amongst members of the Hes/Her/Hairy family of basic helix-loop-helix (bHLH) transcriptional repressors has been reported in mice, chicken, and zebrafish, providing evidence for conservation of the oscillator in vertebrates [10–13]. A molecular oscillator regulates the Notch, Fgf, and Wnt signaling pathways in which the Notch and Fgf genes oscillate in opposite phase to the Wnt genes [14]. Wnt3a signaling mediated by β-catenin which controls the oscillatory signaling in the Notch pathway [15]. Following periodic activation of Notch 1, Notch intracellular domain (NICD), the cleaved form of the Notch 1 receptor, translocates to the nucleus. NICD activates transcription of multiple target genes including Hairy/Hes/Her genes, Lunatic fringe (Lfng), and Notch-related ankyrn repeat protein (Nrap) [14, 16, 17].

A stripe of expression of genes occurs in response to the periodic clock signal at a region referred to as the determination front, which is defined by opposing retinoic acid (RA), FGF, and Wnt signaling gradients, posteriorly regressing as the embryo elongates along the anterior-posterior axis [15, 18, 19] Figure 3. The exposure of cells in the posterior presomitic mesoderm to high levels of FGF and Wnt activity enables the maintenance of an undifferentiated state [20, 21]. Below the determination front, cells are capable of responding to the segmentation clock through the activation of boundary specific genes Mesp2 and Riply [21–23]. Wnt3a provides a crucial function in both the clock and wavefront portions associated with somitogenesis and through Msgn1 plays a major role in the segmentation clock through regulation of Notch and Wnt signaling pathways [24]. As a result of active Wnt signaling, active Wnt signaling, Msgn1 and Wnt targets are expressed. A phase lag allows for Msgn1 to activate Notch related genes. RA plays an important role in the preservation of spine symmetry through its buffering action of the Left-Right pathway which creates asymmetry through the action of Nodal [25]. Since the majority of patients with IS exhibit a spinal curve to the right, an underlying defect in left-right asymmetry has been hypothesized [26].

4. Teratogens Associated with CVM

Various maternal exposures during pregnancy including alcohol use [27], anticonvulsant medications such as valproic acid [28–30], hyperthermia [31], maternal insulin-dependent diabetes mellitus, and gestational diabetes [32–34] have been observed to be associated with the occurrence of CVM in animal models and humans. Single nucleotide polymorphisms in glucose metabolizing genes including *GLUT1*, *HK1*, and *LEP* are postulated to be related to the occurrence of malformations observed in diabetic embryopathy. The occurrence of reactive oxygen species (ROS) has been proposed as a mechanism for altered somitogenesis in diabetic embryopathy [35]. Mutations in the planar cell polarity gene, *CELSR1* (*Caherin, EGF Lag Seven Pass G-Type Receptor 1-3)*, have been identified in patients with either neural tube defects or caudal agenesis [36]. Mutations in planar cell polarity genes are associated with a shortened body axis, widened neural plate, and neural tube defects [37]. CVM have been observed in laboratory animals exposed to I (Kr)-blockers (class III anti-arrhythmic agent), zinc deficient diet, the organophosphate pesticide chlopyrifos fumonisins (environmental toxins produced *Fusarium moniliforme* (*F. verticilliodes*), *F. proliferatum*, and other *Fusarium* species of molds), during pregnancy [38–40].

Fish with vertebral deformities and abnormal mechanical vertebral properties were produced following exposure of juvenile fourhorn sculpin, *Myoxocephalus quadricornis* L. to tetrachloro-1, 2-benzoquinone, a component in bleached kraft mill effluents [41]. Exposure to carbon monoxide[42] and boric acid are associated with alterations in HOX-mediated gene expression [43]. Retinoic acid, a vitamin A analogue, has been observed to cause homeotic transformations in mice and axial skeletal truncation in the *Dominant hemimelia (dh)* mouse, suggesting a possible relationship between retinoic acid signaling and the *dh* gene [44]. Increased axial skeletal defects and apoptosis were associated

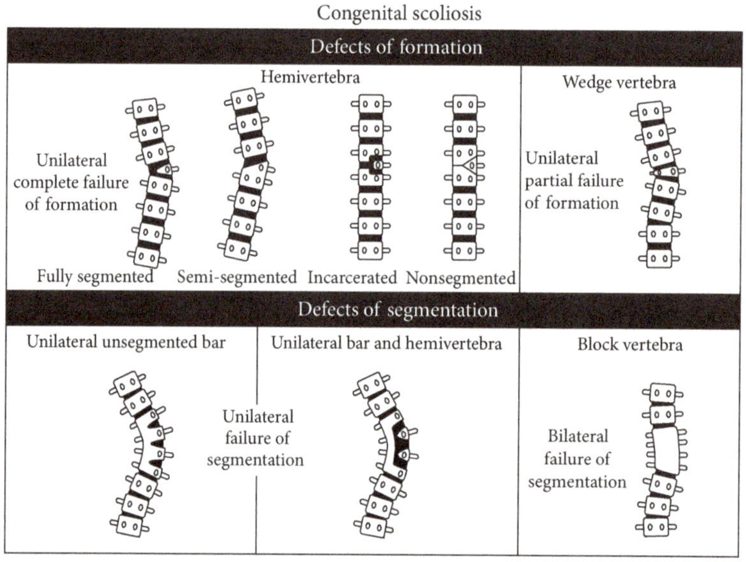

FIGURE 1: Diagram of spine illustrating defects of formation (wedge and hemivertebrae) and segmentation (vertebral bar and block vertebrae). Reprinted with permission from McMaster [6].

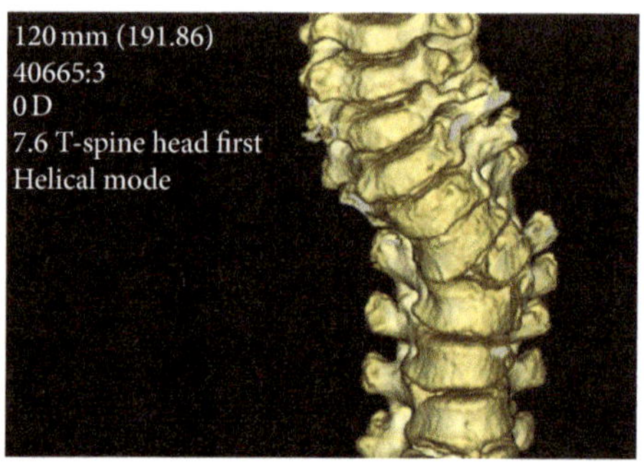

FIGURE 2: 3D reconstruction illustrating congenital scoliosis. Left T4 hemivertebrae displayed. Courtesy of Dr. Kenneth Noonan.

with inhibition of nitric oxide (NO) production or the addition of NO to developing chick embryos [45]. Low birth weight, decreases in successive births, and behavioral deficits replicated by carbon monoxide alone in animal models have been reported to occur in conjunction with cigarette smoking during pregnancy [46, 47]. Cigarette smoke generation of ROS resulting in somite anoxic damage could potentially contribute to the development of CVM.

The occurrence of CS in monozygotic twins [48] is consistent with an observed increased risk for congenital malformations in both monozygotic and dizygotic twins [49]. Congenital malformations and syndromes including Prader-Willi, Angelman, and Beckwith-Wiedemann syndromes have been linked to assisted reproductive technology (ART) [50]. Methyl donor content of the growth media has been suggested as a possible mechanism of CVM occurrence in ART-assisted pregnancies, and nutritional factors have been implicated for their occurrence in non-ART pregnancies, suggesting a possible relationship between epigenetic factors and CVM. Similar to other birth defects, CVM often represent sporadic occurrences making epigenetic factors another plausible mechanism for investigation.

Hyperthermia has been associated with CVM development. Heat shock proteins are recruited when there is exposure to nonteratogenic doses of heat (<2°C) which provide protection for proteins against subsequent damage by teratogenic doses of heat (>2°C). Heat shock proteins attach to uncovered active sites, thus preventing their binding with other functionally impaired aggregate proteins [51]. Hyperthermia results in inhibition of the cell cycle and induces apoptosis. Although the exact mechanism responsible for altered somitogenesis associated with heat is uncertain, Notch/Delta signaling pathway proteins may undergo alteration(s) and result in abnormal vertebral patterning.

Presently there are no reported studies which describe the relative contribution of maternal exposures to CVM development. In a series of 206, 244 live births, still births, and elective terminations, a total of 5 cases of isolated hemivertebrae, and 22 cases of hemivertebrae with other birth defects were identified [52]. The most common maternal exposure associated with CVM was maternal diabetes (5 cases) followed by twinning (2 cases).

5. Classification of CVM

A classification scheme for CVM which is simple and unified is essential for clinicians and researchers to describe individual and collective CVM from both a phenotypic and genetic etiologic vantage point. A number of classification schemes for CVM have been proposed which have individually focused upon different components associated with CVM, an occurrence including a developmental basis for CVM, [53, 54] syndromic diagnosis of CVM (i.e. spondylocostal

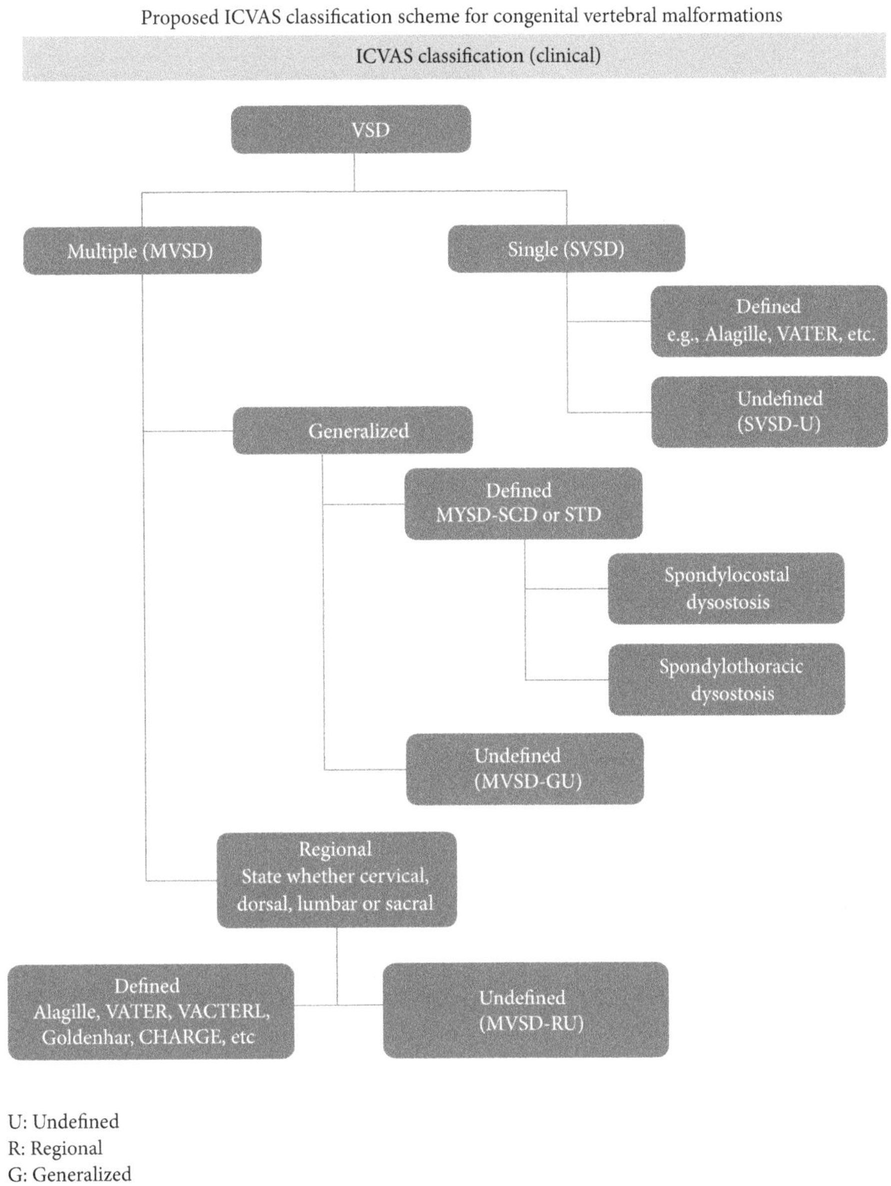

FIGURE 3: Algorithm for International Consortium for Vertebral Anomalies and Scoliosis (ICVAS) classification of congenital vertebral malformation. Reproduced with permission Expert opinion in [7]. Reproduced from Expert Opinion in *Expert Opin. Med. Diagn. (2008) 2(10):1107-1121* with permission of Informa UK Ltd.

dysostosis, Klippel-Feil, etc.) [54–56], and mode of inheritance [57]. Recently a proposed pilot classification system by the International Consortium for Vertebral Anomalies (CVM) and Scoliosis (ICVAS) was outlined algorithmically in Figure 4 [58]. A category of vertebral segmentation defects (VSDs) may be defined as a single (SVSD) or multiple (MVSD). Known syndromes such as hemifacial microsomia or VACTERL may be associated with an SVSD. MVSDs are defined as generalized when there is involvement of 10 or greater contiguous vertebral bodies and may represent a defined phenotype such as spondylocostal dysostosis or spondylothoracic dysostosis, or an undefined phenotype. Alternatively, MSVD may have a regional distribution and be associated with a defined or undefined phenotype. Since prior usage of the term "Jarcho Levin syndrome" has been associated with a wide range of inconsistent skeletal features, and has been used indiscriminately, ICVAS has recommended that this term not be used. A high degree of inter observer reliability has been noted with the proposed classification system, which provides a basis for future cohort genetic analysis of similar CVM phenotypes.

6. Monogenic CVM

Mutations in Notch signaling genes have been identified in two monogenic forms of CVM. Spondylocostal dysostosis (SCD) is an autosomal recessive disorder, with occasional

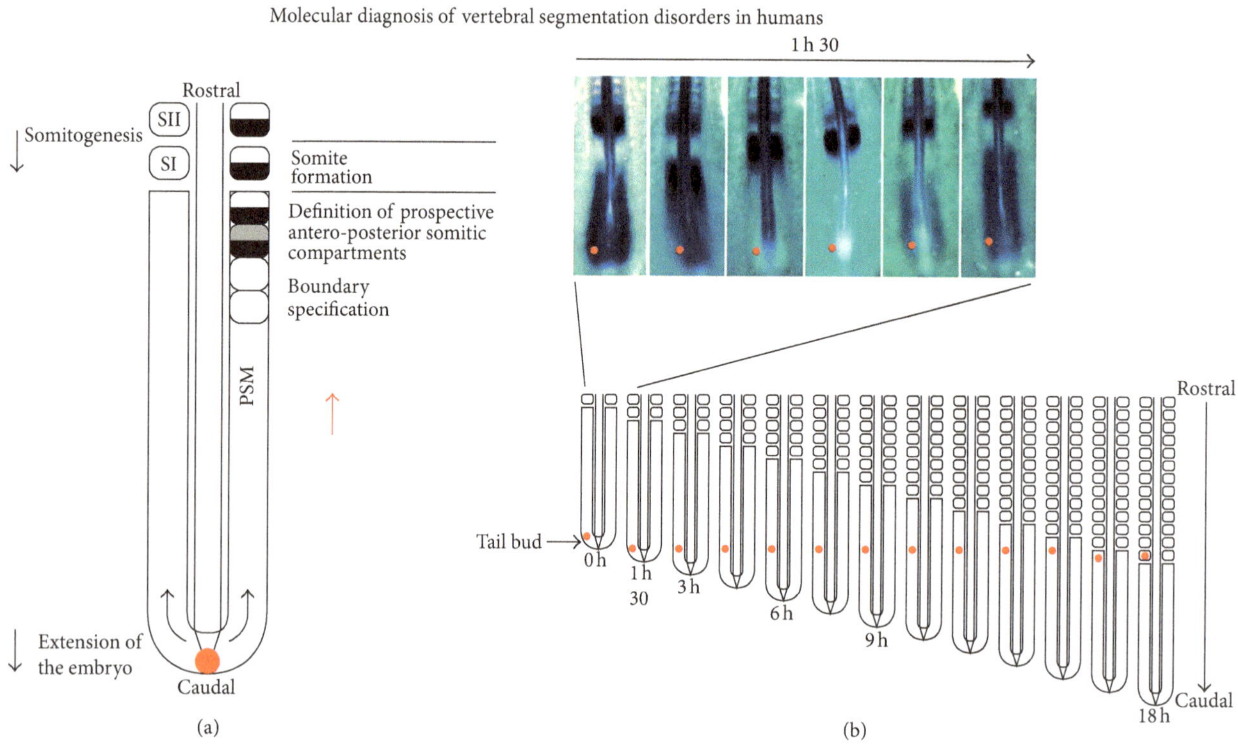

Figure 4: Illustration of somite formation from the presomitic mesoderm (PSM) in the chick embryo. Paired somites are formed every 90 minutes in a periodic fashion every 90 minutes shown in (a). (b) A molecular clocked linked to segmentation by dynamic and periodic expression of the cyclic genes in the PSM. Top: Lunatic Fringe mRNA expression appears as a wave sweeping across the whole PSM once during each somite formation as illustrated by in situ hybridization in this 17-somite-old chick embryo. During each somite formations, PSM cells illustrated by the dot undergo a phase of upregulation of the cycling genes followed by a phase of down regulation of these genes. Bottom: As shown in this schematic representation of the progression of somitogenesis in the embryo, the cycles of expression of the cyclic genes will last while the cells remain in the PSM, which corresponds approximately to the time to form 12 somites in the chick embryo. These PSM cells undergo 12 oscillations of the expression of the cycling genes. Reproduced with permission Expert Opinion in [9]. Reproduced from Expert Opinion in *Expert Opin. Med. Diagn. (2008) 2(10):1107-1121* with permission of Informa UK Ltd.

autosomal dominant inheritance. Radiographically, SCD is characterized by contiguous vertebral segmentation defects in addition to rib abnormalities Figure 5. Affected individuals have disproportionate short stature, characterized by a shortened trunk and protuberant abdomen. Associated features include scoliosis and mild respiratory compromise. Mutations in *DLL3*, a Notch pathway signaling gene, were identified in Arab-Israeli and Pakistani kindreds using synteny conversion analysis [59]. Mutations in Notch signaling pathway genes, including *MESP2* [60], *LFNG* [61], and *HES7*, have subsequently been identified [62]. The term "pebble beach" sign refers to morphologically abnormal vertebral bodies characterized by a smooth, round contour, usually associated with the presence of a *DLL3* mutation [63]. Hypoplasia of the left vertebral artery has been reported in one affected individual with a compound heterozygous mutation in *HES7* (158D/V186Y).

Spondylothoracic dysostosis (STD) is an autosomal recessive disorder of vertebral segmentation with a clinical phenotype of disproportionate short stature, with increased thoracic anterior posterior diameter. STD has a radiographic appearance characterized by the presence of posterior rib fusion, also referred to as a "crab like thorax," as illustrated in Figure 6 [64]. There is some degree of respiratory compromise due to the presence of the short thoracic cage. STD is caused by mutations in the MESP2 gene, and has a prevalence of 1/12,000 in the Puerto Rican population, with a suggestion of a founder effect of the E103X (p.Glu103X) mutation among Puerto Ricans [65]. Only 25% of affected children with STD survive into adolescence and adulthood, indicating that the degree of respiratory compromise is more severe in STD as compared to SCD. Thoracic insufficiency syndrome is associated with STD and is associated with underlying diminished lung volume and chest wall stiffness. CVM can be associated with a variety of syndromes as shown in Table 1.

7. Sporadically Occurring CVMs

Because CVM and associated syndromes usually represent sporadic occurrences, even within a particular family, it is difficult to identify causal genetic factors. A panel of genes associated with vertebral patterning defects including *PAX1*, *DLL3*, *SLC35A3*, *WNT3A*, *TBX6*, and *T (Brachyury)* were sequenced by our group in 50 patients with heterogeneous

Table 1: Some syndromes that include congenital vertebral malformations.

Syndrome	OMIM reference	Corresponding gene(s)
Acrofacial dysostosis*	263750	
Aicardi*	304050	
Alagille	118450	*JAGGED1, NOTCH2*
Anhalt*	601344	
Atelosteogenesis III	108721	*FLNB*
Campomelic dysplasia	114290	*SOX9*
Casamassima-Morton-Nance*	271520	
Caudal regression*	182940	
Cerebro-facio-thoracic dysplasia*	213980	
CHARGE	214800	*CHD7*
"Chromosomal"		
Currarino	176450	*HLXB9*
DeLa Chapelle*	256050	
DeGeorge/Sedlackova	188400	Microdeletion, 10p13-p14, 22q11.2,
Dysspondylochondromatosis*		
Femoral hypoplasia-unusual facies*	134780	
Fibrodysplasia ossificans progressive	135100	*ACVR1*
Fryns-Moerman*		
Goldenhar* (Oculo-auriculo-vertebral spectrum)	164210	
Incontinentia Pigmenti	308300	*NEMO*
Kabuki	147920	*MLL2*
Kaufman-McKusick	236700	*MKKS*
KBG Syndrome*	148050	
Klippel-Feil*	118100	*?PAXl, GDF6*
Larsen	150250	*FLNB*
Lower mesodermal agenesis*		
Maternal diabetes*		
MURCS Association*	601076	
Multiple Pterygium Syndrome	265000	*CHRNG*
OEIS Syndrome*	258040	
Phaver*	261575	
Rapadilino	266280	*RECQL4*
Robinow	268310	*ROR2*
Rolland-Desbuquois*	224400	
Rokitansky Sequence*	277000	*?WNT4*
Silverman	224410	*HSPG2*
Simpson-Golabi-Behmel	312870	*GPC3*
Sirenomelia*	182940	
Spondylocarpotarsal Synostosis	272460	*FLNB*
Spondylocostal Dysostosis	277300	*DLL3, MESP2, LFNG*
Spondylothoracic Dysotosis*	277300	*MESP2*
Thakker-Donnai*	227255	
Toriello*		
Urioste*		
VATER/VACTERL*	192350	
Verloove-Vanhorick*	215850	
Wildevanck*	314600	
Zimmer*	273395	

*Underlying cause not known. Reproduced from *Expert Opinion in Expert Opin. Med. Diagn. (2008) 2(10):1107-1121* with permission of Informa UK Ltd.

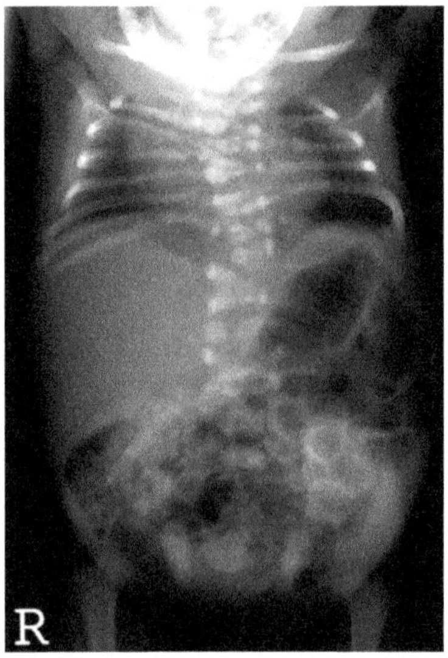

Figure 5: Radiographic features of spondylocostal dystostosis including contiguous vertebral malformations with asymmetric rib malformations. Photograph courtesy of Peter D. Turnpenny M.D., Royal Devon and Exeter Hospital.

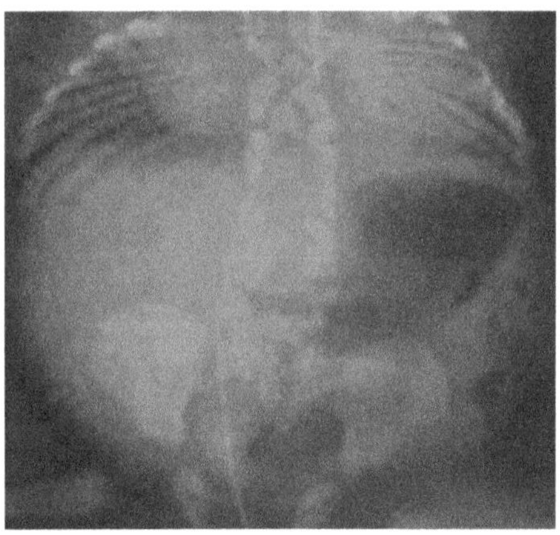

Figure 6: Radiograph features of spondylothoracic dysostosis demonstrating contiguous vertebral malformations with symmetric posterior rib fusion. Reproduced with permission Expert Opinion in [9].

types of CVMs [66–70]. A mutation (c.1013C>T) resulting in an alanine to valine change was found at amino acid position 338 in the *T (Brachyury)* gene in three affected patients, in this cohort that was not present among 886 chromosomes in the CEPH diversity panel [66]. Collectively these patients had maternal pregnancy exposure histories of diabetes, valproic acid, and clomiphene. The third affected individual did not have any history of maternal exposure during pregnancy. The phenotypes of these patients were all distinct and included cervical and thoracic CVM and sacral agenesis. This mutation had previously been described in another individual with sacral agenesis with no history of maternal diabetes during pregnancy [71]. Although no mutations in *TBX6* were identified in the previously described patient series, polymorphisms of the somite patterning gene *TBX6*, specifically rs2289292 (located at exon 8) and rs380962 (located at the $5'$UTR), may have an important role in the pathogenesis of congenital scoliosis in the Chinese Han population [72].

CVM may mediated through complex interactions of genetic, environmental and epigenetic factors. Gestational hypoxia in $Hes7^{+/-}$ and $Mesp2^{+/-}$ mice results in an increase in severity of CVM in mice. This effect mediated by abnormal FGF signaling results in altered somitogenesis and provides evidence that an environmental trigger such as hypoxia can potentiate a CVM occurrence in a genetically susceptible background [73]. The observation that the phenotypic expression of tail kinks in the axin fused mouse ($Axin^{Fu}$) can be altered by increased DNA methylation supports an epigenetic contribution to CVM occurrence [74].

Whole exome sequence (WES) and whole genome sequence (WGS) platforms represent suitable platforms for the identification of candidate gene sequence variants and copy number variants (CNV). WES analyzes approximately 1% of the entire genome and highlights identification of sequence variation in the coding and splice site regions in annotated genes identifying approximately 20,000 sequence variants. WGS is capable of uncovering all genetic and genomic variations, including single nucleotide variants (SNV) and CNV identifying approximately 3.5 million sequence variants [75]. A variety of filtering algorithms, including elimination of sequence variants, present in databases such as dbSNP and the 1,000 Genomes Project database, are implemented to narrow down potential candidate genes. Among coding variants decreasing priority is given to nonsense, frameshift, splice-site, and missense mutations. Inheritance modeling (dominant, recessive) computer prediction in conjunction with disease specific information helps to enable further refinement.

Evidence for localization of vertebral patterning genes identified in mice, Xenopus, and chickens, in synteny blocks supports a hypothesis for conservation of vertebral patterning genes among amniotes [76]. SNV identified in patterning genes previously identified in model organisms should be sought initially, although the advantage of WES and WGS is the ability to identify novel genes and pathways associated with disease. Following identification of a narrowed and focused list of candidate genes, functional confirmation is necessary. WES is applicable for the identification of SNV in highly penetrant mendelian disease phenotypes, whereas WGS has applications for both mendelian and complex phenotype identification in addition to sporadic phenotypes which are the result of *de novo* CNVs or SNVs.

8. "Sporadically" Occurring CVM-Related Syndromes

Oculo-auriculo-vertebral spectrum disorders and Klippel-Feil syndrome are two frequently encountered syndromes associated with CVM. Progress has been made in understanding their etiologies and each is discussed below.

8.1. Oculo-Auriculo-Vertebral Spectrum (Hemifacial Microsomia). Major clinical features of oculo-auriculo-vertebral spectrum (OAVS) include unilateral microtia, craniofacial asymmetry, mandibular hypoplasia, ocular epibulbar dermoid, and CVM [77]. Additional features include: cleft lip with or without cleft palate, congenital heart disease, and congenital renal malformations. There is overlap between OAVS and other syndromes including Treacher Collins syndrome (associated with microtia, lower eyelid colobomas, and mandibular hypoplasia), Fanconi Anemia (radial ray abnormalities, short stature, elevated diepoxy butane induced chromosome breakage), and VACTERL syndrome. At the present time there is no common etiology for OAVS, although there is evidence supporting vascular disruption [78], maternal diabetes [79], and other teratogenetic agents including retinoic acid [80] and thalidomide [81]. Using high density oligonucletotide microarray CGH technology, 12 of 86 (14%) patients with hemifacial microsomia studied were identified as having a CNV, including 4 patients with deletions and/or 8 patients with duplications ranging between 2.3–2.8 Mb in size [82]. Of the three patients with CVM who had CNV, one patient had a paternally inherited 9q34.11 duplication. None of the genes involved in the 9q34.11 have any known function with respect to vertebral body development; a second patient had a duplication involving 20p12.2. The *ANKRD5* gene was present within this region and is not known to have any known function in somite formation; the third patient had a coincident isodicentric Y chromosome. These results indicate that CNV represents a minority of genetic causes for hemifacial microsomia and support a hypothesis for genetic heterogeneity of OAVS.

8.2. Klippel Feil Syndrome. The majority of cases of Klippel-Feil syndrome (short neck, low posterior hairline, and fusion of cervical vertebrae) represent sporadic occurrences within a family. However, Klippel-Feil syndrome may represent a familial occurrence in which multiple family members are affected. Autosomal dominant, autosomal recessive, and X-linked forms of Klippel-Feil syndrome have been reported [83]. Wildervank syndrome refers to a constellation of features including Klippel-Feil syndrome, congenital hearing loss, Duane retraction syndrome (limitation of abduction with narrowing of the palpebral fissure and retraction of the globe) [84].

Klippel-Feil syndrome is sometimes associated with mirror movements, or the involuntary movement of the one extremity mimicking the opposite extremity, with a central mirror serving as a reference point, reflecting the image of the voluntary extremity to the opposite side [85–88]. One neuroanatomic basis for mirror movements is hypothesized to be related to variations in the normal pathways of descending corticospinal tracts, including the crossed lateral corticospinal tract (LCT), uncrossed anterior corticospinal tract (ACT), and anterolateral corticospinal tract (ALCT) [88]. Other hypotheses include delayed resolution following a CNS insult or loss of normal control pathways. No coding mutations were identified in a series of genes associated with aberrant ocular motor and corticospinal axon path development in a patient with Wildervanck syndrome, mirror movements and neuroschisis, including *ROBO3*, *CHN1*, *HOXA1*, *DCC*, and *GDF6* [89]. Analysis of additional patients would be helpful to support a hypothesis for mutations in genes associated with corticospinal axon path development.

A mutation at a highly conserved region in the BMP ligand *GDF6* gene c.866T>C was identified in both familial and sporadic forms of Klippel Feil syndrome [90]. The variable expressivity in affected family members and incomplete penetrance observed in *GDF6* knockout mice suggest thresholds of GDF6 necessary for spine development are subject to modification by environmental factors and may vary between individuals and within different spinal regions. An autosomal dominant mutation (R266C) in *GDF3* has been identified in one family with ocular defects including iris and retinal coloboma and CVM [91]. Zebrafish morpholinos for *Gdf1/3* demonstrated retinal colobomas and trunk shortening with vertebral malformations.

9. Idiopathic Scoliosis

9.1. Management. While CS is associated with underlying CVM, the spine in IS has a normal morphologic appearance. The incidence of IS for treatable curves defined as 25° or greater is greater in females than in males with a ratio of 2 : 1, respectively. Gender differences may underlie scoliotic curve progression [92].

Current management of IS in a growing child includes: (1) Observation of curves that are <25°, (2) Bracing fulltime for curves progressing >25°, and (3) surgery (spinal fusion and instrumentation) for curves >40–45°. By age 16, 0.6% of affected people will have required active treatment with a full-time thoracolumbar-sacral orthosis (TLSO) or surgical correction with instrumentation [3]. Bracing involves the wearing of a TLSO 22 hours/day until spinal maturation [93]. Fulltime bracing is 80%–85% effective in holding curves under the surgery range at the completion of growth. However, in spite of full compliance with brace wear, there is a 15%–20% failure of bracing, and surgery is indicated.

Though scoliosis manifests during adolescence, it continues to cause significant medical problems most of late adolescent and adult life. The population of scoliotic teenagers treated in the 1950s and 1960s has now reached adulthood. Those who underwent surgical corrections are now manifesting the late effects of both the underlying scoliosis and interventional outcomes. Those who had no surgical intervention also manifest the later effects of scoliosis: back pain, progression, and significant respiratory and cardiac compromise [94]. These late consequences are not surprising in light of the pathological consequences associated with the disorder. Significant health problems have been reported in association with IS, including chronic back and neck pain, flatback syndrome, disc herniations, osteoarthritis, osteoporosis, kyphosis, disability, cosmetic dissatisfaction, and psychologic distress [95]. Patients with severe scoliosis, that is, curves >70°, are 3 times more likely to die from cardiopulmonary disease than unaffected individuals [96].

9.2. Genetic Etiologies of IS. The mode of inheritance of IS has not been solidly established and is under debate [1, 26,

95, 97–100]. Inheritance patterns reported include autosomal dominant with variable penetrance, autosomal recessive, multifactorial, and X-linked dominant modes. Hypotheses advanced to explain pathogenesis of IS include abnormalities in the composition of the connective tissue matrix, melatonin, calmodulin, neuromuscular imbalance, and altered vestibular function. Previous studies, illustrated in Table 2, demonstrated genetic heterogeneity for IS, although no single gene linked with the development of IS has been identified to date.

Candidate gene analysis of IS has focused on stratification of genes on the basis of their presumed function including: connective tissue, bone formation and metabolism, melatonin signaling pathway, puberty, and growth [115]. Several genes encoding extracellular matrix proteins, including elastin, types I and II collagen (COL1A1, COL1A2, COL2A1), and fibrillin, failed to demonstrate linkage to IS [97, 116]. Melatonin is considered a contributor to IS based on the observation that pinealectomy in newborn chickens leads to a spinal deformity similar to IS in humans [117]. Melatonin signaling was also impaired in patients with IS [118]. However, no evidence for linkage of IS to chromosome 4q, the locus for the human melatonin 1A receptor, has been observed, indicating that scoliosis does not result solely from melatonin deficiency [105, 119].

Linkage to 19p13 was described in two separate studies [102, 108]. Two loci within this region are credible candidates for IS: fibrillin 3 and thromboxane A2 receptor. Fibrillin 3 is a component of the extracellular matrix, which contributes to microfibrillar structure. Since abnormalities in platelet function have been reported in IS [120, 121], attention has turned towards understanding the interaction between calmodulin, myosin, and actin in platelets and subsequent development of IS.

These studies described above were largely based on analysis of strategically spaced genetic markers across the genome in large families with IS in order to identify linkages to a chromosomal region corresponding to the potential genetic basis for IS. Further exploration of candidate gene region(s) demonstrating association with familial IS would be required to determine their relative contribution to isolated sporadic (non familial) cases of IS.

9.3. Genetic Prognostic Factors Associated with IS and Curve Progression. Why and which curves will fail treatment are not known. Theories abound as to hypokyphotic curves, larger magnitude curves, and less flexible curves. There is evidence that genetic factors such as estrogen receptor genotype may predict curve progression in IS [122]. There is also evidence that elevated calmodulin levels contribute to curve progression in IS, possibly through interference with estrogen binding to the estrogen receptor [123]. SNPs have been used to develop an AIS-Prognostic Test (AIS-PT) to identify the curves that will not require bracing or surgery and curves that will fail bracing.

Determining which children with adolescent idiopathic scoliosis (AIS) between the ages of 9 and 13 years will require bracing is a challenge for the treating orthopedic surgeon. An application of genetic knowledge is to use this information in combination with additional clinical information to determine which patients using a series of 52 single nucleotide polymorphisms associated with genetic loci on all chromosomes except 3, 13, 21, and the Y chromosome, in conjunction with a the Cobb angle at the time of initial diagnosis, a logistic regression analysis has been utilized to obtain an AIS Prognostic Test score between 1 and 200 [124]. In three tested populations, low risk scores of <41 were observed to have a negative predictive value of 100%, 99%, and 97%. High risk scores (181–200) would identify the 1-2% of patients most likely to progress to a severe curve. Those patients with intermediate risk scores (51–180) would require close follow up for their curve progression by an orthopedic surgeon. Presently, information regarding the biological function of the genes used for the AIS Prognostic Test score is incomplete. The potential advantage of prognostic testing would be to reduce costs of imaging in those patients who are at a lower risk for scoliosis curve progression.

In addition to previous studies suggesting a genetic component linked to the development of IS as a binary trait, there is evidence that genetic factors may predict curve progression in IS. An association study performed in 304 females with IS demonstrated a significantly greater Cobb angle at the time of growth maturation among patients with estrogen receptor genotype XX and Xx compared to patients with genotype xx ($P = 0.002$) [122]. A higher risk for operative treatment was observed among patients with genotype XX and Xx, compared to patients with genotype xx. There is also evidence that elevated calmodulin levels contribute to curve progression in IS, possibly through interference with estrogen binding to the estrogen receptor [123].

The single-nucleotide polymorphism SNP-418G/C in the tissue inhibitor of metalloproteinase-2 gene promoter region was associated with thoracic scoliosis curve severity [125]. Downregulation of *TIMP-2* transcriptional activity resulting in increased vascular proliferation and enhanced anterior spine endochondral ossification during adolescence could result in disproportionate spinal growth and result in thoracic scoliosis. The promoter polymorphism (rs11063714) in the neurotrophin 3 (*NTF3*) gene is associated with curve severity for IS in the Chinese Han population. Individuals affected with IS having an AA genotype had lower mean maximum Cobb angle as compared to patients with AG and GG genotypes [126]. Patients who were skeletally mature and had an AA genotype had greater success for treatment with bracing as compared to patients with GG genotype. Egr $3^{-/-}$ mice fail to express NTF3 and have proprioceptive dysfunction due to muscle spindle agenesis, apoptosis of proprioceptive neurons, proprioceptive neuron apoptosis, and disruption of synaptic connectivity between muscle sensory and motor neurons. A reduction in the number of muscle spindles and malfunction has been demonstrated in spinal muscle obtained from patients with IS, examined histologically and histochemically [127]. There is also increased expression of NTF3 messenger RNA in paravertebral muscle in IS [119]. These observations in addition to a strong linkage signal on chromosome 12p13 [111], the *NTF3* locus provide support for a role of *NTF3* in the pathogenesis of IS.

Table 2: Summary of prior genetic linkage studies for IS.

Study	No. of Families/Individuals	Region(s)	Model	Comments
Wise et al. [101]	1/14	6q distal 10q 18q	Autosomal dominant	Genome wide search in one family of French Acadian and English descent (7 affected members), with validation of "hot spots" in a second large family
Chan et al. [102]	7/52	19p13.3	Autosomal dominant	Recruited Asian patients in whom scoliosis developed in adolescence
Baghernajad Salehi et al. [103]	1/17	17p.11	Autosomal dominant	3 generation Italian family
Justice et al. [104]	202/1198	Xq23 Xq26.1	X-linked dominant	Maximum lod score of 1.69 (theta = 0.2) identified at marker GATA172D05. A lod score of 2.23 for this marker was found in one family with six affected individuals
Morcuende et al. [105]	47/176	4q35	N/A	No linkage to *MTNR1A* (Melatonin Receptor 1A) and no mutations in *MTNR1A*
Bashiardes et al. [106]	7 individuals	8p23.2-8q11.21	Autosomal dominant	Pericentric inversion in chromosome 8 disrupts *SNTG1* (syntrophin). Five of 7 individuals in family have *SNTG1* deletion
Miller et al. [107]	202/1198	6, 9, 16 and 17	Autosomal dominant	Model independent linkage analysis
Alden et al. [108]	202/1198	19p11.3	Autosomal dominant	Threshold of curvature set at 30°. Fibrillin 3, thromboxane A2 receptor, possible candidates
Baghernajad Salehi et al. [103]	1500 individuals	Chromosome 3 Chromosome 7	Autosomal dominant	Patients' familial relationships established through database
Gao et al. [109]	52	8q	N/A	CHD7 Gene polymorphisms are associated with susceptibility to idiopathic scoliosis
Ocaka et al. [110]	25/208	9q31.2-q34.2; 17q25.3-qter	Autosomal dominant	Confirmation of 9q [107]
Raggio et al. [111]	7/48	12p13.3	Autosomal dominant; autosomal recessive	All families contribute to recessive model. 5/7 families contribute to the dominant model
Gurnett et al. [112]	1/22	18q	Autosomal dominant	LOD score 3.86 Scoliosis and pectus excavatum
Sharma et al. [113]	419	3p26.3 ($P < 8 \times 10^{-8}$)	N/A	GWAS study. *CHL1, DSCAM, CNTNAP2* genes involved in axon guidance
Takahashi et al. [114]	1050	*LBX1* ($P = 1.24 \times 10^{-19}$)	N/A	GWAS study. LBX1 is determinant of dorsal spinal neurons; altered somatosensory function

The above summary illustrates the difficulty of identifying causative genes for IS lies in extreme phenotypic and genetic heterogeneity. Future research will need to be aimed at improved stratification of clinical cases based on factors such as age of onset, curve progression, severity, responsiveness to bracing, and correlation with mutations in genes identified using next generation sequence platforms such as whole exome and whole genome analysis [115].

10. Relationship between Congenital and Idiopathic Scoliosis

Multiple studies support a common genetic etiology for congenital and idiopathic scoliosis. A family history of IS was observed in 17.3% of 237 families in which an affected proband had congenital scoliosis [128]. In 52 families with IS a significant linkage peak was observed on chromosome 8q12 (multipoint LOD 2.77; $P = 0028$). Over transmission of the CHD7 associated polymorphism, *rs4738824* in patients with IS was observed in a cohort of 52 families. Substitution of the A allele of this polymorphism with the G allele is predicted to disrupt a possible binding site for caudal-type (cdx) homeodomain-containing transcription factors. Mutations in *CHD7*, a chromeodomain helicase DNA binding protein are associated with CHARGE syndrome (coloboma of the eye, heart defects, atresia of the choanae, retardation of growth and/or development, genital and/or urinary abnormalities, and ear abnormalities and deafness) [129]. A hypothesis for the development of idiopathic scoliosis is CHD7 may act postnatally to alter spinal growth during the adolescent growth spurt. Chd7 in zebrafish is expressed in somites, brain, eye, and otic vesicle. *Chd7* enables proper symmetric expression of critically important somitogenesis associated genes located downstream from Wnt including *her7*, *cdx1a*, *dlc*, *mespa*, and *ripply*. Zebrafish morpholinos in which CHD7 was knocked down were noted to have tail kinks and a progressively shortened axis [130]. Chd7 plays an important role in somitogenesis as supported by a lack of distinct somite boundary formation and abnormal expression of *ephrin B2a*, an important segment polarity gene when this gene is knocked down in zebrafish [131]. Knockdown of lysyl oxidases lox11 or lox15b in zebrafish in conjunction with diminished copper availability result in distortion of the notochord formation, suggesting a relationship between genetic and nutritional factors in the etiology of notochord development. However no association between coding or tag SNPs in *LOX, LOXL1, LOXL2, LOXL3, LOXL4,* and idiopathic scoliosis was observed.

11. Summary

While CS and IS represent clinically distinct conditions, there is evidence supporting a hypothesis for a common pathogenetic mechanism. The underlying genetic etiologies and respective environmental contributions have not been delineated. The obstacles which need to be overcome include clinical heterogeneity with respect to diversity of the types of CVM with contribute to CS. Idiopathic scoliosis is also a clinically heterogeneous condition and is associated with different ages of onset and prognoses. Advances in genetic technologies can assist in the identification of sequence variants which may contribute to the occurrence of both conditions. Challenges for both conditions are to evaluate their relative contribution to the development of CVM or IS, in addition to determine how multiple mutations in a single individual may interact with one another and environmental factors. The treatment of both conditions requires a multispecialty approach. Unraveling the genetic contributions for both conditions can help to provide improved genetic counseling, prevention, and treatment strategies for families.

References

[1] E. J. Riseborough and R. Wynne Davies, "A genetic survey of idiopathic scoliosis in Boston, Massachusetts," *Journal of Bone and Joint Surgery—Series A*, vol. 55, no. 5, pp. 974–982, 1973.

[2] A. R. Shands and H. B. Eisberg, "The incidence of scoliosis in the state of Delaware; a study of 50,000 minifilms of the chest made during a survey for tuberculosis," *Journal of Bone and Joint Surgery— Series A*, vol. 37, no. 6, pp. 1243–1249, 1955.

[3] E. J. Rogala, D. S. Drummond, and J. Gurr, "Scoliosis: incidence and natural history. A prospective epidemiological study," *Journal of Bone and Joint Surgery—Series A*, vol. 60, no. 2, pp. 173–176, 1978.

[4] M. C. Brand, "Examination of the newborn with congenital scoliosis: focus on the physical," *Advances in Neonatal Care*, vol. 8, no. 5, pp. 265–273, 2008.

[5] B. R. Davies and M. Durán, "Malformations of the cranium, vertebral column, and related central nervous system: morphologic heterogeneity may indicate biological diversity," *Birth Defects Research Part A—Clinical and Molecular Teratology*, vol. 67, no. 8, pp. 563–571, 2003.

[6] M. J. McMaster, "Congenital deformities of the spine," *Journal of the Royal College of Surgeons of Edinburgh*, vol. 47, no. 2, pp. 475–480, 2002.

[7] P. F. Giampietro, S. L. Dunwoodie, K. Kusumi et al., "Molecular diagnosis of vertebral segmentation disorders in humans," *Expert Opinion on Medical Diagnostics*, vol. 2, no. 10, pp. 1107–1121, 2008.

[8] O. Pourquié, "Vertebrate segmentation: from cyclic gene networks to scoliosis," *Cell*, vol. 145, no. 5, pp. 650–663, 2011.

[9] J. Cooke and E. C. Zeeman, "A clock and wavefront model for control of the number of repeated structures during animal morphogenesis," *Journal of Theoretical Biology*, vol. 58, no. 2, pp. 455–476, 1976.

[10] Y. Bessho, H. Hirata, Y. Masamizu, and R. Kageyama, "Periodic repression by the bHLH factor Hes7 is an essential mechanism for the somite segmentation clock," *Genes and Development*, vol. 17, no. 12, pp. 1451–1456, 2003.

[11] S. L. Dunwoodie, M. Clements, D. B. Sparrow, X. Sa, R. A. Conlon, and R. S. P. Beddington, "Axial skeletal defects caused by mutation in the spondylocostal dysplasia/pudgy gene Dll3 are associated with disruption of the segmentation clock within the presomitic mesoderm," *Development*, vol. 129, no. 7, pp. 1795–1806, 2002.

[12] S. A. Holley, R. Geisler, and C. Nüsslein-Volhard, "Control of her1 expression during zebrafish somitogenesis by a Delta-dependent oscillator and an independent wave-front activity," *Genes and Development*, vol. 14, no. 13, pp. 1678–1690, 2000.

[13] C. Jouve, I. Palmeirim, D. Henrique et al., "Notch signalling is required for cyclic expression of the hairy-like gene HES1 in the presomitic mesoderm," *Development*, vol. 127, no. 7, pp. 1421–1429, 2000.

[14] M. L. Dequéant, E. Glynn, K. Gaudenz et al., "A complex oscillating network of signaling genes underlies the mouse segmentation clock," *Science*, vol. 314, no. 5805, pp. 1595–1598, 2006.

[15] A. Aulehla, C. Wehrle, B. Brand-Saberi et al., "Wnt3a plays a major role in the segmentation clock controlling somitogenesis," *Developmental Cell*, vol. 4, no. 3, pp. 395–406, 2003.

[16] S. E. Cole, J. M. Levorse, S. M. Tilghman, and T. F. Vogt, "Clock regulatory elements control cyclic expression of Lunatic fringe during somitogenesis," *Developmental Cell*, vol. 3, no. 1, pp. 75–84, 2002.

[17] W. Sewell, D. B. Sparrow, A. J. Smith et al., "Cyclical expression of the Notch/Wnt regulator Nrarp requires modulation by Dll3 in somitogenesis," *Developmental Biology*, vol. 329, no. 2, pp. 400–409, 2009.

[18] J. Dubrulle, M. J. McGrew, and O. Pourquié, "FGF signaling controls somite boundary position and regulates segmentation clock control of spatiotemporal Hox gene activation," *Cell*, vol. 106, no. 2, pp. 219–232, 2001.

[19] A. Sawada, M. Shinya, Y. J. Jiang, A. Kawakami, A. Kuroiwa, and H. Takeda, "Fgf/MAPK signalling is a crucial positional cue in somite boundary formation," *Development*, vol. 128, no. 23, pp. 4873–4880, 2001.

[20] A. Aulehla and O. Pourquié, "Oscillating signaling pathways during embryonic development," *Current Opinion in Cell Biology*, vol. 20, no. 6, pp. 632–637, 2008.

[21] W. C. Dunty Jr., K. K. Biris, R. B. Chalamalasetty, M. M. Taketo, M. Lewandoski, and T. P. Yamaguchi, "Wnt3a/β-catenin signaling controls posterior body development by coordinating

mesoderm formation and segmentation," *Development*, vol. 135, no. 1, pp. 85–94, 2008.

[22] K. K. Biris, W. C. Dunty Jr., and T. P. Yamaguchi, "Mouse Ripply2 is downstream of Wnt3a and is dynamically expressed during somitogenesis," *Developmental Dynamics*, vol. 236, no. 11, pp. 3167–3172, 2007.

[23] Y. Moritomo, O. Koga, H. Miyamoto, and T. Tsuda, "Congenital anophthalmia with caudal vertebral anomalies in Japanese Brown cattle," *The Journal of Veterinary Medical Science*, vol. 57, no. 4, pp. 693–696, 1995.

[24] R. B. Chalamalasetty, W. C. Dunty Jr., K. K. Biris et al., "The Wnt3a/beta-catenin target gene Mesogenin1 controls the segmentation clock by activating a Notch signalling program," *Nature Communications*, vol. 2, no. 1, article 390, 2011.

[25] J. Vermot and O. Pourquié, "Retinoic acid coordinates somitogenesis and left-right patterning in vertebrate embryos," *Nature*, vol. 435, no. 7039, pp. 215–220, 2005.

[26] U. M. Ahn, N. U. Ahn, L. Nallamshetty et al., "The etiology of adolescent idiopathic scoliosis," *American Journal of Orthopedics*, vol. 31, no. 7, pp. 387–395, 2002.

[27] S. J. Tredwell, D. F. Smith, P. J. Macleod, and B. J. Wood, "Cervical spine anomalies in fetal alcohol syndrome," *Spine*, vol. 7, no. 4, pp. 331–334, 1982.

[28] L. B. Holmes, E. A. Harvey, B. A. Coull et al., "The teratogenicity of anticonvulsant drugs," *The New England Journal of Medicine*, vol. 344, no. 15, pp. 1132–1138, 2001.

[29] E. Menegola, M. L. Broccia, H. Nau, M. Prati, R. Ricolfi, and E. Giavini, "Teratogenic effects of sodium valproate in mice and rats at midgestation and at term," *Teratogenesis Carcinogenesis and Mutagenesis*, vol. 16, no. 2, pp. 97–108, 1996.

[30] C. V. Vorhees, "Teratogenicity and developmental toxicity of valproic acid in rats," *Teratology*, vol. 35, no. 2, pp. 195–202, 1987.

[31] J. G. Breen, T. W. Claggett, G. L. Kimmel, and C. A. Kimmel, "Heat shock during rat embryo development in vitro results in decreased mitosis and abundant cell death," *Reproductive Toxicology*, vol. 13, no. 1, pp. 31–39, 1999.

[32] A. Åberg, L. Westbom, and B. Källén, "Congenital malformations among infants whose mothers had gestational diabetes or preexisting diabetes," *Early Human Development*, vol. 61, no. 2, pp. 85–95, 2001.

[33] M. L. Martinez-Frias, E. Bermejo, E. Rodriguez-Pinilla, L. Prieto, and J. L. Frias, "Epidemiological analysis of outcomes of pregnancy in gestational diabetic mothers," *American Journal of Medical Genetics*, vol. 78, pp. 140–145, 1998.

[34] E. Passarge and W. Lenz, "Syndrome of caudal regression in infants of diabetic mothers: observations of further cases," *Pediatrics*, vol. 37, no. 4, pp. 672–675, 1966.

[35] P. G. Alexander and R. S. Tuan, "Role of environmental factors in axial skeletal dysmorphogenesis," *Birth Defects Research Part C—Embryo Today*, vol. 90, no. 2, pp. 118–132, 2010.

[36] R. Allache, P. De Marco, E. Merello, V. Capra, and Z. Kibar, "Role of the planar cell polarity gene CELSR1 in neural tube defects and caudal agenesis," *Birth Defects Research Part A—Clinical and Molecular Teratology*, vol. 94, no. 3, pp. 176–181, 2012.

[37] M. Simons and M. Mlodzik, "Planar cell polarity signaling: from fly development to human disease," *Annual Review of Genetics*, vol. 42, pp. 517–540, 2008.

[38] W. Hickory, R. Nanda, and F. A. Catalanotto, "Fetal skeletal malformations associated with moderate zinc deficiency during pregnancy," *Journal of Nutrition*, vol. 109, no. 5, pp. 883–891, 1979.

[39] A. C. Sköld, K. Wellfelt, and B. R. Danielsson, "Stage-specific skeletal and visceral defects of the IKr-blocker almokalant: further evidence for teratogenicity via a hypoxia-related mechanism," *Teratology*, vol. 64, no. 6, pp. 292–300, 2001.

[40] Y. Tian, H. Ishikawa, T. Yamaguchi, T. Yamauchi, and K. Yokoyama, "Teratogenicity and developmental toxicity of chlorpyrifos: maternal exposure during organogenesis in mice," *Reproductive Toxicology*, vol. 20, no. 2, pp. 267–271, 2005.

[41] B. E. Bengtsson, A. Larsson, A. Bengtsson, and L. Renberg, "Sublethal effects of tetrachloro-1,2-benzoquinone—a component in bleachery effluents from pulp mills—on vertebral quality and physiological parameters in fourhorn sculpin," *Ecotoxicology and Environmental Safety*, vol. 15, no. 1, pp. 62–71, 1988.

[42] F. A. Farley, R. T. Loder, B. T. Nolan et al., "Mouse model for thoracic congenital scoliosis," *Journal of Pediatric Orthopaedics*, vol. 21, no. 4, pp. 537–540, 2001.

[43] N. Wéry, M. G. Narotsky, N. Pacico, R. J. Kavlock, J. J. Picard, and F. Gofflot, "Defects in cervical vertebrae in boric acid-exposed rat embryos are associated with anterior shifts of box gene expression domains," *Birth Defects Research Part A—Clinical and Molecular Teratology*, vol. 67, no. 1, pp. 59–67, 2003.

[44] M. H. Owen, L. M. Ryan, and L. B. Holmes, "Effects of retinoic acid on Dominant hemimelia expression in mice," *Birth Defects Research Part A—Clinical and Molecular Teratology*, vol. 85, no. 1, pp. 36–41, 2009.

[45] P. G. Alexander, L. Chau, and R. S. Tuan, "Role of nitric oxide in chick embryonic organogenesis and dysmorphogenesis," *Birth Defects Research Part A—Clinical and Molecular Teratology*, vol. 79, no. 8, pp. 581–594, 2007.

[46] K. S. Bnait and M. J. Seller, "Ultrastructural changes in 9-day old mouse embryos following maternal tobacco smoke inhalation," *Experimental and Toxicologic Pathology*, vol. 47, no. 6, pp. 453–461, 1995.

[47] R. R. Fichtner, K. M. Sullivan, C. L. Zyrkowski, and F. L. Trowbridge, "Racial/ethnic differences in smoking, other risk factors, and low birth weight among low-income pregnant women, 1978–1988," *MMWR. CDC Surveillance Summaries*, vol. 39, no. 3, pp. 13–21, 1990.

[48] A. Kaspiris, T. B. Grivas, and H. R. Weiss, "Congenital scoliosis in monozygotic twins: case report and review of possible factors contributing to its development," *Scoliosis*, vol. 3, no. 1, article 17, 2008.

[49] G. Corsello and E. Piro, "The world of twins: an update," *Journal of Maternal-Fetal and Neonatal Medicine*, vol. 23, supplement 3, pp. 59–62, 2010.

[50] E. L. Niemitz and A. P. Feinberg, "Epigenetics and assisted reproductive technology: a call for investigation," *American Journal of Human Genetics*, vol. 74, no. 4, pp. 599–609, 2004.

[51] G. D. Bennett, "Hyperthermia: malformations to chaperones," *Birth Defects Research Part B*, vol. 89, no. 4, pp. 279–288, 2010.

[52] L. B. Holmes, "Vertebral anomalies: hemivertebrae," in *Common Malformations*, pp. 283–289, Oxford University Press, 2012.

[53] K. Aburakawa, M. Harada, and S. Otake, "Clinical evaluations of the treatment of scoliosis," *Trauma and Orthopaedic Surgery*, vol. 39, pp. 55–62, 1996.

[54] K. Takikawa, N. Haga, T. Maruyama et al., "Spine and rib abnormalities and stature in spondylocostal dysostosis," *Spine*, vol. 31, no. 7, pp. E192–E197, 2006.

[55] M. Klippel and A. Feil, "Un cas d'absence des vertebres cervicales," *Nouvelle Iconog. de la Salpêtrière*, vol. 25, pp. 223–250, 1912.

[56] M. N. Thomsen, U. Schneider, M. Weber, R. Johannisson, and F. U. Niethard, "Scoliosis and congenital anomalies associated with Klippel-Feil syndrome types I-III," *Spine*, vol. 22, no. 4, pp. 396–401, 1997.

[57] G. R. Mortier, R. S. Lachman, M. Bocian, and D. L. Rimoin, "Multiple vertebral segmentation defects: analysis of 26 new patients and review of the literature," *American Journal of Medical Genetics*, vol. 61, no. 4, pp. 310–319, 1996.

[58] A. Offiah, B. Alman, A. S. Cornier et al., "Pilot assessment of a radiologic classification system for segmentation defects of the vertebrae," *American Journal of Medical Genetics, Part A*, vol. 152, no. 6, pp. 1357–1371, 2010.

[59] M. P. Bulman, K. Kusumi, T. M. Frayling et al., "Mutations in the human Delta homologue, DLL3, cause axial skeletal defects in spondylocostal dysostosis," *Nature Genetics*, vol. 24, no. 4, pp. 438–441, 2000.

[60] N. V. Whittock, D. B. Sparrow, M. A. Wouters et al., "Mutated/MESP2 causes spondylocostal dysostosis in humans," *American Journal of Human Genetics*, vol. 74, no. 6, pp. 1249–1254, 2004.

[61] D. B. Sparrow, G. Chapman, M. A. Wouters et al., "Mutation of the LUNATIC FRINGE gene in humans causes spondylocostal dysostosis with a severe vertebral phenotype," *American Journal of Human Genetics*, vol. 78, no. 1, pp. 28–37, 2006.

[62] D. B. Sparrow, D. Sillence, M. A. Wouters, P. D. Turnpenny, and S. L. Dunwoodie, "Two novel missense mutations in HAIRY-AND-ENHANCER-OF-SPLIT-7 in a family with spondylocostal dysostosis," *European Journal of Human Genetics*, vol. 18, no. 6, pp. 674–679, 2010.

[63] P. D. Turnpenny, N. Whittock, J. Duncan, S. Dunwoodie, K. Kusumi, and S. Ellard, "Novel mutations in DLL3, a somitogenesis gene encoding a ligand for the Notch signalling pathway, cause a consistent pattern of abnormal vertebral segmentation in spondylocostal dysostosis," *Journal of Medical Genetics*, vol. 40, no. 5, pp. 333–339, 2003.

[64] J. E. Moseley and R. J. Bonforte, "Spondylothoracic dysplasia—a syndrome of congenital anomalies," *American Journal of Roentgenology, Radium Therapy, and Nuclear Medicine*, vol. 106, no. 1, pp. 166–169, 1969.

[65] A. S. Cornier, K. Staehling-Hampton, K. M. Delventhal et al., "Mutations in the MESP2 gene cause spondylothoracic dysostosis/Jarcho-Levin syndrome," *American Journal of Human Genetics*, vol. 82, no. 6, pp. 1334–1341, 2008.

[66] N. Ghebranious, R. D. Blank, C. L. Raggio et al., "A missense T(Brachyury) mutation contributes to vertebral malformations," *Journal of Bone and Mineral Research*, vol. 23, no. 10, pp. 1576–1583, 2008.

[67] N. Ghebranious, J. K. Burmester, I. Glurich et al., "Evaluation, of SLC35A3 as a candidate gene for human vertebral malformations," *American Journal of Medical Genetics, Part A*, vol. 140, no. 12, pp. 1346–1348, 2006.

[68] N. Ghebranious, C. L. Raggio, R. D. Blank et al., "Lack of evidence of WNT3A as a candidate gene for congenital vertebral malformations," *Scoliosis*, vol. 2, no. 1, article 13, 2007.

[69] P. F. Giampietro, C. L. Raggio, C. Reynolds et al., "DLL3 as a candidate gene for vertebral malformations," *American Journal of Medical Genetics, Part A*, vol. 140, no. 22, pp. 2447–2453, 2006.

[70] P. F. Giampietro, C. L. Raggio, C. E. Reynolds et al., "An analysis of PAX1 in the development of vertebral malformations," *Clinical Genetics*, vol. 68, no. 5, pp. 448–453, 2005.

[71] C. Papapetrou, F. Drummond, W. Reardon, R. Winter, L. Spitz, and Y. H. Edwards, "A genetic study of the human T gene and its exclusion as a major candidate gene for sacral agenesis with anorectal atresia," *Journal of Medical Genetics*, vol. 36, no. 3, pp. 208–213, 1999.

[72] Q. Fei, Z. Wu, H. Wang et al., "The association analysis of TBX6 polymorphism with susceptibility to congenital scoliosis in a Chinese han population," *Spine*, vol. 35, no. 9, pp. 983–988, 2010.

[73] D. B. Sparrow, G. Chapman, A. J. Smith et al., "A mechanism for gene-environment interaction in the etiology of congenital scoliosis," *Cell*, vol. 149, no. 2, pp. 295–306, 2012.

[74] R. A. Waterland, D. C. Dolinoy, J. R. Lin, C. A. Smith, X. Shi, and K. G. Tahiliani, "Maternal methyl supplements increase offspring DNA methylation at Axin fused," *Genesis*, vol. 44, no. 9, pp. 401–406, 2006.

[75] C. Gonzaga-Jauregui, J. R. Lupski, and R. A. Gibbs, "Human genome sequencing in health and disease," *Annual Review of Medicine*, vol. 63, pp. 35–61, 2012.

[76] P. F. Giampietro, C. L. Raggio, and R. D. Blank, "Use of synteny conversion in identification of candidate genes for somitogenesis in humans," *Open Journal of Orthopedics*, vol. 2, pp. 62–68, 2012.

[77] M. M. Cohen, B. R. Rollnick, and C. I. Kaye, "Oculoauriculovertebral spectrum: an updated critique," *Cleft Palate Journal*, vol. 26, no. 4, pp. 276–286, 1989.

[78] R. Cousley, H. Naora, M. Yokoyama, M. Kimura, and H. Otani, "Validity of the Hfm transgenic mouse as a model for hemifacial microsomia," *Cleft Palate-Craniofacial Journal*, vol. 39, no. 1, pp. 81–92, 2002.

[79] R. Wang, M. L. Martínez-Frías, and J. M. Graham Jr., "Infants of diabetic mothers are at increased risk for the oculo-auriculo-vertebral sequence: a case-based and case-control approach," *Journal of Pediatrics*, vol. 141, no. 5, pp. 611–617, 2002.

[80] E. J. Lammer, D. T. Chen, R. M. Hoar et al., "Retinoic acid embryopathy," *The New England Journal of Medicine*, vol. 313, no. 14, pp. 837–841, 1985.

[81] R. W. Smithells and I. Leck, "The incidence of limb and ear defects since the withdrawal of thalidomide," *The Lancet*, vol. 281, no. 7290, pp. 1095–1097, 1963.

[82] C. Rooryck, N. Souakri, D. Cailley et al., "Array-CGH analysis of a cohort of 86 patients with oculoauriculovertebral spectrum," *American Journal of Medical Genetics, Part A*, vol. 152, no. 8, pp. 1984–1989, 2010.

[83] R. A. Clarke, S. Singh, H. McKenzie, J. H. Kearsley, and M. Y. Yip, "Familial Klippel-Feil syndrome and paracentric inversion inv(8)(q22.2q23.3)," *American Journal of Human Genetics*, vol. 57, no. 6, pp. 1364–1370, 1995.

[84] L. Wildervank, "The cerrvico-oculo-acusticus syndrome," in *Congenital Malformations of the Spine and Spinal Cord Handbook of Clinical Neurology*, P. Vinken, G. Bruyn, and N. Myrianthopoulous, Eds., North Holland, New York, NY, USA, 1978.

[85] W. J. Gardner, "Klippel-Feil syndrome, iniencephalus, anencephalus, hindbrain hernia and mirror movements. Overdistention of the neural tube," *Child's Brain*, vol. 5, no. 4, pp. 361–379, 1979.

[86] C. H. Gunderson and G. B. Solitare, "Mirror movements in patients with the Klippel-Feil syndrome. Neuropathologic observations," *Archives of Neurology*, vol. 18, no. 6, pp. 675–679, 1968.

[87] P. Rasmussen, "Persistent mirror movements: a clinical study of 17 children, adolescents and young adults," *Developmental Medicine and Child Neurology*, vol. 35, no. 8, pp. 699–707, 1993.

[88] S. A. Royal, R. S. Tubbs, M. G. D'Antonio, M. J. Rauzzino, and W. J. Oakes, "Investigations into the association between cervicomedullary neuroschisis and mirror movements in patients with Klippel-Feil syndrome," *American Journal of Neuroradiology*, vol. 23, no. 4, pp. 724–729, 2002.

[89] T. Högen, W.-M. Chan, E. Riedel et al., "Wildervanck's syndrome and mirror movements: a congenital disorder of axon migration?" *Journal of Neurology*, vol. 259, no. 4, pp. 761–763, 2012.

[90] M. Tassabehji, M. F. Zhi, E. N. Hilton et al., "Mutations in GDF6 are associated with vertebral segmentation defects in Klippel-Feil syndrome," *Human Mutation*, vol. 29, no. 8, pp. 1017–1027, 2008.

[91] M. Ye, K. M. Berry-Wynne, M. Asai-Coakwell et al., "Mutation of the bone morphogenetic protein GDF3 causes ocular and skeletal anomalies," *Human Molecular Genetics*, vol. 19, no. 2, pp. 287–298, 2009.

[92] S. Weinstein, "The thoracolumbar spine," in *Turek's Orthopedics: Principles and Their Application*, S. Weinstein and J. Buckwalter, Eds., pp. 447–484, Lippincott Company, Philadelphia, Pa, USA, 1994.

[93] A. L. Nachemson, L. E. Peterson, D. S. Bradford et al., "Effectiveness of treatment with a brace in girls who have adolescent idiopathic scoliosis. A prospective, controlled study based on data from the Brace Study of the Scoliosis Research Society," *Journal of Bone and Joint Surgery—Series A*, vol. 77, no. 6, pp. 815–822, 1995.

[94] D. S. Bradford, B. K. B. Tay, and S. S. Hu, "Adult scoliosis: surgical indications, operative management, complications, and outcomes," *Spine*, vol. 24, no. 24, pp. 2617–2629, 1999.

[95] H. Garland, "Hereditary scoliosis," *British Medical Journal*, vol. 1, no. 3816, article 328, 1934.

[96] W. F. Enneking and P. Harrington, "Pathological changes in scoliosis," *Journal of Bone and Joint Surgery—Series A*, vol. 51, no. 1, pp. 165–184, 1969.

[97] N. H. Miller, "Cause and natural history of adolescent idiopathic scoliosis," *Orthopedic Clinics of North America*, vol. 30, no. 3, pp. 343–352, 1999.

[98] N. H. Miller, B. Mims, A. Child, D. M. Milewicz, P. Sponseller, and S. H. Blanton, "Genetic analysis of structural elastic fiber and collagen genes in familial adolescent idiopathic scoliosis," *Journal of Orthopaedic Research*, vol. 14, no. 6, pp. 994–999, 1996.

[99] G. C. Robin and T. Cohen, "Familial scoliosis. A clinical report," *Journal of Bone and Joint Surgery—Series B*, vol. 57, no. 2, pp. 146–147, 1975.

[100] S. L. Weinstein, L. A. Dolan, J. C. Cheng, A. Danielsson, and J. A. Morcuende, "Adolescent idiopathic scoliosis," *The Lancet*, vol. 371, no. 9623, pp. 1527–1537, 2008.

[101] C. A. Wise, R. Barnes, J. Gillum, J. A. Herring, A. M. Bowcock, and M. Lovett, "Localization of susceptibility to familial idiopathic scoliosis," *Spine*, vol. 25, no. 18, pp. 2372–2380, 2000.

[102] V. Chan, G. C. Y. Fong, K. D. K. Luk et al., "A genetic locus for adolescent idiopathic scoliosis linked to chromosome 19p13.3," *American Journal of Human Genetics*, vol. 71, no. 2, pp. 401–406, 2002.

[103] L. B. Salehi, M. Mangino, S. De Serio et al., "Assignment of a locus for autosomal dominant idiopathic scoliosis (IS) to ohuman chromosome 17p11," *Human Genetics*, vol. 111, no. 4-5, pp. 401–404, 2002.

[104] C. M. Justice, N. H. Miller, B. Marosy, J. Zhang, and A. F. Wilson, "Familial idiopathic scoliosis: evidence of an X-linked susceptibility locus," *Spine*, vol. 28, no. 6, pp. 589–594, 2003.

[105] J. A. Morcuende, R. Minhas, L. Dolan et al., "Allelic variants of human melatonin 1A receptor in patients with familial adolescent idiopathic scoliosis," *Spine*, vol. 28, no. 17, pp. 2025–2029, 2003.

[106] S. Bashiardes, R. Veile, M. Allen et al., "SNTG1, the gene encoding γ1-syntrophin: a candidate gene for idiopathic scoliosis," *Human Genetics*, vol. 115, no. 1, pp. 81–89, 2004.

[107] N. H. Miller, C. M. Justice, B. Marosy et al., "Identification of candidate regions for familial idiopathic scoliosis," *Spine*, vol. 30, no. 10, pp. 1181–1187, 2005.

[108] K. J. Alden, B. Marosy, N. Nzegwu, C. M. Justice, A. F. Wilson, and N. H. Miller, "Idiopathic scoliosis: identification of candidate regions on chromosome 19p13," *Spine*, vol. 31, no. 16, pp. 1815–1819, 2006.

[109] X. Gao, D. Gordon, D. Zhang et al., "CHD7 gene polymorphisms are associated with susceptibility to idiopathic scoliosis," *American Journal of Human Genetics*, vol. 80, no. 5, pp. 957–965, 2007.

[110] L. Ocaka, C. Zhao, J. A. Reed et al., "Assignment of two loci for autosomal dominant adolescent idiopathic scoliosis to chromosomes 9q31.2-q34.2 and 17q25.3-qtel," *Journal of Medical Genetics*, vol. 45, no. 2, pp. 87–92, 2008.

[111] C. L. Raggio, P. F. Giampietro, S. Dobrin et al., "A novel locus for adolescent idiopathic scoliosis on chromosome 12p," *Journal of Orthopaedic Research*, vol. 27, no. 10, pp. 1366–1372, 2009.

[112] C. A. Gurnett, F. Alaee, A. Bowcock et al., "Genetic linkage localizes an adolescent idiopathic scoliosis and pectus excavatum gene to chromosome 18 q," *Spine*, vol. 34, no. 2, pp. E94–E100, 2009.

[113] S. Sharma, X. Gao, D. Londono et al., "Genome-wide association studies of adolescent idiopathic scoliosis suggest candidate susceptibility genes," *Human Molecular Genetics*, vol. 20, no. 7, pp. 1456–1466, 2011.

[114] Y. Takahashi, I. Kou, A. Takahashi et al., "A genome-wide association study identifies common variants near LBX1 associated with adolescent idiopathic scoliosis," *Nature Genetics*, vol. 43, no. 12, pp. 1237–1240, 2011.

[115] J. K. Webb, "Reviewer's comment," *European Spine Journal*, vol. 8, no. 2, p. 117, 1999.

[116] A. J. Carr, D. J. Ogilvie, B. P. Wordsworth, L. M. Priestly, R. Smith, and B. Sykes, "Segregation of structural collagen genes in adolescent idiopathic scoliosis," *Clinical Orthopaedics and Related Research*, no. 274, pp. 305–310, 1992.

[117] J. Dubousset, P. Queneau, and M. Thillard, "Experimental scoliosis induced by pineal gland and dienephalic lesions in young chickens: its relation with clinical findings," *Orthopaedic Transactions*, vol. 7, article 7, 1983.

[118] A. Moreau, D. S. Wang, S. Forget et al., "Melatonin signaling dysfunction in adolescent idiopathic scoliosis," *Spine*, vol. 29, no. 16, pp. 1772–1781, 2004.

[119] R. Wang, Y. Qiu, and B. Rui, "Neurotrophin-3 mRNA expression in paravertebral muscles of patients with idiopathic scoliosis," *Chinese Journal of Spine and Spinal Cord*, vol. 15, pp. 532–534, 2007.

[120] K. Kindsfater, T. Lowe, D. Lawellin, D. Weinstein, and J. Akmakjian, "Levels of platelet calmodulin for the prediction of progression and severity of adolescent idiopathic scoliosis," *Journal of Bone and Joint Surgery—Series A*, vol. 76, no. 8, pp. 1186–1192, 1994.

[121] Y. Floman, M. Liebergall, G. C. Robin, and A. Eldor, "Abnormalities of aggregation, thromboxane A2 synthesis, and 14C serotonin release in platelets of patients with idiopathic scoliosis," *Spine*, vol. 8, no. 3, pp. 236–241, 1983.

[122] M. Inoue, S. Minami, Y. Nakata et al., "Prediction of curve progression in idiopathic scoliosis from gene polymorphic analysis," *Studies in Health Technology and Informatics*, vol. 91, pp. 90–96, 2002.

[123] T. Lowe, D. Lawellin, D. Smith et al., "Platelet calmodulin levels in adolescent idiopathic scoliosis: do the levels correlate with curve progression and severity?" *Spine*, vol. 27, no. 7, pp. 768–775, 2002.

[124] K. Ward, J. W. Ogilvie, M. V. Singleton, R. Chettier, G. Engler, and L. M. Nelson, "Validation of DNA-based prognostic testing to predict spinal curve progression in adolescent idiopathic scoliosis," *Spine*, vol. 35, no. 25, pp. E1455–E1464, 2010.

[125] J. Jiang, B. Qian, S. Mao et al., "A promoter polymorphism of tissue inhibitor of metalloproteinase-2 gene is associated with severity of thoracic adolescent idiopathic scoliosis," *Spine*, vol. 37, no. 1, pp. 41–47, 2012.

[126] Y. Qiu, S.-H. Mao, B.-P. Qian et al., "A promoter polymorphism of neurotrophin 3 gene is associated with curve severity and bracing effectiveness in adolescent idiopathic scoliosis," *Spine*, vol. 37, no. 2, pp. 127–133, 2012.

[127] W. G. Tourtellotte and J. Milbrandt, "Sensory ataxia and muscle spindle agenesis in mice lacking the transcription factor Egr3," *Nature Genetics*, vol. 20, no. 1, pp. 87–91, 1998.

[128] S. B. Purkiss, B. Driscoll, W. G. Cole, and B. Alman, "Idiopathic scoliosis in families of children with congenital scoliosis," *Clinical Orthopaedics and Related Research*, no. 401, pp. 27–31, 2002.

[129] L. E. L. M. Vissers, C. M. A. Van Ravenswaaij, R. Admiraal et al., "Mutations in a new member of the chromodomain gene family cause CHARGE syndrome," *Nature Genetics*, vol. 36, no. 9, pp. 955–957, 2004.

[130] N. L. Jacobs-Mcdaniels and R. C. Albertson, "Chd7 plays a critical role in controlling left-right symmetry during zebrafish somitogenesis," *Developmental Dynamics*, vol. 240, no. 10, pp. 2272–2280, 2011.

[131] S. A. Patten, N. L. Jacobs-McDaniels, C. Zaouter, P. Drapeau, R. C. Albertson, and F. Moldovan, "Role of Chd7 in zebrafish: a model for CHARGE syndrome," *PLoS ONE*, vol. 7, no. 2, Article ID e31650, 2012.

12

Neuroimaging and Neurocognitive Correlates of Aggression and Violence in Schizophrenia

Elisabeth M. Weiss

Department of Psychology, Karl-Franzens University of Graz, University-Platz 2, 8010 Graz, Austria

Correspondence should be addressed to Elisabeth M. Weiss; e.weiss@uni-graz.at

Academic Editors: C. Strazielle and A. Weizman

Individuals diagnosed with major mental disorders such as schizophrenia are more likely to have engaged in violent behavior than mentally healthy members of the same communities. Although aggressive acts can have numerous causes, research about the underlying neurobiology of violence and aggression in schizophrenia can lead to a better understanding of the heterogeneous nature of that behavior and can assist in developing new treatment strategies. The purpose of this paper is to review the recent literature and discuss some of the neurobiological correlates of aggression and violence. The focus will be on schizophrenia, and the results of neuroimaging and neuropsychological studies that have directly investigated brain functioning and/or structure in aggressive and violent samples will be discussed as well as other domains that might predispose to aggression and violence such as deficits in responding to the emotional expressions of others, impulsivity, and psychopathological symptoms. Finally gender differences regarding aggression and violence are discussed. In this context several methodological and conceptional issues that limited the comparison of these studies will be addressed.

1. Introduction

Aggression and violence are declared as leading public health problems and therefore violence in the community has obvious social relevance for political, criminal justice, and health care systems [1]. Epidemiological studies have shown that individuals diagnosed with major mental disorders such as schizophrenia are more likely to be engaged in violent behavior than the general population [2–6]. However, violence committed by persons with schizophrenia is a heterogeneous phenomenon. It is unquestionable that societal influences, such as poverty, discrimination, exposure to violence, and physical abuse, play a key role in the genesis of violence. For example, individuals who are abused as children have increased levels of violence in adulthood [7, 8]. Furthermore, in a recent meta-analysis, Fazel et al. [3] could show that most of the risk for violence appears to be mediated by substance abuse comorbidity. Although aggressive acts can have numerous causes, research about the underlying neurobiology of violence and aggression in schizophrenia can lead to a better understanding of the heterogeneous nature of that behavior and can assist in developing new treatment strategies. In response, a large number of studies have been published to determine the roots of violence and aggression, but the underlying neurobiology is only just beginning to be understood.

The purpose of this paper is to review the recent literature and discuss some of the neurobiological correlates of aggression and violence in the literature. The focus will be on schizophrenia and the results of neuroimaging studies and neuropsychological assessments that have directly investigated brain functioning and/or structure in aggressive and violent schizophrenic samples. Additionally, other domains that might predispose to aggression and violence such as deficits in responding to the emotional expressions of others, impulsivity, and psychopathological symptoms will be discussed. In this context, the relevance of various methodological and conceptual issues on the results of these studies will be emphasized.

2. Evidence from Brain Lesions and Brain Imaging Studies

Over the last years, there has been an increasing body of data on neuropsychiatric disorders that raise the question about a possible relationship between the abnormal function of specific regions of the brain and the occurrence of violent and aggressive behavior. The regions of the brain most often linked to aggression and violence are the temporal cortex/limbic system (amygdale, hippocampus, cingulate gyrus, portions of the thalamus, and hypothalamus and their connections) and the orbitofrontal cortex (for a review, see Volavka [9]).

Since the middle of the nineteenth century, case studies of patients with neurodegenerative disorders or after traumatic brain injury have reported about violent and antisocial behavior, impulsivity, and inability to inhibit responses after damage to the orbitofrontal cortex [10–13]. For example the dramatic case of Phineas Cage, a railroad worker, who had an iron bar driven through the orbito-frontal cortex as a result of an explosion [14]. After the accident he became belligerent, socially inappropriate, unrealistic, and impersistent. The Vietnam Head Injury Study (VHIS) found that subjects with lesions limited to the frontal lobes tended to show about 10% more aggressive and violent behaviors compared with patients with nonfrontal head injury and controls without head injury [15]. Furthermore, persons with frontal network damage acquired before the age of 8 have also been reported to have adult histories of recurrent impulsive, aggressive, and antisocial behavior [16–18]. Moreover, reports have found higher rates of antisocial behavior in patients with frontotemporal dementia, even when compared with equally cognitively impaired patients with Alzheimer's disease [19, 20].

Morphometric neuroimaging studies of aggressive and violent subjects have consistently found frontal lobe abnormalities (for reviews, see [21–25]). However, to date the structural MRI literature produced inconsistent results regarding the volume size abnormalities in aggressive and violent patients, with most studies finding reduced volumes of frontal structures in violent patients (see the meta-analysis of 43 structural and functional imaging studies of Yang and Raine [26]), while others reported increased volumes in these brain regions [27–31]. Furthermore abnormalities in cortical thickness in the ventromedial prefrontal cortex [32] and reduced white matter integrity in the ventral prefrontal cortex, measured with diffusion tension imaging (DTI) [33], were associated with aggressive attitudes and violence.

Only a handful of studies examined differences in grey matter volumes between violent and nonviolent schizophrenic patients. Yang et al. [34] found reduced gray matter volumes in the hippocampus and parahippocampal gyrus in murderers with schizophrenia, in the parahippocampal gyrus in murderers without schizophrenia, and in the prefrontal cortex in nonviolent schizophrenic patients compared to normal controls. Volume reductions in the hippocampus in violent schizophrenic patients were also seen in other studies [35, 36]. Since hippocampal/parahippocampal deficits have been linked to memory impairments and affective dysregulation, Yang et al. [34] hypothesized that volume reductions in the hippocampus may predispose individuals with schizophrenia to be less sensible to social and emotional signs, which might contribute to the generation of conflicts and the inability to recognize signals for solution, leading to conflict escalation. Less consistent patterns of gray matter volume reductions were found in other studies, comparing violent and nonviolent schizophrenic patients. These studies are reporting about reductions in mesial temporal structures [37], in the amygdale [38], in the sensorimotor cortex [35], in orbitofrontal cortex [36], in the cerebellum, and in the region around the supramarginal gyrus [39]. One study [27] found larger left orbitofrontal cortex grey matter volumes in aggressive schizophrenic patients. These inconsistent results in structural brain volumetric studies can be explained by methodological differences between studies including differences in the study samples (inclusion of multiple diagnostic categories such as schizoaffective patients or patients with comorbidity of personality disorders or psychoactive substance misuse) and treatment characteristics.

Studies focusing on the patterns of brain activation using PET, SPECT, and FMRI have documented focal decreases in frontal and temporal cortical activity associated with various neuropsychiatric disorders (for reviews, see [20–25]). They provide data on both resting brain activity and task-related activity.

Using positron emission tomography (PET), Wong et al. [40] reported reduced glucose metabolism in the temporal cortex in violent schizophrenic patients, whereas Raine et al. [41–43] found reduced glucose metabolism in the prefrontal cortex and other regions (superior parietal regions, angular gyrus and corpus callosum) in murderers using the continuous performance tasks to elicit frontal activity. Similarly, in a single photon emission computed tomography (SPECT) Spaletta et al. [44] found reduced prefrontal regional cerebral blood flow in aggressive schizophrenic patients during the Wisconsin Card Sorting Task (WCST). However, one has to keep in mind that the sample size in the few PET and SPECT studies showing an abnormal frontotemporal circuitry in aggressive patients is fairly small and the location of abnormal metabolism varied among patients.

Functional imaging studies (fMRI) on aggression in schizophrenia and other mental disorders produced also inconsistent results, with most studies showing an abnormal activation in the temporoventromedial cortex region, but less consistent patterns in other regions [45–52]. Again, comparison between studies is hampered by methodological differences such as different cognitive activations tasks (e.g., visual verbal working memory tasks, affective words, emotional faces), heterogeneous patient populations, and small sample sizes. Only one study examined the resting state functional connectivity in aggressive schizophrenic patients, showing a significant reduction in functional connectivity between the amygdale and ventral prefrontal cortex [53].

In summary the neuroimaging literature on aggression in schizophrenia and other mental disorders implicates dysfunctions in the frontotemporal circuitry (for reviews, see [21–25, 54]). These findings are consistent with the role of medial temporal and orbitofrontal regions in emotional processing and executive cognitive functioning, which encompasses abilities such as attention, planning, organization, abstract reasoning, self-monitoring, and the ability to use feedback to modulate behavior. This has been speculated to lead to cognitive biases that increase the chances of behaving aggressively in response to stressful and provocative situations [4]. The reported abnormalities in prefrontal size or activity may, therefore, represent a predisposition to affective states relevant to aggressive behavior, without necessarily signifying an incapacity to avoid actual violent acts, and no study has reliably demonstrated a characteristic pattern of frontal network dysfunction predictive of violent crime (for review, see Filley et al. [55]). Although the etiological implications of these prefrontal network dysfunctions are not fully understood, there is converging evidence that cognitive deficits may underlie early school failure, dropouts, alcohol and drug use, and ultimately, encounters with the legal system as violent offenders (for review, see [9, 10]).

3. Evidence from Neuropsychological Assessments

3.1. Deficits in Executive Functions. It is fairly common that the majority of schizophrenic patients have profound deficits on measures of executive functions. At the descriptive level, patients with schizophrenia seem to have difficulties selecting relevant information from their environment and attaching an appropriate meaning to that information. Green [56] provided the following definition of executive function:

"Executive functioning refers to a host of neurocognitive activities that are associated with the prefrontal cortex such as planning, problem solving, shifting cognitive set and alternating between two or more tasks."

Therefore, executive functions allow you to set goals, make and modify mental "models" of actions, organize your activity, focus your attention selectively, and avoid impulses and distractions that could sidetrack you from accomplishing your aims.

Reviews of the literature tend to support a significant association between prefrontal executive dysfunctions measured by neuropsychological testing and increased antisocial and aggressive behavior [54, 57]. Morgan and Lilienfeld [57] found in their meta-analysis that antisocial groups performed .62 standard deviations worse on executive tests than comparison groups, but the strength of the correlation between deficits in executive functions and antisocial behavior varied according to the types of antisocial behaviors exhibited by study subjects, with criminality and delinquency showing a stronger relationship than conduct disorder, psychopathy, or clinically defined antisocial personality disorder.

Only a few studies have examined the relationship between performance on neuropsychological tests and violence among schizophrenic patients (see Table 1). However, the results of these studies have been inconsistent. Several studies [58–62] did not find a difference in neuropsychological test performance between schizophrenic patients with aggressive behavior and those without. In contrast, three studies [63–65] found superior performance on neuropsychological measures among violent schizophrenic patients compared to nonviolent patients with schizophrenia. Roy et al. [63] found, in a sample of 20 inpatients with chronic schizophrenia, that violent patients (defined on the basis of chart review and ward behavior) outperformed nonviolent patients on several subscales of the Wechsler Adult Intelligence Scale Revised (WAIS-R): verbal IQ, digit symbol, and block design. A study by Lapierre et al. [64] found a correlation between enhanced performance on both the Wisconsin Card Sorting Test (WCST) and a verbal fluency test and lifetime "number of aggression against another person" among 31 outpatients with schizophrenia. The low-violence group did not achieve significantly better scores than the violent group on any neuropsychological measure in either study. Rasmussen et al. [65] compared 13 violent schizophrenic inpatients with 13 nonaggressive schizophrenic patients and 13 healthy control subjects. Violent schizophrenic patients outperformed nonviolent schizophrenic patients on the Trail Making Test and showed faster reaction time on all reaction time tests but more failed inhibitions on the Go-NoGo test.

Other authors showed that neuropsychological impairments were associated with violence among inpatients with schizophrenia [66–68]. Krakowski et al. [66] classified schizophrenia inpatients into high ($N = 22$), low ($N = 27$), or no violence ($N = 22$) groups on the basis of ward behavior. Patients in the high-violence group were significantly more impaired in the area of integrative sensory and motor function than those in the nonviolent group, as measured by their scores on the Benton Visual Retention Test and the WAIS-R performance IQ, especially on the subtests: digit symbol test and blocking test. On these subtests, violent patients received higher scores in the study by Roy et al. [63]. Adams et al. [67] found that impairment on the Lubria-Nebraska Neuropsychological Battery was related to history of violent arrest but not to inpatient violence in a sample of 37 incarcerated persons with schizophrenia. Barkataki et al. [68] could show that schizophrenic patients with a history of violence produced poorer performance in an executive task (WCST) than nonviolent schizophrenic patients, with the violent patients making significantly more perseverative errors.

Of the remaining studies none dealt exclusively with schizophrenia. However, in two of the studies a majority of the participants had a diagnosis of schizophrenia. One study compared 23 forensic inpatients, 16 of whom had a diagnosis of schizophrenia, who had committed a violent crime [69]. Impairment on several neuropsychological tests, the judgment of line orientation test, the symbol digit modalities test, the Stroop Interference Test, and the test of nonverbal intelligence, was correlated with the frequency and severity of violent behavior. In a larger study, Krakowski et al. [70] compared 33 inpatients with a history of community violence, as determined by self-report of arrest for violent crime and chart reviews for such arrests, with 69 inpatients who denied arrests for violent crimes. Of the 102 patients included in the study, 72 percent had a diagnosis of schizophrenia or schizoaffective disorder. A history of community violence was significantly related to impairment on some WCST

Table 1: Results of relevant neuropsychological studies in aggressive schizophrenic patients.

Authors	Sample characteristics	Results of relevant neuropsychological studies
Lafayette et al. [58]	96 schizophrenic patients (34 violent arrests, 23 nonviolent arrest, 39 no arrest)	No significant differences between the groups in the WAIS, Wisconsin Card Sortig Test, Trail Making Test, Verbal fluency Test, Stroop Test, American National Adult Reading Test
Krakowski et al. [59]	32 transiently violent schizophrenic patients, 27 persistently violent schizophrenic patients	No difference in the average performance and verbal IQ on the WAIS-R
Wong et al. [60]	20 male schizophrenic patients who had committed several violent offenses, 19 male schizophrenic patients who had committed only 1 violent offense.	No difference in the WAIS performance between the groups
Silver et al. [61]	35 violent patients with chronic schizophrenia or schizoaffective disorder, 35 nonviolent schizophrenic patients, 46 healthy controls	No difference between violent and nonviolent schizophrenic patients in the cognitive test battery
Fullam and Dolan [62]	33 violent and 49 nonviolent male forensic inpatients with schizophrenia	No difference between violent and nonviolent schizophrenic patients in the cognitive test battery but lower IQ scores in the violent schizophrenic patients
Roy et al. [63]	20 chronic, treatment-resistant inpatients with schizophrenia; (11 violent and 9 low-violent men)	Violent patients outperformed nonviolent patients on the verbal IQ, digit symbol test, block design
Lapierre et al. [64]	31 schizophrenic men (outpatients) and 30 healthy control subjects	Higher level of violence in the more cognitively functional individuals on the Wisconsin Card Sorting Test and Controlled Oral Word Association test
Rasmussen [65]	13 inpatients aggressive schizophrenic patients from a maximum security psychiatric unit, 13 nonaggressive schizophrenic patients, 13 healthy controls	Violent schizophrenic patients outperformed nonviolent schizophrenic patients on the Trail Making Test and showed faster reaction time on all reaction time tests but more failed inhibitions on the Go-NoGo test
Krakowski et al. [66]	28 high, 27 low, and 34 nonviolent schizophrenic patients	High-violent patients were more impaired on the Benton Visual Retention Test, digit symbol test, block design and had lower performance IQ scores on the WAIS-R
Adams et al. [67]	37 male schizophrenic patients	History of violent arrests but not inpatients violence was associated with impairment on the Luria Nebraska neuropsychological battery
Barkataki et al. [68]	13 individuals with a history of serious violence and a diagnosis of antisocial personality disorder, 13 individuals with a history of violence and schizophrenia, 15 individuals with schizophrenia without a history of violent behaviour, 15 healthy control subjects	Violent schizophrenic patients had a higher number of errors in the Wisconsin Card Sorting Test
Foster et al. [69]	1 year prospective study of aggression in 23 male forensic psychiatric inpatients	Scores on Stroop Color Word Tasks, Judgment of Line Orientation Test, Symbol Digit Modalities Test only significantly predicted frequency but not severity
Krakowski et al. [70]	33 psychiatric violent inpatients versus 69 nonviolent psychiatric inpatients	History of community violence was related to impairment on some Wisconsin Card Sorting Subtests, finger tapping, Perdue pegboard

WAIS-R: Wechsler Adult Intelligence Scale-revised.

subtests as well as impairment in the finger-tapping test and the Perdue pegboard test (both left handed). Finally, Nestor [71] examined the neuropsychological and clinical correlates of extreme violence retrospectively in young and older inpatients of a forensic psychiatric hospital. The young group exhibited significantly higher rates of learning disabilities and history of childhood conduct disorders, whereas the older group had a significantly higher rate of psychosis.

Three studies [72–74] aimed to determine models for explaining aggressive behavior in relation to executive functions, psychopathological symptoms, and behavioral variables such as anger. In a study of Song and Min [72] the structural equation model revealed a direct, significant path of the emotion anger to aggressive behavior, whereas schizophrenic symptoms and cognitive functions were indirectly related to aggressive behavior through the relationship between the emotion of anger and aggressive behavior, suggesting that executive dysfunction may affect the stimulant of anger by weakening impulse control. Two other studies [73, 74] could show that executive dysfunction predicted aggressive and violent behavior and psychiatric symptomatology. Serper et al. [73] concluded that patients with executive dysfunctions may not possess the behavioral inhibition skills needed to cope with the presence of symptoms and other stressful events that accompany acute psychosis and hospitalization which may result, consequently, in increased manifestations of aggressive behavior. Finally, a recent study Krakowski and Czobor [75] could show that in schizophrenic patients executive function was a strong predictor of response to atypical antipsychotic medication, with clozapine exerting an antiaggressive effect even in the presence of executive dysfunction.

To summarize, a large number of studies have found that dysfunctions of the frontal cortex are associated with limitations in the executive capacity to regulate aggressive behavior (for reviews, see [4, 10, 57]). Therefore, neuropsychological deficits can reduce the number of options an individual perceives or has availablity to respond to a given situation. As a component of the human flight and fight response, aggression may serve as an adaptive mechanism. When cognitive dysfunction is present, however, aggression may dominate the behavioral response and override avoidance or withdrawal. Deficits including defective inhibitory control, impulsivity, difficulty in drawing on past learning to recognize a dangerous course of action, impaired capacity to anticipate future consequences of present behavior, and insufficient self-monitoring, may all conspire to conceal more socially desirable courses of action, which may result, consequently, in increased manifestations of aggressive behavior. Although social and environmental factors have major effects on the expression of aggression and violence, neuropsychological integrity also helps to determine the ability to behave in a social acceptable manner. However, studies investigating the relationship between violence in schizophrenic patients and neuropsychological functioning produced mixed results, with reports of better, similar, and worse performance in violent schizophrenic patients. One reason for these inconsistencies in study results may be that the standard tests of executive functions may not detect orbitofrontal or ventromedial prefrontal dysfunction relevant to aggression and criminal behavior. Furthermore, there is a substantial variation in the neuropsychological test batteries used in different studies.

3.2. Deficits in Responding to the Emotional Expressions of Others. The expression of emotions and the ability to recognize facial expressions of emotions in other people is an important component of interpersonal communication in humans [75]. Certain facial expressions like happiness, sadness, anger, fear, disgust, and surprise are universally recognized, whereas social emotions such as guilt, shame, arrogance, admiration, and flirtatiousness are particular to cultural and ethnical groups [76, 77]. Emotion is normally regulated in the human brain by a complex circuit consisting of the orbital frontal cortex, amygdala, hypothalamus, anterior cingulate cortex, and several other interconnected regions [78]. Impairments in emotion regulation, emotional inexpressiveness, and other emotion-related deficits are regarded as core features of schizophrenia (for a review, see Borod [78]). Abnormal expression of emotional states usually consists of flattening of affects and inappropriate affect and may precede the onset of psychosis by many years [79]. Abnormal experience of emotion ranges from depression to less frequently manic symptoms. Abnormal recognition is described as impaired ability to recognize facial expression of emotion.

Psychological research underscores especially the relation between deficits in regulation of negative emotions and aggressive and violent behavior [80]. Accurate interpretations of non-verbal cues such as facial expressions are important for normal social interaction [81] and deficient abilities to be appropriately guided by the social cues of others and identify one's emotional state may lead to aggressive and violent behavior [82–85]. Flattening of affect as it is seen in schizophrenia may further contribute to aggressive behavior insofar as a failure to express emotions can lead to a reliance on maladaptive ways of expressing emotions, such as through verbal and physical aggression [86].

Violent offenders show deficits in recognizing negative facial expressions of emotions [87, 88], a deficit associated with many other forms of psychopathology such as autism spectrum disorders, schizophrenia, and obsessive compulsive disorder. More specifically, previous studies could show that aggressive individuals show a negative emotional bias for ambiguous facial expressions [89]. Violent schizophrenic patients were more likely to perceive anger in emotionally neutral faces [90] and showed a poorer ability to discriminate between intensity of emotions [61]. Dodge and McNiel et al. [91, 92] predicted that a cognitive style characterized by hostile attributions increases the risk of violence because in ambiguous situations aggressive individuals who attend to fewer emotional cues are biased towards aggressive cues and display deficits in what is described as affective perspective taking. Furthermore, some authors suggest that mentalizing, which is the ability to attribute mental states to oneself and others, can be viewed as an inhibitor of violent and aggressive behavior [93]. Two studies [94, 95] could show that violent schizophrenic patients have deficient emotional but intact cognitive mentalizing abilities.

Another line of research is investigating the relationship between personality traits and aggression. The relationship between antisocial behavior or psychopathy and violence is well established (for a review, see Walsh et al. [96]), and a meta-analysis could show functional impairments in orbitofrontal, dorsolateral frontal, and anterior cingulate cortex in antisocial behavior [97]. Among schizophrenic patients antisocial personality disorder and psychopathy are associated with early onset and persistent violent offending [98, 99].

Bettencourt et al. [100] conducted a comprehensive review to understand the relationship between personality and aggressive behavior, under provoking and non-provoking conditions. The authors could show that trait aggressiveness and trait irritability influenced aggressive behavior under both provoking and neutral conditions but that other personality variables (e.g., trait anger, type A personality, dissipation rumination) influenced aggressive behavior only under provoking conditions. Since aggression is closely linked to hypervigilance towards stimuli that could be perceived as threatening [101, 102] one other important symptom, possibly related to outbreaks of aggression and violence, particularly in adolescents and young adults, may be "gelotophobia" (from gelos, Greek for laughter), which is the fear to being laughed at [103, 104]. Similar to violent individuals persons with higher levels of gelotophobia have deficits in downregulating their negative affect, show a greater anger proneness, and have a tendency to recall interpersonal situations with a higher intensity of negative feelings [105–107]. The suspicion that gelotophobia may be related to aggression and violence had recently been fuelled by anecdotal evidence suggesting that perpetrators of violent acts such as school shootings had a horror of being mocked and may have taken revenge for having been laughed at [108, 109]. However, more research is needed to extrapolate this relationship between gelotophobia or other personality factors and aggressive behavior to schizophrenic patients.

4. Association between Impulsivity and Violence

A further factor mediating the brain-violence relationship which is also linked to the frontal lobe is impulsivity, a complex, multifaceted construct including cognitive, personality, and behavioral components (e.g., sensation seeking, risk taking, and self control) [110]. In general aggression can be distinguished into a goal-directed predatory/premeditated aggression and a reactive/impulsive aggression [111]. Premeditated aggression occurs without provocation and is defined as a planned, conscious, and controlled aggressive act that is instrumental in nature. Impulsive aggression is more reactive and typically described as an emotionally charged aggressive response either unprovoked or out of proportion to the provocation leading to agitation and a loss of behavioral control. Since impulsive individuals have difficulties inhibiting their urges this behavioral style may result in risky behavior, including drug and alcohol abuse [112]. Alcoholintoxication for example, reduces behavioral inhibition and has been linked with aggression in a number of studies [113–116]. Prior research has shown that poor impulse control is associated with aggression and violence in men but not women [117–120]. Dysfunctions of the ventromedial prefrontal region (VMPFC), including the orbitofrontal cortex (OFC), anterior cingulate cortex (ACC), and medial prefrontal cortex, as well as the amygdala were associated with impulsive-aggressive behavior [33, 121–125], whereas individuals with predominantly premeditated aggression showed no prefrontal deficts [125]. Additionally, neuropsychological studies have shown a clear link between impulsive-aggressive behavior and problems in executive functioning [e.g., [126–128]]. Again, some studies could show that individuals who present with marked premediated aggression such as psychopaths do not present with poor performance on general measures of frontal-lobe functioning [129, 130]. Accumulating evidence points towards an important role of several neurotransmitters such as serotonin, dopamine, and noradrenalin in impulsive behavior, and recent findings also implicate glutamate and cannabinoid neurotransmission in impulsivity (for a review, see Pattij and Vanderschuren [131]). Therefore, impulsive behavior may be responsive to pharmacological treatment, and several studies could show that agents with serotonergic-enhancing properties such as serotonin-reuptake inhibitors [132–134] as well as antiepileptic dugs may reduce incidences of impulsive aggression, but not premediated aggression (for reviews, see Huband et al. [135] and Stanford et al. [136]).

4.1. Association between Violence and Psychopathological Symptoms. To some extent the increased risk of violence in patients with schizophrenia may be related to specific psychotic symptoms, such as delusions of thought insertion, thought control, and persecution or to command hallucinations, but the link between violence and psychotic symptoms can be minimal.

Link and Stueve [137] reported that violent behavior was associated with the presence of "threat/control-override symptoms": delusions of domination by external force, thought insertion, and feeling that people wish to harm the patient. However, epidemiological study did not investigate whether there was a temporal linkage between delusions and violence. Junginger et al. [138] concluded that delusional motivation of violence appeared to be rare, though 40% of the violent subjects in that study reported that they had committed at least one serious act of violence that was definitely motivated by delusions. Taylor [139] interviewed 121 incarcerated forensic psychotic (mostly schizophrenic) patients about the motives for the offenses they had committed while living in the community. The author estimated that 82% of their offenses (violent and nonviolent offenses combined) were probably attributable to their illness and that psychotic symptoms probably accounted directly for most of the very violent behavior, but considerable time elapsed between the offenses and the interviews, and the respondent may have had reason to represent their criminal behavior as driven by mental illness.

Some patients may commit violent acts in response to auditory command hallucinations. In a sample of 93 psychiatric inpatients, Junginger [140] rated the level of dangerousness of the most recently reported command hallucinations and the degree to which the patient complied with the command. He concluded that psychiatric patients who experience command hallucinations are at risk for dangerous behavior. However, others have concluded that although experienced by many patients with schizophrenia and often violent in content, command hallucinations may not be important predictors of violence [141, 142]. In a comparison of violent and nonviolent patients with schizophrenia (n = 31 per group) Cheung et al. [143] reported no association between command hallucinations and violence; yet, violent patients were more likely to have had persecutory delusions and were more severely psychotic than the nonviolent patients.

In summary, there is still a controversy regarding the relationship between psychotic symptoms in schizophrenic patients and aggressive behavior with some authors reporting that positive psychotic symptoms such as delusions of thought insertion, thought control and persecution, or command hallucinations were associated with a history of assaults [144, 145], whereas others could not observe association between positive symptoms of schizophrenia and violence [62].

4.2. Gender and Aggression. In healthy people, aggression is arguably the most salient emotional behavior differentiating the sexes with men showing greater abundance [146], including arrests for homicide and violent crimes [147]. Studies of aggression in psychiatric disorders showed variable findings (for a review, see Maccoby and Jacklin [146]). Several studies have suggested that psychiatric disorders, especially schizophrenia, reduce the gender difference and in hospitalized psychiatric patients eliminate it altogether [148–151]. However, in order to understand better gender differences in violence, multiple manifestations of violence must be differentiated and the complexity of the phenomenon must be taken into consideration. For example, Hiday et al. [152] demonstrated that male subjects had a greater prevalence of more serious violence involving weapons or injury in the 4 months preceding hospitalization, but there were no gender differences when measures of violence that were more inclusive (incorporating threats as well as fights not involving weapons or injuries) were used. Additionally, Weiss et al. [153] could show that physical aggression and antisocial behavior in the community were more pronounced in schizophrenic men compared to schizophrenic women. In a study by Krakowski and Czobor [154], women with major psychiatric disorders were more verbally abusive and threatening during their hospitalization than the men. This finding is consistent with the predominance of verbal aggression reported in women showing that in the general population, women throughout life are more likely to use verbal than physical aggression [155]. A meta-analytic review of studies on gender differences in the general population [156] also indicated that the male overrepresentation in aggression is more distinct for severe physical aggression.

5. Conclusions

Violent and criminal behavior in schizophrenic patients is caused by multiple, probably interacting causal factors. Dysfunctions in the frontotemporal circuitry appear to be the most consistent feature in aggressive and violent schizophrenic patients. Limitations in the executive capacity and/or deficits in the interpretation of emotional signals such as facial affects can lead to cognitive biases that increase the chances of behaving aggressively in response to stressful and provocative situations. However, studies elucidating the relationship between neuroimaging results, neurocognitive functioning, personality traits, and antisocial and violent behavior produced inconsistent results. Most studies investigating the neurobiological correlates of aggressive and violent behavior are limited by several methodological problems. Notably, the definition and measurement of violence varied between studies. Most studies focused on community violence, while only few studies examined inpatient violence, which is not necessarily predicted by previous community violence [157]. Additionally, the number of aggressive behavior and violent incidents was assessed differently between the studies reviewed in this paper, with some authors using patients self-reports, while others used psychiatric files, reports by ward staff, or official records of arrests and convictions. Furthermore, inconsistent findings can result from sample heterogeneities such as comorbidity with antisocial personality disorder/psychopathy or substance abuse. Over and above, differences in the medication type and dosage can add to the variance in study results. Atypical antipsychotic medication has shown greater promise in treating neuropsychological deficits than conventional antipsychotic drugs [158]. In addition, atypical antipsychotic medication, particularly clozapine, has been shown to reduce aggressive and violent behavior in schizophrenic patients [75, 159–162]. The failure to take account of type and dosage of antipsychotic medication in some studies may have limited the detection of group differences in neurocognitive performance and aggressive behavior. Further methodological problems in the literature include a lack of prospective data, small samples sizes, nonrepresentative samples for the criminal population, a lack of adequate controls for known violent risk factors such as drug and alcohol misuse, physical and sexual abuse, family break down, and poverty. Future studies are necessary that examine the course of cognitive deficits, psychopathological symptoms, and aggressive behavior in schizophrenic patients at various stages of patient illness. Since several studies found an association between some genes such as the catechol-O-methyltransferase (COMT) and aggression and violence (for review, see Soyka [54]) the combination of neuroimaging, neuropsychological, and genetic studies might broaden our understanding of the neurobiological basis that underlies aggressive and violent behavior. This interdisciplinary research may lead to an earlier identification of likely aggressors and may result in the formation of individualized treatment plans, which can reduce patients' symptoms and the propensity for criminal behavior and aggression.

References

[1] S. Hodgins, J. Alderton, A. Cree, A. Aboud, and T. Mak, "Aggressive behaviour, victimisation and crime among severely mentally ill patients requiring hospitalisation," *British Journal of Psychiatry*, vol. 191, pp. 343-350, 2007.

[2] J. W. Swanson, M. S. Swartz, R. A. Van Dorn et al., "A national study of violent behavior in persons with schizophrenia," *Archives of General Psychiatry*, vol. 63, no. 5, pp. 490–499, 2006.

[3] S. Fazel, G. Gulati, L. Linsell, J. R. Geddes, and M. Grann, "Schizophrenia and violence: systematic review and meta-analysis," *PLoS Medicine*, vol. 6, no. 8, Article ID e1000120, 2009.

[4] K. Naudts and S. Hodgins, "Neurobiological correlates of violent behavior among persons with schizophrenia," *Schizophrenia Bulletin*, vol. 32, no. 3, pp. 562–572, 2006.

[5] A. Stueve and B. G. Link, "Violence and psychiatric disorders: results from an epidemiological study of young adults in Israel," *Psychiatric Quarterly*, vol. 68, no. 4, pp. 327–342, 1997.

[6] B. G. Link and A. Stueve, "New evidence on the violence risk posed by people with mental illness: on the importance of specifying the timing and the targets of violence," *Archives of General Psychiatry*, vol. 55, no. 5, pp. 403–404, 1998.

[7] C. S. Widom, "The cycle of violence," *Science*, vol. 244, no. 4901, pp. 160–166, 1989.

[8] M. G. Maxfield and C. S. Widom, "The cycle of violence: revisited 6 years later," *Archives of Pediatrics and Adolescent Medicine*, vol. 150, no. 4, pp. 390–395, 1996.

[9] J. Volavka, *Neurobiology of Violence*, American Psychiatric, Washington, DC, USA, 2nd edition, 2002.

[10] M. C. Brower and B. H. Price, "Neuropsychiatry of frontal lobe dysfunction in violent and criminal behaviour: a critical review," *Journal of Neurology Neurosurgery and Psychiatry*, vol. 71, no. 6, pp. 720–726, 2001.

[11] D. Tranel, "'Acquired sociopathy': the development of sociopathic behavior following focal brain damage," *Progress in Experimental Personality & Psychopathology Research*, pp. 285–311, 1994.

[12] C. A. Meyers, S. A. Berman, R. S. Scheibel, and A. Hayman, "Case report: acquired antisocial personality disorder associated with unilateral left orbital frontal lobe damage," *Journal of Psychiatry & Neuroscience*, vol. 17, no. 3, pp. 121–125, 1992.

[13] R. J. R. Blair and L. Cipolotti, "Impaired social response reversal. A case of 'acquired sociopathy'," *Brain*, vol. 123, no. 6, pp. 1122–1141, 2000.

[14] J. M. Harlow, "Passage of an iron rod through the head," *Journal of Neuropsychiatry and Clinical Neurosciences*, vol. 11, no. 2, pp. 281–283, 1999.

[15] J. Grafman, K. Schwab, D. Warden, A. Pridgen, H. R. Brown, and A. M. Salazar, "Frontal lobe injuries, violence, and aggression: a report of the Vietnam head injury study," *Neurology*, vol. 46, no. 5, pp. 1231–1238, 1996.

[16] B. H. Price, K. R. Daffner, R. M. Stowe, and M. M. Mesulam, "The comportmental learning disabilities of early frontal lobe damage," *Brain*, vol. 113, no. 5, pp. 1383–1393, 1990.

[17] P. J. Eslinger, L. M. Grattan, H. Damasio, and A. R. Damasio, "Developmental consequences of childhood frontal lobe damage," *Archives of Neurology*, vol. 49, no. 7, pp. 764–769, 1992.

[18] S. W. Anderson, A. Bechara, H. Damasio, D. Tranel, and A. R. Damasio, "Impairment of social and moral behavior related to early damage in human prefrontal cortex," *Nature Neuroscience*, vol. 2, no. 11, pp. 1032–1037, 1999.

[19] E. Stip, "Compulsive disorder and acquired antisocial behavior in frontal lobe dementia," *Journal of Neuropsychiatry and Clinical Neurosciences*, vol. 7, no. 1, p. 116, 1995.

[20] B. L. Miller, A. Darby, D. F. Benson, J. L. Cummings, and M. H. Miller, "Aggressive, socially disruptive and antisocial behaviour associated with fronto-temporal dementia," *British Journal of Psychiatry*, vol. 170, pp. 150–155, 1997.

[21] M. C. Brower and B. H. Price, "Neuropsychiatry of frontal lobe dysfunction in violent and criminal behaviour: a critical review," *Journal of Neurology Neurosurgery and Psychiatry*, vol. 71, no. 6, pp. 720–726, 2001.

[22] L. Bassarath, "Neuroimaging studies of antisocial behaviour," *Canadian Journal of Psychiatry*, vol. 46, no. 8, pp. 728–732, 2001.

[23] J. L. Bufkin and V. R. Luttrell, "Neuroimaging studies of aggressive and violent behavior: current findings and implications for criminology and criminal justice," *Trauma, Violence & Abuse*, vol. 6, no. 2, pp. 176–191, 2005.

[24] T. Z. Palijan, S. Radeljak, M. Kovač, and D. Kovačević, "Relationship between comorbidity and violence risk assesment in forensic psychiatry—the implicaton of neuroimaging studies," *Psychiatria Danubina*, vol. 22, no. 2, pp. 253–256, 2010.

[25] M. J. Hoptman and D. Antonius, "Neuroimaging correlates of aggression in schizophrenia: an update," *Current Opinion in Psychiatry*, vol. 24, no. 2, pp. 100–106, 2011.

[26] Y. Yang and A. Raine, "Prefrontal structural and functional brain imaging findings in antisocial, violent, and psychopathic individuals: a meta-analysis," *Psychiatry Research*, vol. 174, no. 2, pp. 81–88, 2009.

[27] M. J. Hoptman, J. Volavka, E. M. Weiss et al., "Quantitative MRI measures of orbitofrontal cortex in patients with chronic schizophrenia or schizoaffective disorder," *Psychiatry Research*, vol. 140, no. 2, pp. 133–145, 2005.

[28] N. Rüsch, I. Spoletini, M. Wilke et al., "Inferior frontal white matter volume and suicidality in schizophrenia," *Psychiatry Research*, vol. 164, no. 3, pp. 206–214, 2008.

[29] A. L. Glenn, A. Raine, P. S. Yaralian, and Y. Yang, "Increased volume of the striatum in psychopathic individuals," *Biological Psychiatry*, vol. 67, no. 1, pp. 52–58, 2010.

[30] S. A. De Brito, A. Mechelli, M. Wilke et al., "Size matters: increased grey matter in boys with conduct problems and callousunemotional traits," *Brain*, vol. 132, no. 4, pp. 843–852, 2009.

[31] J. Tiihonen, R. Rossi, M. P. Laakso et al., "Brain anatomy of persistent violent offenders: more rather than less," *Psychiatry Research*, vol. 163, no. 3, pp. 201–212, 2008.

[32] V. M. Narayan, K. L. Narr, V. Kumari et al., "Regional cortical thinning in subjects with violent antisocial personality disorder or schizophrenia," *American Journal of Psychiatry*, vol. 164, no. 9, pp. 1418–1427, 2007.

[33] M. J. Hoptman, J. Volavka, G. Johnson, E. Weiss, R. M. Bilder, and K. O. Lim, "Frontal white matter microstructure, aggression, and impulsivity in men with schizophrenia: a preliminary study," *Biological Psychiatry*, vol. 52, no. 1, pp. 9–14, 2002.

[34] Y. Yang, A. Raine, C. B. Han, R. A. Schug, A. W. Toga, and K. L. Narr, "Reduced hippocampal and parahippocampal volumes in murderers with schizophrenia," *Psychiatry Research—Neuroimaging*, vol. 182, no. 1, pp. 9–13, 2010.

[35] I. Barkataki, V. Kumari, M. Das, P. Taylor, and T. Sharma, "Volumetric structural brain abnormalities in men with schizophrenia or antisocial personality disorder," *Behavioural Brain Research*, vol. 169, no. 2, pp. 239–247, 2006.

[36] V. Kumari, I. Barkataki, S. Goswami, S. Flora, M. Das, and P. Taylor, "Dysfunctional, but not functional, impulsivity is associated with a history of seriously violent behaviour and reduced orbitofrontal and hippocampal volumes in schizophrenia," *Psychiatry Research*, vol. 173, no. 1, pp. 39–44, 2009.

[37] L. P. Chesterman, P. J. Taylor, T. Cox, M. Hill, and J. Lumsden, "Multiple measures of cerebral state in dangerous mentally disordered inpatients," *Criminal Behaviour and Mental Health*, vol. 4, no. 3, pp. 228–239, 1994.

[38] M. Wong, P. Fenwick, G. Fenton, J. Lumsden, M. Maisey, and J. Stevens, "Repetitive and non-repetitive violent offending behaviour in male patients in a maximum security mental hospital—clinical and neuroimaging findings," *Medicine, Science and the Law*, vol. 37, no. 2, pp. 150–160, 1997.

[39] B. K. Puri, S. J. Counsell, N. Saeed, M. G. Bustos, I. H. Treasaden, and G. M. Bydder, "Regional grey matter volumetric changes in forensic schizophrenia patients: an MRI study comparing the brain structure of patients who have seriously and violently offended with that of patients who have not," *BMC Psychiatry*, vol. 8, supplement 1, article S6, 2008.

[40] M. T. H. Wong, P. B. C. Fenwick, J. Lumsden et al., "Positron emission tomography in male violent offenders with schizophrenia," *Psychiatry Research*, vol. 68, no. 2-3, pp. 111–123, 1997.

[41] A. Raine, M. S. Buchsbaum, J. Stanley, S. Lottenberg, L. Abel, and J. Stoddard, "Selective reductions in prefrontal glucose metabolism in murderers," *Biological Psychiatry*, vol. 36, no. 6, pp. 365–373, 1994.

[42] A. Raine, M. Buchsbaum, and L. LaCasse, "Brain abnormalities in murderers indicated by positron emission tomography," *Biological Psychiatry*, vol. 42, no. 6, pp. 495–508, 1997.

[43] A. Raine, J. R. Meloy, S. Bihrle, J. Stoddard, L. LaCasse, and M. S. Buchsbaum, "Reduced prefrontal and increased subcortical brain functioning assessed using positron emission tomography in predatory and affective murderers," *Sciences & the Law*, vol. 16, pp. 319–332, 1998.

[44] G. Spalletta, A. Troisi, S. Alimenti et al., "Reduced prefrontal cognitive activation associated with aggression in schizophrenia," *Schizophrenia Research*, vol. 50, no. 1-2, pp. 134–135, 2001.

[45] M. C. Dolan and R. S. Fullam, "Psychopathy and functional magnetic resonance imaging blood oxygenation level-dependent responses to emotional faces in violent patients with schizophrenia," *Biological Psychiatry*, vol. 66, no. 6, pp. 570–577, 2009.

[46] C. C. Joyal, A. Putkonen, A. Mancini-Marïe et al., "Violent persons with schizophrenia and comorbid disorders: a functional magnetic resonance imaging study," *Schizophrenia Research*, vol. 91, no. 1–3, pp. 97–102, 2007.

[47] V. Kumari, M. Das, P. J. Taylor et al., "Neural and behavioural responses to threat in men with a history of serious violence and schizophrenia or antisocial personality disorder," *Schizophrenia Research*, vol. 110, no. 1–3, pp. 47–58, 2009.

[48] K. A. Kiehl, A. M. Smith, R. D. Hare et al., "Limbic abnormalities in affective processing by criminal psychopaths as revealed by functional magnetic resonance imaging," *Biological Psychiatry*, vol. 50, no. 9, pp. 677–684, 2001.

[49] A. Raine, S. Park, T. Lencz et al., "Reduced right hemisphere activation in severely abused violent offenders during a working memory task: an fMRI study," *Aggressive Behavior*, vol. 27, no. 2, pp. 111–129, 2001.

[50] R. Veit, H. Flor, M. Erb et al., "Brain circuits involved in emotional learning in antisocial behavior and social phobia in humans," *Neuroscience Letters*, vol. 328, no. 3, pp. 233–236, 2002.

[51] A. P. Jones, K. R. Laurens, C. M. Herba, G. J. Barker, and E. Viding, "Amygdala hypoactivity to fearful faces in boys with conduct problems and callous-unemotional traits," *American Journal of Psychiatry*, vol. 166, no. 1, pp. 95–102, 2009.

[52] A. A. Marsh, E. C. Finger, D. G. V. Mitchell et al., "Reduced amygdala response to fearful expressions in children and adolescents with callous-unemotional traits and disruptive behavior disorders," *American Journal of Psychiatry*, vol. 165, no. 6, pp. 712–720, 2008.

[53] M. J. Hoptman, D. D'Angelo, D. Catalano et al., "Amygdalofrontal functional disconnectivity and aggression in schizophrenia," *Schizophrenia Bulletin*, vol. 36, no. 5, pp. 1020–1028, 2010.

[54] M. Soyka, "Neurobiology of aggression and violence in schizophrenia," *Schizophrenia Bulletin*, vol. 37, no. 5, pp. 913-920, 2011.

[55] C. M. Filley, B. H. Price, V. Nell et al., "Toward an understanding of violence: neurobehavioral aspects of unwarranted physical aggression: aspen neurobehavioral conference consensus statement," *Neuropsychiatry, Neuropsychology and Behavioral Neurology*, vol. 14, no. 1, pp. 1–14, 2001.

[56] M. F. Green, *Schizophrenia from a Neurocognitive Perspective: Probig the Impenetrable Darkness*, Allyn and Bacon, Boston, Mass, USA, 1998.

[57] A. B. Morgan and S. O. Lilienfeld, "A meta-analytic review of the relation between antisocial behavior and neuropsychological measures of executive function," *Clinical Psychology Review*, vol. 20, no. 1, pp. 113–136, 2000.

[58] J. M. Lafayette, W. G. Frankle, A. Pollock, K. Dyer, and D. C. Goff, "Clinical characteristics, cognitive functioning, and criminal histories of outpatients with Schizophrenia," *Psychiatric Services*, vol. 54, no. 12, pp. 1635-1640, 2003.

[59] M. Krakowski, P. Czobor, J. Libiger et al., "Violence in schizophrenic patients: the role of positive psychotic symptoms and frontal lobe impairment," *American Journal of Forensic Psychiatry*, vol. 18, no. 1, pp. 39–50, 1997.

[60] T. H. Wong, J. Lumsden, G. W. Fenton, and P. B. Fenwick, "Neuroimaging in mentally abnormal offenders," *1997Criminological and Legal Psychology*, vol. 27, pp. 49–58.

[61] H. Silver, C. Goodman, G. Knoll, V. Isakov, and I. Modai, "Schizophrenia patients with a history of severe violence differ from nonviolent schizophrenia patients in perception of emotions but not cognitive function," *Journal of Clinical Psychiatry*, vol. 66, no. 3, pp. 300–308, 2005.

[62] R. S. Fullam and M. C. Dolan, "Executive function and inpatient violence in forensic patients with schizophrenia," *British Journal of Psychiatry*, vol. 193, no. 3, pp. 247–253, 2008.

[63] S. Roy, J. Herrera, M. Parent, and J. Costa, "Violent and nonviolent schizophrenic patients clinical and developmental characteristics," *Psychological Reports*, vol. 61, pp. 855–861, 1987.

[64] D. Lapierre, C. M. J. Braun, S. Hodgins, J. Toupin, S. Leveillee, and C. Constantineau, "Neuropsychological correlates of violence in schizophrenia," *Schizophrenia Bulletin*, vol. 21, no. 2, pp. 253–262, 1995.

[65] K. Rasmussen, S. Levander, and H. Sletvold, "Aggressive and non-aggressive schizophrenics: symptom profile and neuropsychological differences," *Psychology, Crime & Law*, vol. 2, pp. 119–129, 1995.

[66] M. I. Krakowski, A. Convit, J. Jaeger, S. Lin, and J. Volavka, "Neurological impairment in violent schizophrenic inpatients," *American Journal of Psychiatry*, vol. 146, no. 7, pp. 849–853, 1989.

[67] J. J. Adams, J. R. Meloy, and M. S. Moritz, "Neuropsychological deficits and violent behavior in incarcerated schizophrenics," *Journal of Nervous and Mental Disease*, vol. 178, no. 4, pp. 253–256, 1990.

[68] I. Barkataki, V. Kumari, M. Das et al., "A neuropsychological investigation into violence and mental illness," *Schizophrenia Research*, vol. 74, no. 1, pp. 1–13, 2005.

[69] H. G. Foster, M. Hillbrand, and M. Silverstein, "Neuropsychological deficit and aggressive behavior: a prospective study," *Progress in Neuro-Psychopharmacology and Biological Psychiatry*, vol. 17, no. 6, pp. 939–946, 1993.

[70] M. Krakowski, P. Czobor, M. D. Carpenter et al., "Community violence and inpatient assaults: neurobiological deficits," *Journal of Neuropsychiatry and Clinical Neurosciences*, vol. 9, no. 4, pp. 549–555, 1997.

[71] P. G. Nestor, "Neuropsychological and clinical correlates of murder and other forms of extreme violence in a forensic psychiatric population," *Journal of Nervous and Mental Disease*, vol. 180, no. 7, pp. 418–423, 1992.

[72] H. Song and S. K. Min, "Aggressive behavior model in schizophrenic patients," *Psychiatry Research*, vol. 167, no. 1-2, pp. 58–65, 2009.

[73] M. Serper, D. R. Beech, P. D. Harvey, and C. Dill, "Neuropsychological and symptom predictors of aggression on the psychiatric inpatient service," *Journal of Clinical and Experimental Neuropsychology*, vol. 30, no. 6, pp. 700–709, 2008.

[74] M. Hancock, J. L. Tapscott, and P. N. S. Hoaken, "Role of executive dysfunction in predicting frequency and severity of violence," *Aggressive Behavior*, vol. 36, no. 5, pp. 338–349, 2010.

[75] M. I. Krakowski and P. Czobor, "Executive function predicts response to antiaggression treatment in schizophrenia: a randomized controlled trial," *Journal of Clinical Psychiatry*, vol. 73, no. 1, pp. 74–80, 2012.

[76] P. Ekman and W. V. Friesen, *Unmasking the Face*, Prentice-Hall, Englewood Cliffs, NJ, USA, 1975.

[77] C. G. Kohler, T. H. Turner, R. E. Gur, and R. C. Gur, "Recognition of facial emotions in neuropsychiatric disorders," *CNS Spectrums*, vol. 9, no. 4, pp. 267–274, 2004.

[78] J. C. Borod, *The Neuropsychology of Emotion*, University Press, Oxford, UK, 2000.

[79] E. F. Walker, K. E. Grimes, D. M. Davis, and A. J. Smith, "Childhood precursors of schizophrenia: facial expressions of emotion," *American Journal of Psychiatry*, vol. 150, no. 11, pp. 1654–1660, 1993.

[80] R. J. Davidson, K. M. Putnam, and C. L. Larson, "Dysfunction in the neural circuitry of emotion regulation—a possible prelude to violence," *Science*, vol. 289, no. 5479, pp. 591–594, 2000.

[81] B. Corden, H. D. Critchley, D. Skuse, and R. J. Dolan, "Fear recognition ability predicts differences in social cognitive and neural functioning in men," *Journal of Cognitive Neuroscience*, vol. 18, no. 6, pp. 889–897, 2006.

[82] R. J. R. Blair, "Neurobiological basis of psychopathy," *British Journal of Psychiatry*, vol. 182, pp. 5–7, 2003.

[83] B. Montagne, J. van Honk, R. P. C. Kessels et al., "Reduced efficiency in recognising fear in subjects scoring high on psychopathic personality characteristics," *Personality and Individual Differences*, vol. 38, no. 1, pp. 5–11, 2005.

[84] D. W. Walker and C. Leister, "Recognition of facial affect cues by adolescents with emotional and behavioral disorders," *Behavioral Disorders*, vol. 19, pp. 269–276, 1994.

[85] H. J. Grabe, C. Spitzer, and H. J. Freyberger, "Alexithymia and personality in relation to dimensions of psychopathology," *American Journal of Psychiatry*, vol. 161, no. 7, pp. 1299–1301, 2004.

[86] M. Jakupcak, "Masculine gender role stress and Men's fear of emotions as predictors of self-reported aggression and violence," *Violence and Victims*, vol. 18, no. 5, pp. 533–541, 2003.

[87] L. Robinson, M. D. Spencer, L. D. Thomson et al., "Facial emotion recognition in Scottish prisoners," *International Journal of Law and Psychiatry*, vol. 35, no. 1, pp. 57–61, 2012.

[88] P. N. S. Hoaken, D. B. Allaby, and J. Earle, "Executive cognitive functioning and the recognition of facial expressions of emotion in incarcerated violent offenders, non-violent offenders, and controls," *Aggressive Behavior*, vol. 33, no. 5, pp. 412–421, 2007.

[89] N. C. Walz and B. A. Benson, "Labeling and discrimination of facial expressions by aggressive and nonaggressive men with mental retardation," *American Journal on Mental Retardation*, vol. 101, no. 3, pp. 282–291, 1996.

[90] E. M. Weiss, C. G. Kohler, K. A. Nolan et al., "The relationship between history of violent and criminal behavior and recognition of facial expression of emotions in men with schizophrenia and schizoaffective disorder," *Aggressive Behavior*, vol. 32, no. 3, pp. 187–194, 2006.

[91] K. A. Dodge, "Social-cognitive mechanisms in the development of conduct disorder and depression," *Annual Review of Psychology*, vol. 44, no. 1, pp. 559–584, 1993.

[92] D. E. McNiel, J. P. Eisner, and R. L. Binder, "The relationship between aggressive attributional style and violence by psychiatric patients," *Journal of Consulting and Clinical Psychology*, vol. 71, no. 2, pp. 399–403, 2003.

[93] R. Fullam and M. Dolan, "Emotional information processing in violent patients with schizophrenia: association with psychopathy and symptomatology," *Psychiatry Research*, vol. 141, no. 1, pp. 29–37, 2006.

[94] A. Abu-Akel and K. Abushua'leh, "'Theory of mind' in violent and nonviolent patients with paranoid schizophrenia," *Schizophrenia Research*, vol. 69, no. 1, pp. 45–53, 2004.

[95] K. Majorek, W. Wolfkühler, C. Küper, N. Saimeh, G. Juckel, and M. Brüne, "'Theory of mind' and executive functioning in forensic patients with schizophrenia," *Journal of Forensic Sciences*, vol. 54, no. 2, pp. 469–473, 2009.

[96] Z. Walsh, M. T. Swogger, and D. S. Kosson, "Psychopathy and instrumental violence: facet level relationships," *Journal of Personality Disorders*, vol. 23, no. 4, pp. 416–424, 2009.

[97] Y. Yang and A. Raine, "Prefrontal structural and functional brain imaging findings in antisocial, violent, and psychopathic individuals: a meta-analysis," *Psychiatry Research*, vol. 174, no. 2, pp. 81–88, 2009.

[98] T. Laajasalo, S. Salenius, N. Lindberg, E. Repo-Tiihonen, and H. Häkkänen-Nyholm, "Psychopathic traits in Finnish homicide offenders with schizophrenia," *International Journal of Law and Psychiatry*, vol. 34, no. 5, pp. 324–330, 2011.

[99] P. Moran and S. Hodgins, "The correlates of comorbid antisocial personality disorder in schizophrenia," *Schizophrenia Bulletin*, vol. 30, no. 4, pp. 791–802, 2004.

[100] B. A. Bettencourt, A. Talley, A. J. Benjamin, and J. Valentine, "Personality and aggressive behavior under provoking and neutral conditions: a meta-analytic review," *Psychological Bulletin*, vol. 132, no. 5, pp. 751–777, 2006.

[101] K. A. Dodge, "The structure and function of reactive and proactive aggression," in *The Development and Treatment of Childhood Aggression*, D. J. Pepler and K. H. Rubin, Eds., pp. 201–218, Lawrence Erlbaum, Hillsdale, NJ, USA, 1991.

[102] L. Berkowitz, *Aggression: A Social Psychological Analysis*, McGraw-Hill, New York, NY, USA, 1962.

[103] W. Ruch and R. T. Proyer, "The fear of being laughed at: individual and group differences in Gelotophobia," *Humor*, vol. 21, no. 1, pp. 47–67, 2008.

[104] M. Titze, "Gelotophobia: the fear of being laughed at," *Humor*, vol. 22, no. 1-2, pp. 27–48, 2009.

[105] I. Papousek, W. Ruch, H. H. Freudenthaler, E. Kogler, B. Lang, and G. Schulter, "Gelotophobia, emotion-related skills and responses to the affective states of others," *Personality and Individual Differences*, vol. 47, no. 1, pp. 58–63, 2009.

[106] K. R. Edwards and R. A. Martin, "The fear of being laughed at, social anxiety, and memories of being teased during childhood," *Psychological Test and Assessment Modeling*, vol. 52, pp. 94–107, 2010.

[107] E. M. Weiss, G. Schulter, H. H. Freudenthaler, E. Hofer, N. Pichler, and I. Papousek, "Potential markers of aggressive behavior: the fear of other persons' laughter and its overlaps with mental disorders," *PLoS ONE*, no. 5, Article ID e38088, 2012.

[108] C. Holden, "No laughing matter," *Science*, vol. 324, p. 699, 2009.

[109] W. Ruch, "Fearing humor? Gelotophobia: the fear of being laughed at Introduction and overview," *Humor*, vol. 22, no. 1-2, pp. 1–25, 2009.

[110] J. T. Nigg, "On inhibition/disinhibition in developmental psychopathology: views from cognitive and personality psychology and a working inhibition taxonomy," *Psychological Bulletin*, vol. 126, no. 2, pp. 220–246, 2000.

[111] E. S. Barratt and A. R. Felthous, "Impulsive versus premeditated aggression: implications for mens rea decisions," *Behavioral Sciences and the Law*, vol. 21, no. 5, pp. 619–630, 2003.

[112] R. E. Tarter, L. Kirisci, A. Mezzich et al., "Neurobehavioral disinhibition in childhood predicts early age at onset of substance use disorder," *American Journal of Psychiatry*, vol. 160, no. 6, pp. 1078–1085, 2003.

[113] B. J. Bushman, "Effects of alcohol on human aggression. Validity of proposed explanations," *Recent Developments in Alcoholism*, vol. 13, pp. 227–243, 1997.

[114] D. R. Cherek, J. L. Steinberg, and R. V. Vines, "Low doses of alcohol affect human aggressive responses," *Biological Psychiatry*, vol. 19, no. 2, pp. 263–267, 1984.

[115] R. O. Pihl, J. B. Peterson, and M. A. Lau, "A biosocial model of the alcohol-aggression relationship," *Journal of Studies on Alcohol*, vol. 54, no. 11, pp. 128–139, 1993.

[116] C. W. Lejuez, J. F. Magidson, S. H. Mitchell, R. Sinha, M. C. Stevens, and H. De Wit, "Behavioral and biological indicators of impulsivity in the development of alcohol use, problems, and disorders," *Alcoholism*, vol. 34, no. 8, pp. 1334–1345, 2010.

[117] D. R. Cherek and S. D. Lane, "Laboratory and psychometric measurements of impulsivity among violent and nonviolent female parolees," *Biological Psychiatry*, vol. 46, no. 2, pp. 273–280, 1999.

[118] D. R. Cherek, F. G. Moeller, D. M. Dougherty, and H. Rhoades, "Studies of violent and nonviolent male parolees: II. Laboratory and psychometric measurements of impulsivity," *Biological Psychiatry*, vol. 41, no. 5, pp. 523–529, 1997.

[119] M. James and J. A. Seager, "Impulsivity and schemas for a hostile world: postdictors of violent behaviour," *International Journal of Offender Therapy and Comparative Criminology*, vol. 50, no. 1, pp. 47–56, 2006.

[120] V. Kumari, I. Barkataki, S. Goswami, S. Flora, M. Das, and P. Taylor, "Dysfunctional, but not functional, impulsivity is associated with a history of seriously violent behaviour and reduced orbitofrontal and hippocampal volumes in schizophrenia," *Psychiatry Research*, vol. 173, no. 1, pp. 39–44, 2009.

[121] D. A. Gansler, A. K. W. Lee, B. C. Emerton et al., "Prefrontal regional correlates of self-control in male psychiatric patients: impulsivity facets and aggression," *Psychiatry Research*, vol. 191, no. 1, pp. 16–23, 2011.

[122] A. K. W. Lee, M. Jerram, C. Fulwiler, and D. A. Gansler, "Neural correlates of impulsivity factors in psychiatric patients and healthy volunteers: a voxel-based morphometry study," *Brain Imaging and Behavior*, vol. 5, no. 1, pp. 52–64, 2011.

[123] K. Matsuo, M. Nicoletti, K. Nemoto et al., "A voxel-based morphometry study of frontal gray matter correlates of impulsivity," *Human Brain Mapping*, vol. 30, no. 4, pp. 1188–1195, 2009.

[124] A. S. Antonucci, D. A. Gansler, S. Tan, R. Bhadelia, S. Patz, and C. Fulwiler, "Orbitofrontal correlates of aggression and impulsivity in psychiatric patients," *Psychiatry Research*, vol. 147, no. 2-3, pp. 213–220, 2006.

[125] E. F. Coccaro, C. S. Sripada, R. N. Yanowitch, and K. L. Phan, "Corticolimbic function in impulsive aggressive behavior," *Biological Psychiatry*, vol. 69, no. 12, pp. 1153–1159, 2011.

[126] M. Dolan, W. J. F. Deakin, N. Roberts, and I. Anderson, "Serotonergic and cognitive impairment in impulsive aggressive personality disordered offenders: are there implications for treatment?" *Psychological Medicine*, vol. 32, no. 1, pp. 105–117, 2002.

[127] P. N. S. Hoaken, V. K. Shaughnessy, and R. O. Pihl, "Executive cognitive functioning and aggression: is it an issue of impulsivity?" *Aggressive Behavior*, vol. 29, no. 1, pp. 15–30, 2003.

[128] P. R. Giancola, H. B. Moss, C. S. Martin, L. Kirisci, and R. E. Tarter, "Executive cognitive functioning predicts reactive aggression in boys at high risk for substance abuse: a prospective study," *Alcoholism*, vol. 20, no. 4, pp. 740–744, 1996.

[129] D. Lapierre, C. M. J. Braun, and S. Hodgins, "Ventral frontal deficits in psychopathy: neuropsychological test findings," *Neuropsychologia*, vol. 33, no. 2, pp. 139–151, 1995.

[130] D. G. V. Mitchell, E. Colledge, A. Leonard, and R. J. R. Blair, "Risky decisions and response reversal: is there evidence of orbitofrontal cortex dysfunction in psychopathic individuals?" *Neuropsychologia*, vol. 40, no. 12, pp. 2013–2022, 2002.

[131] T. Pattij and L. J. M. J. Vanderschuren, "The neuropharmacology of impulsive behaviour," *Trends in Pharmacological Sciences*, vol. 29, no. 4, pp. 192–199, 2008.

[132] T. Butler, P. W. Schofield, D. Greenberg et al., "Reducing impulsivity in repeat violent offenders: an open label trial of a selective serotonin reuptake inhibitor," *Australian and New Zealand Journal of Psychiatry*, vol. 44, no. 12, pp. 1137–1143, 2010.

[133] R. J. Kavoussi, J. Liu, and E. F. Coccaro, "An open trial of sertraline in personality disordered patients with impulsive aggression," *Journal of Clinical Psychiatry*, vol. 55, no. 4, pp. 137–141, 1994.

[134] E. F. Coccaro and R. J. Kavoussi, "Fluoxetine and impulsive aggressive behavior in personality-disordered subjects," *Archives of General Psychiatry*, vol. 54, no. 12, pp. 1081–1088, 1997.

[135] N. Huband, M. Ferriter, R. Nathan, and H. Jones, "Antiepileptics for aggression and associated impulsivity," *Cochrane Database of Aystematic Reviews*, vol. 2, Article ID CD003499, 2010.

[136] M. S. Stanford, N. E. Anderson, S. L. Lake, and R. M. Baldridge, "Pharmacologic treatment of impulsive aggression with antiepileptic drugs," *Current Treatment Options in Neurology*, vol. 11, no. 5, pp. 383–390, 2009.

[137] B. G. Link and A. Stueve, "Psychotic symptoms and the violent/illegal behavior of mental patients compared to community controls," in *Violence and Mental Disorder. Developments in Risk Assessment*, J. Monahan and H. J. Steadman, Eds., pp. 137–159, The University of Chicago Press, Chicago, Ill, USA, 1994.

[138] J. Junginger, J. Parks-Levy, and L. McGuire, "Delusions and symptom-consistent violence," *Psychiatric Services*, vol. 49, no. 2, pp. 218–220, 1998.

[139] P. J. Taylor, "Motives for offending among violent and psychotic men," *British Journal of Psychiatry*, vol. 147, pp. 491–498, 1985.

[140] J. Junginger, "Command hallucinations and the prediction of dangerousness," *Psychiatric Services*, vol. 46, no. 9, pp. 911–914, 1995.

[141] D. E. McNiel and R. L. Binder, "The relationship between acute psychiatric symptoms, diagnosis, and short- term risk of violence," *Hospital and Community Psychiatry*, vol. 45, no. 2, pp. 133–137, 1994.

[142] S. Zisook, D. Byrd, J. Kuck, and D. V. Jeste, "Command hallucinations in outpatients with schizophrenia," *Journal of Clinical Psychiatry*, vol. 56, no. 10, pp. 462–465, 1995.

[143] P. Cheung, I. Schweitzer, K. Crowley, and V. Tuckwell, "Violence in schizophrenia: role of hallucinations and delusions," *Schizophrenia Research*, vol. 26, no. 2-3, pp. 181–190, 1997.

[144] K. A. Nolan, J. Volavka, P. Czobor et al., "Aggression and psychopathology in treatment-resistant inpatients with schizophrenia and schizoaffective disorder," *Journal of Psychiatric Research*, vol. 39, no. 1, pp. 109–115, 2005.

[145] A. Fresán, R. Apiquian, C. De La Fuente-Sandoval et al., "Violent behavior in schizophrenic patients: relationship with clinical symptoms," *Aggressive Behavior*, vol. 31, no. 6, pp. 511–520, 2005.

[146] E. E. Maccoby and C. N. Jacklin, *The Psychology of Sex Differences*, Stanford University Press, Stanford, Calif, USA, 1974.

[147] A. L. Pastore, Sourcebook of Criminal Justice Statistics, 1999.

[148] S. Hodgins, "Mental disorder, intellectual deficiency, and crime: evidence from a birth cohort," *Archives of General Psychiatry*, vol. 49, no. 6, pp. 476–483, 1992.

[149] J. W. Swanson, C. E. Holzer, V. K. Ganju, and R. T. Jono, "Violence and psychiatric disorder in the community: evidence from the epidemiologic catchment area surveys," *Hospital and Community Psychiatry*, vol. 41, no. 7, pp. 761–770, 1990.

[150] J. N. Lam, D. E. McNiel, and R. L. Binder, "The relationship between patients' gender and violence leading to staff injuries," *Psychiatric Services*, vol. 51, no. 9, pp. 1167–1170, 2000.

[151] R. L. Binder and D. E. McNiel, "The relationship of gender to violent behavior in acutely disturbed psychiatric patients," *Journal of Clinical Psychiatry*, vol. 51, no. 3, pp. 110–114, 1990.

[152] V. A. Hiday, M. S. Swartz, J. W. Swanson, R. Borum, and H. R. Wagner, "Male-female differences in the setting and construction of violence among people with severe mental illness," *Social Psychiatry and Psychiatric Epidemiology*, vol. 33, no. 1, pp. S68–S74, 1998.

[153] E. M. Weiss, J. Marksteiner, H. Hinterhuber, and K. A. Nolan, "Gender differences in aggression in schizophrenia patients," *Neuropsychiatrie*, vol. 20, no. 3, pp. 186–191, 2006.

[154] M. Krakowski and P. Czobor, "Gender differences in violent behaviors: relationship to clinical symptoms and psychosocial factors," *American Journal of Psychiatry*, vol. 161, no. 3, pp. 459–465, 2004.

[155] N. R. Crick and J. K. Grotpeter, "Relational aggression, gender, and social-psychological adjustment," *Child Development*, vol. 66, no. 3, pp. 710–722, 1995.

[156] A. H. Eagly and V. J. Steffen, "Gender and aggressive behavior. A meta-analytic review of the Social Psychological Literature," *Psychological Bulletin*, vol. 100, no. 3, pp. 309–330, 1986.

[157] H. S. Dinakar and R. N. Sobel, "Violence in the community as a predictor of violence in the hospital," *Psychiatric Services*, vol. 52, no. 2, pp. 240–241, 2001.

[158] E. M. Weiss, R. M. Bilder, and W. W. Fleischhacker, "The effects of second-generation antipsychotics on cognitive functioning and psychosocial outcome in schizophrenia," *Psychopharmacology*, vol. 162, no. 1, pp. 11–17, 2002.

[159] J. W. Swanson, M. S. Swartz, and E. B. Elbogen, "Effectiveness of atypical antipsychotic medications in reducing violent behavior among persons with Schizophrenia in community-based treatment," *Schizophrenia Bulletin*, vol. 30, no. 1, pp. 3–20, 2004.

[160] J. W. Swanson, M. S. Swartz, E. B. Elbogen, and R. A. Van Dorn, "Reducing violence risk in persons with schizophrenia: olanzapine versus risperidone," *Journal of Clinical Psychiatry*, vol. 65, no. 12, pp. 1666–1673, 2004.

[161] M. I. Krakowski, P. Czobor, L. Citrome, N. Bark, and T. B. Cooper, "Atypical antipsychotic agents in the treatment of violent patients with schizophrenia and schizoaffective disorder," *Archives of General Psychiatry*, vol. 63, no. 6, pp. 622–629, 2006.

[162] M. I. Krakowski, P. Czobor, and K. A. Nolan, "Atypical antipsychotics, neurocognitive deficits, and aggression in schizophrenic patients," *Journal of Clinical Psychopharmacology*, vol. 28, no. 5, pp. 485–493, 2008.

13

Role of Hydrogen Sulfide in the Pathology of Inflammation

Madhav Bhatia

Department of Pathology, University of Otago, P.O. Box 4345, Christchurch 8140, New Zealand

Correspondence should be addressed to Madhav Bhatia; madhav.bhatia@otago.ac.nz

Academic Editors: M. A. Choudhry, G. Marucci, and B. Rippe

Hydrogen sulfide (H_2S) is a well-known toxic gas that is synthesized in the human body from the amino acids cystathionine, homocysteine, and cysteine by the action of at least two distinct enzymes: cystathionine-γ-lyase and cystathionine-β-synthase. In the past few years, H_2S has emerged as a novel and increasingly important biological mediator. Imbalances in H_2S have also been shown to be associated with various disease conditions. However, defining the precise pathophysiology of H_2S is proving to be a complex challenge. Recent research in our laboratory has shown H_2S as a novel mediator of inflammation and work in several groups worldwide is currently focused on determining the role of H_2S in inflammation. H_2S has been implicated in different inflammatory conditions, such as acute pancreatitis, sepsis, joint inflammation, and chronic obstructive pulmonary disease (COPD). Active research on the role of H_2S in inflammation will unravel the pathophysiology of its actions in inflammatory conditions and may help develop novel therapeutic approaches for several, as yet incurable, disease conditions.

1. Introduction

Hydrogen sulfide (H_2S) is a colorless, flammable, water-soluble gas characterized by a peculiar smell of rotten eggs. The toxic effects of H_2S have been known for more than 300 years, and it has long been believed to be just an environmental pollutant [1]. In recent years, involvement of H_2S is increasingly being recognized in several physiologic processes and disease states. H_2S is produced endogenously in mammals including humans. In particular, cystathionine-β-synthase (CBS) in the central nervous system and cystathionine-γ-lyase (CSE) in the cardiovascular system are the key enzymes mostly responsible for the endogenous generation of H_2S. Both enzymes use L-cysteine as the main substrate and pyridoxal-5′-phosphate as a cofactor [2]. Other enzymes responsible for the synthesis of H_2S include (1) cysteine aminotransferase (CAT, EC 2.6.1.3), which catalyzes the reaction of l-cysteine with a ketoacid (e.g., α-ketoglutarate) to form 3-mercaptopyruvate and an amino acid such as l-glutamate-3-mercaptopyruvate may then be desulfurated by 3-mercaptopyruvate sulfurtransferase (MPST, EC 2.8.1.2) to form H_2S and pyruvate; (2) cysteine lyase (EC 4.4.1.10), which converts l-cysteine and sulfite to l-cysteate and H_2S [3]. As the end product of CBS- and CSE-catalyzed cysteine metabolism, H_2S exerts a negative feedback effect on the activity of these enzymes [1, 4]. H_2S has been shown to act as a modulator of N-methyl-D-aspartate receptor currents and hippocampal long-term potentiation. It also opens adenosine triphosphate-dependent K^+ channel and interacts with other vasoactive gaseous mediators to relax smooth muscle [4–7]. There is evidence for the formation of a novel nitrosothiol from the interaction of H_2S with nitric oxide (NO), a well-known gaseous mediator [8]. This nitrosothiol appears to play an important role in the action of H_2S [9].

H_2S *in vivo* is metabolized rapidly by a multitude of different chemical and enzymatic processes. Of these, the mitochondrial oxidation mechanism represents the most important route of H_2S catabolism. It involves several enzymatic steps catalyzed by quinine oxidoreductase, S-dioxygenase, and S-transferase and, overall, leads to the formation of thiosulfate. Subsequently, thiosulfate is converted to sulfite by rhodanase and finally the major and stable product, sulfate, by sulfite oxidase [10, 11]. In contrast, cytosolic methylation of H_2S by thiol-S-methytransferase to yield methanethiol and dimethylsulfide represents another less important mechanism of H_2S degradation, and therefore accounts for a smaller amount of H_2S [12]. Additionally, H_2S can be scavenged by methaemoglobin to form sulfhaemoglobin or consumed by metallo- or disulfide-containing molecules such as oxidized glutathione [13, 14]. It can also be oxidized by activated neutrophils to form sulfite [15]. Finally, H_2S is an endogenous reducing agent which can be easily consumed by a variety of circulating oxidant species in the vasculature such as peroxynitrite, hypochlorite, superoxide, or hydrogen peroxide [16–19]. It is excreted mainly by the kidney as free or conjugated sulfate [13].

In this paper, recent evidence that points to a key role of endogenously produced H_2S as a novel mediator of inflammation is discussed.

2. Inflammation

Inflammation is a highly orchestrated, tissue-based response to traumatic, infectious, postischemic, toxic, or autoimmune injury. What Celsus defined around AD40 as "rubor, calor, dolor, tumor" (redness, heat, pain, and swelling) is today an intellectually engaging problem in systems biology, as well as a multibillion dollar market for the pharmaceutical industry. When primary pathogenic events are unknown, control of inflammation is sometimes the next best option. Initiated by responsive leukocytes and lymphocytes, a key component of the process is the trafficking of inflammatory cells to the sites of injury or infection. The cytokine/receptor interactions on the surface of these cells culminate in the expression of new gene products that efficiently kill or injure the invading organisms. However, uncontrolled production of inflammatory products is injurious to host cells and even leads to neoplastic transformation. Therefore, endogenous mechanisms have evolved to limit the production of inflammatory molecules and permit the resolution of the inflammatory response. In-depth studies of these mechanisms are important because defects in the pathway may contribute to the progression of chronic inflammatory disorders, and the pathway itself may present targets for novel anti-inflammatory therapeutic strategies [20–24].

Over the years, various studies have indicated a role of H_2S in the inflammatory process. Reactive oxygen species from activated neutrophils could oxidize H_2S to form sulfite, which then acts to upregulate leukocyte adhesion and neutrophil functions, through activation of Mac-1 β2-integrin (CD11b/CD18) and protein kinase C (PKC)/Ca^{2+}-calmodulin pathway, respectively [15, 25–27]. Administration of nicotinamide adenine dinucleotide phosphate (NADPH) oxidase inhibitor suppressed whilst exogenous application of sodium hydrosulfide (NaHS), an H_2S donor, enhanced these responses [26]. In addition, H_2S provoked the short-term survival of granulocytes via inhibition of caspase-3 cleavage and p38 mitogen-activated protein kinase (MAPK) activation and therefore contributed to the bactericidal activity of neutrophils [28].

Recent work in our laboratory and others has shown a key role of H_2S as a mediator of inflammation in different clinical conditions.

3. Acute Pancreatitis and Associated Lung Injury

Acute pancreatitis is a common clinical condition whose incidence has been increasing over recent years [29–33]. In United States alone, >300,000 patients are hospitalized annually with acute pancreatitis, leading to 3,200 deaths. Acute pancreatitis is a contributing factor in an additional 4,000 deaths annually. It also inflicts a heavy economic burden; the direct cost in the United States alone is > \$2 billion annually [29–33]. In a majority of patients the condition is mild but 25% of patients suffer a severe attack and between 30 to 50% of these will die [29–33]. Most cases are secondary to biliary disease or excess alcohol consumption. The events that regulate the severity of acute pancreatitis are, for the most part, unknown. The exact mechanisms by which diverse etiological factors induce an attack are still unclear, but once the disease process is initiated common inflammatory and repair pathways are invoked. There is a local inflammatory reaction at the site of injury, which if marked leads to systemic inflammatory response syndrome (SIRS), and it is this systemic response that is believed to be ultimately responsible for the majority of the morbidity and mortality [29–33].

Since both CBS and CSE, two major H_2S forming enzymes, are highly expressed in pancreatic acinar cells, it is of interest to understand the potential role of H_2S in acute pancreatitis. Our group was the first to show the role of endogenously produced H_2S as a mediator of inflammation [34]. We showed that mRNA for CSE is expressed in mouse pancreas and that pancreas homogenates convert L-cysteine to H_2S *ex vivo*. Also, plasma levels of H_2S are increased in mice upon induction of acute pancreatitis. The conversion of L-cysteine to H_2S in pancreas homogenates was significantly reduced in mice pretreated with DL-propargylglycine (PAG) [34]. In addition, we showed that treatment of animals with PAG (either prophylactic or therapeutic) reduces the severity of pancreatitis as evidenced by a significant attenuation of hyperamylasemia, acinar cell injury/necrosis, and pancreatic myeloperoxidase (MPO) activity and by histological evidence of diminished pancreatic injury. Severe, but not mild, acute pancreatitis is associated also with lung injury, which is characterized by sequestration of neutrophils within the lung (i.e., increased lung MPO activity) and histological evidence of lung injury. In this study [34], we demonstrated that prophylactic/therapeutic administration of PAG additionally protected mice against acute pancreatitis associated lung injury as evidenced by a significant attenuation of lung MPO activity and by histological evidence of diminished lung injury (alveolar thickening and leukocyte infiltration) [34]. These effects of CSE blockade suggested an important proinflammatory role of H_2S in regulating the severity of pancreatitis and associated lung injury and raise the possibility that H_2S may exert similar activity in other forms of inflammation [34]. More recently, we have shown an important role of CBS in the pathogenesis of acute pancreatitis and associated lung injury [35]. In this study [35] we showed the presence of endogenous as well as caerulein stimulated production of H_2S and ammonia (NH_3) in the pancreas and lung. Caerulein increased plasma and tissue H_2S and NH_3 compared to saline control. Prophylactic or therapeutic administration of aminooxyacetate (AOA), a reversible inhibitor of CBS, directly inhibits CBS in the pancreas thereby reducing H_2S and NH_3 production, and protects against acute pancreatitis, further confirming the role of both the enzymes in inflammation in acute pancreatitis [35].

In isolated pancreatic acinar cells, the level of H_2S and CSE mRNA were also significantly elevated in pancreatic acinar cells stimulated by caerulein [36]. Inhibition of H_2S formation by PAG reduced mRNA expression and production of monocyte chemoatractant protein (MCP)-1, macrophage inflammatory protein- (MIP-) 1α, and MIP-2 in caerulein-stimulated mouse pancreatic acinar cells [36, 37]. Caerulein-induced acute pancreatitis was associated with a significant increase in MCP-1, MIP-1α and MIP-2 mRNA in both the pancreas and lungs, suggesting that they are important early mediators in both local as well as distant inflammatory response [37]. Blockade of H_2S biosynthesis with PAG ameliorates the development of inflammatory process in caerulein-induced acute pancreatitis, acting through downregulation of chemokine expression [36, 37].

Furthermore, recent work in our laboratory has shown that H_2S induces intercellular adhesion molecule-(ICAM-) 1 expression and neutrophil adhesion to caerulein-treated pancreatic acinar cells through nuclear factor- (NF-) κB and Src-family kinases (SFK) pathway [38]. Results in this study [38] showed that H_2S enhances ICAM-1 expression in cearulein hyperstimulated pancreatic acini and that this action involves SFK family phosphorylation. H_2S activates SFKs in acinar cells and inhibition of SFKs impairs H_2S-induced ICAM-1 expression secondary to the inhibition of NF-κB activation. The effect of SFK inhibition on NF-κB activation occurs together with IκBα degradation. The results further demonstrate that neutrophil attachment onto H_2S-treated acinar cells is increased and that inhibition of SFK function inhibits H_2S-induced neutrophil attachment onto acinar cells. Taken together, these data indicate that H_2S engages SFKs in order to signal ICAM-1 expression by a mechanism involving induction of NF-κB. Results in this study [38] are consistent with a model wherein H_2S activation of IκBα and SFKs acts in concert to promote NF-κB activity and ICAM-1 expression. Taken together, we proposed the mechanism by which H_2S regulates ICAM-1 production in pancreatic acinar cells. Given the crucial role of ICAM-1 in facilitating the recruitment of neutrophil to acinar cells, targeting SFKs may be a useful strategy for suppressing the H_2S-activated inflammatory response. These results highlight that SFKs may be an attractive therapeutic target for the treatment of acute pancreatitis. Also, results indicate a key role of the phosphatidylinositol 3-kinase-protein kinase B pathway in relation to the action of H_2S on caerulein-induced cytokine production in isolated mouse pancreatic acinar cells [39].

Intraperitoneal administration of NaHS, an H_2S donor, to mice caused a significant increase in circulating levels of substance P in a dose-dependent manner [40]. H_2S, by itself, could also cause lung inflammation, as evidenced by a significant increase in lung MPO activity and histological evidence of lung injury. The maximum effect of H_2S on substance P levels and on lung inflammation was observed 1 h after NaHS administration. At this time, a significant increase in lung levels of tumor necrosis factor (TNF)-α and interleukin (IL)-1β was also observed. In preprotachykinin (PPT)-A$^{-/-}$ mice genetically deficient in substance P, H_2S did not cause any lung inflammation. Furthermore, pretreatment of mice with CP-96345, an antagonist of the neurokinin-1 receptor (NK-1R) protected mice against lung inflammation caused by H_2S. However, treatment with antagonists of NK-2, NK-3, and calcitonin gene related peptide (CGRP) receptors did not have any effect on H_2S-induced lung inflammation. Depleting neuropeptide from sensory neurons by capsaicin significantly reduced the lung inflammation caused by H_2S. In addition, pretreatment of mice with capsazepine, an antagonist of the transient receptor potential vanilloid-1 (TRPV-1), protected mice against H_2S-induced lung inflammation. These results demonstrated a key role of substance P and neurogenic inflammation in H_2S-induced lung injury in mice [40].

Substance P has been shown to play a key role in inflammation in acute pancreatitis [41–51]. Substance P treatment of isolated pancreatic acini results in an activation of chemokine synthesis, in turn resulting in an activation of inflammatory response [52–56]. Furthermore, substance P induces chemokine synthesis from macrophages and neutrophils, both of which are key players in inflammation [57–60].

In acute pancreatitis, PAG, given prophylactically as well as therapeutically, significantly reduced substance P concentrations in plasma, pancreas, and lung [61]. Moreover, prophylactic as well as therapeutic administration of PAG significantly reduced PPT-A mRNA expression and NK-1R mRNA expression in both pancreas and lung when compared with caerulein-induced acute pancreatitis. This reduction in PPT-A mRNA expression and NK-1R mRNA expression was associated with a protection against acute pancreatitis and associated lung injury. The increase in substance P production and NK-1R gene expression in the pancreas and lungs leads to increased inflammation and tissue injury in the pancreas and lung as evidenced by hyperamylasemia, myeloperoxidase (MPO) activities, and histological examination of the tissue injury. In this study [61] although pulmonary H_2S synthesizing activity was not increased in caerulein group, increased plasma H_2S due to increased pancreatic H_2S synthesizing activity may upregulate PPT-A and NK-1R mRNA expression in lung and thereby caused increased production of SP in lung. Although inhibition of CSE enzyme activity had no impact on pulmonary H_2S synthesizing activity, it caused significant reduction in pulmonary SP in acute pancreatitis. These results suggested that the proinflammatory effects of H_2S may be mediated by SP-NK-1R pathway in acute pancreatitis [61]. In isolated pancreatic acini [36], inhibition of endogenous production of H_2S by PAG significantly suppressed caerulein-induced increase in substance P concentration, PPT-A expression, and NK-1R expression. To determine whether H_2S itself provoked inflammation in acinar cells, the cells were treated with NaHS, that resulted in a significant increase in substance P concentration and expression of PPT-A and NK-1R.

Furthermore, we have shown that PPTA deficiency and blockage of H_2S synthesis may play an important role that can regulate the toll-like receptor 4 (TLR4) pathway and subsequent innate immune response in acute pancreatitis, implying an interaction between SP/H_2S occurs via TLR4 and NF-kB pathway. PPT-A gene deletion regulates H_2S-induced TLR 4 signaling pathway in caerulein-treated pancreatic acinar cells, suggesting that in acute pancreatitis, H_2S may upregulate the TLR4 pathway and NF-κB via substance P [62]. The findings with these two proinflammatory mediators H_2S and SP in TLR4 pathway has a crucial role in pro-inflammatory responses is not only important for understanding the basic mechanisms of H_2S/TLR4-mediated gene activation but may also have implications for the development of anti-inflammatory drugs. Elucidation of the role of H_2S/TLR4 in adaptive immunity might also open new opportunities for future treatment modalities in inflammation [62].

4. Sepsis

Sepsis is defined as the presence of bacteria or their toxins in blood or tissue and the systemic response that follows. Sepsis leading to at least one organ failure characterizes severe sepsis and septic shock is defined by severe sepsis accompanied by hypotension unresponsive to fluid resuscitation. Severe sepsis and septic shock are one of the leading causes of mortality among intensive care units and postoperative care patients [63–66]. The incidence of sepsis in North America has been reported to be 3.0 per 1,000 population, which transforms into an annual number of 750,000 cases, with 210,000 of them being fatal and a large socioeconomic burden [63–66]. The incidence of mortality due to sepsis is increasing and the most likely causes are the increased incidence of resistant pathogens and the advances of medical and surgical procedures that save the lives of many patients but leave them immunocompromized and in a state highly susceptible to death from severe sepsis and septic shock [63–66]. Sepsis and the events that follow are stages in a progressive condition—a systemic response to infection brought about by various inflammatory mediators, such as cytokines and chemokines. A relationship between cytokine cascades and sepsis has long been established but new evidence suggests that adhesion molecules also play a key role.

Using a clinically relevant model of cecal-ligation-and-puncture- (CLP-) induced sepsis, we have shown that H_2S acts as a mediator of inflammation in this condition [67]. CLP-induced sepsis significantly increased the plasma H_2S level and the liver H_2S synthesis 8 h after CLP compared with sham operation. Induction of sepsis also resulted in a significant upregulation of CSE mRNA in liver. On the other hand, prophylactic as well as therapeutic administration of PAG significantly reduced sepsis-associated systemic inflammation, as evidenced by decreased MPO activity and histological changes in lung and liver, and attenuated the mortality in CLP-induced sepsis. Injection of NaHS, an H_2S donor, significantly aggravated sepsis-associated systemic inflammation. Therefore, the effect of inhibition of H_2S formation and administration of NaHS suggests that H_2S plays a proinflammatory role in regulating the severity of sepsis and associated organ injury. Subsequent studies have shown the mechanism by which H_2S contributes to inflammation in sepsis. For example, in one study [68] both prophylactic and therapeutic administration of PAG significantly reduced the mRNA and protein levels of IL-1β, IL-6, TNF-α, MCP-1, and MIP-2 in lung and liver, coupled with decreased nuclear translocation and activation of NF-κB in lung and liver. Inhibition of H_2S formation also significantly reduced lung permeability and plasma alanine aminotransferase activity. In contrast, injection of NaHS significantly aggravated sepsis-associated systemic inflammation and increased NF-κB activation. In addition, H_2S-induced lung inflammation was blocked by the NF-κB inhibitor BAY 11-7082. Therefore, H_2S upregulates the production of proinflammatory mediators and exacerbates the systemic inflammation in sepsis through a mechanism involving NF-κB activation. In another study [69], using intravital microscopy, we found that in sepsis, prophylactic and therapeutic administration of PAG reduced leukocyte rolling and adherence significantly in mesenteric venules coupled with decreased mRNA and protein levels of adhesion molecules (ICAM-1, P-selectin, and E-selectin) in lung and liver. In contrast, injection of NaHS upregulated leukocyte rolling and attachment significantly, as well as tissue levels of adhesion molecules in sepsis. Conversely, in normal mice given NaHS to induce lung inflammation, NaHS treatment enhanced the level of adhesion molecules and neutrophil infiltration in lung. These alterations were reversed by pretreatment with BAY 11-7082. Moreover, expression of the chemokine receptor CXCR2 in neutrophils obtained from H_2S-treated mice was upregulated significantly, leading to an elevation in MIP-2-directed migration of neutrophils. Therefore, H_2S acts as an important endogenous regulator of leukocyte activation and trafficking during an inflammatory response. In a more recent study [70], we have shown that H_2S regulates inflammatory response by activating the extracellular signal related kinase (ERK) pathway in polymicrobial sepsis. In this study, CLP-induced sepsis resulted in a time-dependent increase in the synthesis of endogenous H_2S. Maximum phosphorylation of ERK1/2 and degradation of IκBα in lung and liver were observed 4 h after CLP. Inhibition of H_2S formation by PAG significantly reduced the phosphorylation of ERK1/2 in lung and liver 4 h after CLP, coupled with decreased degradation of IκBα and activation of NF-κB. In contrast, injection of NaHS significantly enhanced the activation of ERK1/2 in lung and liver, therefore leading to a further rise in tissue NF-κB activity. As a result, pretreatment with PAG significantly reduced the production of cytokines and chemokines in sepsis, whereas exogenous H_2S greatly increased it. In addition, pretreatment with PD98059, an inhibitor of MEK-1, significantly prevented NaHS from aggravating systemic inflammation in sepsis. This study, therefore, showed that H_2S may regulate systemic inflammatory response in sepsis via the ERK pathway. In human monocyte U937 cells, H_2S stimulates cell activation with the generation of proinflammatory cytokines, and this response is, at least partially, through the ERK-NF-κB signaling pathway [71]. Similar to CLP-induced sepsis, a pro-inflammatory action of H_2S was also observed in lipopolysaccharide (LPS)-induced endotoxemia [72, 73].

As in acute pancreatitis, substance P has been shown to play a key role in inflammation in sepsis [74–79]. An interaction between H_2S and substance P was shown in a study in which PAG pretreatment or posttreatment significantly decreased the PPT-A gene expression and the production of substance P in lung, whereas administration of NaHS resulted in a further rise in the pulmonary level of substance P in sepsis. PPT-A gene deletion and pretreatment with the NK-1R antagonist L703606 prevented H_2S from aggravating lung inflammation. In addition, septic mice genetically deficient in PPT-A gene or pretreated with L703606 did not exhibit further increase in lung permeability after injection of NaHS [80]. These findings showed that in sepsis, H_2S upregulates the generation of substance P that contributes to lung inflammation and lung injury mainly via activation of the NK-1R. In a more recent study, we have shown that H_2S induces systemic inflammation and multiple organ damage characteristic of sepsis via transient-receptor-potential-vanilloid-type-1-(TRPV1-) mediated neurogenic inflammation [81]. When given subcutaneously 30 minutes before CLP, the TRPV1 capsazepine treatment significantly attenuated systemic inflammation and multiple organ damage caused by sepsis, as characterized by lowered lung and liver MPO activities and histological evidence of diminished pulmonary and hepatic injury. Moreover, capsazepine delayed the onset of lethality and protected against sepsis-associated mortality. Administration of NaHS exacerbated but capsazepine reversed these deleterious effects. In the presence of PAG, capsazepine caused no significant changes to the PAG-mediated attenuation of systemic inflammation, multiple organ damage, and mortality in sepsis. More importantly, capsazepine has no effect on endogenous generation of H_2S, suggesting that H_2S is located upstream of TRPV1 activation, and may play a critical role in regulating the production and release of sensory neuropeptides in sepsis. Therefore, this study showed for the first time that H_2S induces systemic inflammation and multiple organ damage characteristic of sepsis via TRPV1-mediated neurogenic inflammation [81]. Recent results [82] have identified the endogenous neural mediator that implicates in H_2S-induced neurogenic inflammation and the molecular mechanisms by which H_2S promotes TRPV1-mediated neurogenic inflammation in sepsis. In this study, capsazepine treatment resulted in a significant attenuation of circulating and pulmonary levels of substance P in septic mice. Capsazepine also inhibited NaHS-augmented substance P production but had no effect on PAG-mediated abrogation of substance P levels in both plasma and lung. Furthermore, capsazepine significantly reduced H_2S-induced inflammatory cytokines, chemokines, and adhesion molecules expression, and protected against lung and liver dysfunction in sepsis. In the absence of H_2S, capsazepine caused no significant changes to the PAG-mediated attenuation of sepsis-associated systemic inflammatory response and multiple organ dysfunction. Additionally, capsazepine greatly inhibited phosphorylation of ERK1/2 and $I\kappa B\alpha$, concurrent with suppression of NF-κB activation even in the presence of NaHS. In contrast, capsazepine had no effect on PAG-mediated abrogation of these levels in sepsis. Taken together, results in this study showed that H_2S regulates TRPV1-mediated neurogenic inflammation in polymicrobial sepsis through enhancement of SP production and activation of the ERK-NF-κB pathway [82]. Also, a recent study has shown that H_2S upregulates cyclooxygenase-2 (COX-2) and prostaglandin E metabolite [PGEM] in sepsis-evoked acute lung injury via TRPV-1 channel activation [83]. Results in this study [83] demonstrated that induction of sepsis by CLP resulted in a concomitant and significant overproduction of COX-2 and PGEM in the lungs. Administration of NaHS further enhanced the biosynthesis of COX-2 and PGEM whereas PAG significantly decreased these levels. The use of two different yet complementary approaches in this work: exogenous administration of NaHS that serves as an H_2S donor and inhibition of endogenous H_2S synthesis by PAG which acts as an irreversible inhibitor of CSE, directly ascertained the involvement of H_2S in augmenting the production of COX-2 and PGEM in sepsis. The use of capsazepine, a selective TRPV1 antagonist, determined that H_2S upregulates COX-2 and PGEM in sepsis by a TRPV1 channel-dependent mechanism. Additionally, since blockade of TRPV1 by capsazepine attenuated H_2S-augmented COX-2 and PGEM response but had no effect on PAG-mediated attenuation of both parameters in septic lungs, we ascertained from our data that sepsis has a significant sensory neurogenic component that is mediated by H_2S in a TRPV1-dependent manner, and that H_2S stimulation of TRPV1 occurs upstream of COX-2 and PGEM in sepsis [83]. Furthermore, COX-2 inhibition with parecoxib significantly attenuated pulmonary neutrophil infiltration, edema formation, production of inflammatory cytokines, chemokines, and adhesion molecules, as well as restored lung histoarchitecture in sepsis, thereby significantly prevented the development of sepsis-evoked acute lung injury. Moreover, the fact that exogenous administration of NaHS to septic mice showed exacerbated acute lung injury compared to mice subjected to CLP alone, and that these pathophysiologic consequences of acute lung injury were significantly abrogated upon treatment with parecoxib confirm the notion that sepsis-evoked acute lung injury was specifically attributable to the interplay between H_2S and COX-2. Intrigued by the strong inhibitory effects of parecoxib on H_2S-induced inflammation and injury in the lungs of septic mice, our results also suggest that selective blockade of COX-2 could constitute an important therapeutic target for the treatment of sepsis-evoked acute lung injury [83]. This report, therefore, showed that H_2S augments the upregulation of COX-2 and PGEM, which orchestrates the neurogenic inflammatory response via activation of TRPV1 channel, and consequently contributes to lung inflammation and injury in a mouse model of sepsis-induced ALI. Additionally, inhibition of COX-2/PGE_2 pathway in the septic lungs significantly ameliorates inflammation, injury and sepsis-associated mortality; thereby provide a potential therapeutic approach for the prevention of ALI in sepsis [83].

5. Burn Injuries

Burn injuries represent one of the most widespread and devastating forms of trauma and are ranked among the leading causes of morbidity and mortality worldwide with one of the highest burn death rates [84–86]. H_2S has recently been shown to act as a critical mediator of severe burn injury-induced inflammation in mice [87]. The result in this study show that burn injury in mice subjected to 25% total body surface area full thickness burn augmented significant increase in plasma H_2S levels, liver, and lung CSE mRNA expression, and liver H_2S synthesizing activity. Furthermore, the enhanced H_2S/CSE pathway correlates with heightened burn-associated systemic inflammation, as evidenced biochemically and histologically by increased MPO activity and worsened histological changes in the lung and liver. Importantly, the development of systemic inflammation and multiple organ damage were mitigated when endogenous H_2S synthesis was blocked by prophylactic or therapeutic treatment of PAG, along with attenuation of plasma H_2S levels, liver, and lung CSE mRNA expression, and liver CSE synthesizing activity. Administration of NaHS at the same time of burn injury resulted in a further rise in MPO activity and more severe tissue injury in the lung and liver. Collectively, these findings have shown for the first time the role of H_2S in contributing to exaggerated inflammatory damage after burn injury [87]. The mechanism by which H_2S contributes to inflammation remains to be investigated, although, in light of the role of substance P in inflammation in burn injuries [88–90], a potential contribution of substance P in H_2S-induced inflammation in burns is highly likely.

6. Joint Inflammation

Joint inflammation, that clinically manifests as arthritis, is a major health problem worldwide [91–94]. The possible role of endogenous H_2S in the development of joint inflammation has recently been investigated. In these studies, edema was induced by carrageenan in rodent hindpaws. An increase in H_2S synthesis in inflamed hindpaws was seen, suggesting a localized overproduction of H_2S during inflammation [95]. Pretreatment with PAG resulted in a dose dependent inhibition of hindpaw edema as well as hindpaw MPO activity. These findings suggest that H_2S is an endogenous mediator of the development of hindpaw local inflammation. This and other studies, however, have been done in experimental animal models of disease or in cell lines and their clinical relevance remains unclear. Recent reports in the literature, albeit with conflicting results, point to a role of H_2S in rheumatoid arthritis [96, 97]. One of these studies [96] confirmed the pro-inflammatory action of H_2S in rheumatoid arthritis, whereas the other [97] suggested an anti-inflammatory effect.

7. Chronic Obstructive Pulmonary Disease (COPD)

In addition to its role in acute inflammatory diseases, a H_2S appears to be an important mediator in chronic inflammatory disease as well. Chronic obstructive pulmonary disease (COPD) is a common clinical condition characterized by progressive airflow obstruction that is only partly reversible, inflammation in the airways, and systemic effects or comorbities. The main cause is smoking tobacco, but other factors have been identified [98]. Serum H_2S levels were significantly increased in patients with stable COPD as compared to age matched control subjects or those with acute exacerbation of COPD (AECOPD) [99]. Serum H_2S levels were negatively correlated with the severity of airway obstruction in patients with stable COPD whereas they were positively correlated with the lung function in all patients with COPD and healthy controls. Patients with AECOPD and increased pulmonary artery pressure (PASP) had lower levels of H_2S than those with normal PASP, suggesting a negative relation between H_2S and PASP in AECOPD patients. Interestingly, they also found that serum H_2S levels were lower in smokers than non-smokers regardless of their health status (COPD or healthy controls). In addition, patients with AECOPD, whose serum H_2S levels were decreased, had greater neutrophil proportion but lower lymphocyte proportion in sputum than patients with stable COPD, suggesting a potential role of H_2S in regulating inflammatory response at different types or stages of COPD. This study [99] demonstrated that endogenous H_2S may participate in the development of airway obstruction in COPD and that the level of endogenous H_2S may be correlated with the progression and severity of COPD.

8. H_2S-Releasing Non-Steroidal Anti-Inflammatory Drugs (NSAIDs) and Slow H_2S-Releasing Drugs: An Anti-Inflammatory Action of H_2S?

S-diclofenac (ACS 15) is H_2S-releasing diclofenac, which comprises a H_2S-releasing dithiol-thione moiety attached by an ester linkage to diclofenac. We have investigated [100] the effect of treatment with the NSAID diclofenac and its H_2S-releasing derivative ACS15 on caerulein-induced acute pancreatitis and the associated lung injury. Although these two drugs did not have any significant effect on the local pancreatic injury in acute pancreatitis, ACS15 afforded significant protection against acute pancreatitis-associated lung injury. The protective action of this drug was apparent when administered either prophylactically or as a therapeutic treatment. ACS15 significantly attenuated the rise in lung MPO activity in severe acute pancreatitis. In addition, histological evidence showed significant protection against acute pancreatitis-associated lung injury [100]. ACS 15 also more effectively inhibited hindpaw swelling and neutrophil infiltration after carrageenan injection as compared to its parent NSAID [101]. Furthermore, in a rat model of LPS-induced endotoxemia, ACS 15 exhibited enhanced anti-inflammatory effect as compared to the parent drug [102]. Although these results suggest the potential for the use of controlled release H_2S donor compounds against inflammation (and some literature may mistakenly suggest this), the protective action of ACS 15 in LPS-induced endotoxemia was associated with an inhibition of endogenous H_2S synthesis [102]. Therefore, protective actions of H_2S releasing compounds may be caused by an inhibition of endogenous H_2S formation, possibly by a negative feedback mechanism caused by very low local levels of H_2S. These results, therefore, further reinforce the pro-inflammatory action of endogenous H_2S. Another H_2S-releasing drug is S-propargyl-cysteine (SPRC), a structural analog of S-allyl cysteine (SAC) with a common cysteine-containing structure [103]. SPRC has been shown to have a good safety profile and cardioprotective action and has been reported to show protective effects against myocardial infarctions in both adult rat hearts and neonatal cardiomyocytes through H_2S pathway [98–102]. Another slow H_2S releasing compound is GYY4137 (morpholin-4-ium-4-methoxyphenyl(morpholino)phosphinodithioate), which has been reported to have antihypertensive and anti-inflammatory action [104–106]. In a recent study, SPRC 10 mg/kg injected 3 h prior to induction of acute pancreatitis ameliorated the disease by reducing the inflammatory cell infiltration in pancreas and lung and by modulating pro- and anti-inflammatory cytokine profile in plasma. Results showed that pancreatic injury, as evidenced by plasma amylase, pancreatic MPO and histology, and pulmonary injury, as evidenced by lung MPO and histology were significantly ameliorated in the mice treated with SPRC 3 h prior to the induction of pancreatitis. Prolonged increase in MPO activity is reported to indicate continued neutrophil activation, with the liberation of cytokines and other biologically active substances like reactive oxygen species. We observed a significant reduction in the pro-inflammatory cytokines (IL-1β and IL-6) in pancreas and lung of mice treated with SPRC 3 h before the induction of AP compared to the mice pretreated with vehicle. Furthermore, pancreatic and pulmonary anti-inflammatory cytokine interleukin-10 (IL-10) levels were significantly increased in mice pretreated with SPRC compared to vehicle treated group. Thus SPRC provides a valuable lead for the treatment of acute pancreatitis [107]. It could be postulated that the beneficial effects of SPRC in AP could be by virtue of its slow release of endogenous H_2S and a possible negative feedback mechanism on CSE.

In some studies, endogenous production and exogenous administration of H_2S has also been reported to be anti-inflammatory in many models of pathologies including asthma [108], synovitis [109], LPS induced inflammation [110], rhinitis [111], ischemia reperfusion [112], neuropathologies [113], and gastric pathologies [114, 115]. The mechanisms of hydrogen sulfide's anti-inflammatory properties are still to be elucidated and may be more indirect than the pro-inflammatory effects, and may occur primarily with administration of lower concentrations and/or slow releasing compounds. Other possible mechanisms include hypothermia and tissue protection [23].

9. The Way Forward

In recent years, substantial basic science research has led to a reasonably clear understanding of the role of H_2S as an inflammatory mediator. Several gaps in knowledge, however, remain. Firstly, a lot of the data on H_2S in inflammation has been generated using inhibitors of H_2S synthesis, such as PAG. While undoubtedly very useful pharmacological tools in a new but rapidly expanding research field, it is unlikely that compounds such as PAG are entirely specific since they target the pyridoxal phosphate binding site of CSE and CBS and other PLP-dependent and -independent enzymes [116–121]. Therefore, there is need to develop inhibitors of H_2S synthesis, which are more selective and have a better safety profile than the ones that are currently available. Approaches using CSE knockout mice [122] would enable further define the role of H_2S in inflammation. Also, clinical studies examining the significance of H_2S in clinical inflammatory conditions are scarce. Despite it being in its infancy stage, early results in this direction have been rather promising and allow us to consider the clinical potential of developing drugs that interfere with H_2S production. Indeed, efforts are underway to determine the therapeutic potential of targeting H_2S in treatment of inflammatory pathologies. Nevertheless, our understanding of the molecular mechanisms by which H_2S contributes to inflammation is still fragmentary. Active research in this direction will lead to further insights into the development of new therapeutic intervention for inflammatory conditions, and most importantly, to facilitate transition of our knowledge from the laboratory to the clinic.

Abbreviations

H_2S: Hydrogen sulfide;
CBS: Cystathionine-β-synthase;
CSE: Cystathionine-γ-lyase;
CAT: Cysteine aminotransferase;
MPST: 3-Mercaptopyruvate sulfurtransferase;
NO: Nitric oxide;
PKC: Protein kinase C;
NADPH: Nicotinamide adenine dinucleotide phosphate;
NaHS: Sodium hydrosulfide;
MAPK: Mitogen-activated protein kinase;
SIRS: Systemic inflammatory response syndrome;
PAG: DL-propargylglycine;
MPO: Myeloperoxidase;
NH_3: Ammonia;
AOA: Aminooxyacetate;
MCP: Monocyte chemoatractant protein;
MIP: Macrophage inflammatory protein;
ICAM: Intercellular adhesion molecule;
NF: Nuclear factor;
SFK: Src-family kinases;
TNF: Tumor necrosis factor;
IL: Interleukin;
PPT: Preprotachykinin;
NK-1R: Neurokinin-1 receptor;
CGRP: Calcitonin gene related peptide;
TRPV-1: Transient receptor potential vanilloid-1;
ERK: Extracellular signal related kinase;
TLR4: Toll-like receptor 4;

COX-2: Cyclooxygenase-2;
PGEM: Prostaglandin E metabolite;
COPD: Chronic obstructive pulmonary disease;
AECOPD: Acute exacerbation of COPD;
PASP: Pulmonary artery pressure;
NSAIDs: Non-steroidal anti-inflammatory drugs;
SAC: S-allyl cysteine
SPRC: S-propargyl-cysteine;
CLP: Cecal ligation and puncture.

Acknowledgments

The author's laboratory is supported by Research Grants from the Lottery Health, Arthritis New Zealand, and University of Otago (Establishment Grant and University of Otago Research Grant).

References

[1] US National Research Council, Subcommittee on Hydrogen Sulfide, Division of Medical Sciences. Hydrogen Sulfide. University Park Press, Baltimore Md, USA, 1979.

[2] M. Bhatia, "Hydrogen sulfide and substance P in inflammation," *Antioxidants and Redox Signaling*, vol. 12, no. 10, pp. 1191–1202, 2010.

[3] L. Li, A. Hsu, and P. K. Moore, "Actions and interactions of nitric oxide, carbon monoxide and hydrogen sulphide in the cardiovascular system and in inflammation—a tale of three gases!," *Pharmacology and Therapeutics*, vol. 123, no. 3, pp. 386–400, 2009.

[4] P. K. Moore, M. Bhatia, and S. Moochhala, "Hydrogen sulfide: from the smell of the past to the mediator of the future?" *Trends in Pharmacological Sciences*, vol. 24, no. 12, pp. 609–611, 2003.

[5] M. Bhatia, "Hydrogen sulfide as a vasodilator," *IUBMB Life*, vol. 57, no. 9, pp. 603–606, 2005.

[6] W. Zhao, J. Zhang, Y. Lu, and R. Wang, "The vasorelaxant effect of H_2S as a novel endogenous gaseous KATP channel opener," *EMBO Journal*, vol. 20, no. 21, pp. 6008–6016, 2001.

[7] K. Abe and H. Kimura, "The possible role of hydrogen sulfide as an endogenous neuromodulator," *Journal of Neuroscience*, vol. 16, no. 3, pp. 1066–1071, 1996.

[8] M. Whiteman, L. Li, I. Kostetski et al., "Evidence for the formation of a novel nitrosothiol from the gaseous mediators nitric oxide and hydrogen sulphide," *Biochemical and Biophysical Research Communications*, vol. 343, no. 1, pp. 303–310, 2006.

[9] M. Y. Ali, C. Y. Ping, Y. Y. P. Mok et al., "Regulation of vascular nitric oxide in vitro and in vivo; a new role for endogenous hydrogen sulphide?" *British Journal of Pharmacology*, vol. 149, no. 6, pp. 625–634, 2006.

[10] T. M. Hildebrandt and M. K. Grieshaber, "Three enzymatic activities catalyze the oxidation of sulfide to thiosulfate in mammalian and invertebrate mitochondria," *FEBS Journal*, vol. 275, no. 13, pp. 3352–3361, 2008.

[11] M. Goubern, M. Andriamihaja, T. Nübel, F. Blachier, and F. Bouillaud, "Sulfide, the first inorganic substrate for human cells," *FASEB Journal*, vol. 21, no. 8, pp. 1699–1706, 2007.

[12] M. D. Levitt, J. Furne, J. Springfield, F. Suarez, and E. DeMaster, "Detoxification of hydrogen sulfide and methanethiol in the cecal mucosa," *Journal of Clinical Investigation*, vol. 104, no. 8, pp. 1107–1114, 1999.

[13] R. O. Beauchamp Jr., J. S. Bus, and J. A. Popp, "A critical review of the literature on hydrogen sulfide toxicity," *Critical Reviews in Toxicology*, vol. 13, no. 1, pp. 25–97, 1984.

[14] R. P. Smith and R. A. Abbanat, "Protective effect of oxidized glutathione in acute sulfide poisoning," *Toxicology and Applied Pharmacology*, vol. 9, no. 2, pp. 209–217, 1966.

[15] H. Mitsuhashi, S. Yamashita, H. Ikeuchi et al., "Oxidative stress-dependent conversion of hydrogen sulfide to sulfite by activated neutrophils," *Shock*, vol. 24, no. 6, pp. 529–534, 2005.

[16] M. Whiteman, J. S. Armstrong, S. H. Chu et al., "The novel neuromodulator hydrogen sulfide: an endogenous peroxynitrite "scavenger"?" *Journal of Neurochemistry*, vol. 90, no. 3, pp. 765–768, 2004.

[17] M. Whiteman, N. S. Cheung, Y. Z. Zhu et al., "Hydrogen sulphide: a novel inhibitor of hypochlorous acid-mediated oxidative damage in the brain?" *Biochemical and Biophysical Research Communications*, vol. 326, no. 4, pp. 794–798, 2005.

[18] L. Chang, B. Geng, F. Yu et al., "Hydrogen sulfide inhibits myocardial injury induced by homocysteine in rats," *Amino Acids*, vol. 34, no. 4, pp. 573–585, 2008.

[19] B. Geng, J. Yang, Y. Qi et al., "H_2S generated by heart in rat and its effects on cardiac function," *Biochemical and Biophysical Research Communications*, vol. 313, no. 2, pp. 362–368, 2004.

[20] B. Mazumder, X. Li, and S. Barik, "Translation control: a multifaceted regulator of inflammatory response," *Journal of Immunology*, vol. 184, no. 7, pp. 3311–3319, 2010.

[21] C. Nathan, "Points of control in inflammation," *Nature*, vol. 420, no. 6917, pp. 846–852, 2002.

[22] A. Hegde and M. Bhatia, "Hydrogen sulfide in inflammation: friend or foe?" *Inflammation and Allergy*, vol. 10, no. 2, pp. 118–122, 2011.

[23] J. R. Rivers, A. Badiei, and M. Bhatia, "Hydrogen sulfide as a therapeutic target for inflammation," *Expert Opinion on Therapeutic Targets*, vol. 16, no. 5, pp. 439–449, 2012.

[24] M. Bhatia and S. Moochhala, "Role of inflammatory mediators in the pathophysiology of acute respiratory distress syndrome," *Journal of Pathology*, vol. 202, no. 2, pp. 145–156, 2004.

[25] C. Ratthe, M. Pelletier, C. J. Roberge, and D. Girard, "Activation of human neutrophils by the pollutant sodium sulfite: effect on cytokine production, chemotaxis, and cell surface expression of cell adhesion molecules," *Cellular Immunology*, vol. 105, no. 2, pp. 169–175, 2002.

[26] I. Beck-Speier, J. G. Liese, B. H. Belohradsky, and J. J. Godleski, "Sulfite stimulates NADPH oxidase of human neutrophils to produce active oxygen radicals via protein kinase C and Ca2+/calmodulin pathways," *Free Radical Biology and Medicine*, vol. 14, no. 6, pp. 661–668, 1993.

[27] T. Shigehara, H. Mitsuhashi, F. Ota et al., "Sulfite induces adherence of polymorphonuclear neutrophils to immobilized fibrinogen through activation of Mac-1 β2-integrin (CD11b/CD18)," *Life Sciences*, vol. 70, no. 19, pp. 2225–2232, 2002.

[28] L. Rinaldi, G. Gobbi, M. Pambianco, C. Micheloni, P. Mirandola, and M. Vitale, "Hydrogen sulfide prevents apoptosis of human PMN via inhibition of p38 and caspase 3," *Laboratory Investigation*, vol. 86, no. 4, pp. 391–397, 2006.

[29] M. Bhatia, F. L. Wong, Y. Cao et al., "Pathophysiology of acute pancreatitis," *Pancreatology*, vol. 5, no. 2-3, pp. 132–144, 2005.

[30] M. Bhatia, M. Brady, S. Shokuhi et al., "Inflammatory mediators in acute pancreatitis," *Journal of Pathology*, vol. 190, no. 2, pp. 117–125, 2000.

[31] M. Bhatia, "Acute pancreatitis as a model of SIRS," *Frontiers in Bioscience*, vol. 14, no. 6, pp. 2042–2050, 2009.

[32] M. Bhatia, "Novel therapeutic targets for acute pancreatitis and associated multiple organ dysfunction syndrome," *Current Drug Targets*, vol. 1, no. 4, pp. 343–351, 2002.

[33] M. Bhatia, J. P. Neoptolemos, and J. Slavin, "Inflammatory mediators as therapeutic targets in acute pancreatitis," *Current Opinion in Investigational Drugs*, vol. 2, no. 4, pp. 496–501, 2001.

[34] M. Bhatia, F. L. Wong, D. Fu, H. Y. Lau, S. M. Moochhala, and P. K. Moore, "Role of hydrogen sulfide in acute pancreatitis and associated lung injury," *FASEB Journal*, vol. 19, no. 6, pp. 623–625, 2005.

[35] M. Kumaraswamy, Z. Jing, and M. Bhatia, "Aminooxyacetate inhibits hydrogen sulfide and ammonium synthesis and protects mice in acute pancreatitis," *International Journal of Integrative Biology*, vol. 8, no. 1, pp. 7–14, 2009.

[36] R. Tamizhselvi, P. K. Moore, and M. Bhatia, "Hydrogen sulfide acts as a mediator of inflammation inacute pancreatitis: in vitro studies using isolated mouse pancreatic acinar cells," *Journal of Cellular and Molecular Medicine*, vol. 11, no. 2, pp. 315–326, 2007.

[37] R. Tamizhselvi, P. K. Moore, and M. Bhatia, "Inhibition of hydrogen sulfide synthesis attenuates chemokine production and protects mice against acute pancreatitis and associated lung injury," *Pancreas*, vol. 36, no. 4, pp. e24–e31, 2008.

[38] R. Tamizhselvi, Y. H. Koh, J. Sun, H. Zhang, and M. Bhatia, "Hydrogen sulfide induces ICAM-1 expression and neutrophil adhesion to caerulein-treated pancreatic acinar cells through NF-κB and Src-family kinases pathway," *Experimental Cell Research*, vol. 316, no. 9, pp. 1625–1636, 2010.

[39] R. Tamizhselvi, J. Sun, Y. H. Koh, and M. Bhatia, "Effect of hydrogen sulfide on the phosphatidylinositol 3-kinase-protein kinase B pathway and on caerulein-induced cytokine production in isolated mouse pancreatic acinar cells," *Journal of Pharmacology and Experimental Therapeutics*, vol. 329, no. 3, pp. 1166–1177, 2009.

[40] M. Bhatia, L. Zhi, H. Zhang, S. W. Ng, and P. K. Moore, "Role of substance P in hydrogen sulfide-induced pulmonary inflammation in mice," *American Journal of Physiology*, vol. 291, no. 5, pp. L896–L904, 2006.

[41] M. Bhatia, A. K. Saluja, B. Hofbauer et al., "Role of substance P and the neurokinin 1 receptor in acute pancreatitis and pancreatitis-associated lung injury," *Proceedings of the National Academy of Sciences of the United States of America*, vol. 95, no. 8, pp. 4760–4765, 1998.

[42] M. Bhatia, J. Slavin, Y. Cao, A. I. Basbaum, and J. P. Neoptolemos, "Preprotachykinin-A gene deletion protects mice against acute pancreatitis and associated lung injury," *American Journal of Physiology*, vol. 284, no. 5, pp. G830–G836, 2003.

[43] H. Y. Lau, F. L. Wong, and M. Bhatia, "A key role of neurokinin 1 receptors in acute pancreatitis and associated lung injury," *Biochemical and Biophysical Research Communications*, vol. 327, no. 2, pp. 509–515, 2005.

[44] J. Sun and M. Bhatia, "Blockade of neurokinin-1 receptor attenuates CC and CXC chemokine production in experimental acute pancreatitis and associated lung injury," *American Journal of Physiology*, vol. 292, no. 1, pp. G143–G153, 2007.

[45] H. Y. Lau and M. Bhatia, "The effect of CP96,345 on the expression of tachykinins and neurokinin receptors in acute pancreatitis," *Journal of Pathology*, vol. 208, no. 3, pp. 364–371, 2006.

[46] H. Y. Lau and M. Bhatia, "Effect of CP-96,345 on the expression of adhesion molecules in acute pancreatitis in mice," *American Journal of Physiology*, vol. 292, no. 5, pp. G1283–G1292, 2007.

[47] Y. H. Koh, S. Moochhala, and M. Bhatia, "The role of neutral endopeptidase in caerulein-induced acute pancreatitis," *Journal of Immunology*, vol. 187, no. 10, pp. 5429–5439, 2011.

[48] E. F. Grady, S. K. Yoshimi, J. Maa et al., "Substance P mediates inflammatory oedema in acute pancreatitis via activation of the neurokinin-1 receptor in rats and mice," *British Journal of Pharmacology*, vol. 130, no. 3, pp. 505–512, 2000.

[49] J. Maa, E. F. Grady, S. K. Yoshimi et al., "Subtance P is a determinant of lethality in diet-induced hemorrhagic pancreatitis in mice," *Surgery*, vol. 128, no. 2, pp. 232–239, 2000.

[50] Z. J. He, J. H. Winston, T. E. Yusuf et al., "Intraductal administration of an NK1 receptor antagonist attenuates the inflammatory response to retrograde infusion of radiological contrast in rats: implications for the pathogenesis and prevention of ERCP-induced pancreatitis," *Pancreas*, vol. 27, no. 1, pp. e13–e17, 2003.

[51] R. D. Ramnath and M. Bhatia, "Substance P treatment stimulates chemokine synthesis in pancreatic acinar cells via the activation of NF-κB," *American Journal of Physiology*, vol. 291, no. 6, pp. G1113–G1119, 2006.

[52] R. D. Ramnath, J. Sun, S. Adhikari, L. Zhi, and M. Bhatia, "Role of PKC-δ on substance P-induced chemokine synthesis in pancreatic acinar cells," *American Journal of Physiology*, vol. 294, no. 3, pp. C683–C692, 2008.

[53] R. D. Ramnath, J. Sun, S. Adhikari, and M. Bhatia, "Effect of mitogen-activated protein kinases on chemokine synthesis induced by substance P in mouse pancreatic acinar cells," *Journal of Cellular and Molecular Medicine*, vol. 11, no. 6, pp. 1326–1341, 2007.

[54] R. D. Ramnath, J. Sun, and M. Bhatia, "Role of calcium in substance P-induced chemokine synthesis in mouse pancreatic acinar cells," *British Journal of Pharmacology*, vol. 154, no. 6, pp. 1339–1348, 2008.

[55] R. D. Ramnath, J. Sun, and M. Bhatia, "Involvement of SRC family kinases in substance P-induced chemokine production in mouse pancreatic acinar cells and its significance in acute pancreatitis," *Journal of Pharmacology and Experimental Therapeutics*, vol. 329, no. 2, pp. 418–428, 2009.

[56] R. D. Ramnath, J. Sun, and M. Bhatia, "PKC δ mediates pro-inflammatory responses in a mouse model of caerulein-induced acute pancreatitis," *Journal of Molecular Medicine*, vol. 88, no. 10, pp. 1055–1063, 2010.

[57] J. Sun, R. D. Ramnath, and M. Bhatia, "Neuropeptide substance P upregulates chemokine and chemokine receptor expression in primary mouse neutrophils," *American Journal of Physiology*, vol. 293, no. 2, pp. C696–C704, 2007.

[58] J. Sun, R. D. Ramnath, L. Zhi, R. Tamizhselvi, and M. Bhatia, "Substance P enhances NF-κB transactivation and chemokine response in murine macrophages via ERK1/2 and p38 MAPK signaling pathways," *American Journal of Physiology*, vol. 294, no. 6, pp. C1586–C1596, 2008.

[59] J. Sun, R. D. Ramnath, R. Tamizhselvi, and M. Bhatia, "Neurokinin A engages neurokinin-1 receptor to induce NF-κB-dependent gene expression in murine macrophages: implications of ERK1/2 and PI 3-kinase/Akt pathways," *American Journal of Physiology*, vol. 295, no. 3, pp. C679–C691, 2008.

[60] J. Sun, R. D. Ramnath, R. Tamizhselvi, and M. Bhatia, "Role of protein kinase C and phosphoinositide 3-kinase-Akt in

substance P-induced proinflammatory pathways in mouse macrophages," *FASEB Journal*, vol. 23, no. 4, pp. 997–1010, 2009.

[61] M. Bhatia, J. N. Sidhapuriwala, S. Wei Ng, R. Tamizhselvi, and S. M. Moochhala, "Pro-inflammatory effects of hydrogen sulphide on substance P in caerulein-induced acute pancreatitis," *Journal of Cellular and Molecular Medicine*, vol. 12, no. 2, pp. 580–590, 2008.

[62] R. Tamizhselvi, P. Shrivastava, Y. H. Koh, H. Zhang, and M. Bhatia, "Preprotachykinin-A gene deletion regulates hydrogen sulfide-induced Toll-like receptor 4 signaling pathway in cerulein-treated pancreatic acinar cells," *Pancreas*, vol. 40, no. 3, pp. 444–452, 2011.

[63] R. Devi Ramnath, S. Weing, M. He et al., "Inflammatory mediators in sepsis: cytokines, chemokines, adhesion molecules and gases," *Journal of Organ Dysfunction*, vol. 2, no. 2, pp. 80–92, 2006.

[64] G. S. Martin, D. M. Mannino, S. Eaton, and M. Moss, "The epidemiology of sepsis in the United States from 1979 through 2000," *New England Journal of Medicine*, vol. 348, no. 16, pp. 1546–1554, 2003.

[65] M. M. Levy, R. P. Dellinger, S. R. Townsend et al., "The surviving sepsis campaign: results of an international guideline-based performance improvement program targeting severe sepsis," *Critical Care Medicine*, vol. 38, no. 2, pp. 367–374, 2010.

[66] M. Bhatia, M. He, H. Zhang, and S. Moochhala, "Sepsis as a model of SIRS," *Frontiers in Bioscience*, vol. 14, no. 12, pp. 4703–4711, 2009.

[67] H. Zhang, L. Zhi, P. K. Moore, and M. Bhatia, "Role of hydrogen sulfide in cecal ligation and puncture-induced sepsis in the mouse," *American Journal of Physiology*, vol. 290, no. 6, pp. L1193–L1201, 2006.

[68] H. Zhang, L. Zhi, S. Moochhala, P. K. Moore, and M. Bhatia, "Hydrogen sulfide acts as an inflammatory mediator in cecal ligation and puncture-induced sepsis in mice by upregulating the production of cytokines and chemokines via NF-κB," *American Journal of Physiology*, vol. 292, no. 4, pp. L960–L971, 2007.

[69] H. Zhang, L. Zhi, S. M. Moochhala, P. K. Moore, and M. Bhatia, "Endogenous hydrogen sulfide regulates leukocyte trafficking in cecal ligation and puncture-induced sepsis," *Journal of Leukocyte Biology*, vol. 82, no. 4, pp. 894–905, 2007.

[70] H. Zhang, S. M. Moochhala, and M. Bhatia, "Endogenous hydrogen sulfide regulates inflammatory response by activating the ERK pathway in polymicrobial sepsis," *Journal of Immunology*, vol. 181, no. 6, pp. 4320–4331, 2008.

[71] L. Zhi, A. D. Ang, H. Zhang, P. K. Moore, and M. Bhatia, "Hydrogen sulfide induces the synthesis of proinflammatory cytokines in human monocyte cell line U937 via the ERK-NF-κB pathway," *Journal of Leukocyte Biology*, vol. 81, no. 5, pp. 1322–1332, 2007.

[72] L. Li, M. Bhatia, Y. Z. Zhu et al., "Hydrogen sulfide is a novel mediator of lipopolysaccharide-induced inflammation in the mouse," *FASEB Journal*, vol. 19, no. 9, pp. 1196–1198, 2005.

[73] M. Collin, F. B. M. Anuar, O. Murch, M. Bhatia, P. K. Moore, and C. Thiemermann, "Inhibition of endogenous hydrogen sulfide formation reduces the organ injury caused by endotoxemia," *British Journal of Pharmacology*, vol. 146, no. 4, pp. 498–505, 2005.

[74] P. Puneet, A. Hegde, S. W. Ng et al., "Preprotachykinin-A gene products are key mediators of lung injury in polymicrobial sepsis," *Journal of Immunology*, vol. 176, no. 6, pp. 3813–3820, 2006.

[75] A. Hegde, H. Zhang, S. M. Moochhala, and M. Bhatia, "Neurokinin-1 receptor antagonist treatment protects mice against lung injury in polymicrobial sepsis," *Journal of Leukocyte Biology*, vol. 82, no. 3, pp. 678–685, 2007.

[76] W. N. Siaw, H. Zhang, A. Hegde, and M. Bhatia, "Role of preprotachykinin-A gene products on multiple organ injury in LPS-induced endotoxemia," *Journal of Leukocyte Biology*, vol. 83, no. 2, pp. 288–295, 2008.

[77] A. Hegde, M. Uttamchandani, S. M. Moochhala, and M. Bhatia, "Plasma cytokine profiles in Preprotachykinin-A knockout mice subjected to polymicrobial sepsis," *Molecular Medicine*, vol. 16, no. 1-2, pp. 45–52, 2010.

[78] A. Hegde, R. Tamizhselvi, J. Manikandan, A. J. Melendez, S. M. Moochhala, and M. Bhatia, "Substance P in polymicrobial sepsis: molecular fingerprint of lung injury in preprotachykinin-A-/- mice," *Molecular Medicine*, vol. 16, no. 5-6, pp. 188–198, 2010.

[79] A. Hegde, Y. H. Koh, S. M. Moochhala, and M. Bhatia, "Neurokinin-1 receptor antagonist treatment in polymicrobial sepsis: molecular insights," *International Journal of Inflammation*, vol. 2010, Article ID 601098, 10 pages, 2010.

[80] H. Zhang, A. Hegde, W. N. Siaw, S. Adhikari, S. M. Moochhala, and M. Bhatia, "Hydrogen sulfide up-regulates substance P in polymicrobial sepsis-associated lung injury," *Journal of Immunology*, vol. 179, no. 6, pp. 4153–4160, 2007.

[81] S. F. Ang, S. M. Moochhala, and M. Bhatia, "Hydrogen sulfide promotes transient receptor potential vanilloid 1-mediated neurogenic inflammation in polymicrobial sepsis," *Critical Care Medicine*, vol. 38, no. 2, pp. 619–628, 2010.

[82] S. F. Ang, S. M. Moochhala, P. A. MacAry et al., "Hydrogen sulfide and neurogenic inflammation in polymicrobial sepsis: involvement of substance P and ERK-NF-κB signaling," *PLoS ONE*, vol. 6, no. 9, Article ID e24535, 2011.

[83] S. F. Ang, S. W. Sio, S. M. Moochhala et al., "Hydrogen sulfide upregulates cyclooxygenase-2 and prostaglandin E metabolite in sepsis-evoked acute lung injury via transient receptor potential vanilloid type 1 channel activation," *Journal of Immunology*, vol. 187, no. 9, pp. 4778–4787, 2011.

[84] D. Church, S. Elsayed, O. Reid, B. Winston, and R. Lindsay, "Burn wound infections," *Clinical Microbiology Reviews*, vol. 19, no. 2, pp. 403–434, 2006.

[85] S. Hettiaratchy and P. Dziewulski, "ABC of burns: pathophysiology and types of burns," *British Medical Journal*, vol. 328, no. 7453, pp. 1427–1429, 2004.

[86] F. W. Endorf and D. Ahrenholz, "Burn management," *Current Opinion in Critical Care*, vol. 17, no. 6, pp. 601–605, 2011.

[87] J. Zhang, S. W. S. Sio, S. Moochhala, and M. Bhatia, "Role of hydrogen sulfide in severe burn injury-induced inflammation in mice," *Molecular Medicine*, vol. 16, no. 9-10, pp. 417–424, 2010.

[88] S. W. S. Sio, M. K. Puthia, J. Lu, S. Moochhala, and M. Bhatia, "The neuropeptide substance P is a critical mediator of burn-induced acute lung injury," *Journal of Immunology*, vol. 180, no. 12, pp. 8333–8341, 2008.

[89] S. W. S. Sio, S. Moochhala, J. Lu, and M. Bhatia, "Early protection from burn-induced acute lung injury by deletion of preprotachykinin-A gene," *American Journal of Respiratory and Critical Care Medicine*, vol. 181, no. 1, pp. 36–46, 2010.

[90] S. W. S. Sio, S. F. Ang, J. Lu, S. Moochhala, and M. Bhatia, "Substance p upregulates cyclooxygenase-2 and prostaglandin

E metabolite by activating ERK1/2 and NF-κB in a mouse model of burn-induced remote Acute lung injury," *Journal of Immunology*, vol. 185, no. 10, pp. 6265–6276, 2010.

[91] M. J. Plant, P. W. Jones, J. Saklatvala, W. E. R. Ollier, and P. T. Dawes, "Patterns of radiological progression in early rheumatoid arthritis: results of an 8 year prospective study," *Journal of Rheumatology*, vol. 25, no. 3, pp. 417–426, 1998.

[92] D. Symmons, G. Turner, R. Webb et al., "The prevalence of rheumatoid arthritis in the United Kingdom: new estimates for a new century," *Rheumatology*, vol. 41, no. 7, pp. 793–800, 2002.

[93] D. L. Scott, D. A. Willoughby, and D. R. Blake, "Molecular insights into rheumatoid arthritis," *Molecular Aspects of Medicine*, vol. 12, no. 5, pp. 341–394, 1991.

[94] D. M. F. M. Van der Heijde, "Joint erosions and patients with early rheumatoid arthritis," *British Journal of Rheumatology*, vol. 34, no. 2, pp. 74–78, 1995.

[95] M. Bhatia, J. Sidhapuriwala, S. M. Moochhala, and P. K. Moore, "Hydrogen sulphide is a mediator of carrageenan-induced hindpaw oedema in the rat," *British Journal of Pharmacology*, vol. 145, no. 2, pp. 141–144, 2005.

[96] B. Kloesch, M. Liszt, D. Krehan et al., "High concentrations of hydrogen sulphide elevate the expression of a series of pro-inflammatory genes in fibroblast-like synoviocytes derived from rheumatoid and osteoarthritis patients," *Immunology Letters*, vol. 141, no. 2, pp. 197–203, 2012.

[97] B. Fox, J. T. Schantz, R. Haigh et al., "Inducible hydrogen sulfide synthesis in chondrocytes and mesenchymal progenitor cells: is H_2S a novel cytoprotective mediator in the inflamed joint?" *Journal of Cellular and Molecular Medicine*, vol. 16, no. 4, pp. 896–910, 2012.

[98] M. Decramer, W. Janssens, and M. Miravitlles, "Chronic obstructive pulmonary disease," *Lancet*, vol. 379, no. 9823, pp. 1341–1351, 2012.

[99] Y. H. Chen, W. Z. Yao, B. Geng et al., "Endogenous hydrogen sulfide in patients with COPD," *Chest*, vol. 128, no. 5, pp. 3205–3211, 2005.

[100] M. Bhatia, J. N. Sidhapuriwala, A. Sparatore, and P. K. Moore, "Treatment with H_2S-releasing diclofenac protects mice against acute pancreatitis-associated lung injury," *Shock*, vol. 29, no. 1, pp. 84–88, 2008.

[101] J. Sidhapuriwala, L. Li, A. Sparatore, M. Bhatia, and P. K. Moore, "Effect of S-diclofenac, a novel hydrogen sulfide releasing derivative, on carrageenan-induced hindpaw oedema formation in the rat," *European Journal of Pharmacology*, vol. 569, no. 1-2, pp. 149–154, 2007.

[102] L. Li, G. Rossoni, A. Sparatore, L. C. Lee, P. Del Soldato, and P. K. Moore, "Anti-inflammatory and gastrointestinal effects of a novel diclofenac derivative," *Free Radical Biology and Medicine*, vol. 42, no. 5, pp. 706–719, 2007.

[103] Q. Wang, H. R. Liu, Q. Mu, P. Rose, and Y. Z. Zhu, "S-propargyl-cysteine protects both adult rat hearts and neonatal cardiomyocytes from ischemia/hypoxia injury: the contribution of the hydrogen sulfide-mediated pathway," *Journal of Cardiovascular Pharmacology*, vol. 54, no. 2, pp. 139–146, 2009.

[104] L. Li, M. Whiteman, Y. Y. Guan et al., "Characterization of a novel, water-soluble hydrogen sulfide-releasing molecule (GYY4137): new insights into the biology of hydrogen sulfide," *Circulation*, vol. 117, no. 18, pp. 2351–2360, 2008.

[105] L. Li, M. Salto-Tellez, C. H. Tan, M. Whiteman, and P. K. Moore, "GYY4137, a novel hydrogen sulfide-releasing molecule, protects against endotoxic shock in the rat," *Free Radical Biology and Medicine*, vol. 47, no. 1, pp. 103–113, 2009.

[106] M. Whiteman, L. Li, P. Rose, C. H. Tan, D. B. Parkinson, and P. K. Moore, "The effect of hydrogen sulfide donors on lipopolysaccharide-induced formation of inflammatory mediators in macrophages," *Antioxidants and Redox Signaling*, vol. 12, no. 10, pp. 1147–1154, 2010.

[107] J. N. Sidhapuriwala, A. Hegde, and A. D. Ang, "Effects of S-propargyl-cysteine (SPRC) in caerulein-induced acute pancreatitis in mice," *PLoS ONE*, vol. 7, no. 3, Article ID e32574, 2012.

[108] Y. H. Chen, R. Wu, B. Geng et al., "Endogenous hydrogen sulfide reduces airway inflammation and remodeling in a rat model of asthma," *Cytokine*, vol. 45, no. 2, pp. 117–123, 2009.

[109] E. Ekundi-Valentim, K. T. Santos, E. A. Camargo et al., "Differing effects of exogenous and endogenous hydrogen sulphide in carrageenan-induced knee joint synovitis in the rat: research paper," *British Journal of Pharmacology*, vol. 159, no. 7, pp. 1463–1474, 2010.

[110] L. L. Pan, X. H. Liu, Q. H. Gong, and Y. Z. Zhu, "S-Propargyl-cysteine (SPRC) attenuated lipopolysaccharideinduced inflammatory response in H9c2 cells involved in a hydrogen sulfide-dependent mechanism," *Amino Acids*, vol. 41, no. 1, pp. 205–215, 2011.

[111] S. Kubo, I. Doe, Y. Kurokawa, and A. Kawabata, "Hydrogen sulfide causes relaxation in mouse bronchial smooth muscle," *Journal of Pharmacological Sciences*, vol. 104, no. 4, pp. 392–396, 2007.

[112] N. R. Sodha, R. T. Clements, J. Feng et al., "Hydrogen sulfide therapy attenuates the inflammatory response in a porcine model of myocardial ischemia/reperfusion injury," *Journal of Thoracic and Cardiovascular Surgery*, vol. 138, no. 4, pp. 977–984, 2009.

[113] M. Lee, C. Schwab, S. Yu, E. McGeer, and P. L. McGeer, "Astrocytes produce the antiinflammatory and neuroprotective agent hydrogen sulfide," *Neurobiology of Aging*, vol. 30, no. 10, pp. 1523–1534, 2009.

[114] S. Fiorucci, E. Antonelli, E. Distrutti et al., "Inhibition of hydrogen sulfide generation contributes to gastric injury caused by anti-inflammatory nonsteroidal drugs," *Gastroenterology*, vol. 129, no. 4, pp. 1210–1224, 2005.

[115] I. Hirata, Y. Naito, T. Takagi et al., "Endogenous hydrogen sulfide is an anti-inflammatory molecule in dextran sodium sulfate-induced colitis in mice," *Digestive Diseases and Sciences*, vol. 56, no. 5, pp. 1379–1386, 2011.

[116] Q. Sun, R. Collins, S. Huang et al., "Structural basis for the inhibition mechanism of human cystathionine γ-lyase, an enzyme responsible for the production of H_2S," *Journal of Biological Chemistry*, vol. 284, no. 5, pp. 3076–3085, 2009.

[117] G. Burnett, P. Marcotte, and C. Walsh, "Mechanism-based inactivation of pig heart L-alanine transaminase by L-propargylglycine. Half-site reactivity," *Journal of Biological Chemistry*, vol. 255, no. 8, pp. 3487–3491, 1980.

[118] E. S. Cho, J. Hovanec-Brown, R. J. Tomanek, and L. D. Stegink, "Propargylglycine infusion effects on tissue glutathione levels, plasma amino acid concentrations and tissue morphology in parenterally-fed growing rats," *Journal of Nutrition*, vol. 121, no. 6, pp. 785–794, 1991.

[119] A. Kawaji, K. Yamauchi, S. Fujii, R. Natsuki, E. Takabatake, and Y. Yamaura, "Effects of mushroom toxins on glycogenolysis; comparison of toxicity of phalloidin, α-amanitin and DL-propargylglycine in isolated rat hepatocytes," *Journal of Pharmacobio-Dynamics*, vol. 15, no. 3, pp. 107–112, 1992.

[120] S. Yu, K. Sugahara, K. Nakayama, S. Awata, and H. Kodama, "Accumulation of cystathionine, cystathionine ketimine, and

perhydro-1,4-thiazepine-3,5-dicarboxylic acid in whole brain and various regions of the brain of D,L-propargylglycine-treated rats," *Metabolism*, vol. 49, no. 8, pp. 1025–1029, 2000.

[121] R. Konno, M. Ikeda, K. Yamaguchi, Y. Ueda, and A. Niwa, "Nephrotoxicity of D-propargylglycine in mice," *Archives of Toxicology*, vol. 74, no. 8, pp. 473–479, 2000.

[122] I. Ishii, N. Akahoshi, H. Yamada, S. Nakano, T. Izumi, and M. Suematsu, "Cystathionine γ-lyase-deficient mice require dietary cysteine to protect against acute lethal myopathy and oxidative injury," *Journal of Biological Chemistry*, vol. 285, no. 34, pp. 26358–26368, 2010.

Role of Angiopoietin/Tie2 in Critical Illness: Promising Biomarker, Disease Mediator, and Therapeutic Target?

Alexander Lukasz,[1] Philipp Kümpers,[2] and Sascha David[1]

[1] *Department of Nephrology & Hypertension, Hannover Medical School, Carl-Neuberg Straße 1, 30625 Hannover, Germany*
[2] *Department of Internal Medicine, Rheumatology and Nephrology, University Hospital Münster, 48149 Münster, Germany*

Correspondence should be addressed to Sascha David; david.sascha@mh-hannover.de

Academic Editors: M. A. Choudhry and B. Rippe

Critical illness is a descriptive, broad term for a serious clinical condition that can result from enormously heterogeneous etiologies. A common end feature these patients regularly suffer from is the so-called multiple organ dysfunction syndrome (MODS), often a consequence of organ hypoperfusion and ischemia, coagulopathies, overwhelming inflammatory responses, immune paralysis and mitochondrial dysfunction. Mechanistically, endothelial injury and particularly microvascular leakage is a major step in the pathophysiology of MODS and contributes to its mortality. The angiopoietin (Angpt)/Tie2 system consists of the endothelial tyrosine kinase Tie2 and its 4 circulating ligands (Angpt1-4). The balance between the agonistic ligand "Angpt-1" and the antagonistic one "Angpt-2" regulates baseline endothelial barrier function and its response to injury and is therefore considered a gatekeeper of endothelial activation. This paper provides a systematic overview of the Angpt/Tie2 system with respect to (1) its role as a global biomarker of endothelial activation in critical ill patients, (2) its contribution to MODS pathophysiology as a disease mediator, and last but not least (3) putative therapeutic applications to modify the activation state of Tie2 in mice and men.

1. Introduction

Critical illness is a serious condition that can arise from countless etiologies and that requires highly specialized intensive care units (ICU) for adequate treatment. Among the most common ICU admission reasons are: poisoning, trauma, shock (septic, cardiac, and hemorrhagic), major surgery, respiratory failure, and cardiac ischemia and arrhythmia [1]. One common complication of all these conditions is the so-called multiple organ dysfunction syndrome (MODS) that has a devastating mortality rate [2, 3]. The pathophysiology of MODS is very complex and remains unclear [4, 5]. Hypotheses are multifactorial and range from theories as simple as critical organ hypoperfusion with consequent ischemia to more complex processes as an overwhelming inflammatory response and later immune paralysis [6, 7]. Moreover, the disseminated intravascular coagulopathy (DIC) [8] as well as mitochondrial dysfunction [9] have been demonstrated to play a critical part in the pathogenesis of the syndrome. The repeated failure of clinical trials suggests that some fundamental knowledge is lacking in our current understanding in the development of MODS. A major opportunity, therefore, exists to pursue novel insights into this condition with the hope of improving outcomes.

2. Role of Endothelium

The endothelium pervades every organ and is responsible for a variety of physiological functions [10], such as regulation of oxygen and nutrients transport, blood pressure, coagulation, inflammatory processes, diapedesis, angiogenesis, and volume control between different compartments [11–13]. Despite spatial and temporal heterogeneity in endothelial cell (EC) responses to the noxious stimuli, each of these functions are altered in critical illness [14, 15]. The net result is that the activated endothelium presents a procoagulant, proadhesive surface; fails to produce its usual profile of vasoconstrictive and vasodilatory compounds; and suffers a loss of normal barrier function. Of these changes, increased vascular permeability may be particularly important because it gives rise to hypovolemia and contributes to hemoconcentration, stasis of blood flow, and shock [16, 17]. In every organ, edema basically increases the distance essential nutrients and oxygen must travel to reach their target cells. Thus, systemic vascular changes have severe consequences for organ function.

On the molecular level vascular leakage is determined by a combination of disassembled junctional complexes (e.g., vascular endothelial (VE)-cadherin), and myosin driven cell contraction, resulting in paracellular gap formation [11, 14].

The clinically relevant consequences of this so-called "systemic capillary leakage syndrome" are profound decrease in systemic vascular tone, collapse of the microcirculation, and subsequent distributive shock, acute pulmonary distress syndrome (ARDS), and eventually multiple organ dysfunction syndrome (MODS) [14, 18–20]. Thus, the "activated" endothelium might play a crucial role in the pathophysiology of MODS [14].

3. The Angiopoietin/Tie2 System

In 1996/1997, Davies et al. discovered the angiopoietin (Angpt)/Tie2 ligand-receptor system as the second class of transmembrane vascular-specific receptor tyrosine kinases (the first being the vascular endothelial growth factor (VEGF)/VEGF-receptor system) [21]. Gaining attention as an important regulator in vessel maturation and remodeling, several studies demonstrated that the Angpt-Tie2 system not only regulates angiogenesis, but also controls endothelial inflammation and permeability in a nonredundant manner [22, 23]. Ligation of Angpt-1—secreted by pericytes and vascular smooth muscle cells—to the extracellular fibrinogen-like domain of the Tie2 receptor, which is almost exclusively expressed on endothelial cells (and some monocytes) [24, 25] leads to phosphorylation of the intracellular tyrosine split domain of the receptors that promotes endothelial-cell migration and survival mainly via the canonical phosphatidyl-inositol 3-kinase (PI3 K)/Akt pathway [26]. Furthermore, Angpt-1 signaling strongly activates Rac1 via the IQ motif-containing GTPase activating protein 1 (IQGAP1) [27] thereby shifting the RhoA-Rac1 balance towards Rac1, which morphologically results in a cortical F-actin formation promoting structural integrity of the cytoskeletal architecture [28]. Anti-inflammatory properties of Tie2 signaling are promoted via inhibition of nuclear factor kappa-light-chain-enhancer of activated B cells (NF-kB) mediated expression of leucocyte adhesion molecules expression like intercellular adhesion molecule-1 (ICAM-1) and vascular cell adhesion molecule-1 (VCAM-1) [29]. Hence, Angpt-1 mediated Tie2 phosphorylation has anti-apoptotic, anti-inflammatory and antipermeability effects and maintains a quiescent status quo of the endothelium (Figure 1).

Consistent with the properties of a classical competitive antagonism, Angpt-2 binding to the shared extracellular Tie2 binding domain results in Tie2 dephosphorylation [23]. Data from genetically modified mice underline the hypothesis of functional antagonistic effects of Angpt-1 and Angpt-2 to the Tie2 receptor. Both, Angpt-1-/and Tie2-deficient mice have a lethal phenotype [30, 31]. Consistently, Angpt-2 transgenic mice phenocopy the lethality due to vascular defects like Angpt-1 −/− and Tie2 −/− mice, which suggests that Angpt-2 is indeed a nonredundant antagonistic ligand of Tie2 [32].

Angpt-2 is stored and rapidly released from endothelial vesicles, the Weibel-Palade bodies (WPB), upon different inflammatory stimuli (e.g., TNF-α, LPS, hypoxia) [33]. Angpt-2 sensitizes EC to activation by inflammatory cytokines like TNF-α [34]. In Angpt-2 deficient mice leucocytes cannot attach to the endothelium because of a negative NFkB regulation of leukocyte adhesion molecules, which may result from the vast Angpt-1 signaling [32, 35]. Angpt-2 signaling disrupts the integrity of the endothelial barrier through a RhoA mediated endothelial cell contraction and consequent gap formation [23, 36]. Summarized Angpt-2 signaling activates the endothelial layer from a resting state to a proinflammatory state including expression of leukocyte adhesion molecules and a loss of vascular integrity (Figure 1).

4. Angiopoietin-2 as a Biomarker and Putative Mediator of Endothelial Activation

So far, several groups including our own have investigated circulating Angpt-1 and Angpt-2 levels in critically ill patients. In humans, the balance between both Tie2 ligands appears to be dramatically shifted in favor of Angpt-2, which at least theoretically means that Tie2 receptor signaling is impaired. In sepsis, those Angpt-2 elevations correlate with the severity of illness as assessed by injury severity score [37], organ failure index [38], physiology and chronic health evaluation II (APACHE II) score and sequential organ failure assessment (SOFA) scores [39–44].

It all started in 2006 when Dr. Parikh and his coworkers presented the first clinical and experimental study investigating the role of circulating Angpt-2 in ICU patients. Their investigation was based on previous findings that disrupted Tie2 signaling could arise in the inflammatory milieu of sepsis [45, 46], which might predominantly occur in the lung because of high Tie2 expression levels [47, 48]. Therefore, they hypothesized that excessive Angpt-2 release resulting in a competitive Tie2 antagonism may occur in sepsis and promote pulmonary vascular leakage. Besides quantifying circulating Angpt-2 in enrolled patients with mild and severe sepsis, they tested the effect of human septic serum on the morphology of EC architecture *in vitro*. In fact they found that circulating Angpt-2 was elevated in septic patients and associated with oxygenation failure indicated by a PaO_2/FiO_2 ratio below 200 (defined as ARDS). In contrast to following studies with a larger number of patients Angpt-2 did not correlate with the APACHE II score, although there was a trend to higher Angpt-2 levels in patients with an APACHE II score >25. *In vitro* experiments with EC showed for the first time that cells incubated with septic patient serum induced actin stress fibers and intercellular gap formation. Recombinant Angpt-2 alone was sufficient to reproduce their earlier findings with septic serum. They concluded that Tie2

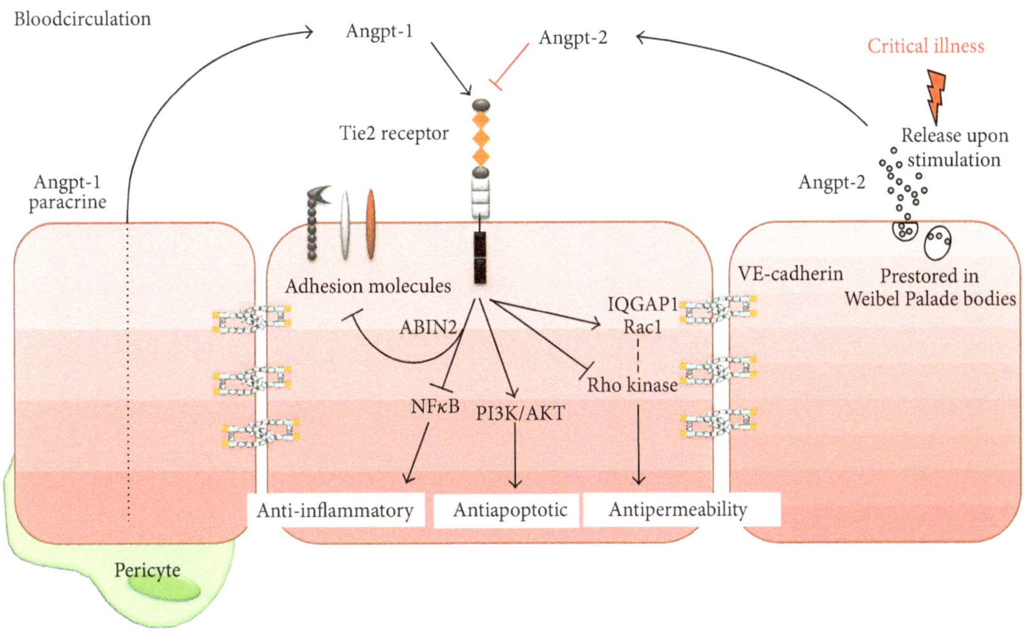

FIGURE 1: Scheme of the endothelial angiopoietin (Angpt)/Tie2 system highlighting fundamental signalling pathways. Angpt-1 ligation phosphorylates and thereby activates the Tie2 receptor promoting an anti-inflammatory signal via inhibition of surface adhesion molecule expression and the transcription factor NfkB. Moreover, the PI3K/Akt pathway promotes an antiapoptotic, prosurvival signal. The antipermeability effects are induced by maintaining the cytoskeletal architecture in a cortical quiescent formation. On a signalling level this is achieved by simultaneous inhibition of the Rho kinase and activation of the small GTPase Rac1 via IQGAP1 binding. Direct effects on the adherens junction protein VE-cadherin via src have also been reported. Upon stimulation, endothelial cells release prestored Angpt-2 from Weibel Palade bodies into the circulation. Angpt-2 competitively antagonizes positive Angpt-1/Tie2 signalling, thus dramatically activating the endothelial cell and priming it for further inflammatory stimuli.

signaling could be impaired as a consequence of excess circulating Angpt-2, which leads to Rho-kinase activation and MLC-p, with the end result being EC contraction, gap formation, and disruption of barrier integrity [36, 49]. This landmark paper was the starting shot for different groups evaluating angiopoietins as biomarkers in sepsis around the globe.

Our own group quantified Angpt-2 in septic ICU patients on admission to a medical ICU. All patients had an invasive hemodynamic monitoring which was performed by the pulse contour continuous cardiac output (PiCCO, Pulsion, Munich, Germany) system to test the hypothesis if high Angpt-2 levels are associated with hemodynamic parameters and surrogates of vascular leakage like the extravascular lung water index (EVLWI). In line with previous reports Angpt-2 concentrations were increasingly higher across strata of the sepsis syndrome (i.e., healthy controls, ICU patients without sepsis, patients with sepsis, and patients with septic shock). Furthermore, Angpt-2 correlated with surrogate markers of pulmonary dysfunction (PaO_2/FiO_2) and tissue hypoxia (serum lactate). Surprisingly, there was no association between Angpt-2 and any hemodynamic parameter including EVLWI.

Likewise van der Heijden et al. detected no association between EVLWI and Angpt-2, which may show the limitation of this method to detect permeability in mechanically ventilated patients. Assessed with the ^{67}Gallium-labelled transferrin method van der Heijden et al. found a correlation between the pulmonary leak index and circulating Angpt-2 [44]. In a multivariate regression model Angpt-2 admission levels outperformed the SOFA and APACHE II score and was an independent marker of 30-day survival [41].

To this point, it was unclear if elevation of circulating Angpt-2 is just an epiphenomena of otherwise activated endothelium (e.g., interleukins) or if it is indeed a direct consequence of the septic stimuli. However, our observation that healthy volunteers subjected to a very small dose of LPS led to a dramatic increase of circulating Angpt-2 within less than 2 hours, even preceding the release of some traditional proinflammatory cytokines, makes a direct endothelial Angpt-2 release upon LPS stimulation likely [51].

Recently published large clinical trials provide further evidence for Angpt-2's potential as a promising biomarker of severity and mortality prediction in a slightly different cohort of patients with acute lung injury (ALI) [52–54]. Calfee and colleagues included an impressive 931 patients with ALI of infectious and noninfectious origin in their study [52]. In non-infection-related ALI, higher baseline Angpt-2 levels were strongly associated with increased mortality. Confusingly, in infection-related ALI there was no Angpt-2 difference in baseline values between survivors and non-survivors. This finding is in contrast with previous findings in which baseline Angpt-2 was consistently associated with outcomes in sepsis (i.e., infection)-related ALI. Calfee and

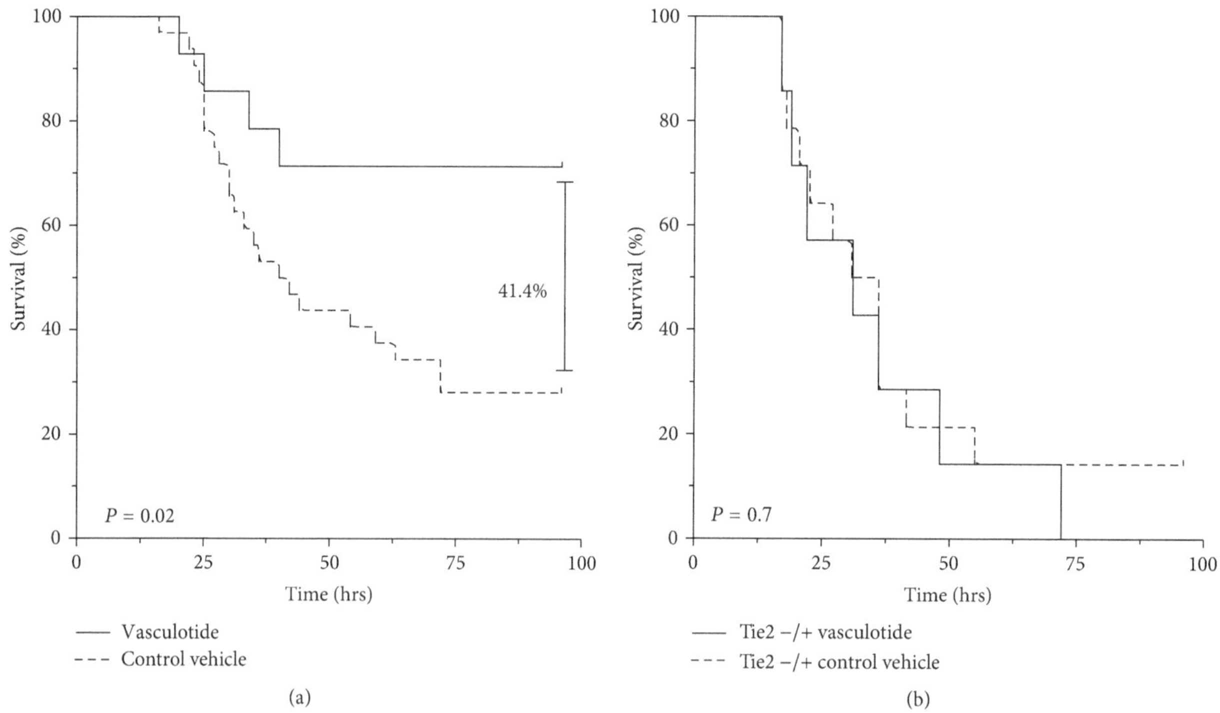

FIGURE 2: Tie2 activation via the synthetic pegylated 7-mer "HHHRHSF" termed Vasculotide (VT) improves survival in experimental murine sepsis. (a) C57BL6 mice were pretreated with 500 ng VT ($n = 15$) or PBS (control, $n = 30$) 7 h prior to injection of a 70% lethal LPS dose. VT improved survival by 41.4% ($P = 0.02$). (b) Male Tie-2 heterozygous (Tie-2 +/−) mice were pretreated with 500 ng VT or PBS 7 h prior to injection of LPS. Survival was indistinguishable ($P = 0.66$) excluding unspecific off target effects of VT. (Modified after: [50].)

colleagues discuss a spectrum bias or differences to previous studies in timing of plasma samples as a possible reason.

In 2010, Ong and colleagues found in a prospective study that the ratio of Angpt-2 to Angpt-1 did predict mortality in 56 ALI patients whereas other factors of endothelial markers (IL-6, IL-8, vWF, thrombomodulin, protein c, icam-1) did not [54]. Given the Tie2 antagonistic concept of Angpt-1 and Angpt-2 this approach using the ratio between both circulating ligands is particularly interesting and deserves careful further analysis.

Acute liver failure (ALF) is a critical condition associated with a severe inflammatory response regularly resulting in massive vascular leakage. We hypothesized that the Angpt/Tie2 system might be involved in this process. Indeed, we observed that Angpt-2 levels in patients with noninfection related primary ALF were associated with the severity of illness. Patients with later transplant free recovery had lower levels of Angpt-2 as those who reached the composite endpoint of death or emergency liver transplantation. Even more interesting, Angpt-2 was identified as an independent predictor of this composite end point. *In vitro* studies underlines the hypothesis of Angpt-2 release from the liver [55].

Together, these results from various clinical and experimental studies demonstrate the potential of Angpt-2 as an endothelial biomarker for severity of illness and outcome prediction in critically ill patients. However, larger prospective trials (in particular in sepsis) are highly desirable to establish Angpt-2 measurements for clinical use.

5. Manipulating the Tie2 Receptor as a Putative Treatment Strategy

5.1. The Ligand Perspective. In 2005, Witzenbichler et al. demonstrated in a fascinating *in vivo* experiment the protective role of Angpt-1 in lipopolysaccharide (LPS) induced endotoxic shock. As a vector to achieve high levels of circulating Angpt-1 they used an adenoviral construct expressing either the human Angpt-1 protein (AdAngpt-1) or a green fluorescent protein (AdGFP) as a control treatment. Hemodynamic function assessed by left heart catheterization was severely depressed in AdGFP compared to AdAngpt-1 treated mice. In detail, mean arterial blood pressure, contractile ability of the heart (initial velocity – dP/dt max), and cardiac output were lower in control mice. Lung water content and activity of pulmonary myeloperoxidase activity as parameters of capillary leakage and lung inflammation were also reduced in the AdAngpt-1 group. The LPS-induced increase in expression levels of pulmonary VCAM-1, ICAM-1, and E-selectin as a marker of endothelial inflammation was markedly lower in AdAngpt-1 mice than in control mice. Furthermore, the survival of AdAngpt-1 mice was slightly superior to control mice (30% overall survival benefit). These experiments showed improved hemodynamic function, reduced lung injury, and a lower inflammatory response accompanied by an improved survival rate in AdAngpt-1 treated mice. Although, adenoviral transduction is generally not feasible in humans and leads to a very high expression of Angpt-1 (up to 1 ug/mL) the authors demonstrated here a potential role of Angpt-1 as an adjunctive agent for the treatment of septic shock [56] and opened a new avenue for specific sepsis therapeutics.

In 2007, Mei et al. provided further evidence for the protective potential of Angpt-1. They showed in a set of *in vivo* experiment the effect of mesenchymal stem cells (MSC) overexpressing Angpt-1 for the prevention of LPS-induced ALI in mice. MSC with or without transfection with the plasmid containing the human Angpt-1 gene (pAngpt-1) were injected in the mice after intratracheal instillation of LPS to induce ALI. Both groups showed a dramatic reduction in LPS-induced pulmonary inflammation quantified by neutrophils and cytokines in the bronchoalveolar space. Of note, the administration of MSC transfected with pAngpt-1 resulted in a nearly complete reversal of LPS-induced pulmonary hyperpermeability, as reflected by reductions in IgM and albumin levels in bronchoalveolar lavage (BAL) [57]. These results underline the potential of a cell-based Angpt-1 gene therapy in the treatment of ALI/ARDS.

In sum, a benefit of upregulating Angpt-1 by different means *in vivo* has been shown in the context of endotoxic shock on the one hand and ALI/ARDS on the other hand. Unfortunately, these approaches using adenoviral gene transfer or modified-stem cell delivery are not feasible to translate in humans yet.

In 2009, Kim et al. determined the positive effect of an increased Angpt-1 signaling in LPS-induced acute kidney injury using a slightly different approach. Mice were pretreated with an engineered variant of native Angpt-1, the so-called Angpt-1 with cartilage oligomeric matrix protein (COMP Angpt-1), which is more potent in phosphorylating Tie2 than native Angpt-1. Three days after COMP Angpt-1 pretreatment mice were challenged with LPS. LPS-induced acute kidney injury (AKI) was ameliorated in the COMP angpt1 group possibly caused by improved renal and systemic hemodynamics, as reflected by an increase of renal blood flow and mean arterial pressure. The inulin-measured glomerular filtration rate was significantly higher in the treated group than in the control group. Again, decreased renal ICAM-1 and VCAM-1 protein expression levels were detected. Furthermore, macrophage infiltration was decreased in COMP Angpt-1 pretreated mice [58]. These results show the protective effect of Angpt-1 signaling, in this case with an engineered variation, COMP Angpt-1, against endotoxic AKI. A comparable experiment with a rescue application of COMP Angpt-1 after LPS infusion to simulate a more realistic setting was not provided but would be highly desirable.

Another way to therapeutically modulate Tie2 phosphorylation is the administration of a PEGylated 7-mer, HHHRHSF, which was recently identified by screening a phage display library for binding to the Tie2 receptor [59]. A polyethylene-oxide clustered version of this peptide is called Vasculotide (VT) and activates Tie2 very effectively and for over 72 hours [60]. In human microvascular endothelial cells (HMVECs), we could show that VT prevented morphological endotoxin-induced gap formation, functional loss of monolayer resistance, and translocation of labeled albumin. These in vitro findings are comparable to Parikh's work from 2006, who showed an analogous protective effect of recombinant Angpt-1 for endothelial cell integrity [36, 50].

From a pharmaceutical point of view VT may hold promise as a drug-like compound. We therefore assessed VT *in vivo* in a model of endotoxemic ALI. And indeed, a single VT injection 7 hours prior to LPS was sufficient to prevent the development of lung vascular leakage, as demonstrated by Evans blue extravasation. Lungs of mice treated with LPS and an empty PEGylated backbone had a 4-fold higher increase in dye extravasation than those treated with VT. VT pretreatment also improved survival of endotoxemia by 41% an effect that was completely abolished in Tie2 heterozygous knockout mice (Figure 2). Indicating the high specificity of VT for Tie2. Rescue experiment with VT given 2 hrs after LPS administration showed only a trend towards improved survival by 33%. Furthermore, echocardiographic evaluations showed also a nonsignificant trend toward improved myocardial performance associated with VT [50]. This finding is discrepant to Witzenbichler's who found improved cardiac performance but might be explained by the differences between Angpt-1 and VT. Again, VT is a 7-mer that specifically (and probably exclusively) binds Tie2. At least in vitro, Suzan Dallabrida demonstrated in 2005 that native, full-length Angpt-1 could also bind integrins on cardiomyocytes thereby improving contractility of this cell type [61].

In another study of our own group Kumpers et al. also provided evidence for the high therapeutic potential of VT in the context of polymicrobial abdominal murine sepsis. Their key finding was that prophylactic as well as therapeutic (i.e., rescue) administration of VT was sufficient to reduce mortality in a clinically relevant experimental murine sepsis model [62]. Both reports provide a proof of principle for the potential use of the Tie2 receptor agonist, VT, as a strategy against vascular leakage thereby improving organ function and survival rates in 2 different models of murine sepsis.

5.2. Perspective of the Antagonist. Given that circulating levels of Angpt-2 (the natural antagonist of Tie2) were so high in different septic clinical populations the question arises if Angpt-2 directly contributes to sepsis severity rather than "just" being a marker of severity. In fact, this question has been asked for a long time but never been answered satisfactory in the "*vascular biology-sepsis community.*"

The first proof of principle Tie2 loss-of-function experiment has been provided by Parikh and coworkers in 2006. Adult mice were pretreated via intraperitoneally injection with a relatively high dose of Angpt-2 or vehicle. The miles assay, an Evans blue extravasation technique, was then used to quantify the vascular leakage. The extravasated dye (that covalently binds to albumin) showed enhanced leakage with a 3-fold increase in lungs and 2-fold increase in livers of Angpt-2 challenged mice compared with vehicle treated controls [36]. These results were the first *in vivo* to demonstrate a putative mechanistic role of Angpt-2 in disrupting the integrity of the endothelium.

Fiedler et al. used an Angpt-2 deficient (−/−) mouse to analyze leucocyte-endothelial interaction in a sterile peritonitis model by intravital microscopy. They could convincingly demonstrate that Angpt-2 deficiency leads to a relevant reduction in adhesion molecules and a consequent failure to firmly adhere to leucocytes [34]. Furthermore, Bhandari et al. found in the same global Angpt-2 knockout mouse that hyperoxia induced ALI is an Angpt-2 driven process that can be ameliorated in the absence of Angpt-2 [63].

Besides these reports so far no data have been published to ultimately prove a mechanistic role of Angpt-2 in the development of MODS in clinically relevant sepsis models.

We therefore designed a series of experiments to investigate the role of Angpt-2 in sepsis morbidity and mortality. In fact, Angpt-2-deficient mice have less organ failure and a survival benefit exceeding 40% in two different murine sepsis models (endotoxin and polymicrobial sepsis) most likely by ameliorating the critical Angpt-2-driven Tie2 deactivation [64]. Moreover, severe morphological changes induced in EC culture by coincubation with serum from septic patients where completely reversible after treatment with an Angpt-2 function-blocking antibody. These *in vivo* and in vitro experiments provide evidence that Angpt-2 directly contributes to the adverse outcomes in sepsis.

A very recent PNAS study from Ghosh et al. comprehensively demonstrated the potential of any Tie2 modulating therapy in another model of critical illness, that is, lethal anthrax infection. Clinically, anthrax infection is dreaded for its dramatic vascular leakage. Therefore, the authors hypothesized that the Angpt/Tie2 system might be involved in this system and found upregulated Angpt-2 in murine and primate models of the disease. They used 2 different knockout models and an Angpt-2 delivering adenovirus (AdAngpt-1) to prove the mechanistic involvement of Angpt/Tie2 in this condition. Interestingly, not only AdAngpt-1, but also Angpt-2 deficient mice showed improved survival in an otherwise 100% lethal anthrax model. Again, as a proof of principle Tie2 deficient mice had a worse outcome using a lower dose of the toxin [65].

6. Conclusion and Future Perspectives

Within the last 5 years, several studies around the globe established the role of elevated circulating Angpt-2 as a biomarker of severity of illness and outcome prediction. Although a promising candidate of global endothelial activation Angpt-2 is not ready for prime time yet. To justify the use of circulating Angpt-2 as an additional routine diagnostic and/or prognostic test large prospective clinical trials are required. In this context, the role of the angiopoietin balance has been given little less attention although theoretically this balance appears to be more important than the absolute levels.

The fundamental role of Tie2 activation as a consequence of alterations in the competitive antagonists Angpt-1 and Angpt-2 in various experimental models of critical illness has been demonstrated by independent groups. Angpt-2 appears to be a disease mediator directly contributing to morbidity and mortality.

Different Tie2 manipulating experimental tools from antibodies to agonistic peptides are available but have not been tested in men. A series of experimental data suggest that both an exogenous Tie2 activating as well as an Angpt-2 inhibition strategy might not only be effective in mice but also generally feasible in men. It is well possible that inhibition of a natural inhibitor (Angpt-2) could reasonably be expected to restore Tie-2 phosphorylation to pre-sepsis levels whereas exogenous receptor activation offers greater titration control, even enabling one to exceed quiescent levels of Tie-2 activation.

In spite of removing activated protein C as the first (and only) specific endothelial targeting sepsis therapeutic from the market, other potential targets make the vasculature a promising target.

Conflict of Interests

The authors have no conflict of interests. Particularly, they have no financial relation with any commercial identity mentioned in the paper.

References

[1] H. K. Simpson, M. Clancy, C. Goldfrad, and K. Rowan, "Admissions to intensive care units from emergency departments: a description study," *Emergency Medicine Journal*, vol. 22, no. 6, pp. 423–428, 2005.

[2] C. Engel, F. M. Brunkhorst, H. G. Bone et al., "Epidemiology of sepsis in Germany: results from a national prospective multicenter study," *Intensive Care Medicine*, vol. 33, no. 4, pp. 606–618, 2007.

[3] R. P. Wenzel, "Treating sepsis," *The New England Journal of Medicine*, vol. 347, no. 13, pp. 966–967, 2002.

[4] R. S. Hotchkiss, P. E. Swanson, B. D. Freeman et al., "Apoptotic cell death in patients with sepsis, shock, and multiple organ dysfunction," *Critical Care Medicine*, vol. 27, no. 7, pp. 1230–1251, 1999.

[5] P. M. Singer, V. De Santis, D. Vitale, and W. Jeffcoate, "Multiorgan failure is an adaptive, endocrine-mediated, metabolic response to overwhelming systemic inaflammation," *The Lancet*, vol. 364, no. 9433, pp. 545–548, 2004.

[6] R. S. Hotchkiss and I. E. Karl, "The pathophysiology and treatment of sepsis," *The New England Journal of Medicine*, vol. 348, no. 2, pp. 138–150, 2003.

[7] R. W. Schrier and W. Wang, "Acute renal failure and sepsis," *The New England Journal of Medicine*, vol. 351, no. 2, pp. 159–169, 2004.

[8] A. Gullo, "Disseminated intravascular coagulation (DIC) in the critical illness," *Minerva Anestesiologica*, vol. 67, no. 12, pp. 831–838, 2001.

[9] M. Tran, D. Tam, A. Bardia, M. Bhasin, G. C. Rowe et al., "PGC-1alpha promotes recovery after acute kidney injury during systemic inflammation in mice," *The Journal of Clinical Investigation*, vol. 121, pp. 4003–4014, 2011.

[10] D. Mehta and A. B. Malik, "Signaling mechanisms regulating endothelial permeability," *Physiological Reviews*, vol. 86, no. 1, pp. 279–367, 2006.

[11] W. C. Aird, "Endothelium as an organ system," *Critical Care Medicine*, vol. 32, no. 5, supplement, pp. S271–S279, 2004.

[12] W. C. Aird, "Phenotypic heterogeneity of the endothelium: I. Structure, function, and mechanisms," *Circulation Research*, vol. 100, no. 2, pp. 158–173, 2007.

[13] W. C. Aird, "Phenotypic heterogeneity of the endothelium: II. Representative vascular beds," *Circulation Research*, vol. 100, no. 2, pp. 174–190, 2007.

[14] W. C. Aird, "The role of the endothelium in severe sepsis and multiple organ dysfunction syndrome," *Blood*, vol. 101, no. 10, pp. 3765–3777, 2003.

[15] M. T. Broman and A. B. Malik, "Cellular and molecular biology for intensivists: a primer—endothelial cells," *Critical Care Medicine*, vol. 33, no. 12, supplement, pp. S517–S519, 2005.

[16] N. M. Goldenberg, B. E. Steinberg, A. S. Slutsky, and W. L. Lee, "Broken barriers: a new take on sepsis pathogenesis," *Science Translational Medicine*, vol. 3, no. 88, Article ID 88ps25, 2011.

[17] C. C. Michel and F. E. Curry, "Microvascular permeability," *Physiological Reviews*, vol. 79, no. 3, pp. 703–761, 1999.

[18] E. Abraham and M. Singer, "Mechanisms of sepsis-induced organ dysfunction," *Critical Care Medicine*, vol. 35, no. 10, pp. 2408–2416, 2007.

[19] S. E. Orfanos, I. Mavrommati, I. Korovesi, and C. Roussos, "Pulmonary endothelium in acute lung injury: from basic science to the critically ill," *Intensive Care Medicine*, vol. 30, no. 9, pp. 1702–1714, 2004.

[20] P. E. Spronk, D. F. Zandstra, and C. Ince, "Bench-to-bedside review: sepsis is a disease of the microcirculation," *Critical Care*, vol. 8, no. 6, pp. 462–468, 2004.

[21] S. Davis, T. H. Aldrich, P. F. Jones et al., "Isolation of angiopoietin-1, a ligand for the TIE2 receptor, by secretion-trap expression cloning," *Cell*, vol. 87, no. 7, pp. 1161–1169, 1996.

[22] N. P. J. Brindle, P. Saharinen, and K. Alitalo, "Signaling and functions of angiopoietin-1 in vascular protection," *Circulation Research*, vol. 98, no. 8, pp. 1014–1023, 2006.

[23] U. Fiedler and H. G. Augustin, "Angiopoietins: a link between angiogenesis and inflammation," *Trends in Immunology*, vol. 27, no. 12, pp. 552–558, 2006.

[24] T. Mustonen and K. Alitalo, "Endothelial receptor tyrosine kinases involved in angiogenesis," *Journal of Cell Biology*, vol. 129, no. 4, pp. 895–898, 1995.

[25] M. A. Venneri, M. De Palma, M. Ponzoni et al., "Identification of proangiogenic TIE2-expressing monocytes (TEMs) in human peripheral blood and cancer," *Blood*, vol. 109, no. 12, pp. 5276–5285, 2007.

[26] I. Kim, H. G. Kim, J. N. So, J. H. Kim, H. J. Kwak, and G. Y. Koh, "Angiopoietin-1 regulates endothelial cell survival through the phosphatidylinositol 3′-kinase/Akt signal transduction pathway," *Circulation Research*, vol. 86, no. 1, pp. 24–29, 2000.

[27] S. David, C. C. Ghosh, A. Mukherjee, and S. M. Parikh, "Angiopoietin-1 requires IQ domain GTPase-activating protein 1 to activate Rac1 and promote endothelial barrier defense," *Arteriosclerosis, Thrombosis, and Vascular Biology*, vol. 31, pp. 2643–2652, 2011.

[28] T. Mammoto, S. M. Parikh, A. Mammoto et al., "Angiopoietin-1 requires p190 RhoGAP to protect against vascular leakage in vivo," *The Journal of Biological Chemistry*, vol. 282, no. 33, pp. 23910–23918, 2007.

[29] D. P. Hughes, M. B. Marron, and N. P. J. Brindle, "The antiinflammatory endothelial tyrosine kinase Tie2 interacts with a novel nuclear factor-κB inhibitor ABIN-2," *Circulation Research*, vol. 92, no. 6, pp. 630–636, 2003.

[30] T. N. Sato, Y. Tozawa, U. Deutsch et al., "Distinct roles of the receptor tyrosine kinases Tie-1 and Tie-2 in blood vessel formation," *Nature*, vol. 376, no. 6535, pp. 70–74, 1995.

[31] C. Suri, P. F. Jones, S. Patan et al., "Requisite role of angiopoietin-1, a ligand for the TIE2 receptor, during embryonic angiogenesis," *Cell*, vol. 87, no. 7, pp. 1171–1180, 1996.

[32] P. C. Maisonpierre, C. Suri, P. F. Jones et al., "Angiopoietin-2, a natural antagonist for Tie2 that disrupts in vivo angiogenesis," *Science*, vol. 277, no. 5322, pp. 55–60, 1997.

[33] U. Fiedler, M. Scharpfenecker, S. Koidl et al., "The Tie-2 ligand angiopoietin-2 is stored in and rapidly released upon stimulation from endothelial cell Weibel-Palade bodies," *Blood*, vol. 103, no. 11, pp. 4150–4156, 2004.

[34] U. Fiedler, Y. Reiss, M. Scharpfenecker et al., "Angiopoietin-2 sensitizes endothelial cells to TNF-α and has a crucial role in the induction of inflammation," *Nature Medicine*, vol. 12, no. 2, pp. 235–239, 2006.

[35] I. Kim, S. O. Moon, S. K. Park, S. W. Chae, and G. Y. Koh, "Angiopoietin-1 reduces VEGF-stimulated leukocyte adhesion to endothelial cells by reducing ICAM-1, VCAM-1, and E-selectin expression," *Circulation Research*, vol. 89, no. 6, pp. 477–479, 2001.

[36] S. M. Parikh, T. Mammoto, A. Schultz et al., "Excess circulating angiopoietin-2 may contribute to pulmonary vascular leak in sepsis in humans," *PLoS Medicine*, vol. 3, no. 3, article e46, 2006.

[37] M. T. Ganter, M. J. Cohen, K. Brohi et al., "Angiopoietin-2, marker and mediator of endothelial activation with prognostic significance early after trauma?" *Annals of Surgery*, vol. 247, no. 2, pp. 320–326, 2008.

[38] J. S. Giuliano Jr., P. M. Lahni, K. Harmon et al., "Admission angiopoietin levels in children with septic shock," *Shock*, vol. 28, no. 6, pp. 650–654, 2007.

[39] D. C. Gallagher, S. M. Parikh, K. Balonov et al., "Circulating angiopoietin 2 correlates with mortality in a surgical population with acute lung injury/adult respiratory distress syndrome," *Shock*, vol. 29, no. 6, pp. 656–661, 2008.

[40] P. Kümpers, C. Hafer, S. David et al., "Angiopoietin-2 in patients requiring renal replacement therapy in the ICU: relation to acute kidney injury, multiple organ dysfunction syndrome and outcome," *Intensive Care Medicine*, vol. 36, no. 3, pp. 462–470, 2010.

[41] P. Kümpers, A. Lukasz, S. David et al., "Excess circulating angiopoietin-2 is a strong predictor of mortality in critically ill medical patients," *Critical Care*, vol. 12, no. 6, article R147, 2008.

[42] A. Lukasz, J. Hellpap, R. Horn et al., "Circulating angiopoietin-1 and angiopoietin-2 in critically ill patients: development and clinical application of two new immunoassays," *Critical Care*, vol. 12, no. 4, article R94, 2008.

[43] S. E. Orfanos, A. Kotanidou, C. Glynos et al., "Angiopoietin-2 is increased in severe sepsis: correlation with inflammatory mediators," *Critical Care Medicine*, vol. 35, no. 1, pp. 199–206, 2007.

[44] M. van der Heijden, G. P. van Nieuw Amerongen, P. Koolwijk, V. W. M. van Hinsbergh, and A. B. J. Groeneveld, "Angiopoietin-2, permeability oedema, occurrence and severity of ALI/ARDS in septic and non-septic critically ill patients," *Thorax*, vol. 63, no. 10, pp. 903–909, 2008.

[45] A. J. Bhatt, G. S. Pryhuber, H. Huyck, R. H. Watkins, L. A. Metlay, and W. M. Maniscalco, "Disrupted pulmonary vasculature and decreased vascular endothelial growth factor, Flt-1, and TIE-2 in human infants dying with bronchopulmonary dysplasia," *American Journal of Respiratory and Critical Care Medicine*, vol. 164, no. 10, pp. 1971–1980, 2001.

[46] A. Papapetropoulos, G. García-Cardeña, T. J. Dengler, P. C. Maisonpierre, G. D. Yancopoulos, and W. C. Sessa, "Direct actions of angiopoietin-1 on human endothelium: evidence for network stabilization, cell survival, and interaction with other angiogenic growth factors," *Laboratory Investigation*, vol. 79, no. 2, pp. 213–223, 1999.

[47] A. I. Su, T. Wiltshire, S. Batalov et al., "A gene atlas of the mouse and human protein-encoding transcriptomes," *Proceedings of the National Academy of Sciences of the United States of America*, vol. 101, no. 16, pp. 6062–6067, 2004.

[48] A. L. Wong, Z. A. Haroon, S. Werner, M. W. Dewhirst, C. S. Greenberg, and K. G. Peters, "Tie2 expression and phosphorylation in angiogenic and quiescent adult tissues," *Circulation Research*, vol. 81, no. 4, pp. 567–574, 1997.

[49] V. Spindler, N. Schlegel, and J. Waschke, "Role of GTPases in control of microvascular permeability," *Cardiovascular Research*, vol. 87, no. 2, pp. 243–253, 2010.

[50] S. David, C. C. Ghosh, P. Kümpers et al., "Effects of a synthetic PEG-ylated Tie-2 agonist peptide on endotoxemic lung injury and mortality," *American Journal of Physiology*, vol. 300, no. 6, pp. L851–L862, 2011.

[51] P. Kümpers, M. van Meurs, S. David et al., "Time course of angiopoietin-2 release during experimental human endotoxemia and sepsis," *Critical Care*, vol. 13, no. 3, article R64, 2009.

[52] C. S. Calfee, D. Gallagher, J. Abbott, B. T. Thompson, and M. A. Matthay, "Plasma angiopoietin-2 in clinical acute lung injury: prognostic and pathogenetic significance," *Critical Care Medicine*, vol. 40, pp. 1731–1737, 2012.

[53] N. J. Meyer, M. Li, R. Feng et al., "ANGPT2 genetic variant is associated with trauma-associated acute lung injury and altered plasma angiopoietin-2 isoform ratio," *American Journal of Respiratory and Critical Care Medicine*, vol. 183, no. 10, pp. 1344–1353, 2011.

[54] T. Ong, D. E. McClintock, R. H. Kallet, L. B. Ware, M. A. Matthay, and K. D. Liu, "Ratio of angiopoietin-2 to angiopoietin-1 as a predictor of mortality in acute lung injury patients," *Critical Care Medicine*, vol. 38, no. 9, pp. 1845–1851, 2010.

[55] J. Hadem, C. L. Bockmeyer, A. Lukasz et al., "Angiopoietin-2 in acute liver failure," *Critical Care Medicine*, vol. 40, pp. 1499–1505, 2012.

[56] B. Witzenbichler, D. Westermann, S. Knueppel, H. P. Schultheiss, and C. Tschope, "Protective role of angiopoietin-1 in endotoxic shock," *Circulation*, vol. 111, no. 1, pp. 97–105, 2005.

[57] S. H. J. Mei, S. D. McCarter, Y. Deng, C. H. Parker, W. C. Liles, and D. J. Stewart, "Prevention of LPS-induced acute lung injury in mice by mesenchymal stem cells overexpressing angiopoietin," *PLoS Medicine*, vol. 4, no. 9, article e269, 2007.

[58] D. H. Kim, Y. J. Jung, A. S. Lee et al., "COMP-angiopoietin-1 decreases lipopolysaccharide-induced acute kidney injury," *Kidney International*, vol. 76, no. 11, pp. 1180–1191, 2009.

[59] R. Tournaire, M. P. Simon, F. le Noble, A. Eichmann, P. England, and J. Pouysségur, "A short synthetic peptide inhibits signal transduction, migration and angiogenesis mediated by Tie2 receptor," *EMBO Reports*, vol. 5, no. 3, pp. 262–267, 2004.

[60] P. Van Slyke, J. Alami, D. Martin et al., "Acceleration of diabetic wound healing by an angiopoietin peptide mimetic," *Tissue Engineering A*, vol. 15, no. 6, pp. 1269–1280, 2009.

[61] S. M. Dallabrida, N. Ismail, J. R. Oberle, B. E. Himes, and M. A. Rupnick, "Angiopoietin-1 promotes cardiac and skeletal myocyte survival through integrins," *Circulation Research*, vol. 96, no. 4, pp. e8–e24, 2005.

[62] P. Kumpers, F. Gueler, S. David et al., "The synthetic Tie2 agonist peptide vasculotide protects against vascular leakage and reduces mortality in murine abdominal sepsis," *Critical Care*, vol. 15, no. 5, article R261, 2011.

[63] V. Bhandari, R. Choo-Wing, A. Harijith et al., "Increased hyperoxia-induced lung injury in nitric oxide synthase 2 null mice is mediated via angiopoietin 2," *American Journal of Respiratory Cell and Molecular Biology*, vol. 46, pp. 668–676, 2012.

[64] S. David, A. Mukherjee, C. C. Ghosh et al., "Angiopoietin-2 may contribute to multiorgan dysfunction and death in sepsis," *Critical Care Medicine*. In press.

[65] C. C. Ghosh, A. Mukherjee, S. David et al., "Impaired function of the Tie-2 receptor contributes to vascular leakage and lethality in anthrax," *Proceedings of the National Academy of Sciences of the United States of America*, vol. 109, pp. 10024–10029, 2012.

15

Congenital Pulmonary Malformation in Children

Montasser Nadeem, Basil Elnazir, and Peter Greally

Paediatric Respiratory Department, The Adelaide and Meath Hospital, Dublin, Incorporating the National Children's Hospital (AMNCH), Tallaght, Dublin 24, Ireland

Correspondence should be addressed to Montasser Nadeem; drnadeem.gad@gmail.com

Academic Editors: H. S. Lai and M. Roth

Congenital Pulmonary Malformations (CPMs) are a group of rare lung abnormalities affecting the airways, parenchyma, and vasculature. They represent a spectrum of abnormal development rather than discrete pathological entities. They are caused by aberrant embryological lung development which occurs at different stages of intrauterine life.

1. Congenital Pulmonary Malformations (CPMs)

CPMs are a group of rare lung abnormalities affecting the airways, parenchyma, and vasculature. They represent a spectrum of abnormal development rather than discrete pathological entities. They are caused by aberrant embryological lung development which occurs at different stages of intrauterine life.

With improved resolution of foetal sonography and Doppler studies, many of these lesions are detected "in utero." Their natural history can be quite variable. Lesions may resolve prior to birth. Some CPMs may present in the early neonatal period with respiratory distress due to a mass effect, while others may be asymptomatic only to be detected in later life on CXRs performed for other reasons. Certain forms of CPM have the potential to undergo malignant change. Conversely, pleuropulmonary blastoma may masquerade as some forms of CPM. When lesions are symptomatic in early life there can be no doubt that surgical resection is the only option. However, the decision-making process becomes more complex when clinicians encounter asymptomatic lesions, in healthy infants, which have been detected either by antenatal USS or incidental chest radiograph.

The presentation, natural history, diagnosis and management of congenital pulmonary airway malformation, congenital lobar emphysema, pulmonary sequestration, bronchogenic cyst, and pleuropulmonary blastoma will be discussed.

2. Congenital Pulmonary Airway Malformation (CPAM)

Congenital pulmonary airway malformation (CPAM) was previously known as congenital cystic adenomatoid malformation (CCAM). Histologically, the lesion of CPAM is characterised by solid adenomatous areas, which consist of closely packed tubular structures resembling terminal bronchioles without mature alveoli [1]. These areas closely resemble normal foetal lung at 16-week gestation [2]. Interspersed with these adenomatous areas are cysts. Postnatally the downstream alveoli can only be ventilated collaterally via the pores of Kohn.

The incidence of CPAM is 1 per 8300 to 35,000 [3], Table 1. It usually affects a single lobe and it is no association with sex predilection [1]. There are five subtypes of CPAM (0–4) depending on the proportion of cysts and adenomatous tissue and the dominant cell types [4]. Types 1 and 2 occur with

TABLE 1: Common congenital pulmonary malformations.

	Incidence/prevalence	Features and presentation	Treatment	Comments
CPAM	Incidence is 1 per 8300 to 35,000 [3]. No sex predilection [1].	Usually limited to one lobe. Many cases are detected by prenatal U/S. CPAM may present in the early neonatal period with respiratory distress. 86% of patients, who were asymptomatic at birth, had become symptomatic by 13 years of age (median age 2 years). Symptoms include pneumonia with or without infected CPAM, respiratory distress, and spontaneous pneumothorax.	Surgical resection is the definitive treatment. Asymptomatic patients can be observed with serial imaging.	Lesions regress antenatally in 59%. Type 4 and type 1 tend to carry a malignancy risk.
CLE	Prevalence rate of 1 in 20,000 live births [12]. Males > females [13].	The left upper lobe is affected in half of the cases. Lesions may be asymptomatic or present with respiratory distress in the newborn period. Those with the lesion may experience dyspnoea or recurring respiratory infection. 15% of cases may have congenital heart disease.	Resection of the affected lobe in symptomatic newborn. Conservative treatment in Asymptomatic patients.	Congenital cardiac anomalies often accompany CLE.
BC	Prevalence rate of 1 per 68,000 [14].	It can occur throughout the tracheobronchial tree. Large cyst presents with respiratory distress and cyanosis in newborns. BC may be detected as incidental findings on chest radiographs. Newborns with large cysts can develop respiratory distress, cyanosis, and feeding difficulty. Compression of the trachea and respiratory arrest has been reported. Wheeze, stridor, atelectasis of the distal lung, dysphagia, and recurrent pneumonia can occur.	Surgery is recommended in all cases.	Typically presented during the second decade of life.
BPS	Incident is 0.29% [15]. Male > female [16].	Lower lobes are mostly affected. Newborn may present with respiratory distress. Patients with ELS may remain asymptomatic. In a case series of 50 patients with ELS, 24% were diagnosed prenatally and 61% were diagnosed by three months of age. Recurrent pneumonia, chest pain, hemoptysis, and shortness of breath, respectively, can occur. The adjacent lung is frequently bronchiectatic in resected ILS specimens.	Symptomatic Patients require surgical intervention. Elective resection is recommended in asymptomatic patients with ILS.	Infection, heart failure, carcinoma, and bleeding can occur in sequestrated lung.

CPAM: congenital pulmonary airway malformation, CLE: congenital lobar emphysema, BC: bronchogenic cysts, BPS: bronchopulmonary sequestration, ILS: intralobar sequestration, ELS: extralobar sequestration.

most frequency [4, 5]. Type 1 lesions are usually unicystic or paucicystic and may contain fluid, they contain little or no adenomatous component. The cysts are greater than 2 cm in diameter and lined with pseudostratified columnar epithelium [4]. Type 2 lesions contain more uniform small cyst of less than 1 cm in diameter [4]. Mucous cells and cartilage are seen in type 1, but not type 2 [4]. Smooth and striated muscle fibres are seen in types 1 and 2, respectively [4]. A coexistent CPAM type 2 has been reported in half of the patients with extralobar sequestration (ELS) [6], however the separation from the lung and the presence of a systemic blood supply are helpful to distinguish between these entities [3]. Type 4 lesions contain large cysts lined with flat alveolar cells, some of which contain surfactant [7]. They involve more peripheral lung. They can present with tension pneumothorax [7]. Type 4 CPAM was considered within type 1, in older publications, as both types are composed of large cysts (up to 10 cm in diameter) [8]. Large cysts are usually observed and pneumothorax can occur in Type 1 PPB [3], which has a histological overlap with type 4 CPAM. It is not easily possible to differentiate between both entities on histology alone [9–11].

2.1. Natural History. The natural history of CPAM can be quite variable. Spontaneous regression during the course of gestation is not uncommon. In 29 patients with CPAM, during fetal life, the size of the lesion decreased in 8 patients, of whom 7 required postnatal surgical resection, and disappeared in 4 patients, of whom 3 required postnatal surgical resection [17]. In children with disappearing fetal lung masses, postnatal CT scans are needed to exclude the persistent abnormalities, which are often subtle or not apparent on plain radiographs [18].

2.2. Prenatal versus Postoperative Pathological Diagnoses. With improved resolution of foetal sonography, many of the CPAM lesions are detected "in utero." However appropriate postnatal investigations, rather than antenatal diagnosis, are essential for surgical decision [19]. No correlation between antenatal ultrasound features and histological diagnosis after surgery has been reported [19, 20]. In one hundred and five complete records of asymptomatic children with prenatally diagnosed lung lesions, the postoperative pathologic diagnoses were different from preoperative radiological findings in 9 patients [21]. In a study of 17 fetuses diagnosed with CPAM by prenatal ultrasound, pathological diagnosis was confirmed in 57% of those with known pathological diagnosis [20]. Tsai et al. showed that, in one hundred and five complete records of asymptomatic children with prenatally diagnosed lung lesions, the postoperative pathologic diagnoses were different from preoperative radiological findings in 9 patients [21].

2.3. Clinical Presentation. CPAM may present in the early neonatal period with respiratory distress due to a mass effect, while others may be asymptomatic only to be detected in later life on CXRs performed for other reasons. Sauvat et al., reported that 3 out of 29 patients with CPAM experience symptoms during the first weeks of life [17]. As many as 86% (18 out of 21) of patients, who were asymptomatic at birth, had become symptomatic by 13 years of age (median age of 2 years) [22]. In patients with CPAM, pneumonia with or without infected CPAM was reported in 43%, respiratory distress in 14%, and spontaneous pneumothorax in 14% [22]. In 31 patients with bronchopulmonary malformations CPAM ($n = 13$), pulmonary sequestrations ($n = 6$), bronchogenic cysts ($n = 3$), congenital lobar emphysemas ($n = 9$), Shanmugam et al. reported that respiratory distress, respiratory infections/pneumonias, and dyspnoea occurred in 9, 22, and 9 out of these 31 patients, respectively [23]. In 16 patients with CPAM, neonatal respiratory impairment, pneumothorax, and recurrent respiratory tract infections occurred in 12, 1, and 3 patients, respectively [24].

2.4. Postnatal Diagnosis. The diagnosis is suggested by CXR, however, a thoracic CT scan is required to confirm the diagnosis [25, 26]. Winters et al. reported that CXR features can be subtle in children with disappearing fetal lung masses, hence postnatal CT scan is needed [18]. In 29 patients with CPAM, postnatal X-ray and CT scan were abnormal in 17 and 25, respectively [17]. CPAM lesions may be confused for a congenital diaphragmatic hernia. Heij et al. showed that 4 out of 16 patients with CCAM had laparotomy for presumed diaphragmatic hernia [24]. In these circumstances, CT scan can be helpful.

2.5. Is There Association between CPAM and Malignancy? An association between type 1 CPAM and bronchoalveolar carcinoma has been reported [27]. In patients with type 1 CPAM, Langston showed that microscopic foci of bronchoalveolar carcinoma and focal mucous cell hyperplasia could occur in up to 5/16 and 2/16 of patients [10]. In those with type 4 CPAM, focal stromal hypercellularity and pleuropulmonary blastoma were documented in 4/8 and 1/8 of patients [10]. The distinction between type 4 CPAMs and grade 1 pleuropulmonary blastomas may not be possible on histology alone [9–11]. Primary pulmonary rhabdomyosarcoma (RMS) has been reported in 13-month-old boy with CPAM [28].

2.6. Maternal Steroid and Fetal Therapy. In 13 patients with predominantly microcystic CPAM, Curran et al. showed that fetuses, who had CPAM volume-to-head ratio >1.6 or nonimmune hydrops, experience an improvement following prenatal betamethasone [29]. In these patients, hydrops and CPAM volume-to-head ratio improved in 77.8% and 61.5% of the patients, respectively. Adzick reported two fetuses (>32-week gestation), with lung lesion and hydrops, experienced an ex utero intrapartum therapy strategy with resection of the lesion and survived [30]. In fetuses with CPAM and hydrops, fetal resection or thoracoamniotic shunt is recommended [31]. Serial fetal thoracocenteses may be an alternative or an adjunct to fetal surgery in selected cases [31]. Adzick et al. showed that hydrops resolution and neonatal survival occurred in 8 out of 13 fetuses, with CPAM and nonimmune hydrops, who experienced fetal surgical resection of the lesions at 21 to 29 week of gestation [32]. Five out of six fetuses, with a very large solitary cyst, who had thoracoamniotic shunting, survived [32]. In 67 fetuses with cystic lung lesions, percutaneous intrauterine laser therapy and thoracoamniotic shunts had been performed in 1 and 3 fetuses, respectively [20].

2.7. Recommendation and Management. Air travel in children suffering from cystic lung lesions is controversial because of the risk of pneumothorax. Most clinicians caution against air travel in children with enlarging cystic lesions. All infants with antenatally diagnosed CPAM should be evaluated. Symptomatic children require surgical resection [33]. When CPAM is asymptomatic some clinicians prefer to observe rather than refer for surgery. However, when one considers the risk of pulmonary compression, infection, and the low risk for malignancy, it is not surprising that many clinicians prefer the operative approach [23, 33]. In the majority of cases, pulmonary resection is indicated as soon as the diagnosis is made, with emergency resection in those with severe respiratory distress.

3. Bronchogenic Cyst (BC)

Bronchogenic cyst is a rare CPM, with a prevalence rate of 1 per 68,000 [14]. BC represents part of the spectrum of broncho-pulmonary foregut malformations [34]. The primitive foregut gives rise through a central outpunching to the trachea-bronchial tree. Between the 5–16th week of gestation the bronchi develop by a process of budding and branching. Buds can develop at any site along the trachea-bronchial tree which, if their development arrests, become BC. The cysts contain tissue normally found in the airways (mucous glands, smooth muscle, elastic tissue, and cartilage). BC may occur in paratracheal, carinal, paraesophageal, hilar, suprasternal notch, and miscellaneous locations [35–37]. The latter occurs when buds detach and migrate to ectopic sites, for example, pericardial, cervical, and abdominal [35–37].

3.1. Diagnosis and Presentation. BC may be detected as incidental findings on chest radiographs and account for 10% of mediastinal masses in children. The postnatal diagnosis of BC may be suspected on chest radiograph but a thoracic CT scan is needed to confirm the diagnosis [38]. In a case series of 33 patients with bronchogenic cysts, the lesions usually presented as spheroid mediastinal masses, near the carina or right paratracheal area [39]. Newborns with large cysts can develop respiratory distress, cyanosis, and feeding difficulty [40]. Compression of the trachea and respiratory arrest has been reported in infant with BC [41]. BC in a bronchial location may present with wheeze and recurrent pneumonia. If the airway obstruction is only partial and gives rise to a ball-valve effect, then hyperinflation of the distal lung will occur which may mimic CLE. Where the obstruction is complete, atelectasis of the distal lung may occur leading to infection. High tracheal BC may present with stridor. Cysts may communicate with the airway and become infected and rupture. Paraesophageal cyst may give rise to dysphagia. Pericardial BC may present with Superior Vena Cava obstruction. In a series of 10 infants and children (age between 16 days and 6 years) with bronchogenic cyst, respiratory distress, cyanosis, chronic cough, and fever and dysphasia were reported in 70%, 40%, 50%, and 20% of patients, respectively [42]. The differential diagnosis depends on location and may include lymphadenopathy, oesophageal duplication cyst, neuroblastoma, cystic hygroma, and dermoid cyst.

3.2. Association between BC and Malignancy. A rare association between BC and neuroblastoma had been reported in 2 children [43]. A recent meta-analysis of bronchogenic cysts found that 45% of 683 asymptomatic adults progressed to develop complications and that there was a small risk 0.7% of malignant transformation within the cyst [44]. Bronchoalveolar cell carcinoma is the most common form of malignancy associated with BC.

3.3. Management. Surgical excision should be considered in all cases because of the likelihood of eventual development of symptoms and malignant change [45].

4. Congenital Lobar Emphysema (CLE)

CLE is relatively rare affecting 1 in 20,000 live births [12]. It occurs more commonly in males [13] and most frequently affects the left upper lobe [46]. Most series report that within the affected lobe the alveoli are anatomically and numerically normal. It is postulated that the condition is caused by either absence or maldevelopment of cartilaginous rings or bronchomalacia of a proximal airway due to extrinsic compression "in utero." However, in 50% of cases the airway appears normal. The net effect is air trapping in the affected lobe [47].

4.1. Presentation and Diagnosis. Lesions may be asymptomatic or present with respiratory distress in the newborn period [48]. Later, infants may experience dyspnoea (57%) or recurring respiratory infection (28%) [48]. On CXR, hyperlucency of the affected lobes is the characteristic feature [48]. The diagnosis may be confirmed on chest CT [49]. The differential diagnosis includes type 1 unicystic CPAM, pneumtothorax, Swyer-James syndrome, bronchogenic cyst, and diaphragmatic hernia.

4.2. Association with Malignancy and Heart Diseases. Type I pleurapulmonary blastoma may mimic CLE. In one report of a patient with asymptomatic CLE, the lesion was resected due to increasing size and pleuro-pulmonary blastoma type I was confirmed on histology [50]. This overlap in the spectrum of diagnoses prompts the surgical view to resect CPM. A cardiac evaluation is required because as many as 15% of cases may have congenital heart disease [48].

4.3. Management. Early surgical excision is required for newborns with respiratory distress [49, 51]. However, infants and older children who are asymptomatic or have minimal symptoms can be treated conservatively [52]. Surgical excision of the affected lobe is the appropriate treatment in all infants under 2 months of age and in infants older than 2 months presenting with severe respiratory symptoms. Infants older than 2 months presenting with mild to moderate respiratory symptoms associated with normal bronchoscopic findings can be treated conservatively [48].

5. Bronchopulmonary Sequestration (BPS)

BPS is a rare congenital malformation of the lower respiratory tract and comprises 0.15 to 6.4% of all CPM. The incident rate of pulmonary sequestration is 0.29% [15]. It is an area of nonfunctioning lung tissue that commonly receives its arterial blood supply from the descending aorta. The sequestered lobe has no communication with the tracheobronchial tree. BPS is classified as either intralobar sequestration (ILS), in which the lesion is located within a normal lobe and lacks its own visceral pleura or extralobar (ELS), in which the lesion is located outside the lung and has its own visceral pleura.

ILS lesions account for 80% of sequestrations [16]. The sequestration commonly occurs in the lower lobe, primarily in the left posterior basal segment [16]. With respect to ILS, the venous drainage is usually to the pulmonary circulation [53]. However, ELS frequently have systemic venous drainage.

Other congenital anomalies occur in 3/18 and 3/4 of ILS and ELS, respectively [54]. In 28 patients with BPS, diaphragmatic hernia, atrial septal defect, dextrocardia, double superior caval vein, and a sliding hernia and an esophageal bronchus communicating with an ELS have been seen in 2 and 1 each, respectively [54]. Gezer et al. reported a case of diaphragmatic hernia in 1 (12.5%) patient with ELS [53]. In one series, the association between ELS and type 2 CPAM has been reported in as many as 50% of patient [6].

5.1. Prenatal and Postnatal Diagnosis. In a previous study of pregnant women with antenatally diagnosed ELS, the lesions regressed before delivery in 28/41 (68%) cases [32]. Postnatal diagnosis of ELS often can be made from chest radiograph appearance. However, ultrasonography with Doppler imaging or thoracic CT with contrast may be used to define the lesion. ELS are often discovered in infants who present with other conditions for example, heart failure, polyhydramnios, or prematurity.

6. Presentation

The age of presentation is variable in children with ELS. In a case series of 50 patients with ELS, 24% were diagnosed prenatally and 61% were diagnosed by three months of age [6]. In 27 patients (age between 3.5 and 51 years) with BPS, 10, 6, 2, and 2 experience recurrent pneumonia, chest pain, hemoptysis, and shortness of breath, respectively [53]. The adjacent lung is frequently bronchiectatic in resected ILS specimens. The differential diagnosis of BPS includes CPAM, congenital diaphragmatic hernia, bronchogenic cyst, and mediastinal tumour.

6.1. Complications. These include haemoptysis, haemothorax, and malignant transformation. Levine et al., documented severe congestive heart failure in 2 infants with BPS and large arterio-venous shunts [55]. A localised carcinoma in the sequestrated lung tissue has also been reported [56].

6.2. Fetal Therapy. In fetuses with BPS and hydrops, open fetal surgery, coagulation of the blood supply, or thoracoamniotic shunting has been recommended [57]. BPS with hydrops has been treated successfully with laser coagulation of the feeding systemic artery of the sequestration under ultrasound guidance [57]. Rammos et al. reported 2 babies, with BPS, who required postnatal thoracotomy performed on the 10th day of life in spite of prenatal amnioperitoneal shunt, pleural drainage, and laser ablation of the feeding artery [58].

6.3. Management. Immediate surgical intervention is required in patients with respiratory distress. In view of the high rate of complications, elective resection is often recommended even in asymptomatic patients with BPS [54]. Ayed and Owayed reported that the age of intervention was 11 weeks (range, 13–43 weeks), in those with pulmonary sequestration [51].

7. Pleuropulmonary Blastoma (PPB)

It is a rare tumor of pleura and lung in young children. The incidence of PPB is 1 in 250,000 live births [59]. There are 3 different types of PPB. Type 1 lesion presents in a cystic form, which is indistinguishable from benign lung cyst. However, nodules within the cystic lesions and solid masses are present in types 2 and 3, respectively. PPB is the most frequent malignancy associated with childhood lung cysts. A quarter of PPBs are associated with a familial predisposition to dysplasia. PPB should be considered in infants and children presenting with lung cysts and pneumothorax, bilateral lung cysts, or a family history of PPB-associated conditions, including renal cystic disease and small bowel polyps. Cerebral metastases had been reported in types 2 and 3 PPB [60]. This suggests routine brain imaging to monitor development of metastasis in patients with PPB.

8. Conclusion

Congenital Lung malformations are becoming more frequently recognised with the advent of improved antenatal imaging. There is considerable debate among clinicians as to the best approach to these lesions in asymptomatic infants as many of the lesions have the potential to involute over time. Further longitudinal studies are needed to address the appropriate approach towards management for each of the CPM discussed.

Abbreviations

CPAM: Congenital pulmonary airway malformation
CLE: Congenital lobar emphysema
BC: Bronchogenic cysts
BPS: Bronchopulmonary sequestration
PPB: Pleuropulmonary blastoma.

References

[1] K. Higby, B. A. Melendez, and H. S. Heiman, "Spontaneous resolution of nonimmune hydrops in a fetus with a cystic adenomatoid malformation," *Journal of Perinatology*, vol. 18, no. 4, pp. 308–310, 1998.

[2] I. Cha, N. S. Adzick, M. R. Harrison, and W. E. Finkbeiner, "Fetal congenital cystic adenomatoid malformations of the lung: a clinicopathologic study of eleven cases," *American Journal of Surgical Pathology*, vol. 21, no. 5, pp. 537–544, 1997.

[3] J. R. Priest, G. M. Williams, D. A. Hill, L. P. Dehner, and A. Jaffé, "Pulmonary cysts in early childhood and the risk of malignancy," *Pediatric Pulmonology*, vol. 44, no. 1, pp. 14–30, 2009.

[4] J. T. Stocker, J. E. Madewell, and R. M. Drake, "Congenital cystic adenomatoid malformation of the lung. Classification and morphologic spectrum," *Human Pathology*, vol. 8, no. 2, pp. 155–171, 1977.

[5] L. Morelli, I. Piscioli, S. Licci, S. Donato, A. Catalucci, and F. Del Nonno, "Pulmonary congenital cystic adenomatoid malformation, type I, presenting as a single cyst of the middle lobe in an adult; case report," *Diagnostic Pathology*, vol. 2, no. 1, article 17, 2007.

[6] R. M. Conran and J. T. Stocker, "Extralobar sequestration with frequently associated congenital cystic adenomatoid malformation, type 2: report of 50 cases," *Pediatric and Developmental Pathology*, vol. 2, no. 5, pp. 454–463, 1999.

[7] J. T. Stocker, "Congenital pulmonary airway malformation: a new name for and an expanded classification of congenital cystic adenomatoid malformation of the lung," *Histopathology*, vol. 41, supplement 2, pp. 424–431, 2002.

[8] J. T. Stocker, "The respiratory tract," in *Pediatric Pathology*, J. T. Stocker and L. P. Dehner, Eds., pp. 445–517, Lippincott Williams & Wilkins, Philadelphia, Pa, USA, 2nd edition, 2001.

[9] F. MacSweeney, K. Papagiannopoulos, P. Goldstraw, M. N. Sheppard, B. Corrin, and A. G. Nicholson, "An assessment of the expanded classification of congenital cystic adenomatoid malformations and their relationship to malignant transformation," *American Journal of Surgical Pathology*, vol. 27, no. 8, pp. 1139–1146, 2003.

[10] C. Langston, "New concepts in the pathology of congenital lung malformations," *Seminars in Pediatric Surgery*, vol. 12, no. 1, pp. 17–37, 2003.

[11] A. Mechoulan, M. D. Leclair, M. Yvinec, H. J. Philippe, and N. Winer, "Pleuropulmonary blastoma: a case of early neonatal diagnosis through antenatal scan screening," *Gynecologie Obstetrique Fertilite*, vol. 35, no. 5, pp. 437–441, 2007.

[12] C. L. Thakral, D. C. Maji, and M. J. Sajwani, "Congenital lobar emphysema: experience with 21 cases," *Pediatric Surgery International*, vol. 17, no. 2-3, pp. 88–91, 2001.

[13] D. R. Kirks, *Practical Pediatric Imaging in Diagnostic Radiology of Infants and Children*, Little Brown, 2nd edition, 1994.

[14] A. P. Schouten van der Velden, R. S. V. M. Severijnen, and T. Wobbes, "A bronchogenic cyst under the scapula with a fistula on the back," *Pediatric Surgery International*, vol. 22, no. 10, pp. 857–860, 2006.

[15] S. G. Gao, G. Y. Cheng, K. L. Sun, and J. He, "Diagnosis and surgical treatment of pulmonary sequestration," *National Medical Journal of China*, vol. 87, no. 23, pp. 1616–1617, 2007.

[16] Y. Wei and F. Li, "Pulmonary sequestration: a retrospective analysis of 2625 cases in China," *European Journal of Cardio-Thoracic Surgery*, vol. 40, no. 1, pp. e39–e42, 2011.

[17] F. Sauvat, J. L. Michel, A. Benachi, S. Emond, and Y. Revillon, "Management of asymptomatic neonatal cystic adenomatoid malformations," *Journal of Pediatric Surgery*, vol. 38, no. 4, pp. 548–552, 2003.

[18] W. D. Winters, E. L. Effmann, H. V. Nghiem, and D. A. Nyberg, "Disappearing fetal lung masses: importance of postnatal imaging studies," *Pediatric Radiology*, vol. 27, no. 6, pp. 535–539, 1997.

[19] M. Davenport, S. A. Warne, S. Cacciaguerra, S. Patel, A. Greenough, and K. Nicolaides, "Current outcome of antenally diagnosed cystic lung disease," *Journal of Pediatric Surgery*, vol. 39, no. 4, pp. 549–556, 2004.

[20] J. A. Miller, J. E. Corteville, and J. C. Langer, "Congenital cystic adenomatoid malformation in the fetus: natural history and predictors of outcome," *Journal of Pediatric Surgery*, vol. 31, no. 6, pp. 805–808, 1996.

[21] A. Y. Tsai, K. W. Liechty, H. L. Hedrick et al., "Outcomes after postnatal resection of prenatally diagnosed asymptomatic cystic lung lesions," *Journal of Pediatric Surgery*, vol. 43, no. 3, pp. 513–517, 2008.

[22] A. Wong, D. Vieten, S. Singh, J. G. Harvey, and A. J. A. Holland, "Long-term outcome of asymptomatic patients with congenital cystic adenomatoid malformation," *Pediatric Surgery International*, vol. 25, no. 6, pp. 479–485, 2009.

[23] G. Shanmugam, K. MacArthur, and J. C. Pollock, "Congenital lung malformations—antenatal and postnatal evaluation and management," *European Journal of Cardio-thoracic Surgery*, vol. 27, no. 1, pp. 45–52, 2005.

[24] H. A. Heij, S. Ekkelkamp, and A. Vos, "Diagnosis of congenital cystic adenomatoid malformation of the lung in newborn infants and children," *Thorax*, vol. 45, no. 2, pp. 122–125, 1990.

[25] C. Lanza, V. Bolli, V. Galeazzi, B. Fabrizzi, and G. Fabrizzi, "Cystic adenomatoid malformation in children: CT histopathological correlation," *Radiologia Medica*, vol. 112, no. 4, pp. 612–619, 2007.

[26] W. S. Kim, K. S. Lee, I. O. Kim et al., "Congenital cystic adenomatoid malformation of the lung: CT-pathologic correlation," *American Journal of Roentgenology*, vol. 168, no. 1, pp. 47–53, 1997.

[27] D. West, A. G. Nicholson, I. Colquhoun, and J. Pollock, "Bronchioloalveolar carcinoma in congenital cystic adenomatoid malformation of lung," *Annals of Thoracic Surgery*, vol. 83, no. 2, pp. 687–689, 2007.

[28] C. Ozcan, A. Celik, Z. Ural, A. Veral, G. Kandilo⊠lu, and E. Balik, "Primary pulmonary rhabdomyosarcoma arising within cystic adenomatoid malformation: a case report and review of the literature," *Journal of Pediatric Surgery*, vol. 36, no. 7, pp. 1062–1065, 2001.

[29] P. F. Curran, E. B. Jelin, L. Rand et al., "Prenatal steroids for microcystic congenital cystic adenomatoid malformations," *Journal of Pediatric Surgery*, vol. 45, no. 1, pp. 145–150, 2010.

[30] N. S. Adzick, "Management of fetal lung lesions," *Clinics in Perinatology*, vol. 30, no. 3, pp. 481–492, 2003.

[31] M. F. Brown, D. Lewis, R. M. Brouillette, B. Hilman, and E. G. Brown, "Successful prenatal management of hydrops, caused by congenital cystic adenomatoid malformation, using serial aspirations," *Journal of Pediatric Surgery*, vol. 30, no. 7, pp. 1098–1099, 1995.

[32] N. S. Adzick, M. R. Harrison, T. M. Crombleholme, A. W. Flake, and L. J. Howell, "Fetal lung lesions: management and outcome," *American Journal of Obstetrics and Gynecology*, vol. 179, no. 4, pp. 884–889, 1998.

[33] M. Stanton and M. Davenport, "Management of congenital lung lesions," *Early Human Development*, vol. 82, no. 5, pp. 289–295, 2006.

[34] T. Berrocal, C. Madrid, S. Novo, J. Gutierrez, A. Arjonilla, and N. Gomez-Leon, "Congenital anomalies of the tracheobronchial tree, lung, and mediastinum: embryology, radiology, and pathology," *Radiographics*, vol. 24, no. 1, article e17, 2004.

[35] F. Sauvat, F. Fusaro, F. Jaubert, B. Galifer, and Y. Revillon, "Paraesophageal bronchogenic cyst: first case reports in pediatric," *Pediatric Surgery International*, vol. 22, no. 10, pp. 849–851, 2006.

[36] A. Zvulunov, B. Amichai, M. H. Grunwald, I. Avinoach, and S. Halevy, "Cutaneous bronchogenic cyst: delineation of a poorly recognized lesion," *Pediatric Dermatology*, vol. 15, no. 4, pp. 277–281, 1998.

[37] K. Pujary, P. Pujary, R. Shetty, P. Hazarika, and L. Rao, "Congenital cervical bronchogenic cyst," *International Journal of Pediatric Otorhinolaryngology*, vol. 57, no. 2, pp. 145–148, 2001.

[38] H. P. McAdams, W. M. Kirejczyk, M. L. Rosado-de-Christenson, and S. Matsumoto, "Bronchogenic cyst: imaging features with clinical and histopathologic correlation," *Radiology*, vol. 217, no. 2, pp. 441–446, 2000.

[39] C. DuMontier, E. R. Graviss, M. J. Silberstein, and W. H. McAlister, "Bronchogenic cysts in children," *Clinical Radiology*, vol. 36, no. 4, pp. 431–436, 1985.

[40] J. Dembinski, M. Kaminski, R. Schild, C. Kuhl, M. Hansmann, and P. Bartmann, "Congenital intrapulmonary bronchogenic cyst in the neonate-perinatal management," *American Journal of Perinatology*, vol. 16, no. 10, pp. 509–514, 1999.

[41] C. C. Harle, O. Dearlove, R. W. M. Walker, and N. Wright, "A bronchogenic cyst in an infant causing tracheal occlusion and cardiac arrest," *Anaesthesia*, vol. 54, no. 3, pp. 262–265, 1999.

[42] G. A. Tireli, H. Ozbey, A. Temiz, T. Salman, and A. Celik, "Bronchogenic cysts: a rare congenital cystic malformation of the lung," *Surgery Today*, vol. 34, no. 7, pp. 573–576, 2004.

[43] B. N. Vazquez, J. Mira, C. Navarro et al., "Neuroblastoma and bronchogenic cyst: a rare association," *European Journal of Pediatric Surgery*, vol. 10, no. 5, pp. 340–342, 2000.

[44] B. Kirmani, B. Kirmani, and F. Sogliani, "Should asymptomatic bronchogenic cysts in adults be treated conservatively or with surgery?" *Interactive Cardiovascular and Thoracic Surgery*, vol. 11, no. 5, pp. 649–659, 2010.

[45] F. Borgnat, P. Lupu Bratiloveanu, C. Gyenes, and Y. Le Bescond, "Bronchogenic cervical cyst in a child," *Revue de Stomatologie et de Chirurgie Maxillo-Faciale*, vol. 112, no. 1, pp. 54–56, 2011.

[46] V. Mikhaĭlova, "Congenital lobar emphysema in childhood," *Khirurgiia*, vol. 49, no. 3, pp. 8–12, 1996.

[47] I. J. Doull, G. J. Connett, and J. O. Warner, "Bronchoscopic appearances of congenital lobar emphysema," *Pediatric Pulmonology*, vol. 21, no. 3, pp. 195–197, 1996.

[48] I. Karnak, M. E. Senocak, A. O. Ciftci, and N. Buyukpamukcu, "Congenital lobar emphysema: diagnostic and therapeutic considerations," *Journal of Pediatric Surgery*, vol. 34, no. 9, pp. 1347–1351, 1999.

[49] G. Rocha, I. Azevedo, J. C. Pinto, C. S. Moura, and H. Guimarães, "Congenital lobar emphysema of the newborn. Report of four clinical cases," *Revista Portuguesa de Pneumologia*, vol. 16, no. 5, pp. 849–857, 2010.

[50] S. Walsh, A. E. Wood, and P. Greally, "Pleuropulmonary blastoma type I following resection of incidentally found congenital lobar emphysema," *Irish Medical Journal*, vol. 102, no. 7, article 230, 2009.

[51] A. K. Ayed and A. Owayed, "Pulmonary resection in infants for congenital pulmonary malformation," *Chest*, vol. 124, no. 1, pp. 98–101, 2003.

[52] S. Ceran, B. Altuntas, G. Sunam, and I. Bulut, "Congenital lobar emphysema: is surgery routinely necessary," *African Journal of Paediatric Surgery*, vol. 7, no. 1, pp. 36–37, 2010.

[53] S. Gezer, I. Tasepe, M. Sirmali et al., "Pulmonary sequestration: a single-institutional series composed of 27 cases," *Journal of Thoracic and Cardiovascular Surgery*, vol. 133, no. 4, pp. 955–959, 2007.

[54] D. van Raemdonck, K. de Boeck, H. Devlieger et al., "Pulmonary sequestration: a comparison between pediatric and adult patients," *European Journal of Cardio-Thoracic Surgery*, vol. 19, no. 4, pp. 388–395, 2001.

[55] M. M. Levine, D. B. Nudel, and N. Gootman, "Pulmonary sequestration causing congestive heart failure in infancy: a report of two cases and review of the literature," *Annals of Thoracic Surgery*, vol. 34, no. 5, pp. 581–585, 1982.

[56] P. Gatzinsky and S. Olling, "A case of carcinoma in intralobar pulmonary sequestration," *Thoracic and Cardiovascular Surgeon*, vol. 36, no. 5, pp. 290–291, 1988.

[57] R. S. G. M. Witlox, E. Lopriore, F. J. Walther, E. R. V. M. Rikkers-Mutsaerts, F. J. C. M. Klumper, and D. Oepkes, "Single-needle laser treatment with drainage of hydrothorax in fetal bronchopulmonary sequestration with hydrops," *Ultrasound in Obstetrics and Gynecology*, vol. 34, no. 3, pp. 355–357, 2009.

[58] K. S. Rammos, C. N. Foroulis, C. K. Rammos, and A. Andreou, "Prenatal interventional and postnatal surgical therapy of extralobar pulmonary sequestration," *Interactive Cardiovascular and Thoracic Surgery*, vol. 10, no. 4, pp. 634–635, 2010.

[59] A. Nasr, S. Himidan, A. C. Pastor, G. Taylor, and P. C. W. Kim, "Is congenital cystic adenomatoid malformation a premalignant lesion for pleuropulmonary blastoma?" *Journal of Pediatric Surgery*, vol. 45, no. 6, pp. 1086–1089, 2010.

[60] J. R. Priest, J. Magnuson, G. M. Williams et al., "Cerebral metastasis and other central nervous system complications of pleuropulmonary blastoma," *Pediatric Blood and Cancer*, vol. 49, no. 3, pp. 266–273, 2007.

Permissions

The contributors of this book come from diverse backgrounds, making this book a truly international effort. This book will bring forth new frontiers with its revolutionizing research information and detailed analysis of the nascent developments around the world.

We would like to thank all the contributing authors for lending their expertise to make the book truly unique. They have played a crucial role in the development of this book. Without their invaluable contributions this book wouldn't have been possible. They have made vital efforts to compile up to date information on the varied aspects of this subject to make this book a valuable addition to the collection of many professionals and students.

This book was conceptualized with the vision of imparting up-to-date information and advanced data in this field. To ensure the same, a matchless editorial board was set up. Every individual on the board went through rigorous rounds of assessment to prove their worth. After which they invested a large part of their time researching and compiling the most relevant data for our readers. Conferences and sessions were held from time to time between the editorial board and the contributing authors to present the data in the most comprehensible form. The editorial team has worked tirelessly to provide valuable and valid information to help people across the globe.

Every chapter published in this book has been scrutinized by our experts. Their significance has been extensively debated. The topics covered herein carry significant findings which will fuel the growth of the discipline. They may even be implemented as practical applications or may be referred to as a beginning point for another development. Chapters in this book were first published by Hindawi Publishing Corporation; hereby published with permission under the Creative Commons Attribution License or equivalent.

The editorial board has been involved in producing this book since its inception. They have spent rigorous hours researching and exploring the diverse topics which have resulted in the successful publishing of this book. They have passed on their knowledge of decades through this book. To expedite this challenging task, the publisher supported the team at every step. A small team of assistant editors was also appointed to further simplify the editing procedure and attain best results for the readers.

Our editorial team has been hand-picked from every corner of the world. Their multi-ethnicity adds dynamic inputs to the discussions which result in innovative outcomes. These outcomes are then further discussed with the researchers and contributors who give their valuable feedback and opinion regarding the same. The feedback is then collaborated with the researches and they are edited in a comprehensive manner to aid the understanding of the subject.

Apart from the editorial board, the designing team has also invested a significant amount of their time in understanding the subject and creating the most relevant covers. They scrutinized every image to scout for the most suitable representation of the subject and create an appropriate cover for the book.

The publishing team has been involved in this book since its early stages. They were actively engaged in every process, be it collecting the data, connecting with the contributors or procuring relevant information. The team has been an ardent support to the editorial, designing and production team. Their endless efforts to recruit the best for this project, has resulted in the accomplishment of this book. They are a veteran in the field of academics and their pool of knowledge is as vast as their experience in printing. Their expertise and guidance has proved useful at every step. Their uncompromising quality standards have made this book an exceptional effort. Their encouragement from time to time has been an inspiration for everyone.

The publisher and the editorial board hope that this book will prove to be a valuable piece of knowledge for researchers, students, practitioners and scholars across the globe.

List of Contributors

Rajiv D. Machado
School of Life Sciences, Faculty of Science, University of Lincoln, Brayford Pool, Lincoln LN6 7TS, UK

M. Neale Weitzmann
Atlanta Department of Veterans Affairs Medical Center, Decatur, GA 30033, USA
Division of Endocrinology and Metabolism and Lipids, Department of Medicine, Emory University School of Medicine, 101Woodruff Circle, 1305 WMRB, Atlanta, GA 30322, USA

Alexey V. Kondyurin, Pourandokht Naseri, Jennifer M. R. Tilley, Neil J. Nosworthy, Marcela M. M. Bilek and David R. McKenzie
Applied and Plasma Physics, School of Physics, University of Sydney, A28, Sydney, NSW 2006, Australia

Lilly Zborowski-Naveh
Deptartment of Ophthalmology, MOR Institute for Medical Data, 51108 Bnei Brak, Israel
Department of Ophthalmology, Wolfson Medical Center, 58100 Holon, Israel

Rita Ehrlich
Department of Ophthalmology, Rabin Medical Center, Beilinson Hospital, 49100 Petach Tikva, Israel

Moshe Luski, Dov Weinberger and Dan D. Gaton
Deptartment of Ophthalmology, MOR Institute for Medical Data, 51108 Bnei Brak, Israel
Department of Ophthalmology, Rabin Medical Center, Beilinson Hospital, 49100 Petach Tikva, Israel
Sackler Faculty of Medicine, Tel Aviv University, 69978 Tel Aviv, Israel

Mona Boaz
Department of Epidemiology, Wolfson Medical Center, 58100 Holon, Israel

Fabrizio Fabrizi
Division of Nephrology and Dialysis, Maggiore Hospital and IRCCS Foundation, Pad. Croff, Via Commenda 15, 20122 Milano, Italy

Gerald M. Higa
Schools of Pharmacy and Medicine and the Mary Babb Randolph Cancer Center, West Virginia University, Morgantown, WV 26506, USA

Jason Hicks and Christopher Isabella
School of Pharmacy, West Virginia University, Morgantown, WV 26506, USA

Philip P. Goodney
Section of Vascular Surgery, Dartmouth-Hitchcock Medical Center, 1 Medical Center Drive, Lebanon, NH 03766, USA
Dartmouth-Hitchcock Medical Center, The Dartmouth Institute for Health Policy and Clinical Practice, Hanover, NH 03765, USA

Katarzyna A. Rejniak
Department of Integrated Mathematical Oncology, H. Lee Moffitt Cancer Center and Research Institute, 12902 Magnolia Drive, Room SRB-4 24000G, Tampa, FL 33612, USA
Department of Oncologic Sciences, College of Medicine, University of South Florida, Tampa, FL 33612, USA

José M. Álvarez-Castro and Gonzalo Alvarez
Department of Genetics, University of Santiago de Compostela, Avenida Carvalho Calero s/n, 27002 Lugo, Galiza, Spain

Richard C. Petersen
Department of Biomaterials and Biomedical Engineering, The University of Alabama at Birmingham, SDB 539, 1919 7th Avenue South, Birmingham, AL 35294, USA

Philip F. Giampietro
Waisman Center, University of Wisconsin-Madison, 1500 Highland Avenue, Madison, WI 53705, USA

Elisabeth M. Weiss
Department of Psychology, Karl-Franzens University of Graz, University-Platz 2, 8010 Graz, Austria

Madhav Bhatia
Department of Pathology, University of Otago, P.O. Box 4345, Christchurch 8140, New Zealand

Alexander Lukasz and Sascha David
Department of Nephrology & Hypertension, Hannover Medical School, Carl-Neuberg Straße 1, 30625 Hannover, Germany

Philipp Kümpers
Department of Internal Medicine, Rheumatology and Nephrology, University Hospital Münster, 48149 Münster, Germany

Montasser Nadeem, Basil Elnazir and Peter Greally
Paediatric Respiratory Department, The Adelaide and Meath Hospital, Dublin, Incorporating the National Children's Hospital (AMNCH), Tallaght, Dublin 24, Ireland